SI Derived Units with Special Names

Quantity	Name	Symbol	SI Unit Expression in Terms of Other Units	SI Unit Expression in Terms of SI Base Units
Frequency	Hertz	Hz		$1/s$
Force	Newton	N		$m\ kg/s^2$
Pressure, stress	Pascal	Pa	N/m^2	kg/ms^2
Energy, work, quantity of heat	Joule	J	$N\ m$	$m^2\ kg/s^2$
Power	Watt	W	J/s	$m^2\ kg/s^3$
Electric charge	Coulomb	C		$s\ A$
Electric potential	Volt	V	W/A	$m^2\ kg/As^3$
Capacitance	Farad	F	C/V	$sA^2/m^2\ kg$
Electric resistance	Ohm	Ω	V/A	$m^2\ kgA^2/s^3$
Conductance	Siemens	S	A/V	$s^3A^2/m^2\ kg$
Magnetic flux	Weber	Wb	$V\ s$	$m^2\ kg/s^2A$
Magnetic field (B)	Tesla	T	Wb/m^2	kg/s^2A
Luminous flux	Lumen	lm		$cd\ sr$

Summary of New and (Old) Radiologic Units

Quantity	Name	Symbol	Expression Other Units	Expression SI Base Units
Activity	Becquerel (curie)	Bq (Ci)	3.7×10^{10} Bq	$1/s$
Absorbed dose	Gray (rad)	Gy (rad)	J/kg (10^{-2} Gy)	m^2/s^2
Dose equivalent	Sievert (rem)	Sv (rem)	J/kg (10^{-2} Sv)	m^2/s^2
Exposure	Coulomb per kilogram (roentgen)	C/kg (R)	C/kg (2.58×10^{-4} C/kg)	sA/kg

Universal Constants

Constant	Unit
Plank's constant	$h = 6.62 \times 10^{-27}$ erg-s $= 6.62 \times 10^{-34}$ J-s $= 4.15 \times 10^{-15}$ eV-s
Velocity of light	$c = 3 \times 10^8$ m/s $= 3 \times 10^{10}$ cm/s
Base of natural logarithms	$e = 2.7183$
Pi	$\pi = 3.1416$

RADIOLOGIC SCIENCE FOR TECHNOLOGISTS

PHYSICS, BIOLOGY, AND PROTECTION 6TH EDITION

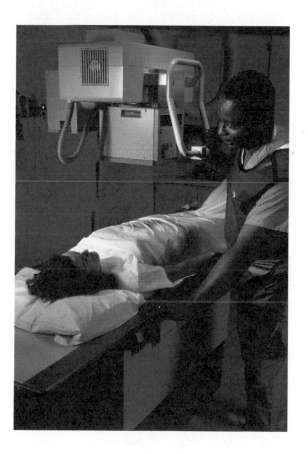

RADIOLOGIC SCIENCE FOR TECHNOLOGISTS

PHYSICS, BIOLOGY, AND PROTECTION 6TH EDITION

STEWART C. BUSHONG, Sc.D., FACR, FACMP

Professor, Department of Radiology
Baylor College of Medicine
Houston, Texas

with 693 illustrations

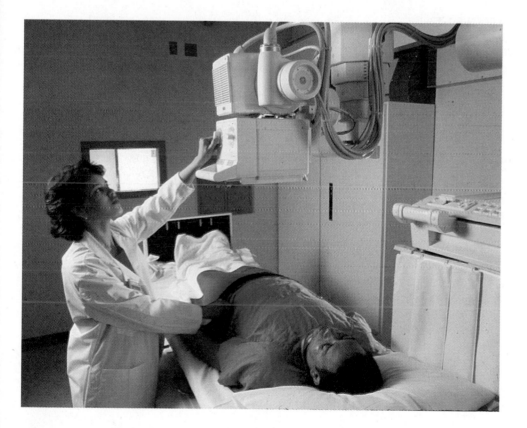

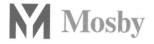 Mosby

A Harcourt Health Sciences Company

St. Louis   London   Philadelphia   Sydney   Toronto

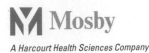
A Harcourt Health Sciences Company

Vice President and Publisher: Don Ladig
Senior Editor: Jeanne Rowland
Senior Developmental Editor: Lisa Potts
Developmental Editor: Linda Woodard
Project Manager: Mark Spann
Production Editor: Julie Eddy
Designer: Judi Lang
Manufacturing Supervisor: Karen Boehme

Cover Photos: Custom Medical Stock Photos, Inc.

Part Opener Photos: Custom Medical Stock Photos, Inc.

SIXTH EDITION

Printed in the United States of America

Mosby, Inc.
11830 Westline Industrial Drive
St. Louis, MO 63146

Library of Congress Cataloging-in-Publication Data
Bushong, Stewart C.
    Radiologic science for technologists: physics, biology, and
protection / Stewart C. Bushong.—6th ed.
      p.   cm.
    Includes bibliographical references and index.
    ISBN 0-8151-1579-2
    1. Radiology, Medical. 2. Medical physics. 3. Radiology,
Medical—Safety measures. I. Title
    [DNLM: 1. Technology, Radiologic. 2. Radiation Protection.
3. Radiation.   WN 160 B979r 1997]
R895.B86   1997
616.07'57—dc21
DNLM/DLC   .   96-29488
00 01 / 9 8 7 6 5 4 3 2

Preface

Imagine a radiographer evaluating body habitus and disease process and selecting technical factors on the x-ray tube control panel. Imagine a radiographer examining a patient using ionizing radiation. Imagine a radiographer evaluating the finished radiograph for diagnostic quality. Imagine if this radiographer had never studied physics. Physics is the basic science for understanding how ionizing radiation fits into the electromagnetic spectrum, how x-rays are formed from the interaction of electrons and the tungsten target of and x-ray tube, and for explaining the effect of ionizing radiation on matter. A radiographer without a background in the fundamentals of physics is not able to make the decisions required in the diagnostic imaging workplace. Radiologists, radiology managers, and patients depend on radiographers to make informed decisions and educated assessments of technical factors and diagnostic image quality. Much is learned from experience but even more is gained from accredited radiography programs with clinical assignments and classwork including extensive study of radiologic physics. The principle purpose of this textbook is to convey a working knowledge of radiologic physics while preparing radiography students as painlessly as possible for the certification examination by the American Registry of Radiologic Technologists (AART). This book will also be a valuable resource for the practicing technologist.

This textbook resulted from lectures from radiologic science courses for students and radiographers in the programs of the University of Houston, the Houston Community College, and for radiology residents at Baylor College of Medicine. These students receive their clinical training in one of the several hospitals and assemble together for much of the instruction. This textbook, therefore, is designed to meet the needs of students who may be receiving clinical training in a wide spectrum of environments and whose classwork may be presented on several levels of difficulty.

HISTORICAL PERSPECTIVE

The practice and the equipment of diagnostic radiology remained relatively stable during the first seven decades following the discovery of x-rays. Truly great changes during that time can be counted on the fingers of one hand: the Crookes tube, the Potter-Bucky diaphragm, and image intensification.

However, since the publication of the first edition of this book in 1975, several great and innovative types of examinations have come into routine use in medical imaging: computed tomography, computed radiography, digital fluoroscopy, and most recently spiral computed tomography. These examinations have been made possible by our truly spectacular technology—computer advances, new x-ray tube designs, and improved image receptors. These developments have transformed radiology into an imaging science.

NOMENCLATURE

Although the United States has not formally adopted the International Systems of Units (SI units), this textbook presents SI units. With this system come the corresponding units of radiation and radioactivity. The roentgen, the rad, and the rem are being replaced by the coulomb/kilogram (C/kg), the gray (Gy), and the sievert (Sv), respectively. Radioactivity is to be expressed in bequerels (Bq). Consequently, throughout this sixth edition, where there has been reference to units other than SI, the SI equivalent will follow in parentheses. A summary of SI and the factors necessary to convert from conventional to SI units is given in the inside front cover of the text.

Additional nomenclatures are continually being introduced into diagnostic radiology, and where appropriate, newer forms are used in this text. SID (source-to-image receptor distance), PBL (positive beam limitation), linearity, reproducibility, and HU (Hounsfield unit) are examples of some of the new vocabulary. In many instances, when conversion from English to metric is made, the result is rounded off. For example, 40 inches target-to-film distance (TFD) is actually 101.6 cm, but it is identified throughout as being equivalent to 100 cm SID.

NEW TO THIS EDITION
Learning Aids

Those readers who have used previous editions of *Radiologic Science for Technologists* will find some significant improvements in this new edition. The most important goal in preparing the sixth edition has been to make the text even more accessible to radiography students. The language used to present information is direct, concise, and easy to understand. To encourage and to make the text reader-friendly, each chapter opens with a list of learning objectives, an outline, and an introduction that overviews the chapter. Each chapter ends with a chapter summary that recaps the major points presented in the chapter. Answering the review questions provided at the end of each chapter can help the reader assess his or her comprehension of the chapter's contents. Because radiologic science cannot be totally separated from mathematics, there are many formulas to learn. In this book formulas and easy-to-understand mathematic equations are clearly highlighted in the text and are followed by problems with clinical significance using these equations. The answers to the problems are calculated line by line to lead the student through to the answer. The review questions at the end of the chapter also include math problems. Key concepts are highlighted in colored boxes throughout the book.

The sixth edition also contains an important new chapter on spiral CT, an innovation of computed tomography that is now routinely used. Other recent innovations in medical imaging described in the textbook are digital fluoroscopy, computed radiography, and advances in film and intensifying screen technology.

Improved Organization

The overall organization of the book is intended to lead the student from less complex subject matter in the beginning to more complex subject matter at the end. The learning is progressive. Chapter introductions and outlines allow the student to survey the material before reading the chapter. Chapter outlines refer to specific headings throughout the chapter so information can be found quickly. Important information in the chapter is boxed and highlighted to allow for quick reference and increased retention of information. Each chapter is concisely reviewed in the chapter summary and is followed by lists entitled "Additional Reading," to encourage the reader to research topics of interest.

New Illustrations

One of the most exciting new features of this new book is the addition of full-color art, which provides better graphic demonstration of the difficult concepts of radiologic science while making the text more attractive and interesting.

ANCILLARIES
Student Workbook

A completely revised edition of *Radiologic Science Workbook and Laboratory Manual* is available. It contains worksheets, fill-in-the blank questions, multiple choice questions, matching items, word problems, and crossword puzzles. All the questions in the accompanying workbook are correlated directly with the text. Use of the workbook will enhance learning and enjoyment of radiologic science.

Related Multimedia

Instructional materials to support teaching and learning radiologic physics have been developed by Mosby and may be obtained by contacting the publisher directly. Multimedia presentations of basic physics, imaging, radiobiology, and radiation protection are available in both slide/audiotape and CD-ROM formats.

Stewart C. Bushong

Acknowledgments

For the preparation of the sixth edition, I am indebted to the many readers of the earlier editions who submitted suggestions, criticisms, corrections, and compliments. For this edition I enlisted the help of many clinical radiographers and educators. I am grateful to the following people: Karen Brown, St. Joseph's Medical Center; Quinn B. Carroll, Midland College; Geoffrey Clarke, UT Health Science Center; Charles Collins, San Diego Mesa College; Patricia Duffy, College of Health Related Professions; Pamela Eugene, Delgado Community College; Kae Fleming, Columbia State Community College; Regina Freidman, Mercy Medical Center; Richard Gwilt, Indian Health Service; Jim Heck, Angelina College; Wayne Hedrick, Aultman Hospital; Carolyn Holdsworth, Portland Community College; John Lampignano, Gateway Community College; Suzanne McIntire, Mercy Hospital Center; Rod Roemer, Triton College; Lil Rossadillo, Pima Medical Institute; Euclid Seesam, British Columbia Institute of Technology; Linda Shields, El Paso Hospital Center; Mel Siedbaud, University of Wisconsin; Sandra Strickland, Pima Medical Institute; Rues Stuteville, Oregon Institute of Technology; Christl Thompson, El Paso Community College; Jean Toth-Allen, CDRH-MQSA; and Judy Williams, Grady Memorial Hospital.

Mosby would also like to thank the following reviewers and consultants: William J. Callaway, Lincoln Land Community College; Wayne R. Hedrick, Northeastern Ohio University College of Medicine and Aultman Hospital; Eugene D. Frank, Mayo Medical School; Kevin C. Sisler, Mayo Medical School; John Lampignano, Gateway Community College; Eric Anderson, Avila College; Cheri Dyke, St. Luke's Hospital; Andrew Shappell, Lima Technical College; Elwin Tilson, Armstrong State College; Adam Bede, College of St. Catherine; Alberto Bell, Jr., Oregon Institute of Technology; Richard Hone, Oregon Institute of Technology; Steve Bollin, El Paso Community College; TerriAnne Linn-Watson, Chaffey College; Deborah Martin, Rapid City Regional Hospital; Tina Phillips, Brandywine Hospital; Douglas Hughes, Mountain State Tumor Institute; Starla Mason, Laramie County Community College; John Clouse, Owensboro Community College; Nancy Perkins, Bakersfield College; David Lahman, Midwestern State University; Robert Luke, Boise State University; Linda Pearson, Midwestern State University; Robert Parelli, Cypress College; Debra Reese, A-B Tech; Joe Dielman, Triton College; Gloria Strickland, Armstrong State College; Joseph Bittengle, University of Arkansas for Medical Science; Mary Reagan, Meridian Technology Center; Paul Bober, Labette Community College; Suzanne Sturdivant; Christopher Gould, San Jacinto College; Nadia Bugg, Midwestern State University, and John Hartwein, St. Louis Community College at Forest Park.

Art Haus, Eastman Kodak Company, and Lee Kitts, Sterling Diagnostic Imaging, were very helpful with the material concerning image receptors and image quality. Their expertise is much appreciated.

I am particularly appreciative of the exceptional effort by Joanna Bligh, M.Ed., R.T.(R). Ms. Bligh reviewed the entire manuscript and did much to adjust the reading level. The pedagogical additions, including chapter outlines, introductions, objectives, summaries, and review questions were written by her. Ms. Bligh wishes to thank Adolphe, the one person who encouraged her to undertake the work on this book. Others who helped her include Janet Salerno, typist, of Waterbury, CT; Jim Merello of Dupont; Lois Powell and Phil Bunch of Kodak; Dr. Peck of the Arthritis Center and John Smith, photographer, of Waterbury, CT; James Thorne, Concord Hospital, Concord NH; Napoleon Martin, Fairview Hospital, Great Barrington, MA; and her daughters, Amanda and Kate. She would also like to thank Lisa Potts, developmental editor, of Mosby. She is indebted to Lisa for her infectious enthusiasm and ability to laugh amid difficulty.

I am deeply indebted to my associates Robert Parry, Sharon Glaze, and Benjamin Archer, who have assisted me with this revision. The illustrations are the work of Crystal Depew, who worked exceptionally hard to render all illustrations in full color. The cartoons by Kraig Emmert help ease any pain associated with physics.

I am also particularly indebted to Judy Matteau Faldyn for the many times she had to struggle through my handwritten notes and unfamiliar symbols and equations. I appreciate her conscientious approach in preparing the final manuscript.

"Physics is fun" is the motto of my radiologic science courses, and I believe this text will help make physics enjoyable for the student radiographer.

Contents

PART ONE: RADIOLOGIC PHYSICS

1. Basic Concepts of Radiation Science, 3
2. Radiographic Definitions and Mathematics Review, 12
3. Fundamentals of the Physics of Radiation Science, 19
4. The Atom, 28
5. Electromagnetic Radiation, 43
6. Electricity, 56
7. Magnetism, 68
8. Electromagnetism, 75

PART TWO: THE X-RAY BEAM

9. The X-ray Unit, 91
10. The X-ray Tube, 107
11. X-ray Production, 126
12. X-ray Emission, 139
13. X-ray Interaction with Matter, 149

PART THREE: THE RADIOGRAPHIC IMAGE

14. Radiographic Film, 165
15. Processing the Latent Image, 177
16. Intensifying Screens, 189
17. Scatter Radiation and Beam-Restricting Devices, 204
18. The Grid, 214
19. Radiographic Quality, 229
20. Radiographic Exposure, 251
21. Radiographic Technique, 258

PART FOUR: SPECIAL X-RAY IMAGING

22. Alternative Film Procedures, 281
23. Mammography, 293
24. Mammography Quality Control, 305
25. Fluoroscopy, 321
26. Introduction to Angiography and Interventional Radiology, 333
27. Computer Science, 341
28. Digital X-ray Imaging, 357
29. Computed Tomography, 377
30. Spiral Computed Tomography, 395
31. Quality Assurance and Quality Control, 407
32. Film Artifacts, 419

PART FIVE: RADIATION PROTECTION

33. Human Biology, 429
34. Fundamental Principles of Radiobiology, 441
35. Molecular and Cellular Radiobiology, 449
36. Early Effects of Radiation, 463
37. Late Effects of Radiation, 477
38. Health Physics, 495
39. Designing for Radiation Protection, 509
40. Radiation Protection Procedures, 523

APPENDICES

A. Sources for Supplementary Teaching Materials, 543
B. Important Dates in the Development of Modern Radiology, 544
C. Answers to Review Questions, 545

Glossary, 558
Index, 563

RADIOLOGIC SCIENCE FOR TECHNOLOGISTS

PHYSICS, BIOLOGY, AND PROTECTION 6TH EDITION

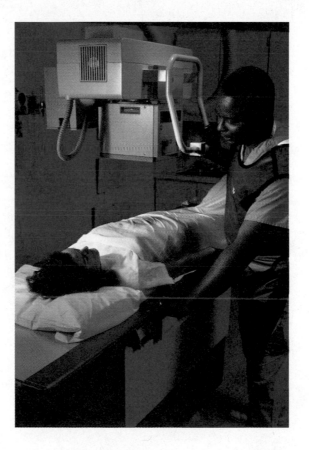

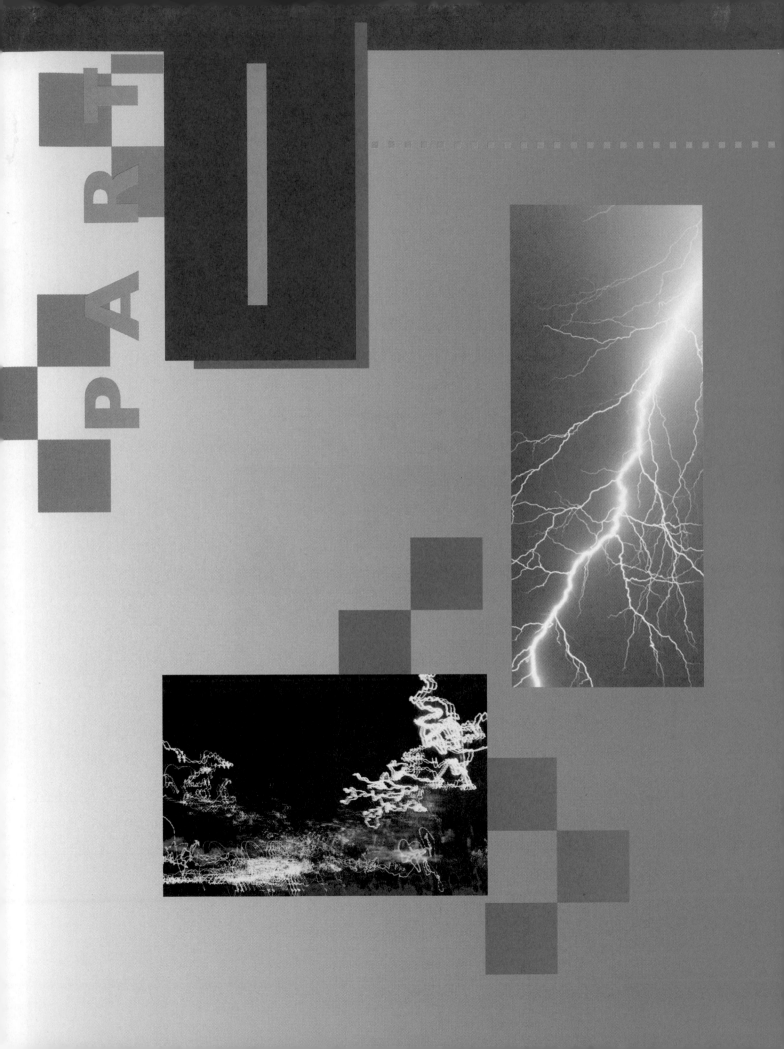

RADIOLOGIC PHYSICS

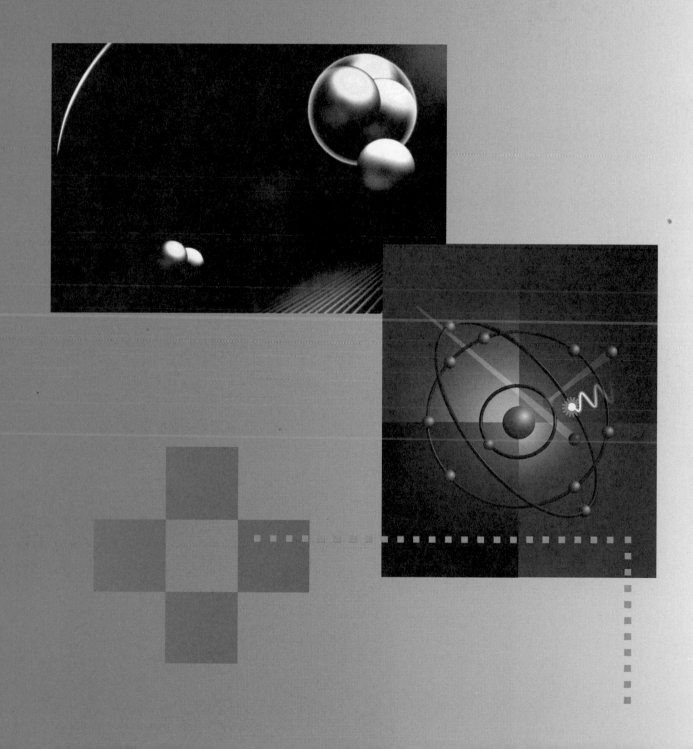

Basic Concepts of Radiation Science

OBJECTIVES

At the completion of this chapter the student will be able to:

1. Identify the difference between matter and energy
2. Define electromagnetic radiation and, specifically, ionizing radiation
3. Explain how x-rays were discovered accidently
4. Discuss human injury caused by radiation
5. List basic radiation protection equipment
6. Describe a brief history of modern radiography and discuss what behaviors are required of a radiographer

OUTLINE

Matter and Energy
    Matter and mass
    Energy

Ionizing Radiation
    Natural sources of ionizing radiation
    Medical x-ray

C hapter I explores the basic concepts underlying the science of radiography. These basic concepts include the study of matter, energy, and the electromagnetic spectrum, of which ionizing radiation is a part. The production of ionizing radiation and its use as a diagnostic tool is the basis of radiography. Radiographers have a great responsibility in performing x-ray examinations using established radiation protection standards with consideration for the safety of patients and medical personnel.

Radiography is a career choice with diverse opportunities. Welcome to the field of diagnostic imaging.

MATTER AND ENERGY
Matter and Mass

Matter is anything that occupies space. It is the material substance with form and shape composing physical objects. The fundamental, complex building blocks of matter are **atoms** and **molecules**. The primary characteristic of matter is **mass,** which is defined as the quantity of matter contained in a physical object.

> Mass or the quantity of matter within a physical object is constant within the universe.

The term *weight* is used to describe the mass of an object in a gravitational field. In other words, weight is the force exerted by a physical object under the influence of gravity. On earth a person weighs 200 pounds because of the mutual attraction or gravity between the earth's mass and the mass of the person; however, on the moon, which has a mass one sixteenth that of the earth, the person would weigh 34 pounds ($\frac{1}{6}$ = 0.17; 0.17 × 200 pounds = 34 pounds). The mass of the person remains the same. It is only the weight of the person that is less on the moon. Mass remains unchanged in another instance. Mass remains unchanged when matter changes from one form to another. Consider a block of ice. The shape of the ice changes as it melts into a puddle of water. If the puddle dries, the water disappears. The ice is transformed from a solid to a liquid to water vapor. If all the particles making up the ice, water, and water vapor were measured separately, the quantity of particles in each form would be the same. Each form has the same mass, although the shape may be different. Mass is constant. It does not change under the influence of gravity or when matter changes state.

Energy

> **Energy**
> The ability to do work.

Like matter, energy can exist in many forms. The following is a list of the forms of energy:

1. **Potential energy** is the capacity to do work because of the position of an object. In Figure 1-1 the heavy guillotine blade held in the air by a rope and pulley is an example of an object possessing potential energy. If the rope is cut, the blade will descend and do its ghastly task. Work was required to get the blade to its high position. Because of this position, the blade has potential energy. Other examples of potential energy include a roller coaster on the top of the incline and the stretched spring of an open screen door.

2. **Kinetic energy** is the energy of motion. An automobile in motion, a turning windmill wheel, or the falling guillotine blade are all examples of kinetic energy. These systems all do work because of their motion.

3. **Chemical energy** is the energy released in a chemical reaction. One way to illustrate the release of chemical energy is to consider the violent burst resulting from the lighting of dynamite. Nitroglycerine and ammonium nitrate combine in the presence of heat or a flame. The violent chemical reaction increases the internal pressure in the dynamite tubes, causing the explosion or energy release.

4. **Electrical energy** is the work done when an electron (negative particle) moves through a wire. This is discussed further in Chapter 5. All electric appli-

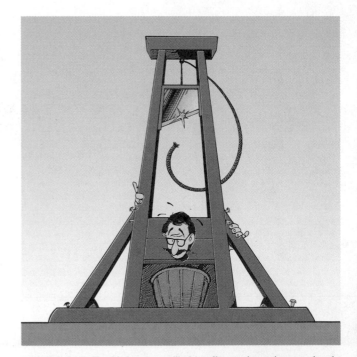

FIGURE 1-1 The blade of a guillotine offers a dramatic example of both potential and kinetic energy. When the blade is pulled to its maximum height and locked in place, it has potential energy. When the blade is allowed to fall, kinetic energy is released.

ances like heaters, dryers, stoves, and refrigerators use electrical energy.

- **Thermal energy** is the energy of motion at the molecular level. It is the kinetic energy of molecules. Thermal energy or heat is measured by temperature. The faster the molecules of matter are moving, the more thermal energy the matter contains and the higher the temperature of the substance.

- **Nuclear energy** is the energy contained in the nucleus of atom. The atomic bomb is an example of the power of nuclear energy.

- **Electromagnetic energy** is the most important form of energy in radiography because it is the type of energy in the x-ray beam and used in magnetic resonance imaging.

In addition to x-rays used in radiography and radio waves used in magnetic resonance imaging, electromagnetic energy spectrum includes microwaves and visible light. Just as matter can be transformed from one form or shape to another, so can energy. For example, the electrical energy in the x-ray unit produces electromagnetic energy in the form of an x-ray beam, which is then converted into light and chemical energy, resulting in an image on the x-ray film. Electromagnetic energy emitted by a source and transferred through space is called *electromagnetic radiation*. Examples of radiation emitted by a source are ultraviolet rays from the sun, heat from a stove, and radio waves from a radio tower.

Albert Einstein combined the concepts of mass and energy in his famous theory of relativity. He won the Nobel Prize in physics in 1921 by describing the mass-energy equivalence. The cornerstone of that theory is the equation $E = mc^2$ where E is energy, m is mass, and c is the speed of light.

IONIZING RADIATION

There are special types of electromagnetic radiation like x-rays, which can **ionize** matter.

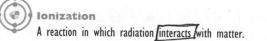

Ionization

A reaction in which radiation interacts with matter.

As radiation passes through matter, it is capable of removing an orbital electron from an atom within the substance (Figure 1-2). As radiation passes close enough to an orbital electron of an atom, it may transfer energy to that electron, causing the atom to escape from its orbit. This free electron may further destabilize surrounding atoms by transferring energy to them. The free electron is a **negative ion**. The destabilized atom is a **positive ion**. The orbital electron and the atom from which it was separated are called an *ion pair*. X-rays and gamma rays are the only forms of electromagnetic radiation with enough energy to ionize matter, although

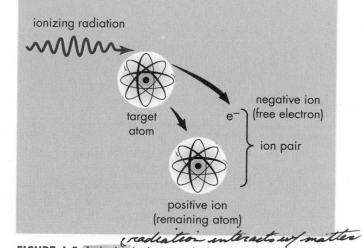

FIGURE 1-2 Ionization is the removal of an electron from an atom. The ejected electron and the resulting positively charged atom are called an *ion pair*.

some fast-moving particles like **alpha** and **beta** are also capable of ionization.

Many types of radiation are harmless, like radio waves and light waves, although ultraviolet light can cause harmful sunburn. Ionizing radiation, however, can seriously injure humans; thus radiographers study radiation protection and radiation biology to learn ways to protect themselves and to limit patient exposure. There are two main sources of radiation harmful to humans—natural sources and man-made sources.

Natural Sources of Ionizing Radiation

Natural environmental radiation comes from three sources—cosmic rays, terrestrial radiation, and naturally occurring radionuclides (radioactive nucleus) in the human body. Cosmic rays are particles that are emitted by the sun and stars. The intensity of cosmic rays increases with the increase in altitude from the earth and the increase in latitude on the earth, that is, toward the poles. Terrestrial radiation is emitted from deposits of uranium, thorium, and other radioactive substances in the earth. The intensity of the terrestrial radiation depends on the geology of the area where deposits are located. The largest component of terrestrial radiation is **radon.** Radon, a **radioactive** gas that emits alpha particles, is produced by the natural decay of uranium and is present in trace quantities in the ground. All ground-based materials such as concrete, bricks, and gypsum wallboard contain radon. Radon gas can be harmful if inhaled in sufficient quantities. Radionuclides, mainly potassium-40, are part of the human metabolism and have been part of the environmental radiation source as long as man has been on earth—100,000 years. Human evolution has undoubtedly been influenced by this natural environmental radiation.

Some genetic scientists contend that evolution, or changes in the genetic substance of organisms, was influenced by ionization of **DNA** (deoxyribonucleic acid.) If this is true, radiation workers and medical personnel must be highly concerned with unnecessary medical radiation exposure.

2 Medical X-ray

Medical x-rays constitute the largest source of man-made ionizing radiation. The medical benefits of x-rays are indisputable; however, the controlled use of radiation is equally as important. **Radiographers, radiologists,** and **biomedical engineers** have equal responsibility in reducing the radiation dosage to personnel and to patients. Other sources of man-made radiation include nuclear power plants and industrial sources, which contribute only insignificantly to the human population's annual radiation dose. Consumer items like watch dials, smoke detectors, televisions, and airport surveillance systems actually contribute more significantly to the annual radiation dose (Figure 1-3).

The ionizing radiation dose to humans is measured in **rads** or **mrads** ($\frac{1}{1000}$ rad). The rad is the unit of radiation absorbed dose or the quantity of radiation absorbed by the human body. Most recently the unit rad has been changed to an international unit called a gray (Gy).

Natural radiation sources contribute approximately 360 mrad to the average **absorbed dose** to each human. Medical x-rays on average contribute 40 mrad.

What percentage of the average radiation exposure to a human is due to medical x-rays?

$$\frac{40 \text{ mrad}}{360 \text{ mrad}} = 0.128 \text{ or } 13\%$$

Even though only 13% of all radiation exposure is due to medical x-ray and medical procedures, radiation workers still need to be concerned about limiting the radiation to personnel and to patients.

Discovery of x-rays. X-rays were not developed. They were discovered by accident. During the 1870s and 1880s, university physics professors were investigating the conduction of **cathode rays** (electrons) through a glass tube that was only partially filled with gasses. The glass tube was called a *Crookes' tube* after an Englishman, Sir William Crookes, who led one of the many experiments. The Crookes' tube is the forerunner of the modern fluorescent light. Experimenting with a Crookes' tube, Wilhelm Roentgen accidently discovered x-rays.

On November 8, 1895, Roentgen was working in his laboratory at Würzburg University in Germany. So that he could better see the effects of the cathode rays in the Crookes' tube, he darkened his laboratory. Several feet away on a bench was a photographic plate coated with **barium platinocyanide,** a fluorescent material. Roentgen covered the Crookes' tube with paper so no visible light escaped from it. Then he activated the

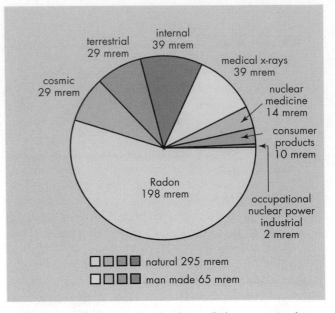

FIGURE 1-3 The contribution of various radiation sources to the total average U.S. population dose equivalent (mrem).

Crookes' tube and noticed that the plate on the nearby bench glowed. The intensity of the glow or **fluorescence** increased as the plate was brought closer to the tube. There was little doubt about the origin of the fluorescence, but the kind of light was unclear. Roentgen called the rays *x-light* because it was an unknown ray. He feverishly continued his investigation for several weeks. His initial investigation was extremely thorough, and he was able to report his experimental results to the scientific community before the end of 1895. In 1901, he received the Nobel Prize in physics. He also published the first medical x-ray—an image of his wife Bertha's hand (Figure 1-4).

Figure 1-5 is a photograph of what is reported to be the first x-ray examination in the United States. It was conducted in early February 1896 in the physics laboratory at Dartmouth College, Hanover, New Hampshire.

The discovery of x-rays ranks high among the amazing events of human history. First of all, x-rays were discovered by accident. Secondly, at least twelve of Roentgen's contemporaries had observed x-rays but none had recognized their significance. Thirdly, Roentgen studied his discovery with such scientific vigor that within little more than a month he had described all the properties of x-rays that are recognized today.

Reports of radiation injury to humans. Unfortunately, in the early years radiation injuries from overexposure occurred fairly frequently. Most injuries were skin damage (**erythema**), loss of hair (**alopecia**), and low red-cell blood count (**anemia**). Physicians and, more commonly, patients were injured because of the low-energy radiation produced by the early tubes and the long exposure times required to get an acceptable radiograph. By

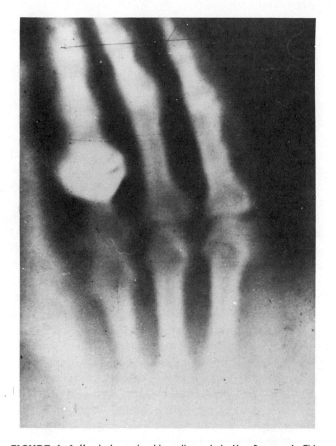

FIGURE I-4 Hand shown in this radiograph is Mrs. Roentgen's. This was the first indication of the possible medical applications of x-rays and was made within a few days of their discovery. *(Courtesy Deutsches Roentgen Museum.)*

1910, with the introduction of the Coolidge tube and the Snook transformer, which decreased the low-energy radiation in the x-ray beam and decreased the exposure times, reports of injury to patients and physicians decreased as well. However, years later, radiologists were developing blood disorders (aplastic anemia and leukemia) more frequently than the rest of the medical community. Because of these reports, radiation protective devices and apparel where developed for use by radiologists. The protective apparel includes lead gloves and aprons. Today, radiologists and radiographers are monitored for radiation exposure with special film badges and are taught radiation control and radiation protection procedures to protect themselves, other medical personnel, and patients.

> The risk of radiation exposure in diagnostic imaging departments is minimal. Radiography is now considered a radiation-safe occupation.

Basic radiation protection. In 1987 the National Council on Radiation Protection and Measurements (NCRP) established limits of radiation exposure for workers in radiation areas and for nonradiation workers. The basic radiation protection goal of the council was to minimize the potential for harm to all individuals exposed to man-made radiation. The following are

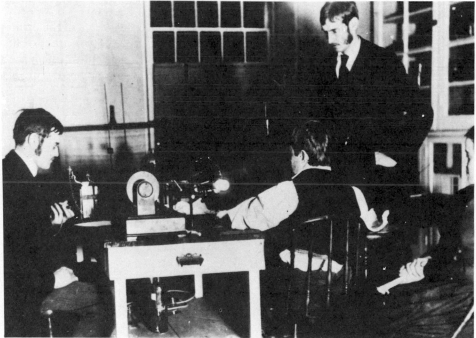

FIGURE I-5 This photograph records the first medical x-ray examination in the United States. A young patient, Eddie McCarthy of Hanover, New Hampshire, broke his wrist while skating on the Connecticut River and submitted to having it photographed by the "x-light." With him are *(left to right)* Professor E.B. Frost, Dartmouth College; his brother, Dr. G.D. Frost, Medical Director, Mary Hitchcock Hospital; and Mrs. G.D. Frost, the hospital's first head nurse. The apparatus was assembled by Professor F.G. Austin in his physics laboratory in Reed Hall, Dartmouth College, on February 3, 1896. *(Courtesy Dartmouth Hitchcock Medical Center.)*

two effects of radiation that are of concern to those who write radiation standards:

1. Early effects occur immediately after the overdose of radiation, which include blood changes and decreased sperm count.
2. Latent effects develop a long time after the exposure incident and can cause cancer changes and possibly genetic effects to offspring.

In 1966, another group concerned with radiation safety, the International Council of Radiation Protection (ICRP), introduced the goal of **ALARA** for all radiation workers. The acronym stands for as low as reasonably achievable. The concept has no specific numerical guidelines, however, the basic tenets follow:

1. Radiation exposure must have a specific benefit
2. All exposure should be kept as low as reasonably achievable *ALARA*
3. Dose of individuals shall not exceed limits for appropriate circumstances

As radiographers and student radiographers become familiar with their work environment within the radiology or diagnostic imaging department, complacency may develop about radiation protection. It is critical to the safety of all radiation workers and to the safety of patients that *radiation protection must be the first consideration* during every x-ray examination or procedure.

"The radiographer utilizes equipment and accessories, employs techniques and procedures, performs services in accordance with an accepted standard of practice, and demonstrates expertise in limiting the radiation exposure to the patient, self, and other members of the health care team"
American Society of Radiographers, *Code of Ethics, #7*

Basic radiation protection for the radiographer is summarized in the following simple list :

1. Time
2. Distance
3. Shielding

The radiographer and other personnel and patients to which he or she is responsible must follow these simple rules outlined above. Reduce or limit the *time* spent near the *radiation source*. Move away or keep as much *distance* as possible from the radiation source. If the radiographer, other personnel, or family members must be near the radiation source, *shielding* must be used as a barrier between the source and the individual. There are other procedures that should be followed as well. Always know and practice the radiation protection policies required at the workplace. For example, abdominal x-rays of females should never be taken in the first trimester of pregnancy unless absolutely necessary. Also, reduce repeated x-rays because each repeat doubles the exposure to the patient. Encourage doctors and office staff to reconsider ordering x-rays for screening purposes (except for mammography). In other words, if the patient has no symptoms, perhaps the x-ray is not necessary. Furthermore, patients who require assistance during an x-ray examination should *never* be held by radiographers or radiography students. It is best to request help by a member of the patient's family, nursing staff, or medical staff (always remember to screen any family member or personnel for pregnancy before allowing them to be in the x-ray room during an exposure).

Some of the primary devices for minimizing radiation exposure are as follows (Figure 1-6):

- **Filtration** in the x-ray tube is generally a metal (aluminum) plate inserted between the tube and the pa-

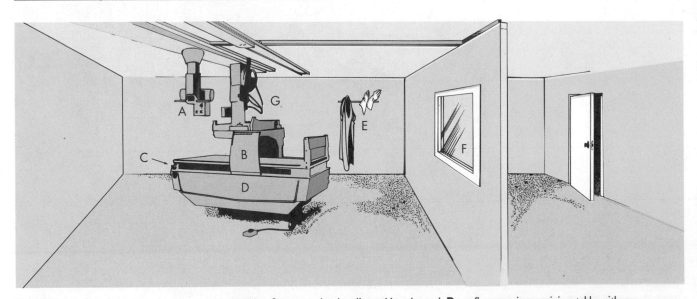

FIGURE 1-6 The general purpose x-ray room includes **A,** an overhead radiographic tube and **D,** a fluoroscopic examining table with an x-ray tube under the table. Some of the more common radiation protection devices are **B,** lead curtain, **C,** Bucky slot cover, **E,** leaded apron and gloves, and **F,** protective viewing window. The location of the image intensifier, **G,** and associated imaging equipment is also shown.

tient. Using the aluminum filter reduces the low energy x-rays, which have little value in forming the x-ray image.

2 ▪ **Collimation** restricts the x-ray beam to only that body part requiring examination and spares the adjacent tissue from radiation exposure. Collimation reduces scattered radiation and improves the visibility of the image.

3 ▪ **Intensifying screens** reduce the exposure to the patient by more than 95% compared with examinations done without screens. The x-ray film is sandwiched between the intensifying screens in the x-ray cassette.

4 ▪ **Protective barriers** are the lead-lined walls or lead-glass windows behind which the radiographer stands during the x-ray exposure (Figure 1-6, *F*).

5 ▪ **Protective apparel** is covered with lead-impregnated material. The material is used for aprons, gloves, and thyroid shields for radiation workers and half-shields and gonadal shields for patients.

6 ▪ **Gonadal shielding** needs special mention. Gonadal shielding or shielding of the sex organs *must* be used on patients of childbearing age if the sex organs are in or near the x-ray beam. Shielding breast tissue is also important. However, lead shields must not interfere with the value of the examination. In other words, if the shield covers the area of interest, do not shield. Otherwise, shield everyone of childbearing age.

Radiation protection is covered in more detail in a later chapter. For now, the following is a list of the important aspects of radiation protection that serves as a summary and a quick reference. A radiographer should:

1. Understand and apply the cardinal principles of radiation control—time, distance, and shielding.
2. Not allow familiarity to result in poor radiation protection procedures.
3. Never stand in the primary beam.
4. Always wear protective apparel or stand behind a protective barrier.
5. Always wear a radiation badge or monitor and position it outside the lead apron on the collar.
6. Never hold a patient during an exposure.
7. If personnel and/or family holds a patient, they *must* wear lead-protective devices.
8. Use gonadal shielding on all persons of childbearing age, and breast shielding when it will not interfere with the area of interest.
9. Avoid radiographic examination of the pelvis and abdomen of a pregnant woman, especially during the first trimester.
10. Always collimate to the smallest field size appropriate for the examination.

Development of modern radiography. During Roentgen's time, electric current and potential were so limited as to require exposures of 30 minutes or more for a satisfactory examination. The development of intensifying screens helped reduce exposure time. Micheal Pupin first used fluorescent screens in conjunction with glass photographic plates in 1896. Only years later did the invention receive adequate recognition and use. In 1904, Charles Leonard found that by exposing two glass plates with the emulsion surfaces together halved the exposure time and improved the image. This double-emulsion film did not become commercially available until 1918. During World War I, when the supply of high-quality glass from Belgium was interrupted, radiologists began to use flexible film rather than glass plates. The film was made from **cellulose nitrate** and it quickly became a better product than the original glass plates.

The fluoroscope was invented by Thomas Edison in 1898 (Figure 1-7). Edison's original fluorescent material was **barium platinocyanide,** a widely used laboratory material. He investigated the use of over 1800 materials including **zinc cadmium sulfide** and **calcium tungstate,** materials in use until the advent of **rare-earth intensifying screens** in the 1970s. Edison abandoned his research when his assistant and longtime friend suffered amputation of both arms because of overexposure to radiation. Clarence Dally, Edison's assistant, died in 1904 and is considered the first fatality from man-made radiation exposure in the United States.

Before the turn of the century, William Rollins, a Boston dentist, found that restricting the x-ray beam by placing a lead sheet with a hole in it over the beam improved the quality of his patients' dental x-rays. He also found that placing an aluminum sheet over the beam further improved his x-rays. Rollins discovered collimation and filtration, which is used in every x-ray machine today.

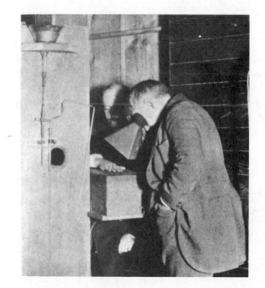

FIGURE 1-7 Thomas Edison is seen viewing the hand of his assistant, Clarence Dally through a fluoroscope of his own design. Dally's hand rests on the box containing the x-ray tube. (From Eisenberg RL: *Radiology: an illustrated history,* St. Louis, 1992, Mosby.)

Early in the 1900s, x-rays became a valuable, large-scale speciality mostly because of the introduction of the Snook transformer and the Coolidge tube. In 1907, H.C. Snook introduced a substitute high-voltage power supply for the static machines and **induction coils** then in use. The capacity of the transformer greatly exceeded the capacity of the Crookes' tube still in use. In 1913,

William Coolidge unveiled his hot-cathode x-ray tube, and it was immediately recognized as far superior to the Crookes' tube. The Coolidge tube was a vacuum tube that allowed x-ray intensity and energy to be accurately selected. The modern era of radiography is dated from the matching of the Coolidge tube with the Snook transformer. In 1921 the Potter-Bucky grid was developed, which greatly improved the visibility of the x-ray image

---

Clinical Skills Performed by Radiographers

Evaluate the need for and use protective shielding.

Take appropriate precautions to minimize radiation exposure to patients.

Restrict beam to limit exposure area, improve image quality, and reduce radiation dose.

Set kVp, mA, and time or automated exposure system to achieve optimal image quality, safe operating conditions, and minimum radiation dose.

Prevent all unnecessary persons from remaining in area during x-ray exposure.

Take appropriate precautions to minimize occupational radiation exposure.

Wear a personal monitoring device while on duty.

Review and evaluate individual occupational exposure reports.

Warm-up x-ray tube according to manufacturer's reccomendations.

Prepare and adjust radiographic unit and accessories.

Prepare and adjust the fluoroscopic unit and accessories.

Recognize and report malfunctions in the radiographic or fluoroscopic unit and ancillary accessories.

Perform basic evaluations of radiographic equipment and accessories (e.g., lead aprons, collimator accuracy).

Inspect and clean screens and cassettes.

Perform start-up or shutdown procedures on automatic processor.

Recognize and report malfunctions in the automatic processor.

Process exposed film.

Reload cassettes by selecting film of proper size and type.

Store film or cassette in a manner that will reduce the possibility of artifact production.

Select appropriate film-screen combination and/or grid.

Determine appropriate exposure factors using calipers, technique charts, and tube rating charts.

Modify exposure factors for circumstances such as involuntary motion, casts and splints, pathological conditions, or patient's inability to cooperate.

Use radiopaque markers to indicate anatomic side, position, or other relevant information.

Evaluate patient and radiographs to determine if additional projections or positions should be recommended.

Evaluate radiographs for diagnostic quality.

Determine corrective measures if radiograph is not of diagnostic quality and take appropriate action.

Select equipment and accessories for the examination requested.

Remove all radiopaque materials from patient or table that could interfere with the radiographic image.

Patient Care Performed by Radiographers

Explain breathing instructions before making the exposure.

Position patient to demonstrate the desired anatomy using body landmarks.

Explain patient preparation (e.g., diet restrictions, preparatory medications) before an imaging procedure.

Properly sequence radiograph procedures to avoid residual contrast material affecting future examinations.

Examine radiographic requisition to verify accuracy and completeness of information.

Use universal precautions.

Confirm patient's identity.

Question female patients of childbearing age about possible pregnancy.

Explain procedures to patient or patient's family.

Evaluate patient's ability to comply with positioning requirements for the requested examination.

Observe and monitor vital signs.

Use proper body mechanics and/or mechanical transfer devices when assisting patients.

Provide for patient comfort and modesty.

Select immobilization devices, when indicated, to prevent patient movement and/or ensure patient safety.

Verify accuracy of patient film identification.

Maintain confidentiality of patient information.

Use sterile or aseptic technique to prevent contamination of sterile trays, instruments, or fields.

Prepare contrast media for administration.

Before administration of contrast agent, gather information to determine if the patient is at increased risk of adverse reaction.

Perform venipuncture.

Observe patient after administration of contrast media to detect adverse reactions.

Recognize need for prompt medical attention and administer emergency care.

Document required information on patient's medical record.

Clean, disinfect, or sterilize facilities and equipment, and dispose of contaminated items in preparation for next examination.

Follow appropriate procedures when in contact with a patient in reverse/protective isolation.

Monitor medical equipment attached to the patient (e.g., intravenous lines, oxygen) during the radiographic procedure.

Position patient, x-ray tube, and image receptor to produce radiographs.

on film. In 1921, Bell Telephone Laboratories invented an amplifier tube, which was adapted for use in fluoroscopy.

Each recent decade has seen remarkable improvement in diagnostic imaging. Figure 1-6 shows the modern radiographic and fluoroscopic (RaF) x-ray room. Ultrasound appeared in the 1960s; computed tomography (CT) and positron emission tomography (PET) were developed in 1970s, and magnetic resonance imaging (MRI) became an accepted modality in the 1980s. Appendix B has a complete list of the important dates in the development of modern radiography.

Joining the team in diagnostic imaging. To become part of this exciting profession a student must complete the prescribed academic courses, obtain clinical experience, and pass the national certification examination given by the American Registry of Radiologic Technologists (ARRT). Both academic expertise and clinical skills are required of radiographers. The boxes on p. 10 are a complete list of the clinical and patient care skills required by an individual who can put the initials **RT** after his or her name.

SUMMARY

Radiography offers a career involving study in many areas of medicine and physics. This first chapter weaves the history and development of radiography with an introduction to physics. Physics includes the study of matter, energy, and the electromagnetic spectrum of which ionizing radiation is a part. It is the production of ionizing radiation and its safe, diagnostic use that is the basis of the diverse field of radiography. As well as emphasing the importance of radiation safety, this chapter also specifies with a detailed list the high level of clinical and patient care skills required by the graduate radiographer.

REVIEW QUESTIONS

1. Matter is defined as _____.
2. Energy is defined as _____.
3. Mass is constant. True or False
4. Describe how weight is different from mass.
5. List and define the seven forms of energy.
6. Name two examples of electromagnetic radiation.
7. In the interaction with matter, how are x-rays different from other electromagnetic radiation?
8. Describe the process that results in the formation of a negative ion and a positive ion.
9. Name the largest component of terrestrial radiation.
10. Define *rad* and name its equivalent term in international units.
11. What percentage of average radiation exposure to a human is due to medical x-rays?
12. What glass tube was the forerunner of the modern fluorscent light?
13. List the three reasons why the discovery of x-rays was one of the amazing events in human history.
14. Why is radiography now considered a radiation-safe occupation?
15. In the early years of the medical use of x-rays, radiation injuries were common. What were the three most common injuries?
16. The acronym ALARA stands for what phrase?
17. Basic radiation protection for the radiographer is summarized in a list of three rules. Name the three rules.
18. Name the six primary devices for minimizing radiation exposure to the patient and the operator.
19. Briefly describe the development of x-ray film.
20. What is the significance of the Snook transformer and the Coolidge tube in the development of the medical use of x-rays?

Additional Reading

Brady C: Accountability and the role-development radiographer, *Radiography (Lond)* 1(2)127, October 1995.

Broda K, Hubbard R: Teamwork in the radiology department, *Images* 9(2):11, Spring 1990.

Cullinan J, Cullinan A: The x-ray's discovery and early uses, part 1, *Radiol Technol* 66(1):47, September-October 1994.

Doherty-Simon MM: Is training for technologists necessary to ensure proper nursing care in the radiology department? *Images* 13(2):3, Summer 1994.

Klempfner G: The centenary of x-rays: celebrating the past and anticipating the future, *Med J Aust* 163(9):455, November 1995.

Mayers A, Wintch K: Administrators evaluate bachelor's degrees for R.T.s, *Radiol Technol* 64(5):292, May-June 1993.

Michael KK: The evolution of continuing education in allied health, *Appl Radiol* 22(4):38, April 1993.

Thomalla K: ASRT's resources place emphasis on member-driver requirements . . . American Society of Radiologic Technologists, *ASRT Scanner* 28(2):3, November 1995.

Wandling KW: Importance of effective communication in radiology: president's message, *Images* 12(3):25, Summer 1993.

Yochum TR: 1895-1995: diagnostic imaging in its first century, *J Manipulative Physiol Ther* 18(9):618, November-December 1995.

2

Radiographic Definitions and Mathematics Review

OBJECTIVES

At the completion of this chapter the student will be able to:

1. Name scientific exponential notation and the associated prefixes
2. List and define units of radiation measurement and absorbed dose
3. Calculate problems using fractions, exponents, and algebraic equations

OUTLINE

Definitions of Radiography
    Numeric prefixes and introduction
      to exponential notation
    Units of ionizing radiation

Mathematics and Algebra Review
    Number systems
    Algebra
    Graphing

This chapter contains the list of definitions used in radiography. Also included in this chapter is a basic mathematics and algebra review.

. . . .

DEFINITIONS IN RADIOGRAPHY
Numeric Prefixes and Introduction to Exponents

Every area of technical knowledge has its own language. Radiography is no exception. Radiography is the study of the **diagnostic** use of ionization radiation, and radiographers use specific units for radiation measurement as their technical language. Some of these units can be very large or very small and require special multiples called *exponents*. Table 2-1 shows the exponential notation relating to numbers that are all multiples of ten. The table also lists prefixes and prefix symbols relating to the multiples of ten.

Standard scientific notation was developed to express very large and very small units without writing out all the zeros. Two basic units used in radiography are **milliamperes** (milliamps) and **kilovolts**. The notation is made simpler if, for example, 0.015 amperes (amps) is written as 15 mA (milliamps) and 75,000 volts is written as 75 kV (kilovolts). Problems using this notation follow:

How many kilovolts are 80,000 volts?

1000 volts = 1 kilovolt
80,000 volts = 80 kV

Write 80,000 volts in scientific notation (exponential form).

8×10^4 (volts)

Units of Ionizing Radiation

In 1981 the International Commission on Radiologic Units (ICRU) issued standard units of measurement for ionizing radiation. Figure 2-1 relates four of the units in hypothetical situations in which the units would be measured. The units are called *SI units* from the French title of Systems Internationale des Units and they are listed and defined in the following sections: *1 C/kg = 100 R*

Roentgen (R) or coulomb/kilogram (C/kg). Traditionally known as the *roentgen (R)*, this is the unit of radiation intensity in air. It is equal to the radiation intensity that will create 2.08×10^9 ion pairs in a cubic centimeter of air. The definition is actually in terms of electric charge per unit mass of air. The charge refers to the electrons liberated by ionization. The output of x-ray units is specified in milliroentgens (mR). The relationship between roentgens and coulombs per kilogram is as follows:

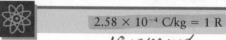
2.58×10^{-4} C/kg = 1 R

1 Gy = 100 rad

Rad or gray (Gy). Traditionally known as the *rad (radiation absorbed dose)*, this is the unit describing the

TABLE 2-1			
Standard Scientific Notation, Prefixes, and Symbols			
Notation		Prefix	Symbol
10^{18}		exa-	E
10^{15}		peta-	P
10^{12}		era-	T
10^{9}		giga-	G
10^{6}		**mega-**	**M**
10^{3}	1000	**kilo-**	**k**
10^{2}	100	hecto-	h
10^{1}	10	deka-	da
10^{-1}	0.1	deci-	d
10^{-2}	0.01	**centi-**	**c**
10^{-3}	0.001	**milli-**	**m**
10^{-6}	0.000001	**micro-**	**μ**
10^{-9}		nano-	n
10^{-12}		pico-	p
10^{-15}		femto-	f
10^{-18}		atto-	a

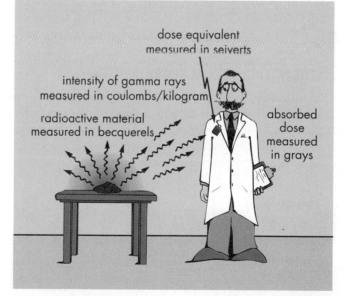

FIGURE 2-1 Radiation is emitted by radioactive material. The quantity of radioactive material is measured in becquerels. Radiation quantity is specified in coulombs/kilogram, grays, or seiverts, depending on the conditions under which it is measured and the use of the measurement. In diagnostic imaging, we may consider 1 R equal to 1 rad equal to 1 rem.

quantity of radiation received by a patient. It is expressed as follows:

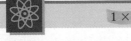

$$1 \times 10^{-2} \text{ Gy} = 1 \text{ rad}$$

1 Sv = 100 rem

Rem or sievert (Sv). Traditionally known as the *rem (radiation equivalent man)*, this is the unit used to express the quantity of radiation received by radiation workers including, in modern times, not only radiographers but also nuclear power plant personnel. Some types of radiation produce more damage than x-rays, and the **biologic effectiveness** factor is calculated into the seivert or rem and accounts for the differences in different levels of biologic damage. The following is the equation for 1 rem:

$$1 \times 10^{-2} \text{ Sv} = 1 \text{ rem}$$

denotes instability of nucleus

Curie or becquerel (Bq). Traditionally known as the *curie (Ci),* this unit expresses the quantity of radioactive material and has nothing to do with the radiation emitted. These quantities are used in the field of **nuclear medicine**, which is a subspeciality in the diagnostic imaging department. The equation for 1 Ci follows:

$$3.7 \times 10^{10} \text{Bq} = 1 \text{ Ci}$$

Table 2-2 lists radiation units and their symbols. The traditional units and the SI units are included.

To summarize, there are four traditional and international units used for the measurement of ionizing radiation. For in-air exposure, the unit is coulomb per kilogram or roentgen. For absorbed dose, the unit is gray or rad. For dose equivalent, the unit is sievert or rem, and for radioactivity, the unit is becquerel or curie.

(does not turn off

MATHEMATICS AND ALGEBRA REVIEW

The following sections review the basic concepts in mathematics and algebra, which are fundamental to further study in radiography. First, number systems, fractions, and decimals are reviewed. Then, algebraic equations and graphing are discussed.

TABLE 2-2		
Radiation Units		
Traditional Units	**SI Units**	**Quantity**
roentgen (R)	coulomb/kilogram (C/kg)	exposure
rad	gray (Gy)	absorbed dose
rem	sievert (Sv)	dose equivalent
curie (Ci)	becquerel (Bq)	radioactivity

Number Systems

The system of numbers based on the multiples of ten is called the *decimal system.* The origin of the decimal system is unknown, but there are theories (Figure 2-2). Numbers in the decimal system can be represented in four ways as shown on Table 2-3. Numbers can be represented as fractions, as decimals, as exponents, or in logarithmic form. It may seem that the logarithmic form has limited use in radiography, but it is used to describe the characteristics of x-ray film, and you will see a logarithmic graph again.

Exponents. Exponents are the superscripts on the number tens in the "Exponential Form" column on Table 2-3. The exponential form or *scientific notation,* as it is called, allows very large and very small numbers to be written simply and calculations of these large or small numbers to be made with ease. To express a number in exponential form, first write the number as a decimal. Then, determine how many spaces the decimal point needs to be moved to express a **whole number.** Spaces to the right of the decimal point indicate negative exponents and spaces to the left indicate positive exponents. For example, in March of 1995 the national debt was approximately:

5 trillion dollars = 5,000,000,000,000.00 dollars

To express this in scientific notation, position the decimal point after the five and count the number of spaces in the direction the decimal point was moved. The decimal point was moved to the left twelve places. So the number is written as follows:

$$5 \times 10^{12} \text{ dollars}$$

A string on Garth Brooks' guitar has a diameter of 0.00075 meters (m). To determine its diameter in scientific notation, position the decimal point between the seven and the five. Next, count the number of spaces the

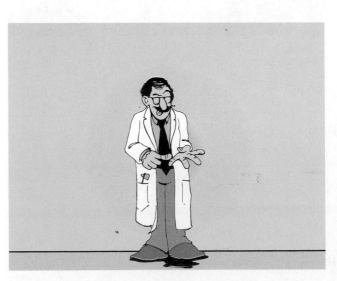

FIGURE 2-2 The probable origin of the decimal number system.

TABLE 2-3

Various Ways to Represent Numbers in the Decimal System

1 Fractional Form	2 Decimal Form	3 Exponential Form	4 Logarithmic Form
10,000	10,000	10^4 *scientific notation*	4.000
1000	1000	10^3	3.000
100	100	10^2	2.000
10	10	10^1	1.000
1	1	10^0	0.000
1/10	0.1	10^{-1}	−1.000
1/100	0.01	10^{-2}	−2.000
1/1000	0.001	10^{-3}	−3.000
1/10,000	0.0001	10^{-4}	−4.000

decimal point moved and in what direction. The decimal point was moved four places to the right. So the notation is written as follows:

$$0.00075 \text{ m} = 7.5 \times 10^{-4} \text{ m}$$

The advantage of using exponential form is the ease of doing calculations. The rules for calculation using exponents are in Table 2-4. Practice the following examples:

$$(2 \times 10^2) \text{ multiplied by } (3 \times 10^3) = 6 \times 10^5$$
$$(4 \times 10^4) \text{ divided by } (2 \times 10^2) = 2 \times 10^2$$
$$(5 \times 10^2)^2 = 25 \times 10^4$$

A **Fractions.** A fraction is a numerical value expressed by dividing one number by another. A fraction is a quotient of two numbers and has a **numerator** and a **denominator.**

Fractions

$$\frac{x}{y} = \frac{\text{numerator}}{\text{denominator}}$$

If the quotient is less than one, the value is a **proper fraction**. If the quotient is greater than one, the value is an **improper fraction.**

Proper Fractions <1	**Improper Fractions** >1
$\frac{1}{2}$ $\frac{3}{5}$ $\frac{9}{10}$	$\frac{3}{2}$ $\frac{6}{5}$ $\frac{10}{7}$

1) *Addition and subtraction.* To add or subtract fractions, first find a **common denominator** then add or subtract the **numerators.**

Addition and Subtraction

$$\frac{2}{3} + \frac{3}{2} = \frac{4}{6} + \frac{9}{6} = \frac{13}{6} \text{ or } 2\frac{1}{6}$$
$$\frac{3}{2} - \frac{2}{3} = \frac{9}{6} - \frac{4}{6} = \frac{5}{6}$$

2) *Multiplication.* To multiply fractions, simply multiply numerators and denominators.

Multiplication

$$\frac{2}{5} \times \frac{7}{4} = \frac{14}{20} = \frac{7}{10}$$

3) *Division.* To divide fractions, invert the second fraction then multiply.

Division

$$\frac{5}{2} \div \frac{7}{4} = \frac{5}{2} \times \frac{4}{7} = \frac{20}{14} = \frac{10}{7} \text{ or } 1\frac{3}{7}$$

4) *Ratios.* **Ratios** are a special application of fractions. Ratios express the mathematical relationship between similar quantities such as feet to the mile or pounds to the kilogram. $\left(\dfrac{5260 \text{ ft}}{1 \text{ mile}}\right)$

TABLE 2-4

Rules for Exponential Calculations

Operation	Rule	Example
1 Multiplication	$10^x \times 10^y = 10^{x+y}$	$10^2 \times 10^3 = 10^{2+3} = 10^5$
2 Division	$10^x \div 10^y = 10^{x-y}$	$10^6 \div 10^4 = 10^{6-4} = 10^2$
3 Raising to a power	$(10^x)^y = 10^{xy}$	$(10^5)^3 = 10^{5\times3} = 10^{15}$
4 Inverse	$10^{-x} = \frac{1}{10^x}$	$10^{-3} = \frac{1}{10^3} = \frac{1}{1000}$
5 Unity	$10^0 = 1$	$3.7 \times 10^0 = 3.7$

Ratios

What is the ratio of feet to the mile?

$$\frac{5260 \text{ feet}}{1 \text{ mile}}$$

Decimals. Fractions that have a denominator that is a power of ten are easily converted to decimals.

Decimals

$$\frac{3}{10} = 0.3 \qquad\qquad \frac{3}{100} = 0.03$$

If the denominator is not a power of ten, then the decimal equivalent can be found by long division or by using a calculator.

Significant figures. Students often ask how many decimal places to calculate in an answer.

Addition and Subtraction

Round the answer to the same number of decimal places as the entry with the /least/ number of places to the *right* of the decimal point.

Question: What is the sum of this equation using the method above?

$$\begin{array}{r} 5.23 \\ +3.5 \\ \hline \end{array}$$

Answer: 8.7

Multiplication and Division

Round the answer to the same number of digits as the entry with the *least* number of digits /regardless/ of the number of decimal places.

Question: What is the product of this equation using the method above?

$$\begin{array}{r} 17.24 \\ \times 0.382 \\ \hline 6.58568 \end{array}$$

Answer: 6.58

Because the number with the *least* digits is 0.382 (three digits), then round the answer to three digits as well.

Algebra

Symbols standing for unknown quantities rather than known numbers are often used in equations. Rules of algebra provide definite ways to solve for unknown quantities. The unknowns are designated by alphabetic symbols a, b, and c or x, y, and z. There are three principal rules of algebra used in the solution of problems.

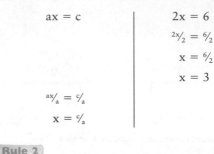

Rule 1
To solve for x
When the unknown x is multiplied by a number, divide both sides of the equation by that number then simplify the equation by solving for x.

Examples:

$ax = c$	$2x = 6$
	$\frac{2x}{2} = \frac{6}{2}$
	$x = \frac{6}{2}$
	$x = 3$
$\frac{ax}{a} = \frac{c}{a}$	
$x = \frac{c}{a}$	

Rule 2
When numbers are added to the unknown, x, subtract that number from both sides of the equation, simplify, and solve for x.

Example:

$$x + a = b$$
$$x + a - a = b - a$$
$$x = b - a$$

Rule 3
When an equation is a fraction, cross-multiply then solve for x.

Examples:

$\frac{x}{a} = \frac{b}{c}$	$\frac{x}{4} = \frac{2}{8}$
$xc = ab$	$\frac{8x}{8} = \frac{8}{8}$
$x = \frac{ab}{c}$	$x = 1$

Proportion. A proportion expresses the relationship of one ratio to another, and it is a special application of fractions and rules of algebra. Fractions can be **directly proportional** or **inversely proportional.**

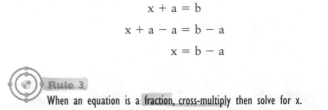

Directly Proportional

$$\frac{a}{b} = \frac{a}{b}$$

Inversely Proportional

$$\frac{a}{b} = \frac{b}{a}$$

Graphs

A graph is a drawing that shows a relationship between two sets of numbers. Most graphs are based on two **axes,** a horizontal or **x-axis** and a vertical or **y-axis.** The point where the two axes meet is called the **origin** (labeled 0 in Figure 2-3).

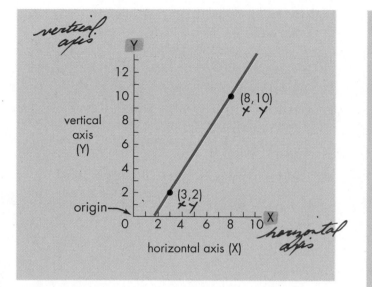

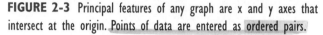

FIGURE 2-3 Principal features of any graph are x and y axes that intersect at the origin. Points of data are entered as ordered pairs.

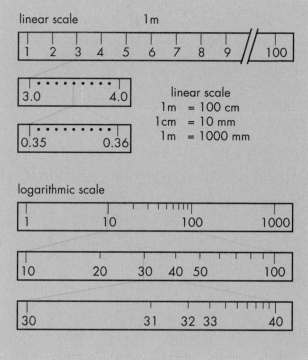

FIGURE 2-4 Linear and logarithmic scales.

Coordinates or sets of numbers are in the form of ordered pairs (x, y), where the first number of the pair represents its place on the x-axis. For example, the ordered pair $(3, 2)$ represents a point three units on the x-axis and two units up the y-axis. The point is plotted in Figure 2-3. If the value of another ordered pair is known, a straight line graph can be constructed with a certain slope and direction to the line or vector.

Sometimes the axes of graphs are not labeled merely x or y but represent specific numerical quantities. The graph demonstrates the relationship between those quantities. Occasionally, the data is in scientific notation and when plotted on the x and y axes, the values extend over a very large range. In these situations a linear scale is not useful, instead a logarithmic scale must be used (Figure 2-4). Semilogarithmic graph combines linear and logarithmic scales. The y-axis is logarithmic and the x-axis is linear.

EXAMPLE: The following data was obtained, which shows the amount of lead thickness required to reduce x-ray intensity from the x-ray tube from 330 mR to 6 mR.

DATA:

mm lead (mm)	0	2	4	6	8
x-ray intensity (mR)	330	140	58	25	11

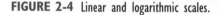

Plot these ordered pairs on linear and semilog paper and estimate the thickness of lead required. One scale is a very small range of values (0 to 8 mm) and is placed on the linear or x-axis. The other scale has a large range of values (330-10 mR) and can be plotted on the logarithmic or y-axis.

ANSWER: (See graph below)
From the semilog plot, the answer is 8.2 mm Pb.

SUMMARY

The technical aspects of radiography are complex. A basic knowledge of mathematics and algebra is required, as well as memorization of the units of radiation measurements and their definitions. Use the chart on p. 18 to answer the questions and calculate the problems in the Review Questions.

REVIEW QUESTIONS

1. Write 100,000 volts in scientific notation.
2. List the conventional units of ionizing radiation and the SI unit equivalents.
3. The output intensity of an x-ray unit is 100 mR. What is this value in SI units?
4. Convert 4050 to scientific notation.
5. Simplify the fraction $^{22}/_{25}$.
6. Given $a = 6.62 \times 10^{-27}$ and $b = 3.766 \times 10^{12}$ what is $a \times b$?
7. What is the value of $^2/_3 + ^4/_5$?
8. What is the value of $^5/_2$ divided by $^7/_4$?
9. Find the decimal equivalent of $^3/_{1000}$.

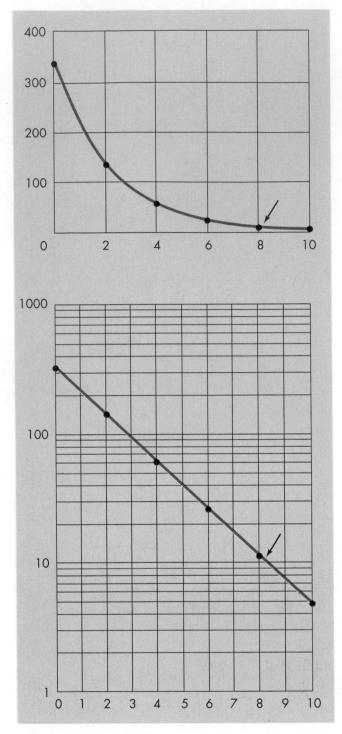

10. What is the decimal equivalent of $^5/_{12}$?

11. What is the product of 17.24 and 0.382? Round off to the appropriate decimal places.

12. In the equation $^x/_5 = \,^3/_8$, solve for x.

13. In the equation ab (x + c) = d, solve for x.

14. Gas mileage is inversely proportional to automobile weight. What is the expected mileage for a 3600 pound car if a 1650 pound car gets 34 miles per gallon?

15. Radiation exposure is directly proportional to the technical factor mAs. At 50 mAs the skin exposure is 240mR. What will be the exposure if the mAs is increased to 60?

Equal lengths of linear scale have equal value. The logarithm scale allows a large range of values to be plotted. Semilogarithmic graphs are often used for plotting radiologic data.

3

Fundamentals of the Physics of Radiation Science

OBJECTIVES

At the completion of this chapter the student will be able to:

1. Discuss the derivation of scientific systems of measurement
2. List the three systems of measurement
3. Identify nine categories of mechanics

OUTLINE

Units of Measurements
  Base quantities and derived
  quantities
Standards of Measurement
  Length
  Mass
  Time
Systems of Measurement
  MKS, CGS, and British systems

Mechanics
  Velocity
  Acceleration
  Motion
  Weight
  Momentum
  Work
  Power
  Energy
  Kinetic energy
  Heat
  Potential energy

n Chapter 1, matter and energy were defined. **Mechanics,** which involves matter in motion, will be discussed in Chapter 2.

The instant the modern x-ray tube produces an x-ray beam, all the laws of physics and mechanics introduced in this text are evident. The **cathode ray** hits the **tungsten** target producing an x-ray beam. X-rays, then, interact with biologic or human tissue. Finally, an image is formed on a sheet of x-ray film. The physics of radiography deals with the interaction between the x-ray beam and matter.

Physics is traditionally grouped into fields such as **thermodynamics, optics, acoustics, mechanics,** and **electromagnetism.** Modern developments have branched physics into other fields including atomic and nuclear physics. In radiography, however, physics is limited to mechanics and electromagnetism. Before the discussion of mechanics, however, the units of measurement in physics and their derivation is introduced.

All scientists strive for exactness in describing **phenomena.** They try to remove the uncertainties by eliminating subjective descriptions of events. To do so, scientists use measurements that can ultimately be represented by numbers. The following discussion describes the building blocks of physics.

UNITS OF MEASUREMENT
Base quantities and derived quantities

There are only three measurable quantities that are the building blocks of all others. The **base quantities** are length, mass, and time. Figure 3-1 illustrates the fundamental role these base quantities play in deriving other quantities used in physics. Secondary quantities or **derived quantities** are a combination of one or more of the base quantities. For example, volume is length to the third power or length cubed (l^3), density is mass divided by volume (m/l^3) and velocity is length divided by time ($1/t$). There are additional measurements used in specialized sciences called *special quantities*. The special quantities in radiation science are units of **exposure, dose, dose equivalent,** and **radioactivity.** Once fundamental quantities are established, they must then relate to a well-defined, invariable standard. **Standards** are usually defined by international organizations or committees and are redefined when progress requires a need for greater precision.

STANDARDS OF MEASUREMENT

The meter, the standard unit of length, was accepted for many years to be the distance between the engraved lines on a **platinum-iridium** bar at the International Bureau of Weights and Measures in Paris, France. In 1960 the need for a more accurate standard led to the redefinition of 1 meter.

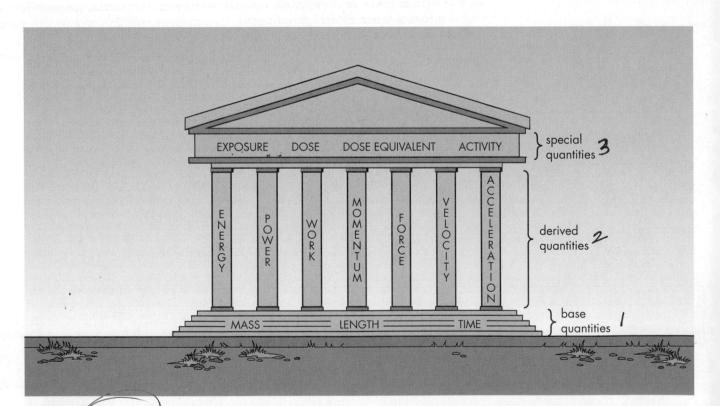

FIGURE 3-1 Base quantities support derived quantities, which in turn support the special quantities of radiologic science.

Length

The meter is now defined as 1,650,763.73 wavelengths of orange light. In the same vault in Paris where the standard meter is kept is the cylinder that represents the standard unit of mass.

Unit of Length

One meter (m) is now defined as the **wavelength** of orange light emitted from an **isotope** of **krypton (86 Kr)**.

Mass

The standard unit of time is the second. Originally, the second was defined in terms of a **mean solar day,** the rotation of the earth on its axis. However, in 1956, the second was redefined as a fraction of the year 1900, which had 365.2422 solar days. In 1964 the second was again redefined as a measurement on an atomic clock.

Unit of Mass

A cylinder of platinum-iridium represents the standard **kilogram** (kg).

Time

Measurement of Time

The second is measured on an **atomic clock,** which is based on the vibrations of **cesium** atoms.

SYSTEMS OF MEASUREMENT

Every measurement has two parts—**magnitude** and a **unit.** For example, in the x-ray room the standard x-ray tube to x-ray film distance is 100 centimeters. The magnitude or the amount 100 is meaningless without a designated unit, the centimeter.

MKS, CGS, and British Systems

The **MKS system** is meters, kilograms, and seconds. The **CGS system** is centimeters, grams, and seconds. The **British system** of feet, pounds, and seconds is not widely used in the world today. The most modern system, the **International System (SI),** in an extension of the MKS system.

Remember: When calculating physics and radiologic problems, the same systems of units must be used.

Table 3-1 illustrates four **systems of units** representing the base quantities of length, mass, and time.

MECHANICS

Mechanics is the segment of physics that deals with the motion of objects. Motion often has direction. A quantity with direction and magnitude is known as a **vector.** Another quantity with magnitude but no direction is a **scalar.** A vector description of a distance is 36 kilometers north. A scalar is simply 36 kilometers.

Velocity

The motion of an object is described in two ways—**velocity** and **acceleration.** Velocity or **speed** is the rate of the change of position of the object over time. The velocity of a car is measured in miles per hour (kilometers per hour). Units of velocity in SI units are meters per second.

Often the velocity of an object changes as its position changes. In the example of a person driving a car a certain distance, the car is always speeding up or slowing down, but the average velocity for the trip could be calculated using the formula:

Average Velocity

$$v = d/t$$
$$d = \text{distance}$$
$$t = \text{time}$$

The **instantaneous velocity** is the velocity at a particular moment, which in this same example is the velocity registered on the car's speedometer at any particular instant.

Acceleration

The rate of change of velocity over time is **acceleration.** Acceleration is, in other words, velocity divided by time or in the MKS system meters per second squared (m/s^2).

	SI Units*	MKS	CGS	British
Length	meter (m)	meter (m)	centimeter (cm)	foot (ft)
Mass	kilogram (kg)	kilogram (kg)	gram (g)	pound (lb)†
Time	second (s)	second (s)	second (s)	second (s)

TABLE 3-1

Systems of Units

*The SI units includes four additional base units.
†The pound is actually a unit of force but is related to mass.

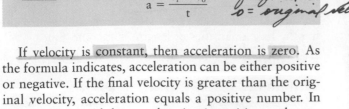

Average Acceleration

$$a = \frac{v_f - v_o}{t}$$

f = final velocity
o = original velocity

If velocity is constant, then acceleration is zero. As the formula indicates, acceleration can be either positive or negative. If the final velocity is greater than the original velocity, acceleration equals a positive number. In this case, it is said that acceleration is positive or that an object is speeding up. If, however, v_f is less than v_o, subtracting v_f from v_o yields a negative number, which physicists refer to as *negative acceleration*. Negative acceleration describes an object that is slowing down.

Refer to the example in Figure 3-2. The acceleration of the dragster is as follows:

$$a = \frac{80 \text{ m/s} - 0 \text{ m/s}}{10.2 \text{ s}}$$

$$a = 7.8 \text{ m/s}^2$$

Motion

In the year 1686 the English mathematician, Sir Isaac Newton, formulated three principles that are recognized even today as fundamental **Laws of Motion.**

Newton's First Law: Inertia

A body will remain at rest or will continue moving at a constant velocity in a straight line unless acted on by an external force.

Newton's first law states that if no force acts on an object, there will be no acceleration.

Figure 3-3 illustrates **inertia.** A portable x-ray machine will not move until forced by a push. Once in motion, it will continue to move unless acted on by an opposing force. That opposing force is **friction.**

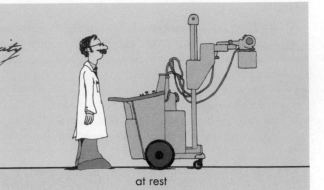

at rest

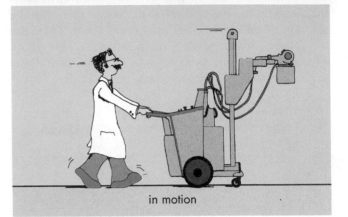

in motion

FIGURE 3-3 Newton's first law states that a body at rest will remain at rest and a body in motion will continue in motion until acted on by an outside force.

Newton's Second Law: Force

The force acted on an object with acceleration is equal to the mass times the acceleration.

$$F = m \times a$$

(mass) × (acceleration)

Force can be thought of as the push or pull on an object. Figure 3-4 illustrates Newton's second law. The SI unit of force is the **newton (N).**

Newton's Third Law: Action/Reaction

For every action there is an equal and opposite reaction.

According to this law, when pushing a heavy block, the block will push back with the same force applied. On the other hand the physics professor in Figure 3-5 is unable to push with enough force against the students who are closing the walls of the clamp room.

Weight

Weight is the force of an object caused by the downward pull of gravity. Objects falling to the earth accel-

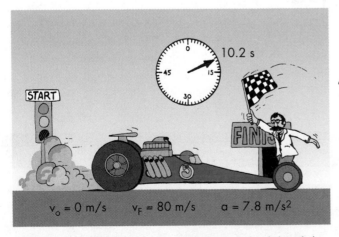

FIGURE 3-2 Drag racing provides a familiar example of the relationships among initial velocity, final velocity, acceleration, and time.

$v_o = 0$ m/s $v_F = 80$ m/s $a = 7.8$ m/s^2

START   10.2 s   FINISH

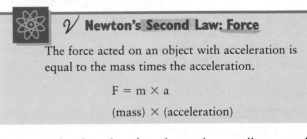

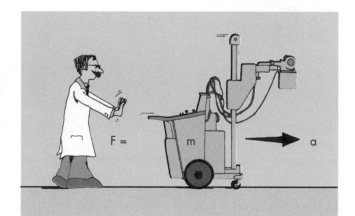

FIGURE 3-4 Newton's second law states that force applied to move an object is equal to the mass of the object times the acceleration.

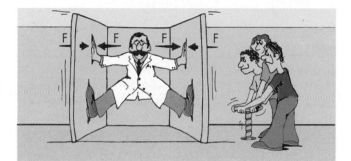

FIGURE 3-5 Student technologists performing a routine physics experiment.

erate at a constant rate. This rate, termed the *acceleration of gravity,* is represented by the symbol g and equals on earth 9.8m/s² in SI units and 32 ft/s² in British units. Recall from Chapter 1 that the value of acceleration of gravity on the moon is one sixth that of the earth. In outer space, weightlessness is due to the absence of gravity. The units of weight are the same as for force—Newtons in SI units or pounds in the British system (Table 3-2). It is important to remember that the weight of an object varies according to gravity, but the mass of the object does not change. In addition, gravity affects all objects the same regardless of mass. A bowling ball and a golf ball have different weights because of the difference in mass; however, gravity will make both accelerate at the same rate. The weight of an object is equal to the product of its mass and the acceleration of gravity.

$$\text{Weight} = \text{mass} \times \text{gravity}$$

5) Momentum

The product of the mass of an object and its velocity is called *momentum* represented by **p.** The greater the velocity of an object, the greater its momentum.

Momentum = p

$$p = m \times v$$

$$(\text{momentum}) = (\text{mass}) \times (\text{velocity})$$

The **conservation of momentum law** states:

Conservation of Momentum
The total momentum before any interaction is equal to the total momentum after the interaction.

To illustrate this principle see Figure 3-6. in which the moving cue ball collides with two stationary billiard balls. The total momentum before the collision is the mass times the velocity of the cue ball. After the collision the momentum is shared by all three balls. Thus the original momentum of the cue ball is conserved (meaning not lost or depleted) after the collision.

6) Work

In physics, **work** has specific meaning. The work applied to an object is equal to the force used over a distance.

Work

$$W = F \times d$$

$$(\text{work}) = (\text{force}) \times (\text{distance})$$

The unit of work in SI units is the **joule (J).** In the diagnostic imaging department, lifting a radiographic cassette is work. As defined in physics, no work is done, however, when the cassette is held motionless.

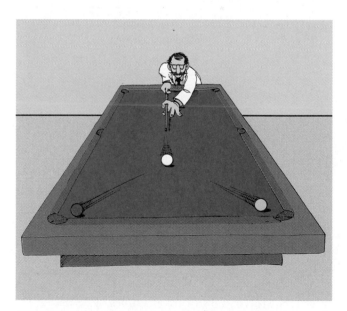

FIGURE 3-6 The conservation of momentum occurs with every pool shot.

7) Power

Power is the rate of doing work, that is, the work performed over time. The equation for power is as follows:

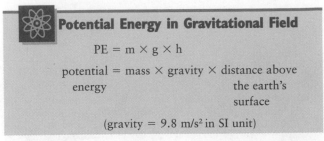

Power

$$P = W \div t$$

$$(\text{power}) = (\text{work}) \div (\text{time})$$

The SI unit for power is joules/second (J/s) or **watt (W)**. The British unit of power is **horsepower (hp)**.

$$1 \text{ hp} = 746 \text{ W}$$

$$1000 \text{ W} = 1 \text{ kilowatt (kW)}$$

8) Energy

Energy is the ability to do work. The forms of energy are discussed in Chapter 1.

Law of Conservation of Energy *and Matter*

Energy cannot be created or destroyed but can be transformed from one form to another.

In other words the total amount of energy in the universe is constant. The SI units of energy are joules, which are the same units for work. **Mechanical energy** is subdivided into **kinetic energy** and **potential energy.**

9) Kinetic Energy

Kinetic energy **(KE)** is the energy of motion or mass times velocity squared.

Kinetic Energy

$$KE = \tfrac{1}{2} (m \times v^2)$$

$$\text{kinetic energy} = \tfrac{1}{2} (\text{mass} \times \text{velocity}^2)$$

10) Potential Energy

Potential energy **(PE)** is the stored energy of position. A textbook on a desk has PE because of its height above the floor. It has the ability to do work by falling to the ground. Gravitational potential energy can be calculated from the following equation:

$$PE = m \times g \times h$$

In this equation, h is the distance above the earth's surface. A coiled spring, a stretched rubber band, and a skier at the top of a jump are examples of PE because of their position. **Gravitational potential energy** is calculated as follows:

Potential Energy in Gravitational Field

$$PE = m \times g \times h$$

$$\begin{aligned}\text{potential} &= \text{mass} \times \text{gravity} \times \text{distance above} \\ \text{energy} & \qquad\qquad\qquad\qquad \text{the earth's} \\ & \qquad\qquad\qquad\qquad \text{surface}\end{aligned}$$

$$(\text{gravity} = 9.8 \text{ m/s}^2 \text{ in SI unit})$$

If a scientist held a ball at the top of the leaning tower of Pisa (Figure 3-7) the ball would have only potential energy. When the ball begins to fall from the tower and the height decreases, the potential energy, depending on the height above the earth's surface, decreases also. Just before impact, since the ball has no height, the potential energy becomes zero. All the initial potential energy has been converted to kinetic energy during acceleration of gravity and the fall toward the earth.

11) Heat

Heat is defined as the kinetic energy of the random motion of molecules. The more rapid and disordered the motion, the more heat a body contains. The **calorie**, the unit of heat, is the energy necessary to raise the temperature of 1 gram (g) of water 1° on the **celsius scale.** The SI unit of heat is the **kilocalorie (kcal)**. It is defined as

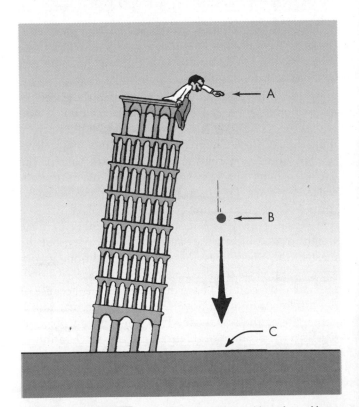

FIGURE 3-7 Potential energy results from the position of an object. Kinetic energy is the energy of motion. **A,** Maximum potential energy; no kinetic energy. **B,** Potential energy and kinetic energy. **C,** Maximum kinetic energy; no potential energy.

the amount of heat required to raise the temperature (T) of 1000 grams (1 kg) of water 1° C. The same amount of heat may have different effects on different substances. For example, only 0.05 calorie is required to change the temperature of 1 gram (g) of silver 1° celsius.

Heat is transferred in the following three ways:

1. **Conduction** is heat transferred by touching. When a high-temperature object touches a low-temperature object, the temperature of both equalize.

    Consider a cast iron skillet on a stove. The heat from the fire is transferred to the molecules at the bottom of the skillet. The molecules begin to move more rapidly with the added energy. This additional energy is passed along from molecule to molecule not just on the bottom of the skillet but up the sides and down the handle as well.

    The same thing happens with a coffee cup filled with hot coffee. The heat from the coffee inside the cup is conducted to the outside by the transference of energy from molecule to molecule from the inside out. This is why a hot cup of coffee makes such an excellent hand warmer on a cold day.

2. **Convection** is the mechanical transfer of rapidly moving or hot molecules in a gas or liquid to another place or object. A steam radiator or a forced-air furnace heats a room by convection. The heat from a radiator is an example of **natural convection**. The air around the radiator is heated. It then rises and cooler air takes its place. This circulation of hot and cool air is natural convection. A forced-air furnace blows heated air into a room, providing forced circulation to complement natural convection.

3. **Thermal** radiation is the reddish glow emitted from hot objects. It is the transfer of heat by **infrared emission**, a type of electromagnetic radiation.

Heat is measured on a **thermometer** calibrated with the following two reference points: (1) the freezing point of water and (2) the boiling point of water. Figure 3-8 shows the three scales—celsius (C), Fahrenheit (F), and Kelvin (K), which measure temperature. These scales are interrelated using the following formulas:

Celsius	$T_c = \frac{5}{9}(T_f - 32)$
Fahrenheit	$T_f = \frac{9}{5} \times T_c + 32$
Kelvin	$T_k = T_c + 273$

Magnetic resonance imaging, a subspecialty of diagnostic imaging, uses very cold liquids to cool the super-conducting magnet. The liquids or **cryogens** have extremely low boiling points. The boiling point

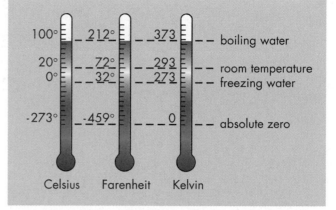

FIGURE 3-8 Three principal scales used to represent temperature. Celsius is the universally adopted scale for reporting purposes.

of liquid nitrogen is −320° F and of liquid helium, −452° F.

SUMMARY

Table 3-2 summarizes the concepts addressed in this chapter.

Practice the Review Questions using the table as a reference.

REVIEW QUESTIONS
Systems of Units

1. The dimensions of a box are 30 cm × 86 cm × 4.2 m. Find the volume using the formula

    v (volume) = l (length) × w (width) × h (height).

    Because the dimensions are listed in different systems of units, the numbers must be converted to the same system first to calculate the proper answer.

    So, 30 cm = 0.3 m

    86 cm = 0.86 m

    Therefore

    v = 0.3 m × 0.86 m × 4.2 m

    = 1.1 m³ (the units are multiplied also)

2. What is the volume of a rectangular-sided radiographic positioning sponge that measures 5 inches by 5 inches by 10 inches?

Velocity

3. What is the velocity of a ball that travels 50 meters in 4 seconds?

TABLE 3-2

Summary of Quantities, Equations, and Units Used in Mechanics

| | | | Units | |
Quality	Symbol	Defining Equation	SI	British
Velocity	v	$v = d/t$	m/s	ft/s
Average velocity	$\bar{v}$	$\bar{v} = \dfrac{v_0 + v_f}{2}$	m/s	ft/s
Acceleration	a	$a = \dfrac{v_f - v_0}{t}$	m/s²	ft/s²
Force	F	$F = m \times a$	N	lb
Weight	Wt	$Wt = m \times g$	N	lb
Momentum	p	$p = m \times v$	kg-m/s	ft-lb/s
Work	W	$W = F \times d$	J	ft-lb
Power	P	$P = W/t$	W	hp
Kinetic energy	KE	$KE = \frac{1}{2} m \times v^2$	J	ft-lb
Potential energy	PE	$PE = m \times gh$	J	ft-lb

$$v \text{ (velocity)} = \frac{d \text{ (distance)}}{t \text{ (time)}}$$

$$v = \frac{50 \text{ m}}{4 \text{ s}}$$

$$= 12.5 \text{ m/s (meters per second)}$$

4. What is the velocity of the portable machine in the hospital elevator if the elevator travels 20 meters to the next floor in 30 seconds?

Average Velocity

5. A Corvette can reach a velocity of 88 mph in ¼ mile. What is the average velocity?

$$v = \frac{v_0 + v_f}{2}$$

$$\text{average velocity} = \frac{\text{initial velocity} + \text{final velocity}}{2}$$

$$v = \frac{0 \text{ mph} + 88 \text{ mph}}{2}$$

$$v = 44 \text{ mph}$$

6. Moving down a ramp, the C-arm fluoroscopy unit reaches a velocity of 1 ft every 5 seconds. What is the average velocity?

Acceleration

7. A 5L Mustang can accelerate to 60 miles per hour in 5.9 seconds. What is its acceleration in SI units?

$$v_f = 60 \text{ mi/hr} \times 1609 \text{ m/mi} \times 1/3600 \text{ hr/s} = 26.8 \text{ m/s}$$

$$a = \frac{26.8 \text{ m/s} - 0 \text{ m/s}}{5.9 \text{ s}}$$

$$a = 4.5 \text{ m/s}^2$$

Force

8. Find the force on a 55-kilogram object accelerated at 14 m/s².
Force equals mass times acceleration.
The SI unit of force is the newton (N).

9. In order for a 3600-pound (1636-kilogram) car to accelerate at 15 m/s², what force is required?

Weight

10. A professor has a mass of 75 kg. What is his weight on the earth? On the moon?

Work

11. Find the work done lifting an infant patient weighing 90 N to a height of 1.5 m.

$$\text{Work} = \text{force} \times \text{distance}$$

Power

12. A radiographer lifts a 0.8-kilogram cassette from the floor to the top of a 1.5-meter table with an acceleration of 3 m/s². What is the power exerted if it takes 1.2 seconds? This is a multistep answer. Remember that work equals force times distance ($w = F \times d$) and force equals mass times acceleration ($F = m \times a$). First find force, then calculate back to the formula for finding power: $P = \text{work/time}$.

13. A rushed radiographer pushes a 35-kilogram portable down a 25-meter hall in 9 seconds with a final velocity of 3 m/s. How much power did this require?

Potential Energy and Kinetic Energy

14. A radiographer holds an 6-kilogram x-ray tube 1.5 meters above the ground. What is its potential energy?

Temperature Conversion

15. Liquid helium with a boiling point of 4° K is used to cool superconducting magnetic resonance imagers. What is its temperature in Fahrenheit?

16. Convert 77° Fahrenheit to degrees Celsius.

17. Convert 80° Fahrenheit to degrees Celsius.

Additional Reading

Laughlin JS: Origins of the science of radiation physics and of the field of radiology, *Med Phys* 22(11):A7, November 1995.

Mould RF: The early history of x-ray diagnosis with emphasis on the contributions of physics 1895-1995, *Phys Med Biol* 40(11):1741, November 1995.

4 The Atom

OBJECTIVES

At the completion of this chapter the student will be able to:

1. Relate the history of the atom from as early as 200 BC
2. Identify the structure of the atom
3. Describe electron shells and instability within atomic structure
4. Discuss radioactivity and the characteristics of alpha and beta particles that can ionize matter
5. Explain the difference between two forms of ionizing radiation—particulate and electromagnetic.

OUTLINE

Centuries of Discovery
  Greek atom
  Dalton atom
  Thompson atom
  Bohr atom
Combinations of Atoms
Fundamental Particles
  Covalent bonding
  Ionic bonding

Atomic Nomenclature
Atomic Structure
  Electron arrangement
Radioactivity
  Radioisotopes
Types of Ionizing Radiation
  Particulate radiation
  Electromagnetic radiation

T his chapter diverges from the study of energy and force to return to the basis of matter itself. What composes matter? What is the magnitude of matter?

From the inner space of the atom to outer space in the universe, there is an enormous range in the size of matter. Over forty orders of magnitude are needed to identify objects as small as the atom and as large as the universe. Because matter spans such large magnitude, powers of 10 are needed to measure objects. Figure 4-1 shows the orders of magnitude and how matter in our surroundings varies in size.

The atom is the smallest unit of matter. As the smallest unit of matter, descriptions of the atom and its structure are essential.

The atom is the building block of the radiographer's understanding of the interaction between ionizing radiation and matter. This chapter explains what happens when energy in the form of x-rays hits or penetrates human tissue. Although human tissue has an extremely complex structure, it is made up of atoms and combinations of atoms. Examining the structure of atoms helps uncover what happens when parts of the atom's structure is changed. The discussion begins with the development of thought about the most elemental part of matter—the atom.

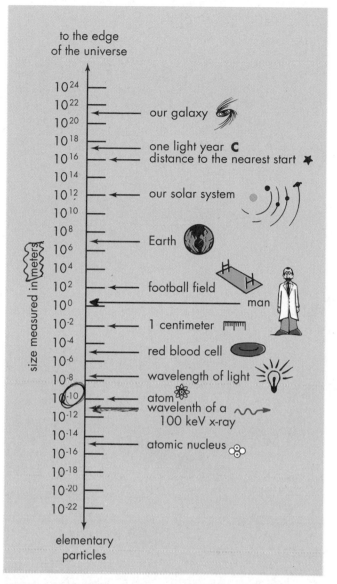

FIGURE 4-1 Matter in our surroundings is composed of objects whose size varies enormously. So wide is the size range that it could hardly be represented with arithmetic nomenclature. Power-of-ten notation is used because over 40 orders of magnitude are necessary to encompass the range of matter as we know it.

CENTURIES OF DISCOVERY
Greek Atom

The earliest recorded reference to the atom comes from the Greeks around 200 BC. The Greeks thought all matter was composed of four substances—earth, water, air, and fire. According to them, all matter could be described as combinations of these four basic substances in various proportions. These substances were modified by four basic essences—wet, dry, hot, and cold. Figure 4-2 represents this theory of matter.

For the Greeks, the term atom, meaning indivisible, described the smallest part of the four basic substances. Each type of Greek atom was represented by a symbol (Figure 4-3, A). Today 108 substances or elements have been identified; 92 are naturally occurring, and the additional 16 have been artificially produced in high-energy particle accelerators.

The Atom ✳

The atom is the smallest part of an element that has all the properties of that element.

There are, however, particles much smaller than the atom known as *subatomic particles*.

Dalton Atom

The Greek description of the structure of matter persisted for hundreds of years and was the theoretical basis for the vain efforts by medieval alchemists to transform lead into gold. It was not until the nineteenth century that the foundation for modern atomic theory was laid. In 1808, John Dalton, an English schoolteacher, published a book summarizing his experiments, which showed that the elements could be classified according to integral values of **atomic mass**. According to Dalton, an element was composed of identical atoms, each re-

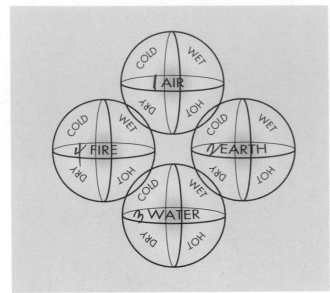

FIGURE 4-2 Symbolic representation of the substances and essences of matter as viewed by the ancient Greeks.

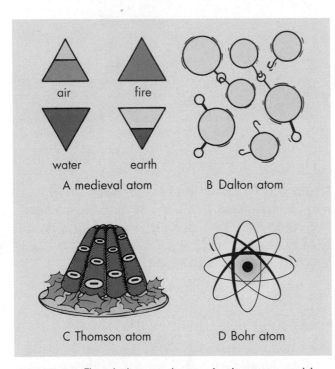

FIGURE 4-3 Through the years the atom has been represented by many symbols. **A,** The Greeks envisioned four different atoms, representing air, fire, earth, and water. These triangular symbols were adopted by medieval alchemists. **B,** Dalton's atoms had hooks and eyes to account for chemical combination. **C,** Thomson's model of the atom has been described as a plum pudding, with the plums representing electrons. **D,** The Bohr atom has a small, dense, positively charged nucleus surrounded by electrons in precise energy levels.

acting the same way in chemical reactions. For example, all oxygen atoms were alike. They looked alike, they were constucted alike, and they reacted alike. They were, however, very different from atoms of any other element. The physical combination of one type of atom with another was interpreted as being a hook-and-eye affair (Figure 4-3, *B*). The size and number of the hooks and eyes were different for each element.

Some 50 years after Dalton's work, a Russian scholar, Dmitri Mendeleev, showed that if the elements were arranged in order of increasing atomic mass, a repetition of similar chemical properties occurred. At that time, about 65 elements had been identified. Mendeleev's work resulted in the first **periodic table of elements**. Although there were many holes in Mendeleev's table, it showed that all the then-known elements could be placed in one of eight groups.

Figure 4-4 is the modern periodic table of elements. Each block represents an element. The superscript is the **atomic number**. The subscript is the **elemental mass**.

All elements in the same group or column react chemically in a similar fashion and have similar physical properties. Except for hydrogen, the elements of group I, called the **alkali metals**, are soft metals that combine readily with oxygen and react violently with water. The elements of group VII, called **halogens**, are gases, are easily vaporized, and combine with metals to form water-soluble salts. Group VIII elements, called the **noble gases**, are highly resistant to reaction with other elements.

Thomson Atom

After the publication of Mendeleev's periodic table, additional elements were identified and the periodic table slowly became filled. Knowledge of the structure of atoms, however, remained scanty. Before the turn of the century atoms were considered indivisible. The only difference between the atoms of one element and the atoms of another was their mass. Through the efforts of many scientists, it became apparent that there was an electrical nature to the atomic structure of matter.

In the late 1890s, while investigating the physical properties of **cathode rays**, J.J. Thomson concluded that electrons were an integral part of all atoms. He described the atom as looking something like a plum pudding, where the plum represented negative electric charges and the pudding was a shapeless mass of uniform positive electrification (see Figure 4-3, *C*). The number of electrons was thought to equal the quantity of positive electrification because the atom was known to be electrically neutral. In 1911, through a series of ingenious experiments, Ernest Rutherford disproved Thomson's model of the atom. Rutherford introduced the **nuclear model**, which described the atom as containing a small, dense, positively charged center

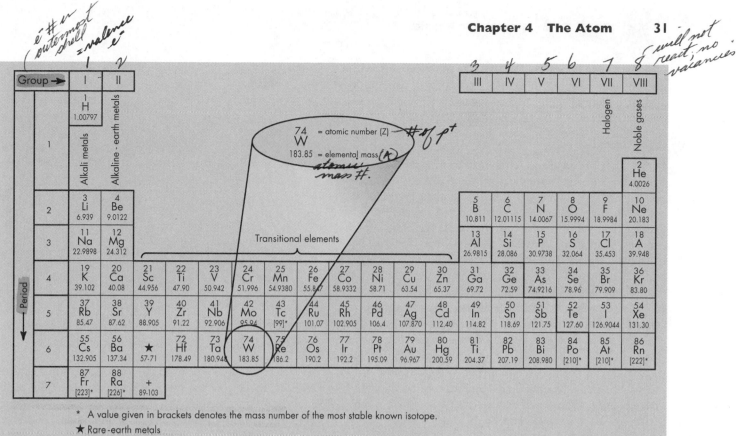

FIGURE 4-4 Periodic table of elements. Tungsten has an atomic number of 74 and an elemental mass of 183.85 atomic mass units.

surrounded by a negative cloud of electrons. He called the center of the atom the *nucleus.*

Bohr Atom

In 1913, Niels Bohr improved Rutherford's description of the atom. Bohr's model was a miniature solar system in which the electrons revolved about the nucleus in prescribed orbits or energy levels. For our purposes, the Bohr atom (see Figure 4-3, *D*) represents the best way to picture the atom, although the details of atomic structure are more accurately described by a newer model derived from **quantum mechanics.** Simply put, the Bohr atom contains a small, dense, positively charged nucleus surrounded by negatively charged electrons that revolve in fixed, well-defined orbits around the nucleus. In the neutral atom the number of electrons is equal to the number of positive charges in the nucleus.

COMBINATION OF ATOMS

Atoms of various elements may combine to form structures called **molecules.**

Molecules in turn may combine to form even larger combinations. For example, hydrogen atoms combine to form a molecule of hydrogen (H_2). The subscript 2 indicates that two hydrogen atoms are present in the

molecule. Oxygen atoms combine also. A molecule of oxygen is written as O_2. Consequently, two molecules of hydrogen ($2H_2$) can combine with one molecule of oxygen (O_2) to form two molecules of water.

$$2H_2 + O_2 = 2H_2O$$

An atom of sodium (Na) can combine with an atom of chlorine (Cl) to form a molecule of sodium chloride (NaCl), which is common table salt:

$$Na + Cl = NaCl$$

Both of these molecules are common in the human body.

A **chemical compound** is the new substance that is formed when two or more atoms of different elements combine.

The formula NaCl represents one molecule of the compound sodium chloride. Sodium chloride has properties that vary more than either sodium or chlorine.

Atoms combine with each other to form compounds (chemical bonding) in two main ways. The examples of H_2O and NaCl can be used to describe these two bonds.

Covalent bonding

Oxygen has six electrons in its outermost shell. It has room for two more electrons, so in a water molecule two hydrogen atoms share their single electrons with the oxygen. The hydrogen electrons orbit both the H and O, thus binding the atoms together. Covalent bonding is characterized by the sharing of electrons.

2) Ionic bonding

Sodium has one electron in its outermost shell. Chlorine has space for one more electron in its outermost shell. The sodium atom will give up its electron to the chlorine. When it does, it becomes ionized because it has lost an electron and now has an imbalance of electrical charges. The chlorine atom also becomes ionized because it has gained an electron and then has more electrons than protons. The result is the two atoms are attracted to each other because they have opposite charges. They are bound to each other by the attraction of their charges.

Sodium, hydrogen, carbon, and oxygen atoms can combine to form a molecule of sodium bicarbonate ($NaHCO_3$). A measurable quantity of sodium bicarbonate constitutes a chemical compound commonly called *baking soda*. The interrelations between atoms, elements, molecules, and compounds are orderly.

> The smallest particle of an element is an atom; the smallest particle of a compound is a molecule.

Although over 100 different elements are known, most elements are rare. Approximately 95% of the earth and its atmosphere consists of only a dozen elements. Similarly, hydrogen, oxygen, carbon, and nitrogen compose over 95% of the human body. Water molecules of hydrogen and oxygen make up about 80% of the mass of the human body.

This organizational scheme is what the ancient Greeks were trying to describe with their substances and essences. Figure 4-5 is a diagram of this modern scheme of matter.

FUNDAMENTAL PARTICLES

Our understanding of the atom today is essentially that which Bohr presented nearly a century ago. With the development of high-energy particle accelerators, or *atom smashers* as they are called, the structure of the nucleus of an atom is slowly being mapped and identified. Nearly 100 subatomic articles have been detected and described by physicists working with these machines. The superconduction supercollider in Waxahachie, Texas (code-named SuperClyde) has led to the discovery of even more subatomic particles. Nuclear structure is now well defined.

> The three primary constituents of an atom—the **electron,** the **proton,** and the **neutron**—are the **fundamental particles** (Table 4-I).

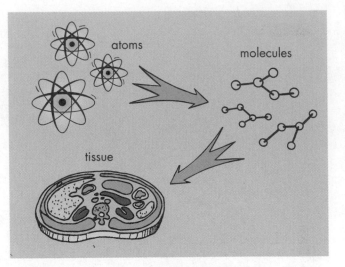

FIGURE 4-5 Matter has many levels of organization. Atoms combine to make molecules, and molecules combine to make tissues.

The atom can be viewed as a miniature solar system with its nucleus as the sun and its electrons as the planets. The arrangement of the electrons around the nucleus determines the manner in which atoms interact. Electrons are very small particles carrying one unit of negative electric charge. Their mass is only 9.1×10^{-31} kilograms. They can be pictured as revolving around the nucleus at nearly the speed of light in precisely fixed orbits, like the planets in our solar system revolve around the sun.

Because atomic particles are extremely small, their mass is expressed in atomic mass units (amu) for convenience. One amu is equal to one twelfth the mass of a carbon-12 atom. The electron mass is 0.000549 amu. When precision is not necessary, a system of whole numbers called *atomic mass numbers* is used. The atomic mass number of an electron is 0.

> The nucleus contains particles called *nucleons,* of which there are two types—**protons** and **neutrons.**

Both protons and neutrons have nearly 2000 times the mass of an electron. The mass of a proton is 1.673×10^{-27} kilograms, and the neutron is just slightly heavier at 1.675×10^{-27} kilograms. The atomic mass number of each is 1. The primary difference between a proton and a neutron is electric charge. The proton carries one unit of positive electric charge. The neutron carries no charge. It is electrically neutral. Table 4-1 lists important characteristics of the electron, proton, and neutron.

ATOMIC NOMENCLATURE

Often an element is indicated by an alphabetic abbreviation called a *chemical symbol.* Table 4-2 lists some important elements and their chemical symbols. The chemical properties of an element are determined by the number and arrangement of electrons in the orbits

TABLE 4-1

Important Characteristics of the Fundamental Particles

Particle	Location	Relative	Mass Kilogram	Amu	Number	Charge	Symbol
1 Electron −	Shells	1	9.109×10^{-31}	0.000549	1/1830	−1	−
2 Proton +	Nucleus	1836	1.673×10^{-27}	1.00728	1	+1	+
3 Neutron 0	Nucleus	1838	1.675×10^{-27}	1.00867	1	0	0

(handwritten: atomic mass unit above Amu; atomic mass # above Number)

TABLE 4-2

Characteristics of Some Radiographic Important Atoms

Element	Chemical Symbol	Atomic Number (Z)	Atomic Mass Number (A)*	Number of Naturally Occurring Isotopes	Elemental Mass (amu)†	K-shell Electron Binding Energy (keV)
Beryllium	Be	4	9	1	9.0122	0.111
Carbon	C	6	12	3	12.0111	0.284
Oxygen	O	8	16	3	15.9994	0.532
Aluminum	Al	13	27	1	26.9815	1.560
Calcium	Ca	20	40	6	40.080	4.038
Iron	Fe	26	56	4	55.847	7.112
Copper	Cu	29	63	2	63.546	8.979
Molybdenum	Mo	42	98	7	95.940	20.00
Ruthenium	Ru	44	102	7	101.07	22.12
Silver	Ag	47	107	2	107.868	25.68
Tin	Sn	50	120	10	118.69	29.20
Iodine	I	53	127	1	126.91	33.17
Barium	Ba	56	138	7	137.34	37.44
Tungsten	W	74	184	5	183.85	69.53
Gold	Au	79	197	1	196.97	80.73
Lead	Pb	82	208	4	207.19	88.00
Uranium	U	92	238	3	238.03	115.6

*Most abundant isotope.
†Average of naturally occurring isotopes.

around the nucleus. In the electrically neutral atom the number of electrons equals the number of protons, and the number of protons is called the *atomic number* represented by Z. Table 4-2 shows that the atomic number of barium is 56, indicating that 56 protons are in the barium nucleus. The number of protons plus the number of neutrons in the nucleus of an atom is called the *atomic mass number* symbolized by A.

A shorthand notation that incorporates the chemical symbol with subscripts and superscripts is used to identify atoms.

$$\text{Mass number A} \atop \text{Atomic number Z} \quad \text{X (chemical symbol)}$$

The chemical symbol (X) is positioned between two subscripts and two superscripts. The subscript and superscript to the left of the chemical symbol represent the atomic number and atomic mass number, respectively. The subscript and superscript to the right are values for the number of atoms per molecule and the **valence** state or energy level of the atom, respectively.

We are concerned only with the scripts to the left of X.

With this nomenclature the atoms of Figure 4-6 would have the following symbolic representation:

$$^{1}_{1}\text{H}, \,^{4}_{2}\text{He}, \,^{7}_{3}\text{Li}, \,^{238}_{92}\text{U}$$

Because the chemical symbol also indicates the atomic number, the subscript is often omitted as follows:

$$^{1}\text{H}, \,^{4}\text{He}, \,^{7}\text{Li}, \,^{238}\text{U}$$

Atoms that have the same atomic number but different atomic mass numbers are called *isotopes*. Isotopes of a given element contain the same number of protons but varying numbers of neutrons. Most elements have more than one stable isotope. The following are the seven natural isotopes of barium:

$$^{130}\text{Ba}, \,^{132}\text{Ba}, \,^{134}\text{Ba}, \,^{135}\text{Ba}, \,^{136}\text{Ba}, \,^{137}\text{Ba}, \,^{138}\text{Ba}$$

Question: How many protons and neutrons are in each of the seven naturally occurring isotopes of barium?

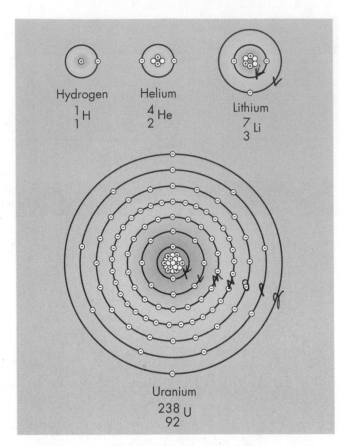

FIGURE 4-6 Atoms are composed of neutrons and protons in the nucleus and electrons in specific orbits surrounding the nucleus. Shown here are the three smallest atoms and the largest naturally occurring atom, uranium.

Answer: The number of protons in each isotope is 56. The number of neutrons is equal to A−Z. The following are examples:

^{130}Ba: 130 − 56 = 74 neutrons
^{132}Ba: 132 − 56 = 76 neutrons
^{134}Ba: 134 − 56 = 78 neutrons

Atomic nuclei that have the same atomic mass number but different atomic numbers are called *isobars*. Isobars are atoms that have different numbers of protons and neutrons but the same total number of nucleons.

Atoms that have the same number of neutrons but different numbers of protons are called *isotones*. Isotones are atoms with different atomic numbers and different mass number but a constant value for the quantity A−Z.

The final category of atomic configuration is the *isomer*. Isomers have the same atomic number and the same atomic mass number. In fact, isomers are identical atoms except that they exist at different energy states because of differences in nuclear arrangement.

Table 4-3 is a summary of the characteristics of these nuclear arrangements.

Question: From the following list of atoms pick out those that are isotopes, isobars, and isotones.
$^{131}_{54}$Xe, $^{130}_{53}$I, $^{132}_{55}$Cs, $^{131}_{53}$I

Answer: ^{130}I and ^{131}I are isotopes. ^{131}I and ^{131}Xe are isobars. ^{130}I, ^{131}Xe, and ^{132}Cs are isotones.

ATOMIC STRUCTURE

The classical representations of the atom, which generally appeared like Figure 4-3, *D* are a beehive of subatomic activity. In fact, the atom, oversimplified in Figure 4-3, *D* is mostly empty space. The nucleus of an atom is very small. It contains nearly all the mass of the atom. If a basketball represented the size of the uranium nucleus, the largest naturally occurring atom, the path of the orbital electrons would take them over 8 miles away. Less than 0.001% of the volume of an atom is occupied by matter. The atom is indeed mostly empty space. The nucleus containing the neutrons and protons of the atoms contains most of its mass. For example, the nucleus of an uranium atom contains 99.998% of the entire mass of the atom. The electron orbits are grouped into different shells. The arrangement of electrons in these shells determines how an atom reacts chemically, that is, how it combines with other atoms. Specifically, the number and arrangement of electrons in the outermost shell determine the chemical behavior of an atom. The number of protons determine the chemical element.

The periodic table of the elements (see Figure 4-4) lists all matter in order of increasing complexity beginning with hydrogen (H). An atom of hydrogen contains one proton in its nucleus and one electron outside the nucleus. Helium (He), the second atom in the table, contains two protons, two neutrons, and two electrons. The third atom, lithium (Li), contains three protons, four neutrons, and three electrons. Two of these electrons are in the same orbital shell, the K shell, as the electrons of hydrogen and helium. The third electron is in the next farther orbital shell from the nucleus, the L shell. Electrons can exist only in certain shells, which

TABLE 4-3

Characteristics of Various Nuclear Arrangements

Arrangement	Atomic Number	Atomic Mass Number	Neutron Number
Isotope	Same	Different	Different
Isobar	Different	Same	Different
Isotone	Different	Different	Same
Isomer	Same	Same	Same

represent different electron binding energies or energy levels. For identification purposes the electron orbital shells are given codes K, L, M, N, O, P, and Q, to represent the relative binding energies of electrons from closest to the nucleus to farthest from the nucleus. The closer an electron is to the nucleus, the higher its binding energy.

The next atom on the periodic table, beryllium (Be), has four protons and five neutrons in the nucleus. Two electrons are in the K shell, and two are in the L shell. The complexity of the electron configuration of atoms increases as one progresses through the periodic table to the most complex naturally occurring element, uranium (U). Uranium has 92 protons and 146 neutrons. The electron distribution is as follows: 2 in the K shell, 8 in the L shell, 18 in the M shell, 32 in the N shell, 21 in the O shell, 9 in the P shell, and 2 in the Q shell. Figure 4-6 is a schematic representation of four atoms. Although these atoms are mostly empty space, they have been diagrammed on one page. If the actual size of the helium nucleus were that in Figure 4-6, the K-shell electrons would be several city blocks away.

In their normal state, atoms are electrically neutral. The electric charge on the atom is 0. The total number of electrons in the orbital shells is exactly equal to the number of protons in the nucleus. If an atom has an extra electron or has had an electron removed, it is ionized. An ionized atom is not electrically neutral but carries a charge equal in magnitude to the difference between the number of electrons and protons. Atoms cannot be ionized by addition or subtraction of protons, since that changes the atom from one element to another. An alteration in the number of neutrons does not ionize an atom because the neutron is electrically neutral.

Figure 4-7 represents the interaction between an x-ray and a carbon atom, a primary constituent of tissue.

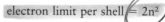

Ionization occurs when the x-ray photon transfers its energy to an orbital electron and ejects that electron from the atom.

This process, called *ionization*, requires approximately 34 eV (electron volts) of energy. The x-ray ceases to exist and an **ion pair** is formed. The remaining atom is now a positive ion, since it contains one more positive charge than negative charge.

In all except for the lightest atoms the number of neutrons is always greater than the number of protons. The larger the atom, the greater the abundance of neutrons over protons. Mendeleev's original periodic table was based on atomic mass. The deviation from sequential mass in this early table was presumed to be caused by inaccurate measurements. The varying neutron-to-proton ratio of the nucleus accounts for this deviation from sequential mass numbers.

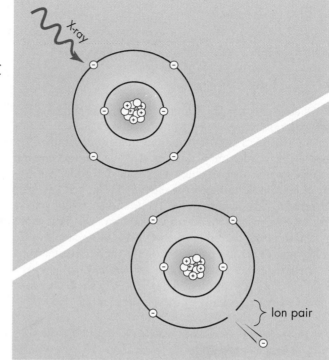

FIGURE 4-7 Ionization of a carbon atom by an x-ray leaves the atom with a net electric charge of +1. The ionized atom and the released electron are called an *ion pair*.

Electron Arrangement

The maximum number of electrons that can exist in each shell increases with the distance of the shell from the nucleus (Table 4-4). The electron limit per shell can be calculated from the following formula, where n is the shell number:

n = shell #

$$\text{electron limit per shell} = 2n^2$$

Question: What is the maximum number of electrons that can exist in the O shell?

$2(5)^2 = 50$

TABLE 4-4

Maximum Number of Electrons That Can Occupy Each Electron Shell

Shell Number	Shell Symbol	Number of Electrons
1	K	2
2	L	8
3	M	18
4	N	32
5	O	50
6	P	72
7	Q	98

Answer: The O shell is the fifth shell from the nucleus; therefore:

$$n = 5$$
$$2n^2 = 2(5)^2$$
$$2n^2 = 2(25)$$
$$2n^2 = 50 \text{ electrons}$$

Physicists call the shell number (n) the **principal quantum number.** Every electron in every atom can be precisely identified by the principal quantum number. The observant reader may have noticed a relationship between the number of shells in an atom and its position on the periodic table of the elements. Oxygen has eight electrons; two occupy the K shell, and six occupy the L shell. Oxygen is in the second period and the sixth group of the the periodic table (Figure 4-4). Aluminum has the following electron configuration: K shell, two electrons; L shell, eight electrons; M shell, three electrons. Therefore aluminum is in the third period (M shell) and third group (three electrons) of the periodic table.

The number of the outermost occupied electron shell of an atom is equal to its **period** in the periodic table.

The number of electrons in the outermost shell is equal to its **group.**

The number of electrons in the outermost shell is the valence of the element. It determines chemical reactivity.

Question: Refering to Figure 4-4, what are the period and group for the gastrointestinal contrast agent, barium?

Answer: Period 6 and group II.

The periodic table shows elements repeating similar chemical properties in groups of eight. In addition to the limitation on the maximum number of electrons allowed in any shell, no outer shell can contain more than eight electrons. All atoms having one electron in the outer shell lie in group I of the periodic table; atoms with two electrons in the outer shell fall in group II; and so on. When eight electrons are in the outer shell, the shell is filled. Atoms with filled outer shells lie in group VIII and are very stable chemically. The orderly scheme of atomic progression from smallest to largest atom is interrupted in the fourth period. Instead of simply adding electrons to the next outer shell, electrons are added to an inner shell. The atoms associated with this phenomenon are called the *transitional elements.* Even in these elements, no outer shell ever contains more than eight electrons. The chemical properties of the transitional elements depend on the number of electrons in the two outermost shells.

An electron does not spontaneously fly off from the nucleus like a ball twirling at the end of a string flies off when the string is cut because electrons are negatively charged and protons are positively charged. The attraction between them is described in a basic law of electricity, which states that opposite charges attract each other.

Centripetal Force   Electrons revolve around the nucleus in fixed orbits or shells. The electrostatic attraction produces a **centripetal force** or center-seeking force that just matches the force of motion or velocity.

The electrons also do not drop into the nucleus because of the strong electrostatic attraction.

Centrifugal Force   In the normal atom the centripetal force just balances the **centrifugal force** or flying-out-from-the-center force.

The opposing forces cause electrons to maintain their distance from the nucleus, and thus electrons travel in a circular or elliptical path. In Figure 4-8 a speeding race car illustrates these principles.

The strength of attachment of an electron to the nucleus, called the *electron binding energy,* is designated E_b. The closer an electron is to the nucleus, the more tightly it is bound. K-shell electrons have higher binding energies than L-shell electrons, L-shell electrons are more tightly bound to the nucleus than M-shell electrons and so on. Not all K-shell electrons of all atoms are bound with the same binding energy. The greater the total number of electrons in an atom, the more tightly each is bound. To put it differently, the larger and more complex the atom, the higher the E_b for electrons in any given shell. Since electrons of large atoms are more tightly bound to the nucleus than those of small atoms, it generally takes more energy to ionize a large atom

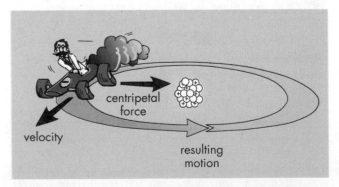

FIGURE 4-8 Electrons revolve about the nucleus in fixed orbits, or shells. The electrostatic attraction produces a centripetal force that just matches the force of motion or velocity, resulting in a specific electron path about the nucleus.

than a small atom. Figure 4-9 represents the binding energies of electrons of several atoms. The metal tungsten (W) is the primary constituent of the target of an x-ray tube. Barium (Ba) is used extensively in radiographic and **fluoroscopic** contrast studies.

Question: How much energy is required to ionize tungsten by removal of a K-shell electron?

Answer: The minimum energy must equal E_b, or 69.5 keV. Less than that and the atom cannot be ionized.

Carbon (C) is an important component of human tissue. E_b for the outer shell of electrons of carbon is only about 10 eV. Yet it has been shown that approximately 34 eV is necessary to ionize atoms in tissue. The difference of 24 eV is deposited as electron excitations, which ultimately results in heat. The value 34 eV to ionize tissue is called the **ionization potential.** $eV = e\text{-}volt$

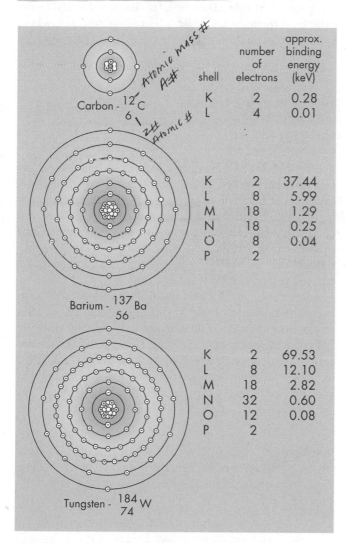

Carbon - $^{12}_{6}$C   *Atomic mass #   A#   z#   Atomic #*

Barium - $^{137}_{56}$Ba

Tungsten - $^{184}_{74}$W

shell	number of electrons	approx. binding energy (keV)
K	2	0.28
L	4	0.01
K	2	37.44
L	8	5.99
M	18	1.29
N	18	0.25
O	8	0.04
P	2	
K	2	69.53
L	8	12.10
M	18	2.82
N	32	0.60
O	12	0.08
P	2	

FIGURE 4-9 Atomic configurations and approximate electron-binding energies for three radiologically important atoms. As atoms get bigger, electrons in a given shell become more tightly bound.

Question: How much more energy is necessary to ionize barium than to ionize carbon by removal of K-shell electrons?

Answer:

$$E_b (Ba) = 37,441 \text{ eV}$$
$$E_b (C) = -284 \text{ eV}$$

$$= 37,157 \text{ eV or } 37.2 \text{ keV (kiloelectron volts)}$$

RADIOACTIVITY

Some atoms exist in an abnormally excited state characterized by an unstable nucleus. To reach stability, the nucleus spontaneously emits particles and energy and transforms itself into another atom. This process is called *radioactive disintegration* or *radioactive decay.* The atoms involved are **radionuclides.** Any nuclear arrangement is called a **nuclide,** but only nuclei that undergo radioactive decay are radionuclides.

Radioisotopes

Many factors affect nuclear stability. Perhaps the most important is the number of neutrons. When a nucleus contains either too few or too many neutrons, the atom can disintegrate radioactively. The end result brings the number of neutrons and protons into a stable and proper ratio. In addition to stable isotopes, many elements have radioactive isotopes, or **radioisotopes.** Artificially produced radioisotopes have been identified for nearly all elements. These may be artificially produced in machines such as particle accelerators or nuclear reactors. Seven radioisotopes of barium have been discovered, all of which are artificially produced. In the following list of barium isotopes, the radioisotopes are in boldface:

^{127}Ba, **^{128}Ba**, **^{129}Ba**, ^{130}Ba, **^{131}Ba**, **^{132}Ba**, **^{133}Ba**, ^{134}Ba, ^{135}Ba, ^{136}Ba, ^{137}Ba, ^{138}Ba, **^{139}Ba**, ^{140}Ba

A few elements have naturally occurring radioisotopes as well. There are two primary sources of these naturally occurring radioisotopes. Some originated at the time of the formation of the earth and are still decaying very slowly. An example is uranium, which decays to radium, which, in turn, decays to radon. These and other products of uranium decay are also radioactive. Others, such as ^{14}C (carbon 14) are continuously produced in the upper atmosphere by the action of cosmic radiation.

Alpha and Beta Emission. Radioactive decay occurs in two ways—**beta emission** and **alpha emission.**

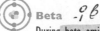 Beta $-^{0}_{-1}\beta$ $n' \rightarrow p^+$

During beta emission, a neutron undergoes conversion into a proton. Simultaneously, an electron-like particle is ejected from the nucleus, escaping from the atom with considerable kinetic energy.

The net result of beta emission therefore is to increase the atomic number by one, whereas the atomic mass number remains the same. This nuclear transformation therefore results in an atom changing from one type of element to another (Figure 4-10).

Radioactivity decay by alpha emission is a much more violent process.

Alpha $_2^4\alpha$

The **alpha particle** consists of two protons and two neutrons bound together. Its atomic mass number is 4.

A nucleus must be extremely unstable to emit an alpha particle, but when it does, it loses two units of positive charge and four units of mass. The transformation is significant because the resulting atom is not only chemically different but is also lighter by 4 amu (Figure 4-11). Beta emission occurs much more frequently than alpha emission. Virtually all radioisotopes are capable of transformation by beta emission, but only heavy radioisotopes are capable of alpha emission. Some radioisotopes are pure beta emitters or pure alpha emitters. Most radioisotopes emit **gamma rays** simultaneously with the particle emission.

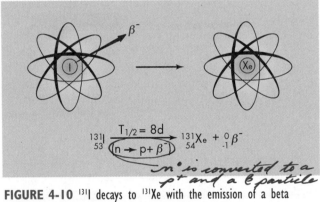

$$_{53}^{131}I \xrightarrow{T_{1/2} = 8d} _{54}^{131}Xe + _{-1}^{0}\beta^-$$
$$(n \rightarrow p + \beta^-)$$

n° is converted to a p⁺ and a ℓ particle

FIGURE 4-10 ^{131}I decays to ^{131}Xe with the emission of a beta particle.

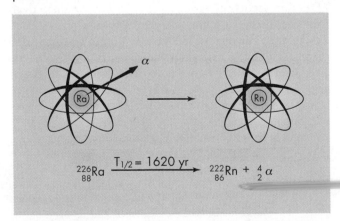

$$_{88}^{226}Ra \xrightarrow{T_{1/2} = 1620 \text{ yr}} _{86}^{222}Rn + _2^4\alpha$$

FIGURE 4-11 The decay of ^{226}Ra to ^{222}Rn is accompanied by alpha emission.

Question: $_{56}^{139}Ba$ is a radioisotope that decays by beta emission. What will be the value of A and Z for the atom that results from this emission? $_{56}^{139}Ba \rightarrow _{-1}^{0}\beta + _{57}^{139}$

Answer: In beta emission a neutron is converted to a proton and a beta particle $n \rightarrow p + b$; therefore $_{56}^{139}Ba \rightarrow _{57}^{139}Ba$. Lanthanum is the element with $Z = 57$; thus $_{57}^{139}La$ is the result of the beta decay of $_{56}^{139}Ba$.

Radioactive Half-Life. Radioactive matter is not here one day and gone the next. Rather, radioisotopes disintegrate into stable isotopes of different elements at an ever-decreasing rate, but the rate and consequently the quantity of radioactive material never quite reach zero. Remember from Chapter 1 that radioactive material is measured in curies (Ci) and that 1 Ci is equal to 3.7×10^{10} atoms disintegrating each second (3.7×10^{10} Bq). The rate of radioactive decay and the quantity of material present at any given time is described mathematically by a formula known as the **radioactive decay law**. From this formula, the quantity known as **half-life ($T_{1/2}$)** is derived.

Radioactive Decay Law

The half-life of a radioisotope is the period of time required for a quantity of radioactivity to be reduced to one half its original value.

Half-lives of radioisotopes vary from less than a second to many years. Each radioisotope has a unique, characteristic half-life. Theoretically, all the radioactivity of a radioisotope never disappears. After each period of time equivalent to one half-life, one half the activity present at the beginning will remain. Therefore, although the quantity of radioisotope progressively decreases, it never quite reaches zero.

Figure 4-12 shows two similar graphs used to estimate the quantity of any radioisotope remaining after any period of time. In these graphs the percent of original radioactivity remaining is plotted against time, measured in units of half-life. To use these graphs, one must express the initial radioactivity as 100% and convert the time of interest into units of half-life. For decay times exceeding three half-lives, the logarithmic form is easier to use.

Question: 65 mCi (2.4×10^9 Bq) of ^{131}I are present at noon on Wednesday. How much will remain 1 week later?

Answer: 7 days $= \frac{7}{8}T_{1/2} = 0.875\ T_{1/2}$. Figure 4-12 shows that at $0.875\ T_{1/2}$ approximately 55% of the initial radioactivity will remain; $55\% \times 65$ mCi (2.4×10^9 Bq) $= 0.55 \times 65 = 35.8$ mCi (1.32×10^9 Bq).

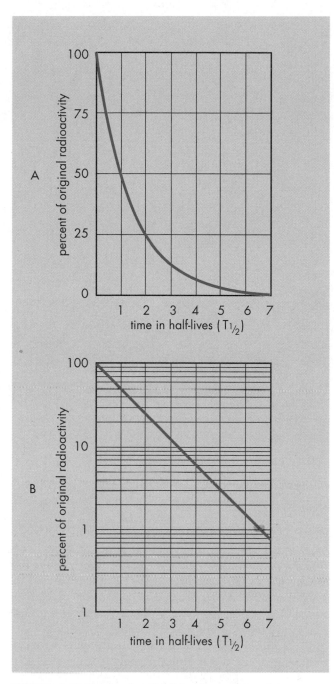

FIGURE 4-12 The quantity of radioisotope remaining after any period of time can be estimated from either, **A**, the linear or, **B**, the semilog graph. The original quantity is assigned a value of 100%, and the time of decay is expressed in units of half-life.

^{14}C is a naturally occurring radioisotope with $T_{1/2}$ (half-life) = 5730 years. The concentration of ^{14}C is incorporated into living material at a constant rate. Trees of the petrified forest contain less ^{14}C than living trees because the ^{14}C of living trees is in equilibrium with the atmosphere. The carbon in a petrified tree was fixed many thousands of years ago and the fixed ^{14}C is reduced with time by radioactive decay (Figure 4-13).

Question: If a piece of petrified wood contains 25% of the ^{14}C that a tree living today contains, how old is the petrified wood?

Answer: The ^{14}C in living matter remains constant as long as the matter is alive because it is constantly exchanged with the environment. In this case the petrified wood has been dead long enough for the ^{14}C to decay to 25% of its original value. That time period represents two half-lives. Consequently, we can estimate that the petrified wood sample is approximately $2 \times 5730 = 11,460$ years old.

Question: How many half-lives are required before a quantity of radioactive material has decayed to less than 1% of its original value?

Answer: A simple approach to this type of problem is to count half-lives.

Half-life number	Radioactivity remaining
1	50%
2	25%
3	12.5%
4	6.25%
5	3.12%
6	1.56%
7	0.78%

A simpler approach finds the answer more precisely. Use the graph on Figure 4-12. The answer is 6.5 half-lives.

Half-life is an essential concept in diagnostic imaging. It is used in nuclear medicine and has an exact parallel in x-ray terminology, the half-value layer, which is the thickness of a material used to reduce x-ray beam intensity to one-half its original intensity.

TYPES OF IONIZING RADIATION

All ionizing radiation can be classified into only two categories—(1) particulate radiation and (2) electromagnetic radiation (Table 4-5). The types of radiation used in diagnostic ultrasound and in magnetic resonance imaging [MRI] are non-ionizing. Ultrasound uses sound radiation, which has different characteristics than electromagnetic radiation. MRI uses electromagnetic radiation, however, the energy of the photons is too low to cause ionization.

Although all ionizing radiation acts on biologic tissue in the same manner, there are fundamental differences between various types of radiation. These differences can be analyzed according to three physical characteristics—mass, charge, and origin (Table 4-5).

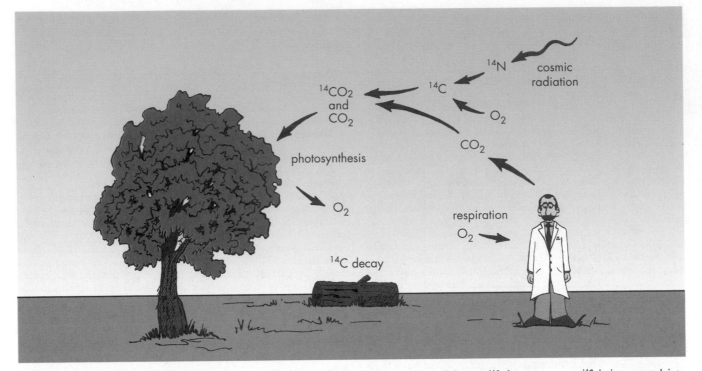

FIGURE 4-13 Carbon is a biologically active element. A small fraction of all carbon is the radioisotope ^{14}C. As a tree grows, ^{14}C is incorporated into the wood in proportion to the amount of ^{14}C in the atmosphere. When the tree dies, further exchange of ^{14}C with the atmosphere does not take place. If the dead wood is preserved by petrification, the ^{14}C content diminishes as it radioactively decays. This phenomenon is the basis for radiocarbon dating.

PARTICULATE RADIATION

Any subatomic particle is capable of causing ionization. Consequently, electrons, protons, and neutrons (even nuclear fragments) can all be classified as particulate, ionizing radiation if they are in motion and possess sufficient kinetic energy. At rest, ionization cannot occur. The principal types of particulate radiation, alpha and beta, are discussed previously in relation to radioactive decay. The alpha particle is equivalent to a helium nucleus. It contains two protons and two neutrons, has a mass of approximately 4 amu, and carries two units of positive electric charge. Compared with an electron, al-

pha particles are emitted only from the nuclei of heavy elements. Light elements cannot emit alpha particles, since they do not have enough excess mass or excess energy. Once emitted from a radioactive atom, the alpha particle travels with high velocity through matter. Because of its great mass and charge, it easily transfers this kinetic energy to orbital electrons of other atoms. Ionization accompanies alpha radiation. The average alpha particle possesses 4 to 7 MeV of kinetic energy and ionizes approximately 40,000 atoms for every centimeter of travel through air. Because of this amount of ionization, the energy of an alpha particle is quickly lost. It

TABLE 4-5

General Classification of Ionizing Radiation

Type of Radiation	Symbol	Atomic Mass Number	Charge	Origin
Particulate				
Alpha radiation	α	4	+2	Nucleus
Beta radiation	β	0	−1	Nucleus
Other particles	*	*	*	Nucleus
Electromagnetic				
Gamma rays	γ	0	0	Nucleus
X-rays	X	0	0	Electron cloud

*Variable

has a very short range in matter. In air, alpha particles can travel about 5 centimeters, whereas in soft tissue the range may be less than 100 microns (μm). Consequently, alpha radiation from an external source is nearly harmless, since the radiation energy is deposited in the superficial layers of the skin. As an internal source of radiation, just the opposite is true. If an alpha-emitting radioisotope is deposited in the body, it can intensely irradiate the local tissue.

Beta particles differ from alpha particles in both mass and charge. They are light particles with an atomic mass number of 0 and carry one unit of negative charge. The only difference between electrons and beta particles is their origins. Beta particles originate in the nuclei of radioactive atoms, and electrons exist in shells outside the nuclei of all atoms. Once emitted from a radioisotope, beta particles traverse air, ionizing several hundred atoms per centimeter. The beta particle has a longer range than an alpha particle. Depending on its energy, a beta particle may traverse 10 to 100 centimeters of air and about 1 to 2 centimeters of soft tissue.

Electromagnetic Radiation

X-rays and gamma rays are forms of electromagnetic ionizing radiation. This type of radiation is covered more completely in the next chapter. X-rays and gamma rays are often called *photons*. Photons have no mass and no charge. They travel at the speed of light (c = 3×10^8 m/s) and are considered energy disturbances in space. Just as the only difference between beta particles and electrons is their origins, so the only difference between x-rays and gamma rays is their origins. Gamma rays are emitted from the nucleus of a radioisotope and are usually associated with alpha or beta emission. X rays are produced outside the nucleus in the electron shells.

X-rays and gamma rays exist either at the speed of light or not at all. Once emitted, they have an ionization rate in air of approximately 100 ion pairs per centimeter, about equal to that for beta particles. Unlike beta particles, however, x-rays and gamma rays have an unlimited range in matter. Total intensity of a beam of photon radiation decreases as the beam passes through layers of tissue, but it never quite reaches zero as does particulate radiation.

In nuclear medicine, beta and gamma radiation are most important. In radiography, only x-rays are important because their energy and quantity can be controlled (Figure 4-14). Because x-rays have a low ionization rate in human tissue, they are particularly useful for **medical imaging** and diagnostic medical use.

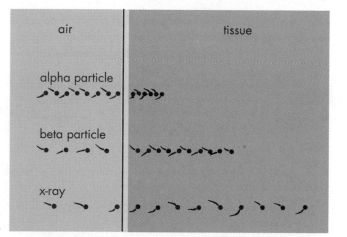

FIGURE 4-14 Different types of radiation ionize matter with different efficiency. Alpha particles are highly ionizing radiation with a very short range in matter. Beta particles do not ionize so readily and have a longer range. X-rays have a low ionization rate and a very long range.

An atom, as described by modern physicists, is the smallest part of an element, and a molecule is the smallest part of a compound, which holds all the properties of that element or compound. The three fundamental particles of the atom are the electron, proton, and neutron. Electrons are negatively charged particles orbiting the nucleus in configurations or shells held in place by the opposing centripetal and centrifugal forces. Chemical reactions occur when outermost orbital electrons are shared or given up to other atoms. Nucleons, neutrons, and protons are each nearly 2000 times the mass of electrons. Protons are positively charged and neutrons have no charge.

Elements are grouped in a periodic table in order of increasing complexity. The groups on the table indicate the number of electrons in the outermost shell. The elements in the periods on the periodic table have the same number of orbital shells. Some atoms have the same number of protons and electrons as other elements but a different number of neutrons, giving the element a different atomic mass unit. These are isotopes. Some atoms, which contain too many or too few neutrons in the nucleus, can disintegrate. This is called *radioactivity*. Two types of radioactive disintegration are alpha emission and beta emission. The half-life of a radioactive element or a radioisotope is the time required for the quantity of radioactivity to be reduced to one half its original value. The age of living material can be determined by ^{14}C dating, in which the half-life of the carbon-14 radioisotope is examined in the material.

Ionizing radiation is either particulate or electromagnetic radiation. Alpha and beta particles are particulate radiation. Alpha particles have four atomic mass units, are positive in charge, and originate from the nucleus of

SUMMARY

As a miniature solar system, the Bohr atom set the stage for the modern interpretation of the structure of matter.

heavy elements. Beta particles have an atomic mass number of zero and have one unit of negative charge. Beta particles originate in the nucleus of radioactive atoms.

X-rays and gamma rays are forms of electromagnetic radiation called photons. These rays have no mass and no charge. X-rays are produced in the electron shells and gamma rays are emitted from the nucleus of a radioisotope.

REVIEW QUESTIONS

1. To the ancient Greeks the term for indivisible was
   a. essences
   b. substances
   c. atom
   d. element
2. Write the modern definition for atom.
3. What did Mendeleev develop?
4. Who developed the concept of the atom as a miniature solar system?
5. Define molecule.
6. What is a chemical compound? Write the chemical equation for common table salt.
7. List the fundamental particles within an atom.
8. Define atomic number. Define atomic mass number.
9. Write the chemical symbols for hydrogen, helium, lithium, and uranium. Include superscripts and subscripts and define each number.
10. Define energy level.
11. Could atoms be ionized by changing the number of positive charges?
12. Describe how ion pairs are formed.
13. What determines the chemical reactivity of an element?
14. List three transitional elements.
15. Why doesn't an electron spontaneously fly off from the nucleus of an atom?
16. Describe the difference between alpha and beta emission.
17. Write the radioactive decay law.
18. How does carbon-14 dating determine the age of petrified wood?
19. What are the two types of ionizing radiation?
20. Describe the properties of photons.

Additional Reading

Balter S: Why (continue to) study physics? *Radiographics* 12(3):609, May 1992.

Mosby's radiographic instructional series: radiologic physics [slide set], St Louis, 1996, Mosby.

CHAPTER

5

Electromagnetic Radiation

OBJECTIVES

At the completion of this chapter the student will be able to:

1. Identify the properties of photons
2. Explain the inverse square law
3. Define wave theory and quantum theory
4. Discuss the electromagnetic spectrum

OUTLINE

Photons
   Velocity and amplitude
   Frequency and wavelength
   Inverse square law
Electromagnetic Spectrum
   Visible light
   Radio frequency
   Ionizing radiation

Wave-Particle Duality
   Wave model: visible light
   Particle model: quantum theory
Matter and Energy Review

P

hotons were first described by the ancient Greeks. Today photons are known as electromagnetic energy, however, these words are commonly used interchangeably. Electromagnetic energy is present everywhere and exists over a wide spectrum of energy levels. X-rays and light energy are examples of photons.

The properties of photons include frequency, wavelength, velocity, and amplitude. In Chapter 5 discussions of visible light, radiofrequency, and ionizing radiation highlight these properties and the importance of electromagnetic radiation in radiography. The **wave equation** and the **inverse square law** are mathematical formulas that further describe how photons behave.

Later in the chapter wave-particle duality of electromagnetic radiation is introduced as **wave theory** and **quantum theory.** Finally, at the end of the chapter, is a summary of matter and energy.

PHOTONS — *electromagnetic energy*

The ancient Greeks recognized the unique nature of light. It was not one of their four basic essences, but it was given important status. They called an atom of light a *photon.* Even today the term *photon* is still used. A photon is the smallest quantity of any type of electromagnetic radiation, just as an atom is the smallest quantity of an element. A photon may be pictured as a small bundle of energy, sometimes called a *quantum,* traveling through space at the speed of light. There are x-ray photons and light photons, as well as other types of electromagnetic photon radiation. The physics of visible light has always been a subject of investigation quite apart from other areas of science. Nearly all the classical laws of optics were described hundreds of years ago. Late in the nineteenth century, James Clerk Maxwell showed that visible light has both electric and magnetic properties, hence the term *electromagnetic radiation.* By the beginning of this century, other types of electromagnetic radiation had been described and a uniform theory evolved.

Velocity and Amplitude

Photons are energy disturbances moving through space at the speed of light (c). Some sources give the speed of light as 186,000 miles per second, but in the SI system of units c = 3×10^8 m/s (meters/second).

Question: What is the value of c in British units or miles per second, given c = 3×10^8 m/s in SI units?

Answer: $c = \dfrac{3 \times 10^8 \text{ meters}}{\text{seconds}} \times \dfrac{\text{miles}}{5280 \text{ ft}} \times \dfrac{3.2808 \text{ ft}}{\text{meters}}$

$= \dfrac{3 \times 3.2808 \times 10^8 \text{ meters-miles-feet}}{5.280 \times 10^3 \text{ seconds-feet-meters}}$

$= 1.864 \times 10^5 \text{ miles/second}$

$= 186,400 \text{ miles/second}$

Photon Velocity

The velocity of electromagnetic photons in British units is 186,400 miles/second or the speed of light. 3×10^8 m/s

Although photons have no mass and therefore no identifiable form, they do have electric and magnetic fields that are continuously moving in a **sinusoidal** fashion. Figure 5-1 shows three examples of a sinusoidal variation. This type of variation is usually called a *sine wave.* Sine waves can be described by a mathematical formula and therefore find application in physics. Sine waves also exist in nature and are associated with many familiar objects (Figure 5-2). Alternating electric current AC consists of electrons moving back and forth sinusoidally through a wire. A long rope fastened at one end vibrates as a sine wave if the free end is moved up and down in whiplike fashion. The arms of a tuning fork vibrate in sinusoidal fashion after being struck on a hard object. The weight on the end of a coil spring varies sinusoidally up and down after the spring has been stretched. The sine waves in Figure 5-1 are identical except for their amplitude; sine wave A has the largest amplitude and sine wave C has the smallest.

Amplitude

Amplitude is one half the range from crest to valley over which the sine wave varies.

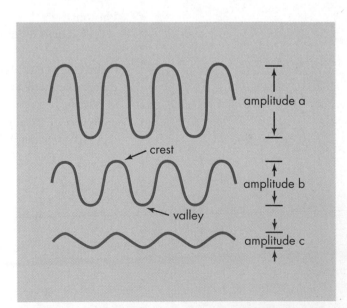

FIGURE 5-1 These three sine waves are identical except for their amplitudes.

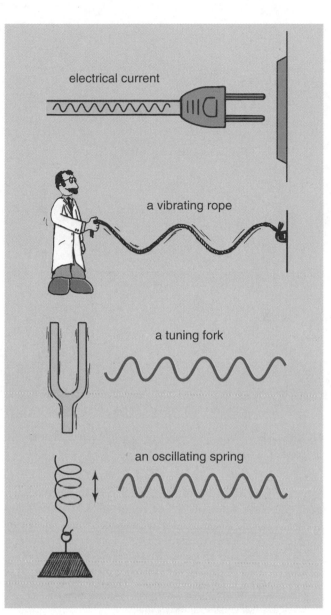

FIGURE 5-2 Sine waves are associated with many naturally occur-ring phenomena in addition to electromagnetic radiation.

Sine-wave amplitude is discussed later in connection with high-voltage generation and rectification in an x-ray unit.

Frequency and Wavelength

The sine-wave model of electromagnetic radiation de-scribes the variations of the electric and magnetic fields as the photon travels with velocity (c). The important properties of this model are **frequency,** represented by f, and **wavelength,** represented by the Greek letter lambda (λ).

Figure 5-3 is another example of a sine wave repre-sented by a vibrating rope. The Texas roadside critter observes the motion of the rope from a point midway between the fastened end and the scientist. If he moves

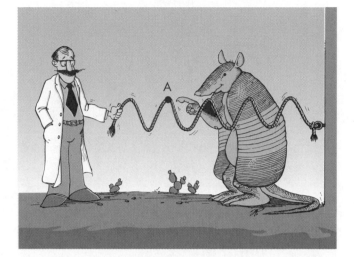

FIGURE 5-3 Moving one end of a rope in a whiplike fashion sets into motion sine waves that travel down the rope to the fastened end. An observer, midway, can determine the frequency of oscillation by counting the crests or valleys that pass a fixed point per unit of time.

his field of view along the rope, he will observe the crest of the sine wave traveling along the rope to the end. If he fixes his attention on one segment of the rope such as point A, he will see the rope rise and fall harmonically as the waves pass. The more rapidly the scientist moves the loose end of the rope up and down, the faster the se-quence of rise and fall.

Frequency

The rate of rise and fall of a sine wave is called **frequency.** It is usually identified as oscillations per second or cycles per second. The unit of measurement is the **hertz (Hz).** One Hz is equal to one cy-cle per second.

The number of crests or the number of valleys that pass the point of an observer per unit time is the frequency. If the observer using a stopwatch counts 20 crests pass-ing in 10 seconds, then the frequency would be 20 cy-cles in 10 seconds or 2 Hz. If the scientist doubles the rate at which he moves the rope up and down, the ob-server would count 40 crests passing in 10 seconds and the frequency would be 4 Hz.

Wavelength

The distance from one crest to another, from one valley to an-other or from any point on the sine wave to the next correspond-ing point, is the **wavelength.**

Figure 5-4 shows sine waves of three different wave-lengths. Wave A repeats every 1 centimeter and there-fore has a wavelength of 1 centimeter. Similarly, wave B has a wavelength of 0.5 centimeter and wave C has a wavelength of 1.5 millimeters. Clearly as the fre-quency is increased, the wavelength is reduced. Three

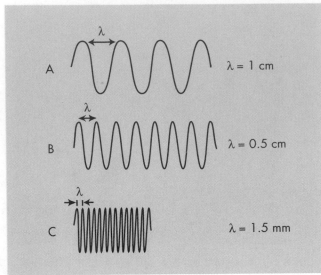

FIGURE 5-4 These three sine waves have different wavelengths. The shorter the wavelength, the higher the frequency.

3 wave parameters—1) velocity, 2) frequency, and 3) wavelength—fully describe a photon of electromagnetic radiation. The relationships among these parameters is important. A change in one affects the value of one or both of the others.

Suppose the physics professor is positioned to observe the flight of the sine-wave arrows to determine their frequency (Figure 5-5). The first is measured and found to have a frequency of 60 Hz. One full oscillation of the sine wave passes every $\frac{1}{60}$ second. The professor-turned-archer now puts an identical sine-wave arrow into his bow and shoots it with less force so that this second arrow has only half the velocity of the first arrow. The observer correctly measures the frequency at 30 Hz, even though the wavelength of the second arrow was the same as that of the first arrow. In other words, as the velocity decreases, the frequency decreases proportionately. The archer then shoots a third sine-wave arrow with precisely the same velocity as the first but with a wavelength twice as long as that of the first. The observed frequency is 30 Hz. Otherwise stated, the wavelength and frequency are inversely proportional at a given velocity.

This illustration demonstrates how the three parameters associated with a sine wave are interrelated. A simple mathematical formula, called the ***wave equation,*** expresses the following relationship:

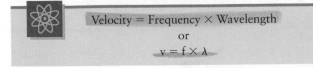

$$\text{Velocity} = \text{Frequency} \times \text{Wavelength}$$
$$\text{or}$$
$$v = f \times \lambda$$

The wave equation is used for both sound and electromagnetic radiation. Keep in mind, however, that

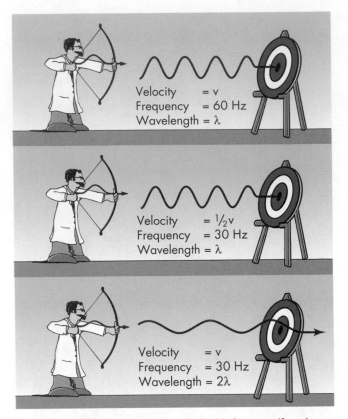

FIGURE 5-5 Relationships among velocity (v), frequency (f), and wavelength (λ) for any sine wave.

sound waves are very much different than electromagnetic photons. The sources of sound are different, they are propogated in different ways, and their velocities vary greatly. Electromagnetic photons travel at the speed of light, and the velocity of sound waves depends on the density of the material it is passing through, that is, sound travels faster through water than air. Sound cannot travel through a vacuum.

Question: The speed of sound in air is approximately 340 m/s. The highest soprano sound that a person can hear is about 20 kHz. What is the wavelength of this sound?

Answer: $v = f \times \lambda$

solve for λ

$\lambda = \dfrac{v}{f}$

$= \dfrac{340 \text{ m/s}}{20 \text{ kHz}}$

$= \dfrac{3.40 \times 10^2 \text{ m}}{s} \times \dfrac{s}{2 \times 10^4}$

$= 1.7 \times 10^{-2} \text{ m}$

$= 1.7 \text{ cm}$

The wavelength of the soprano voice is 1.7 centimeters.

When dealing with electromagnetic radiation, it is possible to simplify the previous equation because all such radiation travels with the same velocity (c) or 186,400 miles/second.

$$c \text{ (velocity)} = f \times \lambda \text{ (frequency} \times \text{wavelength)}$$

The product of frequency and wavelength always equals the velocity of light for electromagnetic radiation. Stated differently, for electromagnetic radiation, frequency and wavelength are inversely proportional. Because frequency and wavelength always equal the velocity of light for electromagnetic radiation as frequency increases, the wavelength decreases and vice versa.

Question: Yellow light has a wavelength of 580 nm. What is the frequency of a photon of yellow light?

Answer: $f = c \div \lambda$

$$= \frac{3 \times 10^8 \text{ m/s}}{580 \text{ nm}}$$

$$= \frac{3 \times 10^8 \text{ m}}{s} \times \frac{1}{580 \times 10^{-9} \text{ m}}$$

$$= \frac{3 \times 10^8 \text{ m}}{s} \times \frac{1}{5.8 \times 10^{-7} \text{ m}}$$

$$= 0.517 \times 10^{15} \text{ cycle/second}$$

$$= 5.17 \times 10^{14} \text{ Hz is the frequency of yellow light}$$

Inverse Square Law

When electromagnetic radiation is emitted from a source such as the sun or a light bulb, the intensity decreases rapidly with the distance from the source. Other electromagnetic energy such as x-rays exhibit precisely the same property. Figure 5-6 shows that as a book is moved farther from a light source, the intensity of light is inversely proportional to the square of the distance of the object from the source. Mathematically this is called the ***inverse square law*** and is expressed as follows:

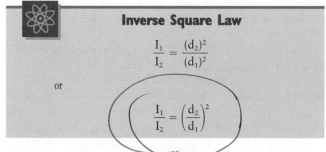

Inverse Square Law

$$\frac{I_1}{I_2} = \frac{(d_2)^2}{(d_1)^2}$$

or

$$\frac{I_1}{I_2} = \left(\frac{d_2}{d_1}\right)^2$$

I_1 is the intensity at distance (d_1) from the source, and I_2 is the intensity at distance (d_2) from the source. The reason for the rapid decrease in intensity with increas-

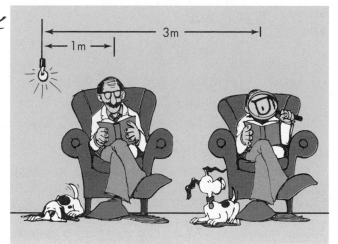

FIGURE 5-6 The inverse square law describes the relationship between radiation intensity and distance from the radiation source.

ing distance is that the total energy emitted is spread out over an increasingly larger area. If the source of radiation is not a point but rather a line, such as a fluorescent lamp, the inverse square law does not hold at distances close to the source. At great distances from the source, the inverse square law can be applied. As a rule, the inverse square law can be applied to distances greater than seven times the longest dimension of the source.

To apply the inverse square law, three of the four parameters must be known. The usual situation involves a known intensity at a fixed distance from the source and an unknown intensity at a greater distance.

Question: The intensity of light from a reading lamp is 100 millilumens (mlm) at a distance of 1 meter. (The lumen is a unit of light intensity.) What is the intensity of this light at 3 meters?

Answer:
$$\frac{I_1}{100 \text{ mlm}} = \frac{1 \text{ m}^2}{3 \text{ m}^2}$$

$$I_1 = (100 \text{ mlm}) \left(\frac{1\text{m}}{3\text{m}}\right)^2$$

$$= (100 \text{ mlm}) (\tfrac{1}{9})$$

$$= 11 \text{ mlm is the intensity of light at 3 meters}$$

This relationship between radiation intensity and distance from the source applies equally well to x-ray intensity.

Question: The intensity of an x-ray beam is 400 mR (103 µC/kg) at 36 in (90 cm). What will the intensity be at 72 in (180 cm)?

Answer: $I_1 = I_2 \left(\dfrac{d_2}{d_1}\right)^2$

$\qquad = (400 \text{ mR}) \left(\dfrac{36 \text{ in}}{72 \text{ in}}\right)^2$

$\qquad = (400 \text{mR}) \, (\frac{1}{2})^2$

$\qquad = (400 \text{mR}) \, (\frac{1}{4})$

$\qquad = 100 \text{mR}$ will be the intensity of the x-ray beam at 72 in

This example illustrates that when the distance from the source is doubled, the intensity of radiation is reduced by one fourth, and conversely, when the distance is halved, the intensity is increased by a factor of four. Often it is necessary to determine the distance from the source at which the radiation has a given intensity. This type of problem is common in diagnostic imaging facilities.

Question: A temporary chest unit is to be set up in a large hall. The intensity is 25 mR (6.5 μC/kg) at 72 in (180 cm). The area behind the chest stand in which the exposure intensity exceeds 1 mR (0.3 μC/kg) is to be cordoned off. How far from the x-ray tube will this area extend?

Answer: $\dfrac{I_1}{I_2} = \dfrac{d_2^2}{d_1^2}$

$\qquad d_2^2 = d_1^2 \left(\dfrac{I_1}{I_2}\right)$

$\qquad d_2 = \left[d_1^2 \left(\dfrac{I_1}{I_2}\right)\right]^{\frac{1}{2}}$

$\qquad\quad = \left[(72^2) \left(\dfrac{25}{1}\right)\right]^{\frac{1}{2}}$

$\qquad\quad = (72^2)^{\frac{1}{2}} \, (25)^{\frac{1}{2}}$

$\qquad\quad = (72)(5)$

$\qquad\quad = 360 \text{ in}$

$\qquad\quad = 30$ feet is the distance from the x-ray source that needs to be cordoned off.

ELECTROMAGNETIC SPECTRUM

The frequency range of electromagnetic radiation extends from approximately 10 to 10^{24} Hz, and the photon wavelengths associated with these ranges of wavelengths are approximately 10^7 to 10^{-16} meters respectively. This wide range of values covers many types of electromagnetic radiation. Grouped together, these ranges of radiation make up the electromagnetic continuum or the **electromagnetic spectrum** (Figure 5-7). The known electromagnetic spectrum has three regions of importance to radiography: (1) visible light, (2) radio frequency and (3) x-radiation. Photons of each of these radiations are essentially the same. Each can be represented as a bundle of energy consisting of varying electric and magnetic fields traveling at the speed of light. The only difference among photons of these various portions of the electromagnetic spectrum is in frequency and wavelength. The electromagnetic spectrum shown in Figure 5-7 contains three different scales; (1) energy, (2) frequency, and (3) wavelength. The velocity of all electromagnetic radiation is constant, but wavelength and frequency are inversely related. In addition, the energy contained in each photon is directly proportional to the frequency.

The earliest investigations in human history concerned visible light. Studies of reflection, refraction, and diffraction showed light to be wavelike, hence the unit of wavelength, the **meter**, was created. Around the 1880s some scientists began experimenting with the radio, which required the oscillation of electrons in a conductor, hence the unit of frequency, the **hertz**, was created. Finally, in 1895 Roentgen discovered x-rays by applying electric energy across a Crookes' tube, hence the unit of energy, the **electron volt**, was created. It should be clear that these three scales are directly related mathematically. If the value of radiation of one scale is known, a value on the other two scales can easily be computed. Scientific investigation of the electromagnetic spectrum has been conducted for over 100 years. Scientists working with radiation in one portion of the spectrum were often unaware of the investigations of others. Consequently, there is no generally accepted, single standard for measuring radiation.

Visible Light

An optical physicist describes photons of visible light in terms of wavelength. When sunlight passes through a prism (Figure 5-8), it emerges not as white light but as the colors of the rainbow. Although photons of visible light travel in straight lines, their course can deviate when they pass from one transparent medium to another. This deviation in line of travel, called **refraction**, is the cause of many peculiar but familiar phenomena, such as a rainbow or the apparent bending of a straw in a glass of water. White light passing through a prism is refracted because it is composed of photons of a range of wavelengths and the prism acts to separate and group the emerging light according to wavelength. The component colors of white light have wavelength values ranging from approximately 400 nanometers (nm) for violet to 700 nm for red. Visible light occupies the smallest segment of the electromagnetic spectrum, but it is the only portion that we can sense directly. Sunlight also contains two types of invisible light—infrared and ultraviolet. **Infrared light** consists of photons with wavelengths longer than those of visible light. Infrared light heats any substance on which it shines. It may be considered **radiant heat**. **Ultraviolet light** is located in the electromagnetic spectrum between visible light and

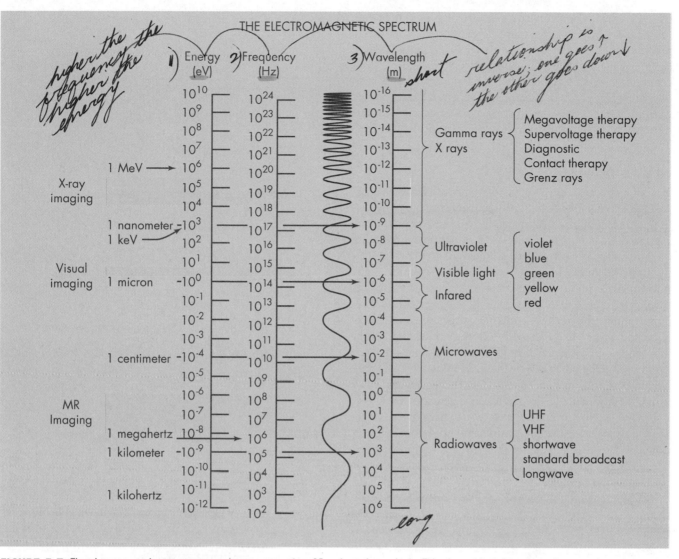

THE ELECTROMAGNETIC SPECTRUM

higher the frequency the higher the energy

short *relationship is inverse; one goes ↑ the other goes down ↓*

1) Energy (eV)	2) Frequency (Hz)	3) Wavelength (m)		
10^{10}	10^{24}	10^{-16}		
10^{9}	10^{23}	10^{-15}		Megavoltage therapy
10^{8}	10^{22}	10^{-14}	Gamma rays	Supervoltage therapy
10^{7}	10^{21}	10^{-13}	X rays	Diagnostic
1 MeV → 10^{6}	10^{20}	10^{-12}		Contact therapy
10^{5}	10^{19}	10^{-11}		Grenz rays
10^{4}	10^{18}	10^{-10}		
1 nanometer 10^{3}	10^{17}	10^{-9}		
1 keV 10^{2}	10^{16}	10^{-8}	Ultraviolet	violet
10^{1}	10^{15}	10^{-7}		blue
1 micron 10^{0}	10^{14}	10^{-6}	Visible light	green
10^{-1}	10^{13}	10^{-5}	Infared	yellow
10^{-2}	10^{12}	10^{-4}		red
10^{-3}	10^{11}	10^{-3}		
1 centimeter 10^{-4}	10^{10}	10^{-2}	Microwaves	
10^{-5}	10^{9}	10^{-1}		
10^{-6}	10^{8}	10^{0}		
10^{-7}	10^{7}	10^{1}		UHF
1 megahertz 10^{-8}	10^{6}	10^{2}	Radiowaves	VHF
1 kilometer 10^{-9}	10^{5}	10^{3}		shortwave
10^{-10}	10^{4}	10^{4}		standard broadcast
1 kilohertz 10^{-11}	10^{3}	10^{5}		longwave
10^{-12}	10^{2}	10^{6}		

X-ray imaging

Visual imaging

MR Imaging

long

FIGURE 5-7 The electromagnetic spectrum extends over more than 25 orders of magnitude. This chart shows the values of energy, frequency, and wavelength and identifies the three imaging windows.

ionizing radiation. It is responsible for molecular interactions that can result in sunburn.

Radio Frequency

A radio or television engineer describes photon emissions in terms of their frequency. For example, radio station WIMP might broadcast at 960 kHz and its associated television station WIMP-TV might broadcast at 63.7 MHz. Communication broadcasts are usually identified by their frequency of transmission and are called *radio frequency* emissions or *RF*. RF comprises a considerable portion of the electromagnetic spectrum. Photons of RF have very low energies and very long wavelengths. **Ham operators** speak of broadcasting on the 10 m band or the 30 m band. These numbers refer to the approximate wavelength of emission. Standard AM broadcast has a wavelength of about 100 m. Television and FM broadcasting occur at a much shorter

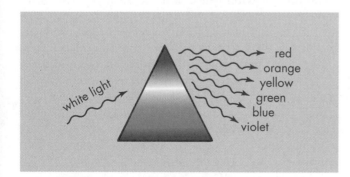

FIGURE 5-8 When white light passes through a glass prism, it is refracted into its component colors. These colors have wavelengths extending from approximately 400 to 700 nm.

wavelength. Because microwaves are also used for communication, there is considerable overlap between what are identified as RF and as microwaves. Short wavelength RF is known as *microwave radiation*. Microwaves have frequencies that vary according to use but are always higher than broadcast RF and lower than infrared. Microwaves have many uses, such as cellular telephone communication, highway speed control, and heating food.

Ionizing Radiation

Unlike radio emissions or visible light, ionizing electromagnetic radiation is usually characterized by the energy contained in a photon. When an x-ray unit is operated at 80 kVp, the x-rays it produces contains energies varying from 0 to 80 keV. An x-ray photon contains considerably more energy than a visible-light photon or a photon from a radio broadcast. The frequency of x-radiation is much higher and the wavelength much shorter than for other types of electromagnetic radiation. The distinction is sometimes made that gamma-ray photons have higher energy than even x-ray photons. In the early days of radiography this was true because of the limited capacity of the available x-ray units. Today, with large particle accelerators available, it is possible to produce x-rays with energies considerably higher than those of gamma-ray emissions. Consequently, the distinction by energy is not appropriate. The only difference between x-rays and gamma rays is their sources of origin.

X-rays are emitted from the electron cloud of an atom that has been artificially stimulated (Figure 5-9). Gamma rays, on the other hand, come from inside the nucleus of a radioactive atom (Figure 5-10). X-rays are produced in electrical machines, whereas gamma rays are emitted spontaneously from radioactive material. Nevertheless, an x-ray and a gamma ray that have equal energy, are alike. This situation is analogous to the difference between beta particles and electrons. These particles are the same, except that beta particles come from the nucleus and electrons come from outside the nucleus.

There are three regions on the electromagnetic spectrum particularly important to radiography. The x-ray region is one. The visible light region is another because radiographers and radiologists view radiographs on a viewbox. And in recent times, the radio frequency range has become important to diagnostic imaging with the advent of **magnetic resonance imaging.**

WAVE-PARTICLE DUALITY

A photon of x-radiation and a photon of visible light are fundamentally the same, except that the former has a much higher frequency and a shorter wavelength than the latter. These differences reflect the way these photons interact with matter. Visible-light photons tend to exhibit more wave nature than particle nature. The op-

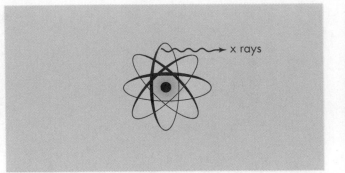

FIGURE 5-9 X-rays are produced outside the nucleus of artificially excited atoms.

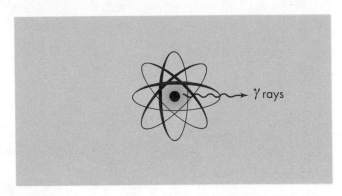

FIGURE 5-10 Gamma rays are produced inside the nucleus of radioactive atoms.

posite is true of x-ray photons, which behave more as particles than waves. In fact, both types of photons exhibit both types of behavior, a phenomenon known as the *wave-particle duality* of radiation. Another way to consider the interaction of electromagnetic radiation with matter is as a function of wavelength. Photons interact with matter most easily when the matter is approximately the same size as the photon wavelength. Consequently, photons of radio broadcast that have wavelengths measured in meters interact with large metal rods or wires called *antennae*. Microwaves, with wavelengths measured in centimeters, interact most easily with objects of the same size such as food products. Visible light has wavelengths measured in micrometers and interacts with living cells such as the rods and cones on the retina of the eye. Ultraviolet light interacts with molecules, and x-rays interact with atoms and subatomic particles. All radiation with wavelengths longer than that of x-radiation interact primarily as a wave phenomenon. X-rays behave as though they were particles.

Wave Model: Visible Light

One of the unique features of human life is the sense of vision. It is interesting that humans have developed organs that sense only a very narrow portion of the enormous spread of the electromagnetic spectrum. This narrow portion is called *visible light.* The visible-light spectrum extends from short-wavelength violet radiation through green and yellow to long-wavelength red radiation. On either side of the visible-light spectrum are ultraviolet and infrared radiation. Neither can be detected by the human eye, but they can be detected by other means such as a photographic emulsion. Visible light interacts with matter very differently from x-rays. When a photon of light strikes an object, it sets molecules of the object into vibration. The orbital electrons of some atoms of some molecules are excited to a higher energy level than normal. This energy is immediately irradiated again as another photon of light. The atomic and molecular structures of the object determine which wavelengths of light are re-radiated. A leaf in the sunlight appears green because all the visible-light photons are absorbed by the leaf but only photons with wavelengths in the green region are re-emitted. Similarly, a balloon may appear red by absorbing all visible photons and re-radiating only the long-wavelength red photons.

Many familiar phenomena of light, such as reflection, absorption, and transmission are explained by using the wave model of electromagnetic radiation. When a pebble is dropped into a still pond, ripples radiate from the center of the disturbance in miniature waves. This situation is similar to the wave nature of visible light. Figure 5-11 shows the difference in the water waves between an initial disturbance caused by a small object and one caused by a large object. The distance between the crests of the waves caused by the large object is much longer than that distance of those waves caused by the small object. The difference in wavelength of these water waves is proportional to the energy introduced into the system. With light, the opposite is true. The shorter the wavelength of light, the greater the photon energy.

If the analogy of the pebble in the pond is extended to a continuous succession of pebbles dropped into a smooth ocean, then at the edge of the ocean the waves will appear straight rather than circular. Light waves behave as though they are straight rather than circular because the distance from the source is great. The manner in which light is reflected from or transmitted through a surface is a consequence of this straight wavelike motion. When the waves of the ocean crash into a vertical bulkhead (Figure 5-12), the reflected waves rebound from the bulkhead at the same angle that the incident waves struck it. When the bulkhead is removed and replaced with a beach, the waves simply crash onto the beach, dissipate their energy, and are absorbed. When an intermediate condition exists in which the bulkhead has been replaced by a line of pilings, the energy of the waves is partially absorbed.

Attenuation
Partial absorption of energy is called *attenuation.*

Visible light can similarly interact with matter. Reflection from the silvered surface of a mirror is common. Examples of transmission, absorption, and attenuation of light are equally easy to identify. When light waves are absorbed, the energy deposited in the absorber reappears as heat. A black asphalt road reflects very little visible light but absorbs a lot of light. In so doing the road surface can become quite hot. Just a slight modification can change the manner in which some materials transmit or absorb light. There are three degrees of interaction between light and an ab-

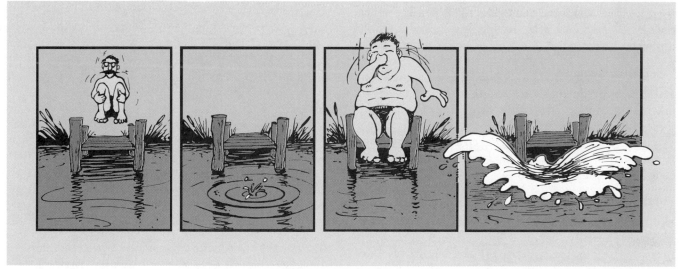

FIGURE 5-11 A small object dropped into a smooth pond creates waves of short wavelength. A large object creates waves of much longer wavelength.

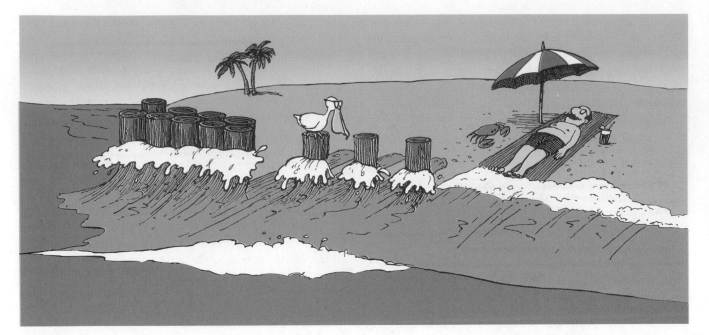

FIGURE 5-12 Energy is reflected when waves crash into a bulkhead. It is absorbed by a beach. Energy is partially absorbed, or attenuated, by a line of pilings. Light is also reflected, absorbed, or attenuated, depending on the composition of the surface on which it is incident.

sorbing material: (1) transparency, (2) translucency, and (3) opacity (Figure 5-13).

Window glass is **transparent.** It allows light to be transmitted through almost unaltered. The glass is clear because the surface is smooth and the molecular structure is tight and orderly. Incident light waves cause molecular and electronic vibrations within the glass. These vibrations are transmitted through the glass and re-emitted almost without change. When the surface of the glass is roughened with sandpaper, light is still transmitted through the glass but is greatly altered and reduced in intensity. Instead of seeing through clearly, there are only shadows. Such glass is translucent. When the glass is painted black, any incidental light is totally absorbed in the paint. Such glass is **opaque** to visible light.

The terms *radiolucent* and *radiopaque* are used routinely in x-ray diagnosis to describe the visual appearance of anatomic structures. Structures that absorb x-rays are called *radiopaque.* Structures that attenuate or partially absorb x-rays are called *radiolucent.* Bone is radiopaque, whereas lung and soft tissue are radiolucent (Figure 5-14).

Particle Model: Quantum Theory

Unlike other portions of the electromagnetic spectrum, x-rays are usually identified by their energy, which is measured in electron volts (eV). The energy of x-ray photons ranges from approximately 1 keV to 50 MeV and higher. The associated wavelength for this range of x-radiation is approximately 10^{-9} to 10^{-12} m. The fre-

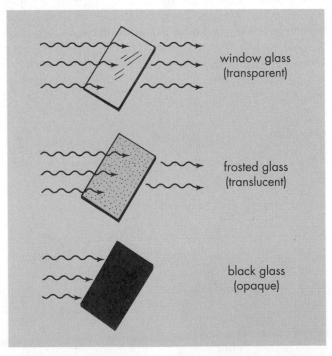

FIGURE 5-13 Objects absorb light in three degrees—not at all (transmission), partially (attenuation), and completely (absorption). The objects associated with these degrees of absorption are called *transparent*, *translucent*, and *opaque*, respectively.

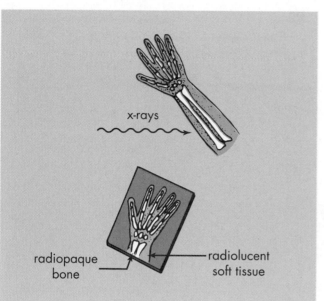

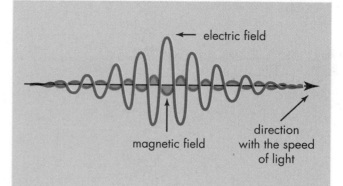

FIGURE 5-15 An x-ray photon can be visualized as two perpendicular sine waves traveling in a straight line at the speed of light. One of the sine waves represents an electric field and the other a magnetic field.

FIGURE 5-14 Structures that absorb x-rays are described as radiolucent or radiopaque, depending on the relative degree of x-ray transmission or absorption, respectively.

quency of these photons varies from approximately 10^{18} to 10^{21} Hz.

Table 5-1 lists the various types of x-rays produced and the general use made of each.

We are primarily interested in the diagnostic range of x-radiation, although what is said for that range holds equally well for other types of x-radiation. The maximum x-ray energy possible is limited only by the size of the x-ray unit. Grenz-ray machines are quite small, whereas some megavoltage units require space equivalent to several rooms.

An x-ray photon can be thought of as containing an electric field and a magnetic field that vary sinusoidally at right angles to each other (Figure 5-15). The wavelength of an x-ray photon is measured as is that of any electromagnetic radiation. The wavelength is the distance from any position on either sine wave to the next

corresponding position. The frequency of an x-ray photon is calculated as is the frequency of any electromagnetic photon using the following equation:

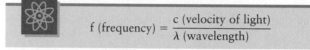

$$f \text{ (frequency)} = \frac{c \text{ (velocity of light)}}{\lambda \text{ (wavelength)}}$$

X-ray photons travel at the speed of light and either exist with velocity (c) or do not exist at all. That is one of the important statements of Planck's quantum theory. Max Planck was a German physicist whose mathematical and physical theories synthesized our understanding of electromagnetic radiation into a uniform model. For this work he received the Nobel Prize in 1918. An important consequence of this theory is the understanding of the relationship between energy and frequency. Photon energy is directly proportional to the photon frequency. The constant of proportionality, known as Planck's constant and symbolized by h, has a numerical value of 4.15×10^{-15} eV-s. Mathematically, the relationship between energy and frequency is expressed as follows:

TABLE 5-1		
Some of the Wide Range of X-rays Produced by Application in Medicine, Research, and Industry		
Type of X-ray	**Approximate Energy**	**Application**
Diffraction	Less than 10kVp	Research: structural and molecular analysis
Grenz rays*	10 to 20 kVp	Medicine: dermatology
Superficial	50 to 100 kVp	Medicine: therapy of superficial tissues
Diagnostic	30 to 150 kVp	Medicine: imaging anatomic structures and tissues
Orthovoltage*	200 to 300 kVp	Medicine: therapy of deep-lying tissues
Supervoltage*	300 to 1000 kVp	Medicine: therapy of deep-lying tissues
Megavoltage	Greater than 1 MV	Medicine: therapy of deep-lying tissues
		Industry: checking integrity of welded metals

*These radiation therapy modalities are no longer in use.

Planck's Constant *relationship between energy and frequency*

$$E(eV) = h \text{ (Planck's constant)} \times f \text{ (photon frequency)}$$

E is the photon energy in eV, h is Planck's constant in eV-s, and f is the photon frequency in hertz.

Question: What is the frequency of a 70 keV x-ray photon?

Answer:
$$E = h \times f$$
$$f = E \div h$$
$$= \frac{7 \times 10^4 \text{ eV}}{4.15 \times 10^{-15} \text{ eV-s}}$$
$$= 1.69 \times 10^{19}/\text{s}$$
$$= 1.69 \times 10^{19} \text{ Hz is the frequency of an x-ray photon at 70 keV}$$

Question: What is the energy contained in one photon of radiation from radio station WIMP, which has a broadcast frequency of 960 kHz?

Answer:
$$E = h \times f$$
$$= (4.15 \times 10^{-15} \text{ eV-s})(9.6 \times 10^5/\text{s})$$
$$= 3.98 \times 10^{-9} \text{ eV is the energy of one photon from the broadcast frequency of 960 kHz}$$

An extension of Planck's equation is the relationship between photon energy and photon wavelength. This relationship is useful in computing equivalent wavelengths of x-rays and other types of radiation. By the equations in the blue box on p. 53 and in the yellow box above, $E = h \times f$ and $f = c \div \lambda$; thus, $E = h\left(\dfrac{c}{\lambda}\right)$ or $E = \dfrac{hc}{\lambda}$.

In other words, photon energy is inversely proportional to photon wavelength. In this relationship the **constant of proportionality** is a combination of two constants, Planck's constant and the speed of light. The longer the wavelength of radiation, the lower the energy of each photon.

MATTER AND ENERGY REVIEW

Everything in existence can be classified as either matter or energy. Furthermore, matter and energy are really manifestations of each other. According to classical physics, matter can be neither created nor destroyed. This law is known as the **law of conservation of matter.** A similar law, the **law of conservation of energy,** states that energy can be neither created nor destroyed. According to Planck's quantum physics and Einstein's physics of relativity, matter can be transformed into energy and vice versa. Nuclear fission, the basis for nuclear generation of electricity, is a familiar example of converting matter into energy. The first equation introduced in Chapter 1 allows the calculation of energy equivalence of matter and the matter equivalence of energy. This equation is a consequence of Einstein's theory of relativity.

$$E = mc^2$$

E in the equation is the energy measured in joules, m is the mass of matter measured in kilograms, and c is the velocity of light measured in meters per second.

Like the electron volt, the joule (J) is a unit of energy. One joule is equal to 6.24×10^{18} eV.

Question: What is the **energy equivalence** of an electron (mass = 9.109×10^{-30} kg), measured in joules and in electron volts?

Answer:
$$E = mc^2$$
$$= (9.109 \times 10^{-31} \text{kg})(3 \times 10^8 \text{ m/s})^2$$
$$= 81.981 \times 10^{-15} \text{ J}$$
$$= (8.1981 \times 10^{-14} \text{ J}) \frac{6.24 \times 10^{18} \text{ eV}}{\text{J}}$$
$$= 51.16 \times 10^4 \text{ eV}$$
$$= 511.6 \text{ keV is the energy of an electron}$$

By using the equation $E = mc^2$ in conjunction with the two equations that relate to electromagnetic radiation (the blue box at the top of p. 47 and the yellow box on this page), one can calculate the **mass equivalence** of a photon when only the photon wavelength or photon frequency is known.

Question: What is the mass equivalence of one photon of 1000 MHz microwave radiation?

Answer:
$$E = h \times f = mc^2$$
$$m = \frac{h \times f}{c^2}$$
$$= \frac{(6.626 \times 10^{-34} \text{ J} \times \text{s})(1000 \times 10^6 \text{ Hz})}{(3 \times 10^8 \text{ m/s})^2}$$
$$= 0.736 \times 10^{-41} \text{ kg}$$
$$= 7.36 \times 10^{-42} \text{ kg is the mass equivalence of a photon of microwave radiation}$$

Question: What is the mass equivalence of a 330 nm photon of ultraviolet light?

Answer:
$$E = \frac{h \times c}{\lambda} = mc^2$$
$$m = \left(\frac{h \times c}{\lambda}\right)\left(\frac{1}{c^2}\right) = \frac{h}{\lambda \times c}$$
$$= \frac{6.626 \times 10^{-34} \text{ J} \times \text{s}}{(330 \times 10^{-9} \text{ m})(3 \times 10^8 \text{ m/s})}$$
$$= 0.00669 \times 10^{-33} \text{ kg}$$
$$= 6.69 \times 10^{-36} \text{ kg is the mass equivalence of a photon of ultraviolet light}$$

Calculations of this type can be used to set up a scale of mass equivalence for the whole electromagnetic spectrum. The mass-energy equivalence scale (Figure 5-16) can be used to check the answers to the above examples.

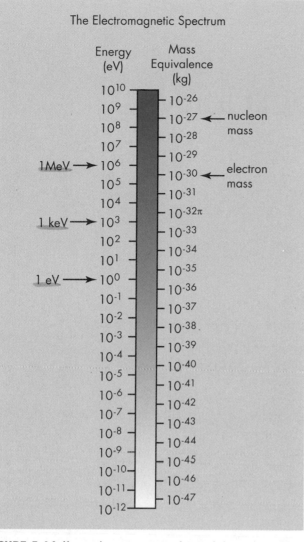

FIGURE 5-16 Mass and energy are two forms of the same medium. This scale shows the equivalence of mass measured in kilograms to energy measured in electron volts.

SUMMARY

Matter and energy can be neither created nor destroyed. Matter and energy are interchangeable.

Radiography focuses on the transference of energy from one form to another in which electrical energy in the x-ray tube creates electromagnetic energy in the form of x-rays. X-rays then interact with matter to form an attenuated beam reaching the image receptor. The film is exposed by light energy, and the radiographic image is formed.

This chapter on electromagnetic radiation presented two of the basic components of radiography, ionizing radiation and visible light.

REVIEW QUESTIONS

1. Photons are _____ moving through space at _____.
2. What is the speed of light in British units?
3. Write the wave equation.
4. How are frequency and wavelength related?
5. Write the inverse square law and describe its meaning in a sentence.
6. The intensity of light from a reading lamp is 100 millilumens (mlm) at a distance of 1 meter (m). What is the intensity of light at 3 meters?
7. As the distance from the source is doubled, the intensity of radiation is _____, and conversely, when the distance from the source is halved, the intensity of radiation is _____.
8. The hertz (Hz) is _____.
9. The known electromagnetic spectrum has three regions of importance to radiography: _____, _____, and _____.
10. What are the range of values of x-ray photons in keV?
11. What is the difference between x-rays and gamma rays?
12. Some regions of the electromagnetic spectrum exhibit wave nature and some regions exhibit particle nature in their interaction with matter. This phemenon is known as _____.
13. Define attenuation.
14. From Table 5-1, the diagnostic range of x-ray energies in kVp is _____.
15. Use Planck's constant to solve the following problem:
    What is the frequency of a 70 keV x-ray photon?
16. Describe the law of the conservation of matter.
17. Describe the law of the conservation of energy.
18. One joule equals _____.
19. Write Einstein's theory of relativity formula.

Additional Reading

Mosby's radiographic instructional series: radiologic physics [slide set], St Louis, 1996, Mosby.

6 Electricity

OBJECTIVES

At the completion of this chapter the student will be able to:

1. Identify the electric charges of protons and electrons
2. Define electrification and state examples
3. List the laws of electrostatics
4. Name examples of conductors and insulators
5. Describe electric circuits and recognize circuit element symbols
6. Define direct and alternating current
7. Identify units of electric potential and electric power

OUTLINE

Electricity
Electrostatics
    Units of electric charge
    Electrification
    Electrostatic laws
    Electric potential (volt)

Electrodynamics
    Conductors and insulators
    Electric circuits
    Direct current and alternating
     current
    Electric power

The x-ray tube and how it operates is part of the study of radiography. This chapter on electricity introduces the basic concepts needed for further study of x-ray tube components.

Because the primary function of the x-ray tube is to convert electric energy into electromagnetic energy or x-rays, the study of electricity is particularly important. This chapter begins by introducing some examples of familiar devices that convert electricity into other forms of energy. Then discussed in detail are the fundamentals of electricity including electrostatics and electrodynamics.

· · · · · · · · · · · · · · · ·

ELECTRICITY

The primary function of an x-ray unit is to convert electric energy into the electromagnetic energy of the x-ray beam (Figure 6-1). Electric energy is supplied to the x-ray unit in the form of a well-controlled electric current. A conversion takes place in the x-ray tube, where electric energy is transformed into x-rays.

Three familiar examples of the conversion of electric energy are as follows. When an automobile battery is recharged, an electric charge restores the chemical energy of the battery. To drive a table saw, electric energy is converted to mechanical energy in an electric motor. A kitchen toaster or an electric range converts electrical energy into thermal energy (Figure 6-2).

Before discussing the conversion of energy in familiar appliances or even in the x-ray tube, basic information must be considered regarding electrostatics.

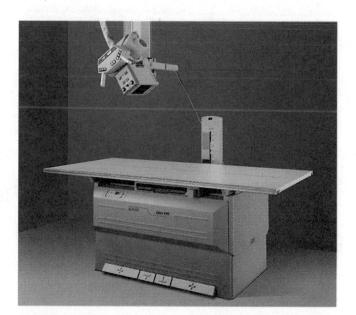

FIGURE 6-1 The x-ray machine converts electrical energy into electromagnetic energy. *(Courtesy Picker International.)*

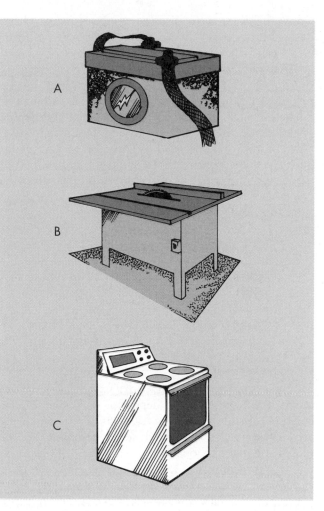

FIGURE 6-2 Electric energy can be converted into other forms by various devices such as **A,** the battery for chemical energy; **B,** the motor for mechanical energy; and **C,** the kitchen range for thermal energy.

ELECTROSTATICS

Matter has been described as having mass, form, and energy equivalence. Matter has another fundamental property as well—electric charge. Electric charge comes in separate units. Each unit is either **positive** or **negative**. The smallest units of electric charge are (1) the electron and (2) the proton. The electron has one unit of negative charge, and the proton has one unit of positive charge.

Units of Electric Charge

The electric charges associated with electrons and protons have the same magnitude but opposite signs. The electron has one unit of negative charge, and the proton has one unit of positive charge.

Because of the way atoms are constructed, electrons are free to travel from the outermost shell of one atom to the next. Protons, however, are fixed inside the nucleus of an atom and are not free to move.

Consequently, nearly all discussions of electric charge deal with negative electric charges associated with the electron.

Electrostatics is the study of electric charges in stationary form. An object is said to be **electrified** if it has too few or too many electrons. The most familiar example of such an electric charge is **static electricity**. When a metal doorknob is touched after having walked across a deep-pile carpet in winter, one gets a shock. Such a shock occurs because electrons are rubbed off the carpet onto one's shoes, causing the person to become electrified. Then the electrons are released onto the doorknob when it is touched.

Electrification Can be Created by the Following:

1. Contact—a connection that causes the flow of electrons.
2. Friction—a buildup of electrons caused by rubbing objects together.
3. Induction—using the electrical field of a charged object to confer a charge on an uncharged object. (Refer to Chapter 8 for further explanation.)

If you run a comb through your hair, electrons are removed from the hair and deposited on the comb. The comb becomes electrified by friction with too many negative charges. An electrified comb can pick up tiny pieces of paper as though it were a magnet (Figure 6-3). Because the comb has excess electrons, it repels some electrons in the paper, causing the closest end of the paper to become slightly positively charged. This results in a small electrostatic attractive force. Similarly, hair is electrified because it has an abnormally low number of electrons and may stand on end because of mutual repulsion. Matter is electrically neutral because in all the

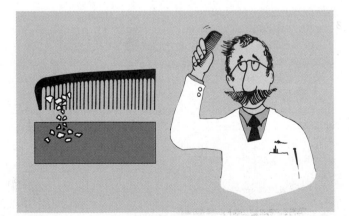

FIGURE 6-3 Running a comb briskly through one's hair may cause both hair and comb to become electrified through the transfer of electrons from hair to comb. The electrified condition may make it possible to pick up small pieces of paper with the comb and may cause hair to stand on end.

universe the total number of negative charges equals the total number of positive charges. The outer-shell electrons of some types of atoms, however, are loosely bound and can easily be removed. Removal of these electrons electrifies the substances from which they were removed and results in static electricity.

Electrification

Electrification occurs when an object becomes charged by the removal or addition of electrons.

Positive electric charges do not move. The transfer of electrons from one object to another causes the first to be positively electrified and the second to be negatively electrified. When a negatively electrified object is brought into contact with an electrically neutral object, the electric charges of the electrified object may be transferred to the neutral object. If the transfer is sufficiently violent, there will be a spark. One neutral object always available to accept electric charges from an electrified object is the earth. The earth behaves as a huge reservoir for stray electric charges. In this capacity, it is called an *electric ground*.

During a thunderstorm, wind and cloud movement can remove electrons from one cloud and deposit them on another. Both clouds become electrified, one negatively and one positively. If the electrification becomes great enough, a discharge between the clouds can occur. Electrons are rapidly transported back to the cloud that is deficient. This phenomenon is called *lightning*. Lightning occurs between clouds, but it can also occur between an electrified cloud and the earth (Figure 6-4).

Another familiar example of electrification is seen in every Frankenstein movie. Usually Frankenstein's laboratory is filled with electric gadgets, wire, and large steel balls with sparks flying in every direction (Figure 6-5). The sparks are created because the various objects, wires, and steel balls are highly electrified. Eventually the storage of electric charges becomes so large that the electrification cannot be sustained. A breakdown occurs by the rapid movement of electrons through the air to an unelectrified object, resulting in the spark, a miniature lightning bolt.

The smallest unit of electric charge is an electron. This charge is much too small to be useful; consequently, the fundamental unit of electric charge is the coulomb (C). One coulomb equals 6.3×10^{18} electron charges.

Question: What is the electrostatic charge of one electron?

Answer: One coulomb is equivalent to 6.3×10^{18} electron charges.

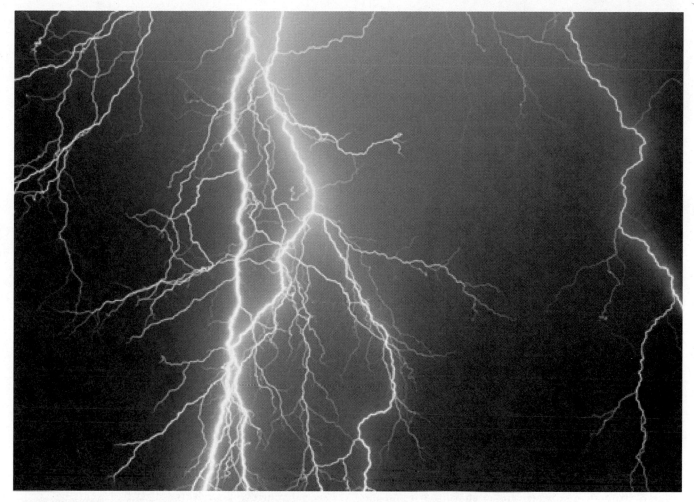

FIGURE 6-4 Electrified clouds are the source of lightning in a storm.

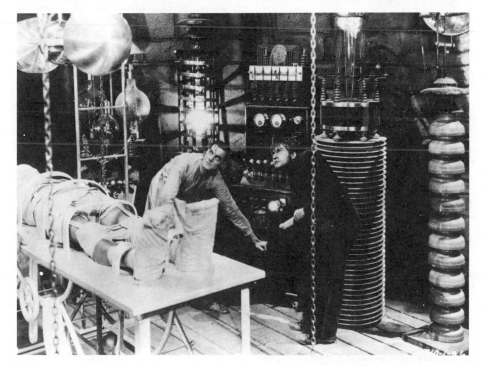

FIGURE 6-5 Early radiologic technologists are shown in this scene from the original *Frankenstein* movie (1931). *(Courtesy The Bettman Archives.)*

$$\frac{1C}{6.3 \times 10^{18} \text{ electron charges}} =$$

$$1.6 \times 10^{-19} \text{ C/electron charge}$$

Question: The electrostatic charge transferred between two people after one has scuffed his feet across a nylon rug is about a microcoulomb. How many electrons are transferred?

Answer: 1 C = 6.3×10^{18} electrons

1 μC = 6.3×10^{12} electrons transferred

Electrostatic Laws

Four general laws of electrostatics describe the way in which electric charges interact with each other and with neutral objects.

Unlike charges attract; like charges repel. (a magnets)

Associated with each electric charge is an **electric field.** The electric field radiates outward from a positive charge and toward a negative charge. Uncharged particles do not have an electric field (Figure 6-6). When two like electric charges, negative and negative or positive and positive, are brought close together, their electric fields are in opposite directions and cause the electric charges to be repelled from each other. When unlike charges, one negative and one positive, are close to each other, the electric fields radiate in the same direction and cause the two charges to be attracted to each other. The force of attraction between unlike charges or repulsion between like charges is due to the electric field. It is called an *electrostatic force*. Uncharged particles exert no electrostatic force and are not acted on by charged particles.

Coulomb's law. The magnitude of the electrostatic force is given by Coulomb's law, as follows:

Coulomb's Law

$$F = k \frac{Q_A \times Q_B}{d^2}$$

Electrostatic force is directly proportional to the product of the charges and inversely proportional to the square of the distance between them.

F is the electrostatic force (newtons), Q_A and Q_B are quantities of electrostatic charge (coulombs), d is the distance between the charges, and k is a constant of proportionality. According to Coulomb's law, the electrostatic force is directly proportional to the product of the electrostatic charges and inversely proportional to the square of the distance between them. The greater the electrostatic charge on either object, the greater the electrostatic force. The electrostatic force is very strong when objects are close but decreases rapidly as objects separate. This **inverse square** relationship for electrostatic force is the same as that for x-ray intensity (see Chapter 5). The equation for electrostatic force has the same form as that for gravitational force, but electrostatic forces act only over short distances, whereas gravitational forces act over very long distances. The electrostatic force can be attractive or repulsive, and the electrostatic force between two charges is unaffected by the presence of a third charge.

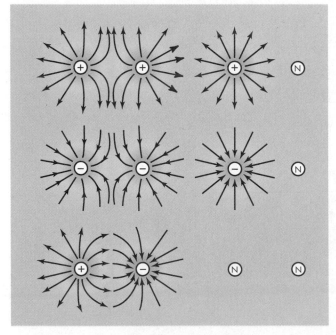

FIGURE 6-6 Unlike charges attract and like charges repel. Uncharged matter (*N*, neutral) is unaffected by charged matter.

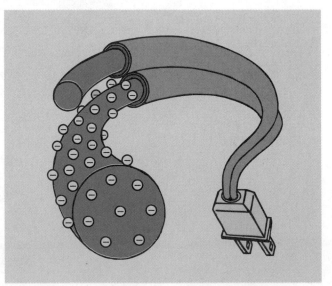

FIGURE 6-7 Cross section of an electrified copper wire, showing that the electrostatic charges reside on the surface of the wire.

Electric-Charge Distribution

When an object becomes electrified, the electric charges are distributed throughout the object.

An example of charge distribution is a thunder cloud. An electrified copper wire is another example. It has its excess electrons spread over the outer surface (Figure 6-7).

Electric-Charge Concentration

Electric charges are concentrated along the sharpest curvature of the surface.

An electrified cattle prod has electric charges equally distributed on the surface of the two electrodes except at each tip where electric charges are concentrated (Figure 6-8). The motto of the manufacturer of this cattle prod is "our business is shocking!"

Electric Potential

In Chapter 1, the relationship between potential energy and work was discussed. Potential energy is stored energy. A system with potential energy has the ability to do work when this energy is released. Electric charges have potential energy. When positioned close to each other, like electric charges have electric potential energy because they can do work when they fly apart. Electrons bunched up at one end of a wire possess electric potential because the electrostatic repulsive force causes some electrons to move along the wire and work can be done.

Potential Energy

The unit of electric potential is the **volt (V).**

Electric potential is sometimes termed *electromotive force (EMF)* or voltage. The higher the voltage, the higher the potential to do work. The electric potential in homes and offices is 110 V. X-ray units usually require 220 V or higher.

ELECTRODYNAMICS

The study of electric charges in motion is called *electrodynamics,* which is recognized as *electricity.* If an elec-

tric potential is applied to objects such as copper wires, then electric charges move along the wire. This is called an *electric current* or electricity. An electric current is the flow of electrons. Electric currents occur in many types of objects and range from the very small currents of the human body measured by electrocardiograms to the very large currents of cross-country electric transmission lines. In addition to electron flow, there is also a direction of electric current. In his early classic experiments, Benjamin Franklin assumed that positive electric charges were conducted on his kite string.

The unfortunate result is the convention that the direction of electric current is always opposite that of electron flow. Electrical engineers work with electric current, whereas physicists are usually concerned with electron flow.

Conductors and Insulators

Matter through which electrons flow easily are electric **conductors.**

Matter that inhibits the flow of electrons are electric *insulators.*

Figure 6-9 shows a section of conventional household electric wire that consists of a metal conducting wire coated with a rubber or plastic insulating material. The insulator confines the electron flow to the conductor. Touching the insulator does not result in a shock, but touching the conductor does. Most metals are good electric conductors. Copper (Co) is the best, but aluminum (Al) is also used. Water is also a good electric conductor because of the salts and other impurities it contains, which is why one should avoid standing in water when operating power tools. Glass, clay, and other earthlike materials are usually good electric insulators. In recent years, materials have been discovered that exhibit both these two different electric characteristics. A **semiconductor** discovered by William Shockley in 1946 is a material that under some conditions behaves as an insulator and under other conditions acts as a conductor. The principal semiconductor materials are silicon (Si) and germanium (Ge). This development led first to the tran-

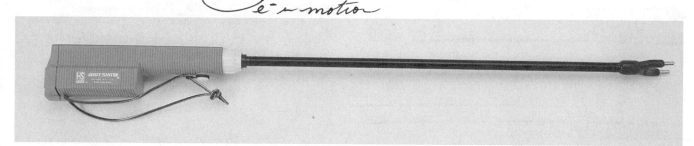

FIGURE 6-8 Electrostatic charges are concentrated on surfaces of sharpest curvature. The cattle prod is a device that takes advantage of this electrostatic law. *(Courtesy Hotshot Products Company.)*

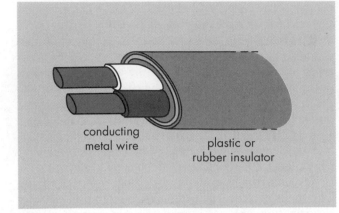

FIGURE 6-9 Conventional electrical wire usually consists of two parts—the metal conductor and the insulator.

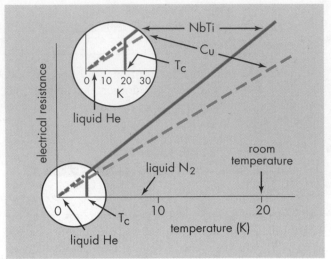

FIGURE 6-10 The electrical resistance of a conductor (Cu) and a superconductor (NbTi) as a function of temperature.

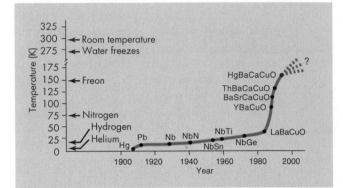

FIGURE 6-11 Recent years have shown a dramatic rise in the initial temperature for superconducting materials.

sistor, then to integrated circuits, and finally to microchips, which are the basis for the present explosion in computer technology.

At room temperature, all material resists the flow of electricity. Resistance decreases, however, as the temperature of material is reduced (Figure 6-10). Some materials exhibit **superconductivity**, which is the property of limited resistance to electron flow below a critical temperature (Tc). Superconductivity was discovered in 1911 but was not developed commercially until the early 1960s. Subsequent scientific investigation has resulted in the demonstration of superconductivity at increasing temperatures (Figure 6-11). In 1987 the Nobel Prize in Physics was awarded to Bednorz and Muller for their work on high temperature superconductivity in a new class of materials. Superconducting materials such as niobium (Nb) and titanium (Ti) allow the flow of electrons without any resistance. Ohm's law and other electrostatic laws described in the next section do not hold true for superconductors. A superconducting circuit is a perpetual motion machine, since current flows without an electric potential or voltage. For material to behave as a superconductor it must be made very cold, which requires energy.

Table 6-1 summarizes the four electrical states of matter.

Electric Circuits

Electrons flow along the outer surface of a wire. Modifying the wire by reducing its cross sectional area (wire gauge) or inserting different material or directions (circuit elements) can increase the resistance to the electron flow (Figure 6-12). When this resistance is controlled and the electrons flow over a closed path, the result is an **electric circuit**. In some respects an electric circuit is similar to a public water system. In a public water system the first step is supplying the water with potential energy by pumping it into a water tower (Figure 6-13).

TABLE 6-1

Four Electrical States of Matter

State	Material	Characteristics
1 Superconductor	Niobium Nb	No resistance to electron flow
	Titanium Ti	No electric potential required
		Must be very cold
2 Conductor	Copper Cu	Variable resistance
	Aluminum Al	Obeys Ohm's law
		Requires a voltage
3 Semiconductor	Silicon Si	Can be conductive
	Germanium Ge	Can be resistive
		Basis for computer technology
4 Insulator	Rubber	Does not permit electron flow
	Glass	Extremely high resistance
		Necessary with high voltage

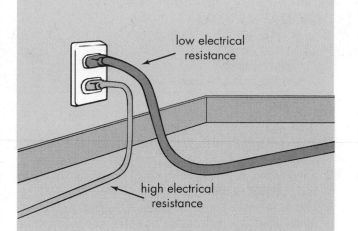

FIGURE 6-12 Electrical resistance is increased with smaller wire and circuit elements.

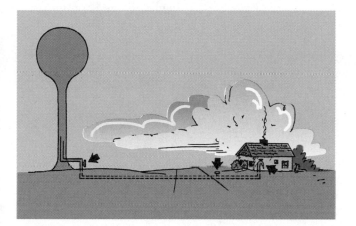

FIGURE 6-13 In some respects a municipal water system is like an electric circuit. Water represents electric current, the water tank represents electric potential, and the valves represent electric resistors.

As the water flows from the water tower through pipes with successively smaller diameters, resistance to its flow increases and the water pressure increases. Similarly, small-diameter wires resist the flow of electric current more than large-diameter wires. A defect somewhere along the water line, such as a faulty valve, creates a large resistance to flow. This is similar to resistive elements built into electric circuits. When the valve is operating properly in the water line, the resistance to the flow of water can be controlled. Similarly, variable resistors in an electric circuit allow control of the flow of electrons. Increasing the resistance decreases the electric current.

After the water has been distributed to homes and is used, it is conveyed along waste water pipes back into the ground. Similarly, electric currents after use can be conducted back to ground or the earth.

Ampere

Electric currents are measured in **amperes (A)**. The ampere measures the number of electrons flowing in the electric circuit.

One ampere is equal to an electric charge of one coulomb flowing through a conductor each second.

Volt

Electric potential is measured in **volts (V)**.

Ohm

Electric resistance is measured in **ohms (Ω)**.

Electrons powered by high voltage have high potential energy and a high capacity to do work. If electrons are inhibited in their flow, the circuit resistance is said to be high.

The manner in which electric currents behave in an electric circuit is described by a relationship known as *Ohm's law.*

Ohm's law states that the voltage across the total circuit or any portion of the circuit is equal to the current times the resistance, or stated mathematically,

$$(volts)\ V = I\ (current) \times R\ (resistance)$$

V is the electric potential in volts, I is the electric current in amperes, and R is the electric resistance in ohms. Variations of this relationship are given in the following two equations:

$$R = \frac{V}{I}$$

$$I = \frac{V}{R}$$

Question: If a current of 0.5 A flows through a conductor that has a resistance of 6 Ω, what is the voltage across the conductor?

Answer: V = I × R

= (0.5 A) (6 Ω)

= 3 V of potential across the conductor

Question: A kitchen toaster draws a current of 2.5 A. If the household voltage is 110 V, what is the electric resistance of the toaster?

Answer: $R = \dfrac{V}{I}$

$= \dfrac{110\ V}{2.5\ A}$

= 44 Ω is the electric resistance of the toaster

Most electric circuits, such as those used in radio, television, or other electronic devices, are very complicated. X-ray circuits are also complicated and contain a number of different types of circuit elements. Table 6-2 identifies some of the important types of circuit elements, the functions of each, and their symbols.

Series and parallel circuits. Usually electric circuits can be described as one of the following two basic kinds: (1) a series circuit (Figure 6-14) or (2) parallel circuit (Figure 6-15).

 Series Circuit

In a **series circuit,** all circuit elements are connected in a line along the same conductor

Rules for series circuits are summarized as follows:

1. The total resistance is equal to the sum of the individual resistances.
2. The current through each circuit elements is the same and is equal to the total circuit current.

3. The sum of the voltage across each circuit element is equal to the total circuit voltage.

Parallel Circuit

A **parallel circuit** contains elements that bridge conductors rather than lie in a line along a conductor.

The basic rules for a parallel circuit are summarized as follows:

1. The sum of the currents through each circuit element is equal to the total circuit current.
2. The voltage across each circuit element is the same and is equal to the total circuit voltage.
3. The total resistance is inversely proportional to the sum of the reciprocals of each individual resistance.

Question: A series circuit contains three resistive elements having values of 8, 12, and 15Ω. If the voltage is 110 V, what is the (1) total resis-

TABLE 6-2		
Electric Circuit Elements; Their Symbol and Function		
Circuit Element	**Symbol**	**Function**
Resistor		Inhibits flow of electrons
Battery		Provides electrical potential
Capacitor (condenser)		Momentarily stores electric charge
Ammeter	Ⓐ	Measures electric current
Voltmeter	Ⓥ	Measures electric potential
Switch		Turns circuit on or off by providing infinite resistance
Transformer		Increases or decreases voltage by fixed amount (AC only)
Rheostat		Variable resistor
Diode		Allows electrons to flow in only one direction
Transistor		Electronic switch that can also amplify signals

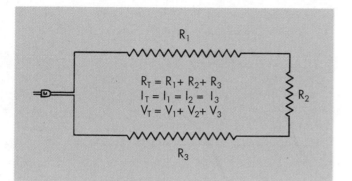

FIGURE 6-14 Series circuit and its basic rules.

$R_T = R_1 + R_2 + R_3$
$I_T = I_1 = I_2 = I_3$
$V_T = V_1 + V_2 + V_3$

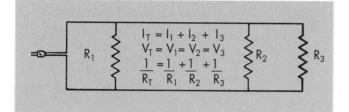

FIGURE 6-15 Parallel circuit and its basic rules.

$I_T = I_1 + I_2 + I_3$
$V_T = V_1 = V_2 = V_3$
$\dfrac{1}{R_T} = \dfrac{1}{R_1} + \dfrac{1}{R_2} + \dfrac{1}{R_3}$

tance and current, (2) the current through each resistor, and (3) the voltage across each resistor?

Answer: Refer to Figure 6-14; let $R_1 = 8\ \Omega$, $R_2 = 12\ \Omega$, $R_3 = 15\Omega$.

1. $R_T = 8\ \Omega + 12\ \Omega + 15\ \Omega = 35\ \Omega$

2. $I_T = I_1 = I_2 = I_3 = V/R = 110/35 = 3.14\ A$

3. $V_1 = (3.14\ A)\ (8\ \Omega) = 25.12\ V$

   $V_2 = (3.14\ A)\ (12\ \Omega) = 37.68\ V$

   $V_3 - (3.14\ A)\ (15\Omega) - 47.10\ V$

Question: Suppose the previous example were a parallel circuit rather than a series circuit. What would be the correct values for total resistance and current, the current through each resistor, and the voltage across each resistor?

Answer: Refer to Figure 6-15.

$$\frac{1}{R_T} = \frac{1}{8\ \Omega} + \frac{1}{12\ \Omega} + \frac{1}{15\ \Omega} =$$

$$\frac{15}{120} + \frac{10}{120} + \frac{8}{120} = \frac{33}{120}$$

$$R_T = \frac{120}{33} = 3.6\ \Omega$$

1. $I_T = 110\ V/3.6\ \Omega = 30.6\ A$

2. $I_1 = 110\ V/8\ \Omega = 13.8\ A$

   $I_2 = 110\ V/12\ \Omega = 9.2\ A$

$I_3 = 110\ V/15\ \Omega = 7.3\ A$

3. $V_1 = V_2 = V_3 = V_T = 110\ V$

Christmas lights are an example of the difference between series and parallel circuits. Christmas lights wired in series have only one wire connecting each lamp. When one lamp burns out, the entire string of lights goes off. Christmas lights wired in parallel, on the other hand, have two wires connecting each lamp. When one lamp burns out, the rest remain lit. Most electric circuits are much more complicated than this. However, for our purposes, electric Christmas lights are a good example. The television monitor in the fluoroscopy room in diagnostic imaging has more than a thousand elements wired into a giant circuit consisting of many subcircuits, each of which is series or parallel or a combination of both.

Direct Current and Alternating Current

Electric current or electricity is the flow of electrons through a conductor.

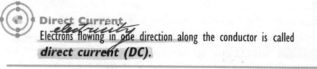

Direct Current
Electrons flowing in one direction along the conductor is called ***direct current (DC).***

Most applications of electricity require that the electrons be controlled so that they flow first in one direction and then in the other.

Alternating Current
Current in which electrons oscillate back and forth is called ***alternating current (AC).***

Figure 6-16 diagrams the phenomena of DC and shows how it can be described by a graph called a ***waveform***.

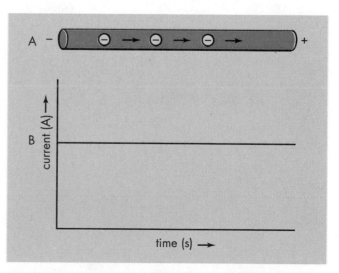

FIGURE 6-16 Representation of direct current. **A,** Electrons flow in one direction only. **B,** The graph of the associated electric waveform is a straight line.

The horizontal or x-axis of the electric waveform represents time. The vertical or y-axis represents the amplitude of the electric current. For DC, the electrons always flow in the same direction with the same velocity. Therefore DC is represented by a horizontal line. The vertical separation between this line and the time axis represents the magnitude of the current. If the line representing the current is above the time axis, it represents the flow of electrons in one direction. Electron flow in the opposite direction is shown by a current line below the time axis. When the current line coincides with the time axis, the magnitude of the current is zero, indicating that no electrons flow.

The waveform for AC is a sine curve (Figure 6-17). Electrons flow first in a positive direction and then in a negative direction. At one instant in time (point 0 in Figure 6-17), all electrons will be at rest. Then they move in the positive direction with increasing potential (segment A). Once they reach maximum potential, represented by the vertical distance from the time axis (point 1), the electrons begin to slow down (segment B). They come to rest again momentarily (point 2) and then reverse motion and flow in the negative direction (segment C), increasing in potential until their velocity in the negative direction is maximum (point 3). Next the potential is reduced to zero (segment D). This oscillation in electron direction occurs in a sinusoidal fashion with each requiring $\frac{1}{60}$ second. Consequently, AC is identified as a 60 Hz (**hertz**) current.

Electric Power

Electric power is measured in **watts (W)**.

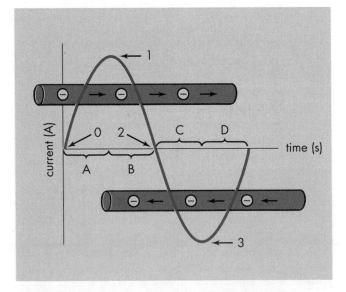

FIGURE 6-17 Alternating current is represented graphically by a sinusoidal electric waveform.

 Electric Power

One watt is equal to 1 A of current flowing through an electric potential of 1 V.

Common household electric appliances such as toasters, blenders, mixers, and radios generally require from 500 to 1500 W of electric power. Light bulbs require from 30 to 150 W of electric power. An x-ray machine may require from 20 to 100 kW of electric power.

Question: If the cost of electric power is 10 cents per kilowatt hour, how much does it cost to operate a 100-watt light bulb an average of 5 hours per day for 1 month?

Answer: Total time on = (30 days/month) (5 hours/day)
= 150 hours/month
Total power consumed = (150 hours/month) (100 W)
= 15,000-W hours/month
= 15 kW-hours/month
Total cost = (15 kW-hours/month) (10 cents/kW-hour)
= $1.50/month to operate a 100 watt light bulb for a month

Electric Power Formula

The basic equation for the computation of electric power is

$$P = I \times V$$

P is the power in watts, I is the current in amperes, and V is the electric potential in volts. Since $V = I \times R$,

$$P = I^2 \times R$$

Either of the previous two equations can be used to compute power.

Question: An x-ray unit that draws 80 A of current is supplied with 220 V. What is the consumed power?

Answer: $P = I \times V$
= (80 A) (220 V)
= 17,600 W
= 17.6 kW of power used by an x-ray unit

Question: The overall resistance of a mobile x-ray unit is 10 Ω. When plugged into a 110 V receptacle, (1) how much current does it draw, and (2) how much power is consumed?

Answer: 1. $I = \dfrac{V}{R} = \dfrac{110}{10} = 11$ A of current drawn by the mobile x-ray unit.

2. $P = I \times V$
= (11 A) (110 V)
= 1210 W
or $P = I^2 \times R$

$$= (11 \text{ A})^2 \times 10\Omega$$

$$= 1210 \text{ W of power used by the mobile x-ray unit.}$$

SUMMARY

The conversion from electrical energy to the electromagnetic energy of the x-ray beam involves study of the components of the x-ray tube. Radiography requires study of the fundamentals of electricity to understand the x-ray tube. Those fundamentals are summarized as follows:

Electrostatics is the study of stationary electric charges.

Electrons and protons have the same unit of charge but opposite signs.

Electrons are negatively charged.

Protons are positively charged.

Electrons are caused to flow from one object to another by contact, by friction, or by induction.

The electrostatic laws are:

1 Like charges attract.

2 Unlike charges repel.

3 Electrostatic force is directly proportional to the product of the charges and inversely proportional to the square of the distance between them. This is known as Coulomb's law and is represented by the following formula:

$$F = k \frac{Q_A \times Q_B}{d^2}$$

4 Electric charge distribution law: when an object becomes electrified the charges are distributed throughout the object.

5 Electric charge concentration law: electric charges are concentrated along the sharpest curvature of the surface of the object.

Potential energy is the ability to do work when energy is released. The unit of electric potential is the volt.

Electrodynamics is the study of electrons in motion, otherwise known as *electricity*.

Conductors are materials through which electrons flow easily.

Insulators are materials that inhibit the flow of electrons.

Electric current is electrons flowing in a closed path with controlled resistance.

Electric current is measured in amperes (A); electric potential is measured in volts (V), and electric resistance is measured in ohms (Ω).

The series circuit has all elements connected along the same conductor. Parallel circuits have elements that bridge the conductor.

Direct current is the flow of electrons in one direction along the conductor. In alternating current, electrons oscillate back and forth along the conductor.

Electric power or 1 W (watt) is equal to 1 A (amp) of current flowing through an electric potential of 1 V (volt).

REVIEW QUESTIONS

1. What is the primary function of the x-ray tube?

2. Name the separate units of electric charge.

3. What does it mean when an object is said to be electrified?

4 What are the three ways electrification can be created?

5. Give an example of an electric ground.

6. What is the fundamental unit of electric charge? What is its value?

7. List the four electrostatic laws.

8. Name the unit of electric potential.

9. Define conductor. Define insulator.

10. What is a semiconductor, and how has it affected modern life?

11. Define electric circuit. — *closed path of e⁻ flow*

12. State Ohm's law.

13. A kitchen toaster draws a current of 2.5 A. If the household voltage is 110 V, what is the electric resistance of the toaster?

14. List the formulas for series circuits and parallel circuits.

15. Define direct current. Define alternating current.

16. An x-ray unit draws 80 A of current and is supplied with 220 V. How much power does it consume?

17. One watt (W) equals _____.

18. Why is it important for radiography students to study electricity?

7

Magnetism

OBJECTIVES

At the completion of this chapter the student will be able to:

1. Discuss the history and discovery of naturally occurring magnetic materials
2. Define magnetic dipole
3. List the three classifications of magnets
4. Identify the interactions between matter and magnetic fields
5. List and discuss the four laws of magnetism

OUTLINE

**History of Naturally Occurring
  Magnetic Materials**
Introduction to Magnetism
Classification of Magnets

Magnetic Laws
  Dipoles
  Attraction and repulsion
  Magnetic induction
  Magnetic force

agnetism has become increasingly important in diagnostic imaging with the recent development and increased use of magnetic resonance imaging (MRI) as a medical diagnostic tool. MRI physics is based on the angular momentum or precession of hydrogen atoms within the body and the effect on the hydrogen atoms by the externally applied magnetic field. Magnetic field safety is an issue in the modern diagnostic imaging workplace.

. . . .

HISTORY OF NATURALLY OCCURRING MAGNETIC MATERIALS

Around 1000 BC shepherds and dairy farmers of the village of Magnesia (what is now Western Turkey) discovered magnetite. **Magnetite** is a magnetic oxide of iron (Fe_3O_4). This rodlike stone would rotate back and forth when suspended by a string. When it came to rest on the string, it supposedly pointed the way to water. It was called a *lodestone* or leading stone. Magnetite was also used as a compass by ancient people. From any spot on earth, magnetite pointed toward the North Pole and following the lodestone north would lead to water.

The word **magnetism** comes from the name of that ancient village Magnesia. Magnetism is a fundamental property of some forms of matter. Ancient observers knew that lodestone or magnetite attracted iron filings. They were also aware of the attraction of small lightweight objects such as paper to an amber rod rubbed with fur. They considered both of these phenomena, magnetism and electrostatics, to be the same.

INTRODUCTION TO MAGNETISM

Magnetism is perhaps more difficult to understand than other characteristic properties of matter such as mass, energy, and electric charge. Magnetism is difficult to detect and to measure. Mass is heavy, energy is seen, and electricity creates shocks, but magnetism cannot be felt or sensed.

Any charged particle in motion creates a magnetic field (Figure 7-1). The magnetic field is perpendicular to the motion of the charged particle and the intensity of magnetism is represented by imaginary lines. If the particle's motion is a closed loop like an electron circling a nucleus, the magnetic field lines will be perpendicular to the plane of motion (Figure 7-2). Electrons circle a nucleus either clockwise or counterclockwise. This motion is related to a property called *electron spin*. The magnetic fields created by a pair of electrons cancel out one another. Therefore atoms having an odd number of electrons in any shell exhibit a net magnetic field. The lines of a magnetic field are always closed loops and are called *bipolar* or *dipolar*. Bipolar or dipolar means there is always a north and a south pole. The small magnet

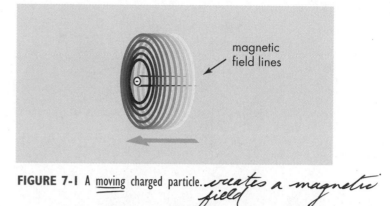

FIGURE 7-1 A moving charged particle. *creates a magnetic field*

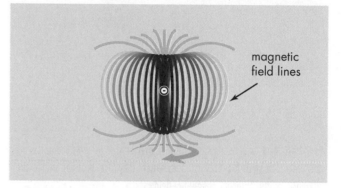

FIGURE 7-2 A moving charged particle induces a magnetic field in a plane perpendicular to its motion.

created by the electron orbit is called a **magnetic dipole**. An accumulation of many atomic magnets with their dipoles aligned creates a **magnetic domain**. If all the magnetic domains in an object are aligned, the object acts like a magnet.

In a hydrogen atom there is a strong magnetic dipole because of the unpaired electron, but in a hydrogen molecule (H_2) the magnetic domains of the two electrons cancel each other out so there is no magnetic dipole. Under normal circumstances, magnetic domains are randomly distributed (Figure 7-3, *A*). When acted on by an external magnetic field the randomly oriented dipoles align to the field (Figure 7-3, *B*). The earth is a case of naturally occurring magnetic field and, as a result, compasses align to the magnetic North Pole.

Spinning electric charges such as the electron also induce a magnetic field (Figure 7-4). The proton in a hydrogen nucleus spins on its axis and creates a nuclear magnetic dipole called a *magnetic moment*. The magnetic moments of hydrogen atoms in the body are the basis of magnetic resonance imaging (MRI).

The magnetic dipoles in a bar magnet generate imaginary lines of the magnetic field (Figure 7-5, *A*). If a nonmagnetic material is brought near such a magnet, there will be no disturbance in these field lines (Figure 7-5, *B*). If **ferromagnetic** material such as soft iron, which is easily magnetized, is brought near the bar magnet, the

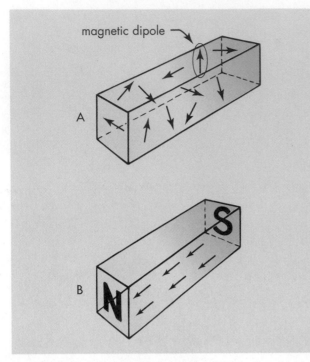

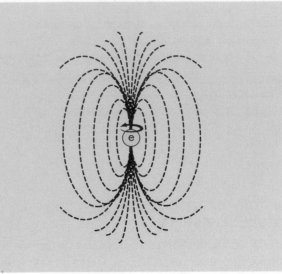

FIGURE 7-4 An electric charge spinning on its own axis will create a magnetic field.

FIGURE 7-3 A, In ferromagnetic material the magnetic dipoles are randomly oriented. **B,** This changes when they are brought under the influence of an external magnetic field.

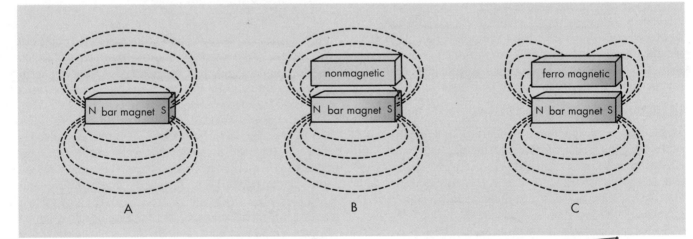

FIGURE 7-5 A, Imaginary lines of force. **B,** These lines of force are undisturbed by nonmagnetic material. **C,** They are deviated by ferromagnetic material.

magnetic field lines will be deviated and concentrated into the ferromagnetic material (Figure 7-5, *C*).

Magnets are classified according to the **origin** of the magnetic property.

CLASSIFICATION OF MAGNETS

There are three principal types of magnets: (1) naturally occurring magnets, (2) artificially induced permanent magnets, and (3) electromagnets. The best example of a **natural magnet** is the earth itself. The earth has a magnetic field because it spins on an axis. Lodestone or magnetite in the earth exhibits strong magnetism, presumably because those substances have remained undisturbed for a long time in the earth's magnetic field. Artificially produced **permanent magnets** are available in many sizes and shapes but principally as bar or horseshoe-shaped magnets usually made of iron. A compass is a prime example of an artificial permanent magnet.

Permanent magnets are typically produced by charging them in the field of an electromagnet (Figure 7-6). Such permanent magnets do not necessarily stay permanent. The magnetic property of a magnet can be destroyed by heating it or even by hitting it with a hammer. The individual magnetic domains are jarred from their alignment and thus become randomly aligned again. Magnetism is then lost. **Electromagnets** consist of wire wrapped around an iron core. When an electric current is conducted through the wire, a magnetic field is created. The intensity of the magnetic field is proportional to the electric current.

All matter can be classified according to the manner in which it interacts with an external magnetic field.

Many materials are unaffected when brought into a magnetic field. Such materials are nonmagnetic and called **dimagnetic**. They cannot be artificially magnetized, and they are not attracted to a magnet. Examples of dimagnetic materials are wood, glass, and plastic. Ferromagnetic materials are iron, cobalt, and nickel. These are strongly attracted by a magnet and can usually be permanently magnetized by exposure to a magnetic field. An alloy of aluminum, nickel, and cobalt called **alnico** is one of the more useful magnets produced from ferromagnetic material. More recently, rare earth ceramics have been developed and are considerably stronger magnets (Figure 7-7). **Paramagnetic** materials lie somewhere between ferromagnetic and nonmagnetic. They are slightly attracted to a magnet and loosely influenced by an external magnetic field. Contrast agents, such as **gadolinium** used in MRI as an injectable substance, are paramagnetic. The degree to which various materials can be magnetized is called *magnetic susceptibility.* Placing wood in the presence of a strong magnetic field will not increase the strength of the field. Wood has low magnetic susceptibility. On the other hand, placing iron in a magnetic field greatly increases the strength of the field. Iron has high magnetic susceptibility.

MAGNETIC LAWS

The physical laws of magnetism are similar to those of electrostatics and gravity. Gravitational, electric, and magnetic forces are fundamental in nature, and their laws are listed on Table 7-1. Note that the equations of force between fields have the same form. There is interest among theoretical physicists to combine these fundamental forces with two others, the strong nuclear force and the weak nuclear interaction, to formulate a **unified field theory.**

Dipoles

Unlike the situation that exists with electricity, there is no smallest unit of magnetism. Dividing a magnet simply creates two smaller magnets, which when divided again create even smaller magnets (Figure 7-8). How do we know that these imaginary lines of the magnetic field exist? They can be demonstrated by the action of iron filings near a magnet (Figure 7-9). If a magnet is placed on a surface with small iron filings, the filings will attach most strongly and with greater concentration to the ends of the magnet. These ends are called *poles* and every magnet has two poles. Magnetic poles exist in two forms: (1) a **north pole** and (2) a **south pole,** which are analogous to positive and negative electrostatic charges.

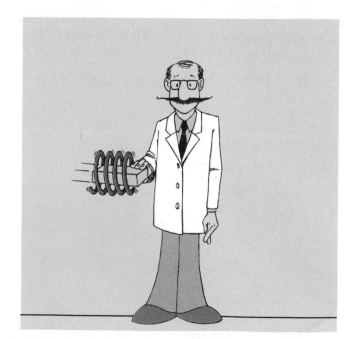

FIGURE 7-6 Permanent magnets are typically produced by charging them in an electromagnet field. *electromagnet*

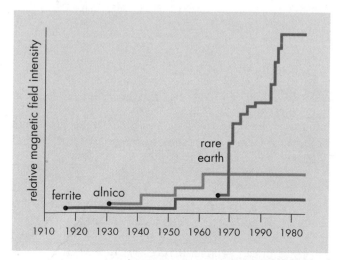

FIGURE 7-7 Rare-earth ceramics create considerably stronger magnets.

TABLE 7-1			
Three Fundamental Forces in Nature			
	Gravitational	Electric	Magnetic
The force:	Attracts only	Attracts and repels	Attracts and repels
It acts in:	A mass, m	A charge, q	A pole, p
Through an associated field:	A gravitational field, g	An electric field, E	A magnetic field, B
With intensity:	$F = m \times g$	$F = q \times E$	$F = p \times B$
The source of the field is:	A mass, M	A charge, Q	A pole, P
The intensity of the field at a distance from the source is:	$g = \dfrac{G \times M}{d^2}$	$E = \dfrac{k \times Q}{d^2}$	$B = \dfrac{kP}{d^2}$
The force between fields is given by:	Newton's law	Coulomb's law	Gauss' law
	$F = -G\,\dfrac{M \times m}{d^2}$	$F = k\,\dfrac{Q_a \times Q_b}{d^2}$	$F = k\,\dfrac{P \times p}{d^2}$
Where:	$G = 6.678 \times 10^{-11}\,\dfrac{N \times m^2}{kg^2}$	$k = 9.0 \times 10^9\,\dfrac{N \times m^2}{C^2}$	$k = 10^{-7}\,\dfrac{W}{A^2}$

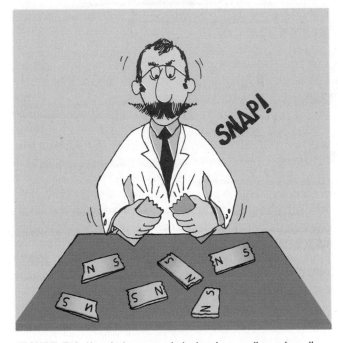

FIGURE 7-8 If a single magnet is broken into smaller and smaller pieces, smaller magnets are produced.

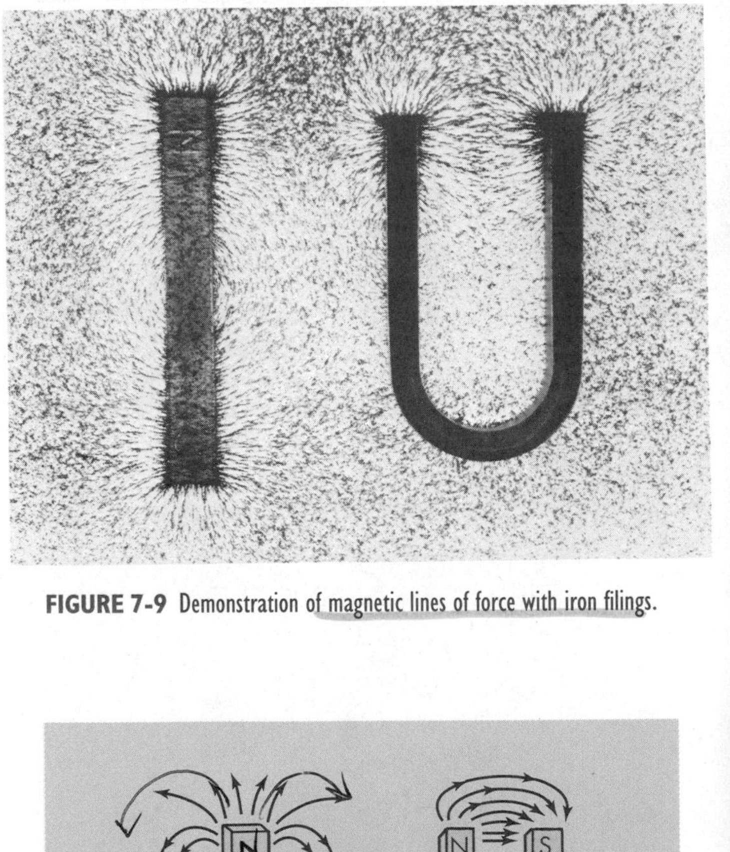

FIGURE 7-9 Demonstration of magnetic lines of force with iron filings.

Attraction and Repulsion

As with electric charges, like magnetic poles repel, unlike magnetic poles attract. Also, by convention, the imaginary lines of the magnetic field leave the north pole of a magnet and return to the south pole (Figure 7-10).

Magnetic Induction

Just as an electrostatic charge can be induced from one material to another, so ferromagnetic material can be made magnetic by induction. Imaginary magnetic field lines are called *magnetic lines of induction*, and the density of the lines is proportional to the intensity of the

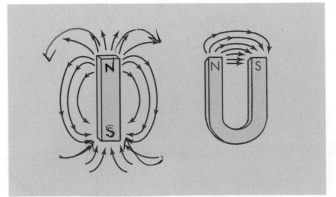

FIGURE 7-10 Imaginary lines of the magnetic field leave the north pole of the magnet and return to the south pole.

magnetic field. When ferromagnetic material such as a piece of soft iron is brought into the vicinity of an intense magnetic field, the lines of induction will be altered by attraction to the soft iron. The iron will be made temporarily magnetic as well (Figure 7-11). If copper, a diamagnetic material, were to replace the soft iron, the diamagnetic material would not affect the field lines nor would the material be made temporarily magnetic. This principle is used with many MRI units that use an iron magnetic shield to reduce the level of the nonuseable fringe magnetic field. Ferromagnetic material acts as a **magnetic sink** by drawing the **fringe lines** of the magnetic field into it. When ferromagnetic material is removed from the magnetic field, it usually does not retain its strong magnetic property. Soft iron, therefore, makes an excellent **temporary magnet**. It is a magnet only while its magnetism is being induced. If properly tempered by heat or exposed to an external field for a long period, some ferromagnetic materials retain their magnetism and become permanent magnets.

Magnetic Force

The force created by a magnetic field behaves similarly to that of the electric field. As a result electric and magnetic forces can be joined in **Maxwell's field theory** of electromagnetic radiation. In Maxwell's field theory force is proportional to the product of the magnetic pole strengths divided by the square of the distance between them. Magnetic force is similar to electrostatic

and gravitational forces that also are inversely proportional to the square of the distance between the objects under consideration. If the distance between two bar magnets is halved, the magnetic force will be increased by four times.

Unit of Magnetic Field Strength
The SI unit of magnetic field strength is the **tesla or gauss.** One tesla (T) = 10,000 gauss (G).

The earth behaves as though it has a large bar magnet embedded in it. The convention of having north and south poles in magnetism actually has its origin in the compass. At the equator, the north pole of a compass points to the earth's North Pole (which is actually the earth's south magnetic pole). As one travels toward the North Pole, the attraction of the compass becomes more intense until the compass needle points directly into the earth, not at the geographic North Pole but at a region in northwestern Canada—the magnetic pole (Figure 7-12). The magnetic pole in the southern hemisphere is in Australia. If a person stood at the south magnetic pole, the compass would point to the sky. The use of a compass might suggest that the earth has a strong magnetic field, but it does not. The earth's magnetic field is approximately 50 µ T at the equator and 100 µ T at the poles. This is 1000 times less than the magnet on a cabinet door latch in an x-ray room.

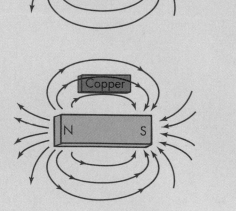

FIGURE 7-11 Iron within the vicinity of lines of induction will be made temporarily magnetic.

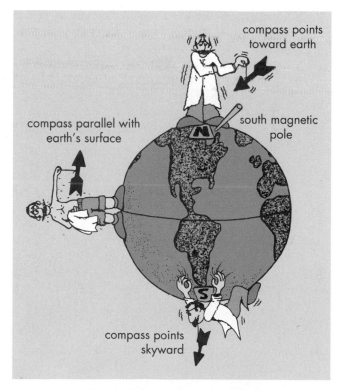

FIGURE 7-12 A free-swinging compass reacts with the earth as though it were a bar magnet.

SUMMARY

The increasing use of magnetic resonance imaging as a medical diagnostic tool emphasizes the importance of magnetism as an area of study for radiography students.

Lodestone or magnetite was observed in the ancient world as having magnetic properties. Matter has magnetic properties because atoms can have an uneven number of electrons in the orbital shells, which gives a charge and a magnetic field to the object.

Magnets are classified according to the origin of their magnetic property. Natural magnets get their magnetism from the earth, permanent magnets are artificially induced magnets, and electromagnets are produced when wires with current flowing are wrapped around an iron core.

Also, matter can be classified by the interaction with an external magnetic field. Substances are either diamagnetic (cannot be magnetized), ferromagnetic (can be easily magnetized), or paramagnetic (exhibit both properties).

The laws of magnetism are listed and described as follows:

1. Magnetic dipoles—every magnet no matter how small has two poles, north and south, equivalent to positive and negative electrostatic charges.
2. Attraction and repulsion—just as with electrostatic charges, like magnetic poles repel and unlike magnetic poles attract.
3. Magnetic induction—a ferromagnetic material can be made magnetic by being placed in the magnetic field lines of a magnet.
4. Magnetic force or Maxwell's field theory—magnetic force is proportional to the product of the magnetic pole strengths divided by the square of the distance between them. The SI units of magnetic field strength are 1 tesla (T) = 10,000 gauss (G).

REVIEW QUESTIONS

1. Why is magnetism an important study in radiography?
2. Where was lodestone discovered and how was it used?
3. Any charged particle in motion will _____.
4. Define magnetic domain.
5. How are magnets classified?
6. List the three principle types of magnets.
7. Describe what makes up an electromagnet.
8. Matter that is not attracted to a magnet is termed _____.
9. Matter that is highly attracted to a magnet is termed _____.
10. Name a contrast agent that is paramagnetic.
11. Define magnetic susceptibility.
12. List the five forces in nature that physicists may combine to form a unified field theory.
13. Magnetic poles exist in two forms: (1) _____ and (2) _____.
14. Describe Maxwell's field theory of electromagnetic radiation.
15. Name the SI unit of magnetic field strength.
16. State the second law of magnetism of attraction and repulsion.
17. What is the third law of magnetism?
18. Describe an example of electrostatics.
19. Explain how a magnetic domain causes an object to behave like a magnet.
20. Is a hydrogen molecule a magnetic dipole? Why or why not?

Additional Reading

Maurino MR: From Thales to Lauterbur, or from the lodestone to MR imaging: magnetism and medicine, *Radiology* 593, 1991.

Taylor BN: New measurement standards for 1990, *Physics Today* 23, August 1989.

8

Electromagnetism

OBJECTIVES

At the completion of this chapter the student will be able to:

1. Discuss the development of the battery as a reliable source of electric current for scientific investigation
2. Relate the experiments of Oersted in defining the relationship between magnetism and electric current
3. Describe the solenoid and the electromagnet
4. Identify the laws of electromagnetic induction
5. Explain the design of the electric generator, the electric motor, the transformer, and the rectifier

OUTLINE

Electromagnetic Force
    Battery
    Electricity and magnetism
Laws of Electromagnetic Induction
    Faraday's law
    Lenz' law
    Self-induction
    Mutual induction

Electromechanical and Electronic Devices
    Electric generator
    Electric motor
    Transformer
    Rectifier

T his chapter combines information from the two previous chapters on electricity and magnetism into a discussion of electromagnetic force. Electromagnetism is the force associated with electrons in motion, otherwise known as *electricity*.

ELECTROMAGNETIC FORCE

Electricity and magnetism are different aspects of the same electromagnetic force. Electromagnetic force is one of the four fundamental forces of nature. The other fundamental forces are gravity, the strong nuclear force, and the weak nuclear interaction. Until the nineteenth century, electricity and magnetism were viewed as separate effects, although many scientists suspected a connection. Scientific research was hampered by the lack of any convenient way to produce and control electricity. The study of electricity in earlier times was limited to the investigation of static charges produced by the friction of rubbing fur on a rubber rod. Charges could be induced to move but only in a sudden discharge such as a spark jumping a gap. During the last century, the development of methods of producing a steady flow of charges or an electric current stimulated the investigation of both electricity and magnetism. The development of the battery led to an increased understanding of electromagnetic phenomena and caused the electric revolution that is so much part of today's technology.

Battery

In the late 1700s an Italian anatomist made a discovery quite by accident. He discovered that a dissected frog leg twitched when touched by two different metals just as if it had been touched by an electrostatic charge. This prompted another Italian, a physicist by the name of Alessandro Volta, to question if an electric current might be produced when two different metals are brought into contact. Using zinc and copper plates, he succeeded in producing a feeble electric current. To increase the current, he stacked the copper-zinc plates similar to a Dagwood sandwich to form what was called the *Voltaic pile,* a precursor of the modern battery. Each zinc-copper sandwich is called a *cell of the battery.* Modern dry cells use a carbon rod as the positive electrode surrounded by an electrolytic paste housed in a negative zinc cylindrical can. The Voltaic pile, the modern battery, and the electronic symbol for the battery are shown in Figure 8-1. The battery is an example of a source of electromotive force (EMF).

Any device that converts some form of energy directly into electric energy is said to be a source of EMF or **stored electric energy.**

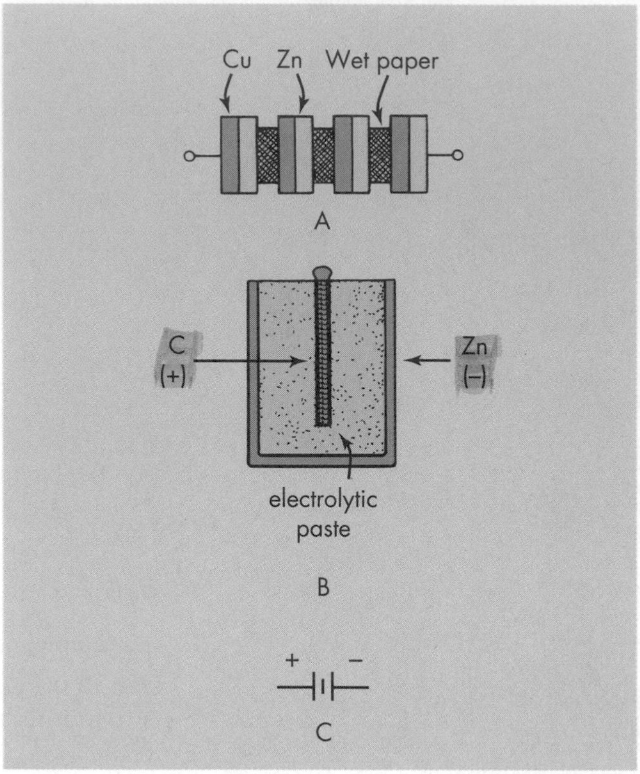

FIGURE 8-1 A, Original Voltaic pile. **B,** A modern dry cell. **C,** The electronic symbol for a battery.

EMF has units of joules per coulomb or volts.

ELECTRICITY AND MAGNETISM

When scientists finally had a source of constant electric current in the battery, they began extensive investigations into the link between electric and magnetic forces. The first such link was discovered in 1820 by **Hans Oersted,** a Danish physicist. Oersted fashioned a long, straight wire supported near a free-rotating magnetic compass (Figure 8-2). With no current flowing through the wire, the magnetic compass pointed north as one would expect. When a current was passed through the wire, however, the compass needle swung to point straight at the wire. This was evidence of a direct link between electric and magnetic phenomena. The electric current evidently produced a magnetic field strong enough to overpower the earth's magnetic field and cause the magnetic compass to point toward the wire.

Any charge in motion induces a magnetic field.

A charge at rest produces no magnetic field. Thus electrons flowing through a wire produce a magnetic field around the wire. The magnetic field is represented by imaginary lines that form concentric circles centered on the wire (Figure 8-3).

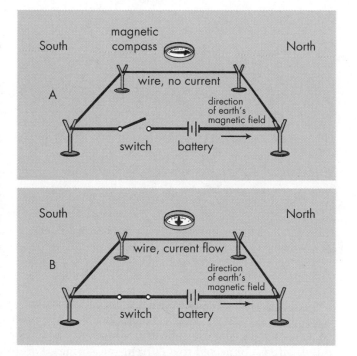

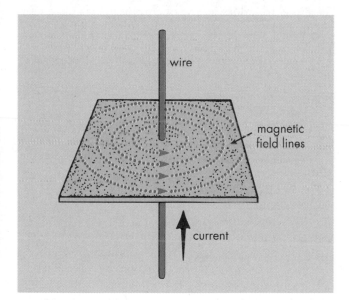

FIGURE 8-2 Oersted's experiment. **A,** With no current in the wire, the compass points north. **B,** With current flowing, the compass points toward the wire.

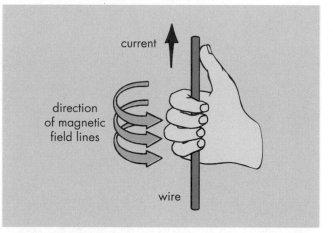

FIGURE 8-4 Determining the direction of the magnetic field around the wire using the right-hand rule.

field lines form concentric circles around each tiny section of the wire. Because the wire is curved, however, these field lines overlap inside the loop. In particular, at the very center of the loop, all the field lines add together to make the magnetic field strong (Figure 8-5). Stacking more loops on top of each other increases the intensity of the magnetic field in the center or **axis** of the stack of loops.

A coil of wire is called a *solenoid.*

The magnetic field is concentrated through the center of the coil (Figure 8-6). The magnetic field can further be intensified by wrapping the coil of wire around ferromagnetic material such as iron. The iron core concentrates the magnetic field. In this case, almost all of the magnetic field lines are concentrated inside the core, escaping only near the ends of the coil.

An **electromagnet** is a ferromagnetic material wrapped in a coil of wire (Figure 8-7).

FIGURE 8-3 Magnetic field lines form concentric circles around the current-carrying wire.

The direction of the magnetic field lines can be determined by using what is called the *right-hand rule.*

Imagine gripping the wire with the right hand. If the thumb is pointed in the direction of the current flow, the fingers of your hand will then curl in the direction of the magnetic field lines (Figure 8-4). These same rules apply if the current is flowing in a circular loop. Magnetic

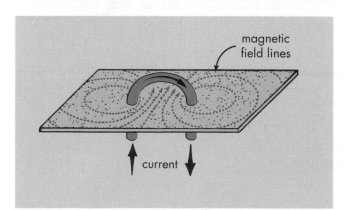

FIGURE 8-5 Magnetic field lines are concentrated on the inside of the loop.

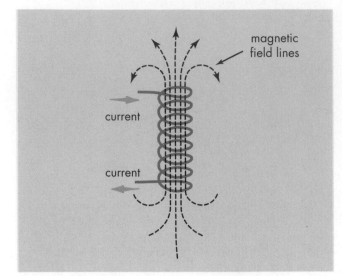

FIGURE 8-6 Magnetic field lines around a solenoid.

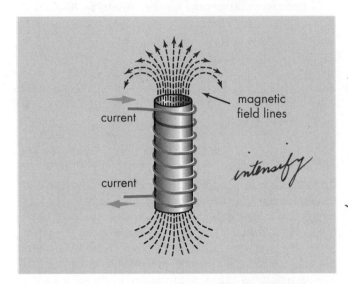

FIGURE 8-7 Magnetic field lines around an electromagnet.

The magnetic field produced by an electromagnet is the same as that produced by a **bar magnet**. That is, if both were hidden from view behind a piece of paper, the pattern of magnetic field lines revealed by iron filings sprinkled on the paper surface would be the same. Of course, the advantage of the electromagnet is that its magnetic field can be adjusted or turned on and off simply by varying the current flow through its coil of wire.

LAWS OF ELECTROMAGNETIC INDUCTION
Faraday's Law

Oersted's experiment demonstrated that electricity can be used to generate magnetic fields. Is the reverse true? Can magnetic fields somehow be used to generate electricity? It took **Michael Faraday,** a self-educated British experimenter, 6 years to find the answer to that question. From a series of experiments, Faraday concluded

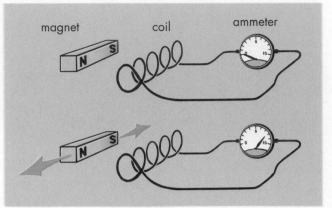

FIGURE 8-8 Schematic description of Faraday's experiment shows how a moving magnetic field includes an electric current.

that an electric current cannot be induced in a circuit merely by the presence of a magnetic field. For example, consider the situation illustrated in Figure 8-8. A coil of wire is connected to a current-measuring device called an **ammeter.** If a bar magnet is set next to the coil, the meter indicates no current in the coil. However, if the magnet is moved, a current flows in the coiled wire. The flow is indicated by the ammeter. Therefore, to induce a flow of current using a magnetic field, the magnetic field cannot be constant but must be changing. This observation is summarized in what is called *Faraday's law,* or the first law of electromagnetic induction.

> Faraday's law says that an electric current will be induced to flow in a circuit if some part of that circuit is in a changing magnetic field.

The magnitude of the induced current depends on the following four factors:

1. The strength of the magnetic field
2. The velocity of the magnetic field as it moves past the conductor
3. The angle of the conductor to the magnetic field
4. The number of turns in the conductor

The changing magnetic field can be produced in many ways. For example, a bar magnet or an electromagnet can be moved near a coil of wire. Conversely, the magnet can be held stationary and the coil of wire moved near it. Alternatively, there need be no motion. An electromagnet can be fixed near a coil of wire. If the current in the electromagnet is then either increased or decreased, its magnetic field will likewise change and induce a flow of current in the coil.

A prime example of electromagnetic induction is radio reception (Figure 8-9). Radio emission consists of waves of electromagnetic radiation. Each wave has an oscillating electric field, and an oscillating magnetic field induces motion in electrons in the radio antennae, re-

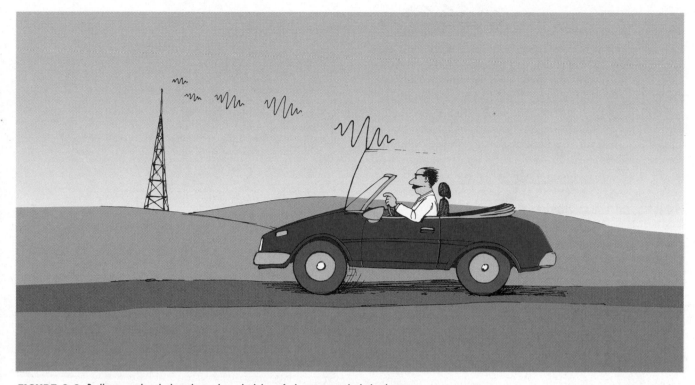

FIGURE 8-9 Radio reception is based on the principles of electromagnetic induction.

sulting in a radio signal. This signal is detected and decoded to produce sound. The essential point in this example is that the intensity of the magnetic field at the wire must be changing to induce a current flow. If the magnetic field intensity is constant, there will be no induced current.

Lenz' Law

In 1834 a Russian scientist, Heinrich Lenz, expanded on Faraday's work. He established the principle for determining the direction induced currents flow. This principle is the second law of electromagnetics or Lenz' law:

Lenz' law states that induced current flows in a direction such that it opposes the action that induces it.

This principle may seem a little confusing at first and is best illustrated by an example (Figure 8-10). The north pole of a magnet is pushed into a coil of wire. Because the magnet is being moved near the coil of wire, we know from the first law of electromagnetics that an induced current flows through the coil of wire. We also know that a coil of wire with a current flowing in it acts as a tiny magnet. One end of the coil will act as a north pole of a magnet and the other end will act as a south pole, but Lenz' law states which end will be which. The action that induces the current in the coil is the motion of the north pole of the magnet toward the coil. According to Lenz' law, to oppose this action, the action

of wire will induce a north magnetic field at its left end (since the coil's north pole will repel, that is, "oppose," the inward motion of the magnet's north pole). To induce a north magnetic pole at the left end of the coil of wire, the induced current must flow as shown in Figure 8-10.

These electromagnetic laws govern the induction of electric currents by magnetic fields of changing intensity. There are two basic types of induction: (1) self-induction and (2) mutual induction. These concepts are fundamental to the later discussions of transformers, electric motors, and generators.

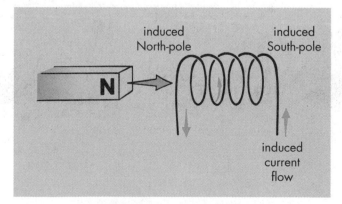

FIGURE 8-10 Demonstration of Lenz' law shows that the current induced in a coil by a moving magnet produces a magnetic field opposing the motion of the magnet.

Self-Induction

(stored electric energy
electromotive force)

If a constant source of EMF (voltage) is connected to a coil of wire, a steady current of electricity will flow through the coil relatively unimpeded and a constant magnetic field will be produced by the coil (Figure 8-11). If a varying source of EMF such as alternating current is connected to the coil, the current flow through the magnetic field produced by the coil will no longer be constant. By Lenz' law an opposing action in the coil will be induced by this changing magnetic field. In this case an induced EMF will be created that opposes the source EMF. If the source EMF increases, the induced-coil EMF opposes it by trying to reduce it. If, on the other hand, the source EMF is falling, then the induced-coil EMF will increase to oppose it.

> **Self-Induction**
> The induction of an opposing EMF in a single coil by its own changing magnetic field is called **self-induction**.

The self-induction of AC circuit components, such as choke coils and transformers, is an important consideration for design of x-ray equipment. In summary a coil passes a steady direct current relatively unimpeded but resists the passage of an alternating current flow because of self-induction in the coil.

Mutual Induction

Faraday showed that it was not necessary to physically move a magnet near a coil to induce a current flow. All that is necessary is that the intensity of the magnetic field change. This can be accomplished by fixing an electromagnet near the coil and varying the current flow through the electromagnet (Figure 8-12). The varying current flow in the electromagnet creates a varying magnetic field, which, when it passes through the coil, induces a current flow in that coil. The first coil through which the varying current is passed is called the *primary coil*. The coil in which the induced current flows is called the *secondary coil*.

(inducing a current in the 2nd coil = mutual induction

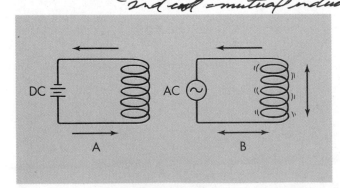

FIGURE 8-11 Demonstration of self-induction. **A,** A coil passes constant current unimpeded. **B,** It will resist the passage of a changing current because of self-induction.

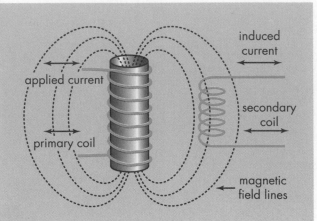

FIGURE 8-12 Inducing a current in the secondary coil is called mutual induction.

> **Mutual Induction**
> The process of inducing a current flow through a secondary coil by passing a varying current through the primary coil is called **mutual induction**.

ELECTROMECHANICAL AND ELECTRONIC DEVICES

Electric motors and generators are practical applications of Oersted's and Faraday's experiments. In the electric motor the electric current produces a mechanical motion. The electric generator works when a magnet is moved near a coil of wire and electricity is induced in the coil of wire. The transformer is another device that makes use of interacting magnetic fields. In the transformer, current and voltage are varied from one side of the device to the other. The rectifier works in a circuit to convert alternating current to direct current. The generator, transformer, and rectifier are specific components of the x-ray tube. Let us now examine these electromechanical and electronic devices in detail.

Electric Generator

mechanical to electric

A simple electric generator is diagrammed in Figure 8-13.

> In a electric generator a coil of wire is placed in a strong magnetic field between two poles of a magnet.

The coil is rotated by mechanical energy. The mechanical energy can be supplied by hand, by water flowing over a water wheel, or by steam flowing past the vanes of a turbine blade in an atomic power plant. Because the coil of wire is moving in the magnetic field, a current is induced in the coil of wire. The induced current, however, is not constant. It varies according to the orientation of the coil's wire in the magnetic field. The induced current flows in the same direction through the coil. The current flow outside the generator changes direction be-

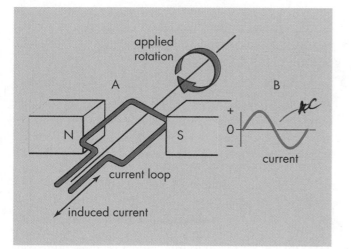

FIGURE 8-13 A, Simple electric generator. **B,** Its output waveform.

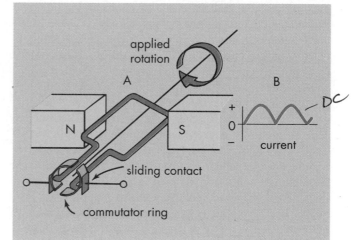

FIGURE 8-14 A, Direct current generator incorporates a commutator ring. **B,** Its output waveform.

cause the slip rings are always in contact with the same side of the coil and the brushes are always in contact with the same slip ring. Since the coil is rotating through the magnetic field, half the time one side is negative. Consequently, the current flowing out of the generator is seen to change direction. Thus this type of simple electric generator produces an **alternating current (AC)**. A **direct current (DC)** generator can be constructed by replacing the slip rings with a simple device called a *commutator ring* (Figure 8-14). The commutator ring acts as a switch, changing the polarity of the contact on the brush wire at precisely those points at which the electrical charge on one side changes. The resulting reversed current, flowing out of the commutator ring assembly, is humped in one direction. The net effect of an electric generator is to convert mechanical energy into electric energy. This conversion process is not 100% efficient because of frictional losses in the mechanical moving parts and heat losses caused by resistances in the electrical components.

Electric Motor
electrical to mechanical

Perhaps a good place to begin a discussion of motors is with an overview of the basic concept that makes motors possible. A motor is an electrical device that converts electrical energy into mechanical energy (motion). Recall that a conductor carrying a current has a magnetic field associated with the current flow. If that conductor were placed within an external magnetic field (e.g., between the north and south poles of a horseshoe magnet), the two magnetic fields would interact. The magnetic field of the conductor would either be (1) attracted to the external magnetic field if the external lines of force were in an opposing direction or (2) repelled by the external magnetic field if the external lines of force were in the same direction. The overall result is that the conductor will be pulled upward or downward as the two magnetic fields

interact. When the current is switched off in the conductor, its magnetic field collapses and it no longer moves. The energy of the electrons moving through the conductor (electrical energy) has been converted to mechanical energy (the motion of the conductor) by the interaction of two magnetic fields.

A simple electric motor has basically the same components as an electric generator (Figure 8-15). In this case, however, the energy source is electric, not mechanical energy.

In an electric motor the electric energy is supplied to the current loop to produce a mechanical motion, that is, the rotation of the loop in the magnetic field.

When a current is passed through the wire loop, a magnetic field is produced, making it a tiny electromagnet. Because it is free to turn, the electromagnet-current loop rotates as it attempts to align itself with the stronger

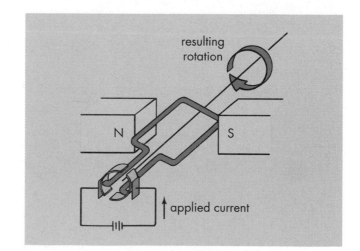

FIGURE 8-15 Simple direct-current electric motor.

magnetic field produced by the external bar magnet. Just as the current loop becomes aligned with the external magnetic field, the commutator ring switches the direction of current flow through the loop and therefore reverses the coil's required alignment. Because of the change in current direction, the electromagnet is no longer aligned with the magnetic field of the bar magnet. It is now opposed to it. The electromagnet-current loop rotates 180 degrees in an attempt to realign itself once again with the bar magnet field. As the electromagnet again nears alignment, the commutator switches the direction of current flow and forces the loop to rotate again. This procedure repeats itself over and over. The electromagnet-current loop is never quite able to align itself with the magnetic field of the bar magnet. The net result is that the current loop rotates continuously. In a practical electric motor, many turns of wire are used for the current loop and many bar magnets are used to create the external magnetic field. The principle of operation, however, is the same. This type of electric motor is called a *direct current motor.*

The type of motor used in some x-ray tubes with rotating anodes is called an *induction motor* (Figure 8-16). In this type of motor the armature is called a **rotor.** Instead of a series of wire loops, the rotor is a cylinder with iron bars placed along its length. The external magnetic field is supplied by several fixed electromagnets called *stators.* No current is passed to the rotor. Instead, current flow is produced in the rotor windings by induction. The electromagnets surrounding the rotor are energized in sequence, producing a changing magnetic field. The induced current flow produced in the rotor windings generates a magnetic field. Just as in a conventional electric motor, this magnetic field attempts to align itself with the magnetic field of the external electromagnets. Because these electromagnets are being energized in sequence, the rotor begins to rotate, trying to bring its magnetic field into alignment. The result is the same as in a conventional electric motor, that is, the rotor rotates continuously. The difference is that electric energy is supplied to the external magnets rather than to the rotor windings.

Transformer

Both electric motors and generators make use of interacting electromagnetic fields produced by electric currents. The generator converts mechanical to electrical energy, and the motor converts electrical to mechanical energy. Another device that makes use of the interacting magnetic fields produced by changing electric currents is the **transformer.** It does not convert one form of energy to another but rather transforms electrical potential and electric current into higher or lower intensities. Recall from the discussion of mutual induction that if two coils are placed near each other and a changing current is applied to one of them (the primary), then a current will be induced to flow in the other coil (the secondary). Recall also that placing a core of magnetic material in the center of the coil greatly increases the strength of the magnetic field passing through its center. The magnetic field lines tend to be concentrated in the magnetic core material and escape mainly at the ends. Imagine, however, that this magnetic core is bent around so that it forms a continuous loop (Figure 8-17). There are no end surfaces from which the magnetic field lines can escape. Therefore the magnetic field tends to be confined to the loop of magnetic core material.

If the secondary coil is then wound around the other side of this loop of core material, almost all the magnetic field produced by the primary coil will also pass through the center of the secondary coil. Thus there is a good **coupling** between the magnetic field produced by the primary coil and the secondary coil. A changing current in the primary coil will induce a changing current in the secondary coil. This type of device is called a *transformer.* Because a transformer operates on the

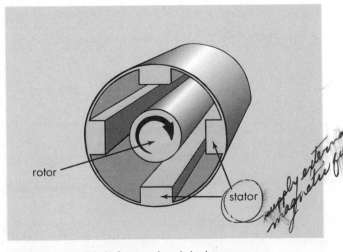

FIGURE 8-16 Principal parts of an induction motor.

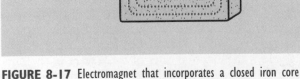

FIGURE 8-17 Electromagnet that incorporates a closed iron core produces a closed magnetic field primarily confined to the core.

principle of mutual induction, it will only operate with a changing electric current (AC). A direct current applied to the primary coil induces no current in the secondary coil.

The transformer is used to change the magnitude of current and voltage in an AC circuit. This change is directly proportional to the ratio of the number of turns (windings) of the secondary coil (N_s) to the number of turns in the primary coil (N_p). If there are ten turns on the secondary coil for every turn on the primary coil, then the voltage generated in the secondary circuit (V_s), will be ten times the voltage supplied to the primary circuit (V_p). Mathematically, the transformer law is represented as follows:

Transformer Law for Voltage

$$\frac{V_s}{V_p} = \frac{N_s}{N_p}$$

V = voltage
N = # of turns/windings

The quantity N_s/N_p is known as the **turns ratio** of the transformer. The voltage change across the transformer is proportional to the turns ratio. A transformer with a turn ratio greater than 1 is said to be a **step-up transformer** because the voltage is increased or stepped up from the primary side to the secondary side. When the turns ratio is less than 1, the transformer is called a **step-down transformer.**

As the voltage changes across a transformer, the current (I) changes also. The transformer law may also be written as follows:

Transformer Law for Current

$$\frac{I_s}{I_p} = \frac{N_p}{N_s}$$

I = current

Transformer Law for Voltage and Current

$$\frac{I_s}{I_p} = \frac{V_p}{V_s}$$

The change in current across a transformer is in the opposite direction from the voltage change but in the same proportion. For example, if the voltage is doubled, the current is halved. In a step-up transformer the current on the secondary side (I_s) is smaller than the current on the primary side (I_p). In a step-down transformer the secondary current is larger than the primary current.

The transformer is not 100% efficient, although the losses in power from the primary side to the secondary side are considered negligible. Nevertheless, there are three principal causes for transformer energy losses: (1) Electric current in the copper wire experiences resis-

tance that results in heat generation. These are called I^2R losses. (2) The alternate reversal of the magnetic field caused by the alternating current meets a resistance known as **hysteresis.** Finally, (3) **eddy currents** can be formed as predicted by Lenz' law. These currents oppose the magnetic field that induced them, creating a loss of transformer efficiency.

Question: There are 125 turns on the primary side of a transformer and 90,000 turns on the secondary side. If 110 V AC is supplied to the primary winding, what will be the voltage induced in the secondary winding?

Answer:

$$\frac{V_s}{V_p} = \frac{N_s}{N_p}$$

$$V_s = V_p \left\{ \frac{N_s}{N_p} \right\}$$

$$= (110 \text{ V}) \left\{ \frac{90,000}{125} \right\}$$

$$= (110)\,(720)\text{V}$$

$$= 79,200 \text{ V}$$

$$= 79.2 \text{ kV is the voltage induced in the secondary winding of the transformer}$$

Question: The turns ratio of a filament transformer is 0.125. What will be the filament current if the current flowing through the primary winding is 0.8 A?

Answer:

$$\frac{I_s}{I_p} = \frac{N_p}{N_s}$$

$$I_s = I_p \left\{ \frac{N_p}{N_s} \right\}$$

$$= (0.8 \text{ A}) \left(\frac{1}{0.125} \right)$$

$$= 6.4 \text{ A is the current flowing through the secondary winding of the filament transformer}$$

Types of Transformers. There are many ways to construct a transformer (Figure 8-18). The type of transformer discussed above is a **closed-core transformer.**

Closed-Core Transformer

The closed-core transformer is a square doughnut of magnetic material as shown in Figure 8-18, A.

The closed-core transformer is not a single piece but rather is a built-up slab of laminated layers of iron. This layering helps reduce energy losses caused by the heat built up by the changing magnetic field in the transformer.

Another type of transformer is called an **autotransformer** (Figure 8-18, B). An autotransformer consists of an iron core with only one winding of wire.

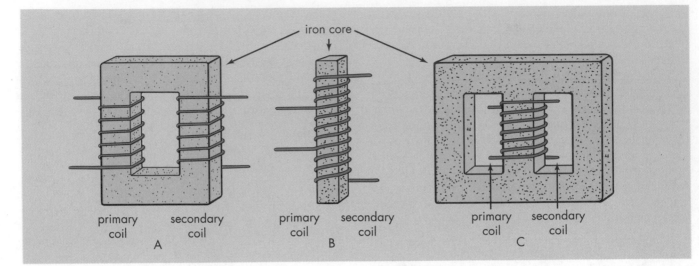

FIGURE 8-18 Types of transformers. **A,** Closed-core transformer. **B,** Autotransformer. **C,** Shell-type transformer.

Autotransformer

An autotransformer consists of an iron core with only one winding of wire.

This single winding acts as both the primary and the secondary winding. The autotransformer is based on self-induction rather than mutual induction. Connections are made at different points on the coil. Because both the primary and the secondary sides are connected to the same wire, it is used when only a small step up or step down in voltage is required. The autotransformer is not suitable for use as the high-voltage transformer in an x-ray machine.

The third type of transformer is the **shell-type transformer** (Figure 8-18, C). Because this type of transformer traps even more of the magnetic field lines of the primary winding, it is more efficient than a closed-core transformer.

Shell-type Transformer

A shell-type transformer traps even more of the magnetic field lines of the primary winding and is thus a more efficient transformer than a closed-core transformer.

It is more efficient than the closed-core transformer. Most transformers in modern use have this type of construction. This is the type of transformer used in modern x-ray equipment.

Rectifier

The electrical devices discussed thus far are important components of modern x-ray systems. Induction motors are used to spin the anodes in most x-ray tubes, and step-up transformers provide the high voltage necessary for the production of x-rays. The specific roles these components play in the x-ray system are discussed in more detail in later chapters. There is one other component related to x-ray production—the **rectifier.**

The current from a common wall plug is alternating current (AC). The current changes direction, back and forth, 60 times each second. However, an x-ray tube requires direct current (DC), so electrons flow in only one direction. Therefore some means must be provided for converting AC to DC. This process of converting AC to DC is called **rectification.** The electronic device that allows current flow in only one direction is a **rectifier.** There are two principal types of rectifiers: (1) vacuum-tube rectifiers and (2) solid-state diodes.

Vacuum-Tube Rectifiers. Consider an evacuated glass tube with a small coil of wire or **filament** at one end (Figure 8-19). If a large current is passed through this filament, it will heat up and "boil" electrons off its surface. This process is called **thermionic emission.** *Therm* refers to heat, *ion* refers to a charged particle, and *emission* means to give off. Thus thermionic emission refers to giving off electrons from a heated surface. This emitter of electrons is the filament and constitutes the **cathode** or negative side of the tube. A cold metallic plate is placed at the other end of the glass envelope. This is the **anode** or positive side. This combination of hot electron-emitting cathode and cold anode enclosed in a vacuum-sealed glass tube is the basis for most electronic tubes, including the x-ray tube.

An electric current is made up of a flow of electrons. Therefore the electrons, thermionically boiling off the hot filament of a vacuum tube, offer the opportunity for a current. If the anode (+) is connected to a positive voltage relative to the cathode (−), the electrons at the cathode (−) will be attracted to the anode (+). They stream across the length of the tube, causing an electron flow through the tube from the cathode to the anode (Figure 8-20). If, however, a higher voltage is

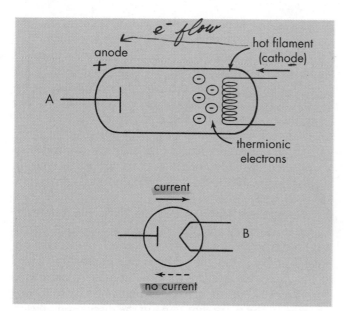

FIGURE 8-19 **A,** Basic vacuum tube. **B,** The electronic symbol.

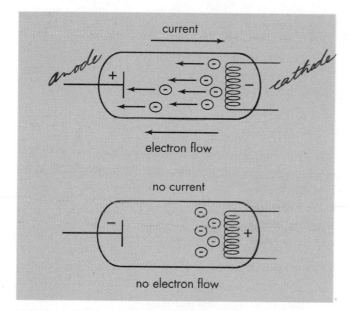

FIGURE 8-20 Vacuum-tube diodes will conduct electrons in only one direction, from cathode to anode.

placed on the cathode than the anode, there will be no reverse current. In summary, then, a simple vacuum tube conducts electrons from the cathode to the anode but not from the anode to the cathode. This type of vacuum tube, sometimes called a *diode* because it has two (di-) electrodes, is a rectifier.

Solid-State Rectifiers. Vacuum-tube devices were first developed in the early part of this century. In the 1950s an entirely new class of electronic **solid state** devices was developed from **semiconductor** material. It has long been known that metals are good conductors of electricity and that other materials such as glass or plastics

are poor conductors of electricity. These poor conductors are called insulators. There is a third class of materials called *semiconductors,* which lies between the range of insulators and conductors in their ability to conduct electricity. Tiny crystals of these semiconductors were found to have some useful electrical properties, and they are the basis of the **solid-state microchip** computers available today.

Semiconductors are classed into two types—**n type** and **p type.** N-type semiconductors have loosely bound electrons that are relatively free to move about inside the material. P-type semiconductors have spaces where there are no electrons, called *holes.* These holes are similar to the space between cars in heavy traffic. As the line of cars moves forward, the space moves backward. Holes are as mobile as electrons. Consider a tiny crystal of n-type material placed in contact with a p-type crystal to form what is called a *p-n junction* (Figure 8-21). If a higher potential is placed on the p side of the junction, then the electrons and holes will both migrate toward the junction and wander across it (Figure 8-22). This flow of electrons and holes constitutes an electric

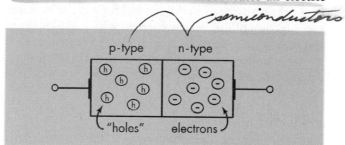

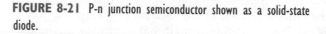

FIGURE 8-21 P-n junction semiconductor shown as a solid-state diode.

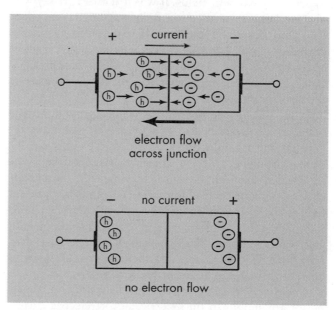

FIGURE 8-22 Solid-state diodes will conduct electrons in only one direction.

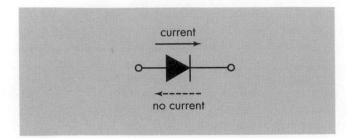

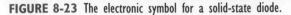

FIGURE 8-23 The electronic symbol for a solid-state diode.

current. If, however, a positive potential is placed on the n side of the junction, both the electrons and holes will be swept away from the junction and there will be no electrons at the junction surface available to form a current. Thus, in this case, there will be no electric current through the p-n junction. Therefore a solid-state p-n junction tends to conduct electricity in only one direction. This type of p-n junction is called a **solid-state diode.** Solid-state diodes, like tubes, are rectifiers because they pass electric current easily in only one direction. The arrowhead in the symbol for a diode indicates the direction of the electric current, which is opposite to the flow of the electrons (Figure 8-23). Rectification in an x-ray unit is essential for the safe and efficient operation of the x-ray tube.

SUMMARY

The development of the battery as a constant electricity source by Alessandro Volta in the 1700s prompted further investigations of the electric and magnetic forces. Hans Oersted demonstrated that electricity can be used to generate magnetic fields. It was Michael Faraday who observed the flow of current in a changing magnetic field and described the first law of electromagnetics (Faraday's law). Heinrich Lenz expanded on Faraday's experiments. The second law of electromagnetics is Lenz' law, which states that current flows opposite to the action that induces it.

Induction, or the production of electricity in a magnetic field, is described in two ways—(1) self-induction and (2) mutual induction. If a steady or direct current flows through a wire, a constant magnetic field will be created around the wire. If, however, the current changes direction as in alternating current, the magnetic field is constant. Self-induction occurs when the changing magnetic field of a single wire induces an opposing electromotive force. Mutual induction occurs when current flows through a secondary coil by passing varying current through an adjacent primary coil.

The practical applications of the laws of electromagnetics are shown in the electric motor (electric current produces mechanical motion); the electric generator (a

magnet is moved near a coil of wire and electricity is induced in the wire); and the transformer (electric potential and electric current are changed to higher or lower intensities.) The transformer law states that current and voltage changes across the transformer are directly proportional to the ratio of the number of turns of wire from the primary to the secondary side.

There are three types of energy losses in a transformer: (1) resistance losses or I^2R losses, (2) hysteresis losses, and (3) eddy currents. There are three types of transformers: (1) closed core, (2) autotransformer, and (3) shell type.

The rectifier is another electronic device used in the x-ray tube circuit. A rectifier changes alternating current to direct current. The x-ray tube is a type of vacuum-tube rectifier. Modern rectifiers are microchips called *semiconductors* and are used in computer hardware. The next chapter on the x-ray unit and the following chapter on the x-ray tube expand the discussion on electronic devices.

REVIEW QUESTIONS

1. Who used zinc and copper plates to create an electric current?

   a. Hans Oersted

   b. Michael Faraday

   c. Alessandro Volta

2. Any charge in motion creates an electric field. Describe the experiment that supports this statement.

3. A solenoid is _____.

4. What is the right-hand rule?

5. Define electromagnet.

6. List and define the first two laws of electromagnetics.

7. Name the four factors which relate to the magnitude of an induced current.

8. Describe the process of mutual induction.

9. Draw and label the parts of an electric motor.

10. Explain how an electric generator works.

11. Show how direct current can be produced in an electric generator.

12. List the components of an induction motor and describe how they work.

13. Write the transformer law for voltage and current.

14. A transformer has 240 turns on the primary side and 200 turns on the secondary side. If the current on the primary side is 2 A, what will be the current on the secondary side?

15. A transformer has 100 turns on the primary side and 1000 turns on the secondary. The voltage on the primary side is 120 V. What is the voltage on the secondary side?

16. The resistance caused by alternating current and the alternating reversal of the magnetic fields is called _____.

17. The transformer that has a single winding that acts as both the primary and secondary winding is called a(n) _____.

18. Converting AC to DC is called _____.

19. Define the root words of the term thermionic emission.

20. Define semiconductor.

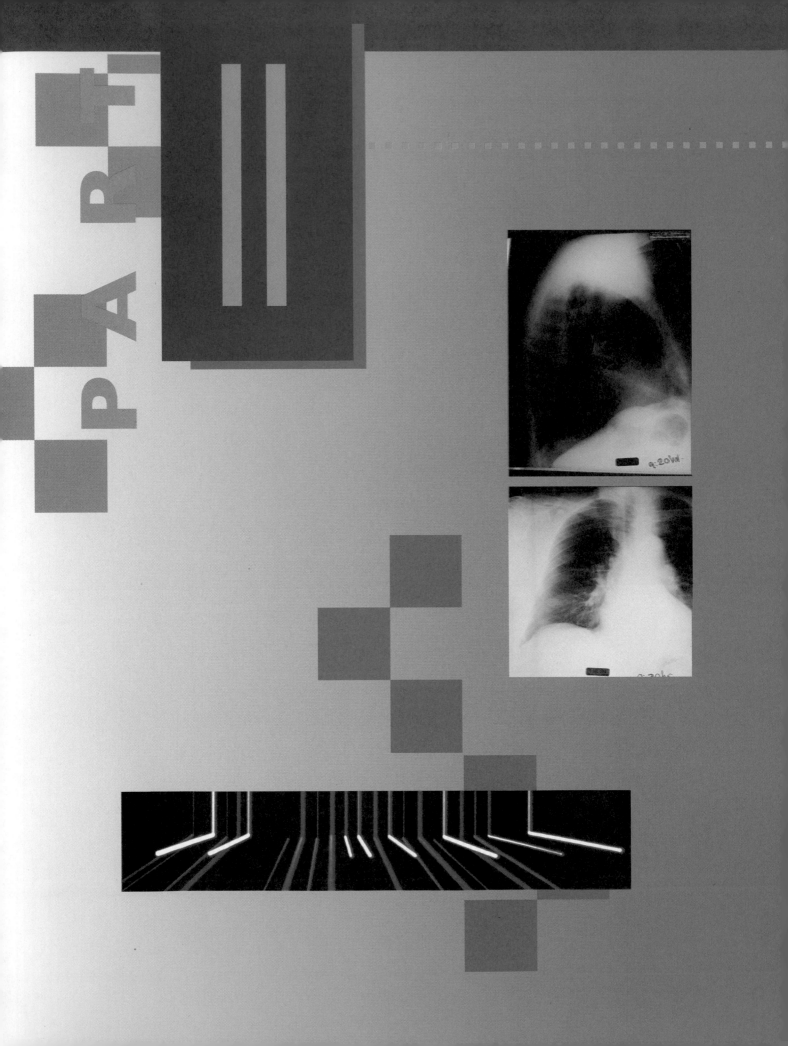

PART II

THE X-RAY BEAM

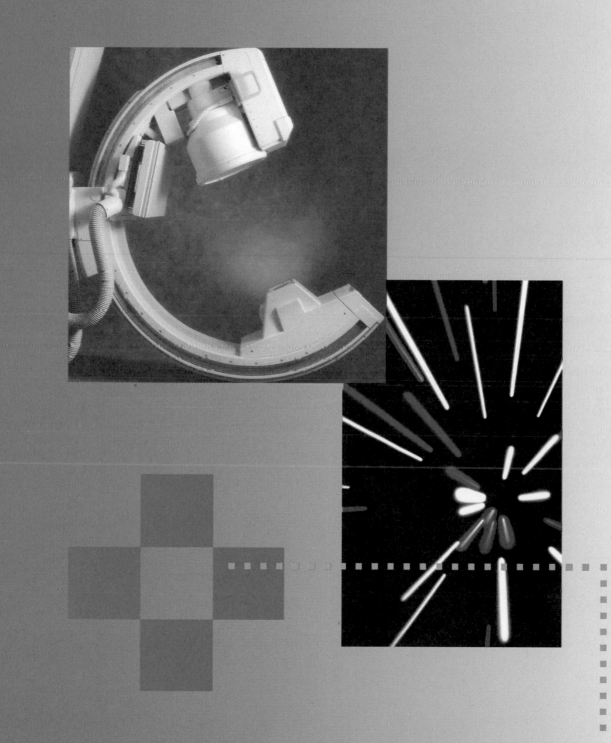

9

The X-ray Unit

OBJECTIVES

At the completion of this chapter the student will be able to:

1. Identify the components of the operator's console or control panel, which is mounted outside the x-ray room
2. Explain the operation of the high-voltage generator, including the autotransformer, the filament transformer, and the rectifiers
3. Relate the important differences between single-phase and three-phase power, including voltage ripple
4. Define the power rating unit in the watt

OUTLINE

X-ray Unit
   Operating console
High-Voltage Generator
   High-voltage transformer
   Voltage rectification
Single-Phase Power

Three-Phase Power
   High-frequency generator
   Voltage ripple
Power Rating
   X-ray circuit

T he following are the three components of the x-ray unit (machine): (1) the x-ray tube, (2) the operating console, and (3) the high-voltage generator. Discussion of the x-ray tube is presented in Chapter 10. This chapter explains in detail the components on the operating console. Discussion of the high-voltage generator, as well as single- and three-phase power, is presented.

X-RAY UNIT

The many different types of x-ray units are identified according to either the energy of the x-rays they produce or the way the x-rays are used. Diagnostic medical x-ray units come in many different shapes and sizes, some of which are shown in Figure 9-1. They are usually operated at kilovoltages ranging from 25 to 150 kVp (**peak kilovoltage**) and at tube currents from 100 to 1200 mA (**milliamps**). The modern, general-purpose x-ray examination room usually contains a **radiographic unit** and **fluoroscopic unit** with an **image intensifier**. The radiographic tube is attached to an overhead movable crane assembly that permits easy positioning of the tube and aiming of the x-ray beam. The fluoroscopic x-ray tube is usually located under the radiographic table. A room equipped with both radiographic and fluoroscopic units is described in Chapter 1 (see Figure 1-6). The room in Figure 1-6 can be used for nearly all radiographic and fluoroscopic examinations. Regardless of the type of x-ray unit used, a radiographic table is required (Figure 9-2). The radiographic table may be flat or curved but must be uniform in thickness and as **radiolucent** to x-rays as possible. Carbon-fiber table tops are strong enough to support patients who weigh up to 300 pounds yet absorb little radiation; thus the x-rays can pass through the table material and expose the x-ray film. Most table tops **float**. They are easily unlocked and moved by the radiographer. Just under the table top is an opening for a **Bucky tray** to hold an x-ray **cassette** and **grid**. If the table is used for fluoroscopy, the tray must be moved to the foot of the table. The Bucky opening is automatically shielded from radiation with a **Bucky slot cover**. Fluoroscopic tables tilt and can be identified by their degree of tilt. For example, a $^{90}/_{30}$ table would tilt 90 degrees to the foot side and 30 degrees to the head side (Figure 9-3).

Each x-ray unit, regardless of its design, has the following three principal parts: (1) the **x-ray tube**, (2) the **operating console**, and (3) the **high-voltage generator**. In some types of x-ray apparatus, such as dental and mobile units, these three components are housed compactly. Most equipment, however, has the x-ray tube located in the x-ray room, the operating console in an adjoining control room, and a protective barrier separating the two. The protective barrier must have a leaded window for viewing the patient during examination. The high-voltage generator may be housed in an equipment cabinet positioned against a wall in the x-ray room. A few installations take advantage of false ceilings, and these generators are located out of sight above the examination room. Newer generator designs using high-frequency circuits require even less space. Figure 9-4 is a drawing of a conventional general-purpose x-ray examination room.

In this chapter a description of the operating console and its many components, as well as an explanation of the high-voltage generator, are presented. The x-ray tube is discussed in detail in the next chapter. The presentation begins with an illustration of the operating console labeled with the parts under discussion. Learn to recognize the controls and find out what they do.

Operating Console

The part of the x-ray machine most familiar to the radiographer is the operating console. This apparatus allows the radiographer to control the x-ray tube current and voltage so that the useful x-ray beam is of proper quantity and quality (Figure 9-5). **Quantity** refers to the number of x-rays or the intensity of the beam usually expressed in mR or mR per mAs (milliroentgens per milliampere seconds). **Quality** refers to the penetrating quality of the x-ray beam and is expressed by **kVp** (peak kilovolts) or **half-value layer** (HVL).

As shown in Figure 9-5, the following are some basic controls that every panel has: (1) the on/off control, (2) mAs selection, (3) kVp selection, (4) table or wall unit activation, and (5) the exposure switch. In addition, the operating console provides adjustment of **line compensation** and occasionally separate mA and **exposure-time** controls. Sometimes a milliampere-second (mAs) meter is also provided. On equipment that incorporates automatic-exposure control (often called phototiming), only mAs controls are present. All the electric circuits connecting the meters and controls that are located on the operating console are low voltage so that the possibility of hazardous shock is minimized. Figure 9-6 is a simplified schematic diagram for a typical operating console. A look inside an operating console indicates the extent to which this schematic drawing is simplified.

Many modern operating consoles are based on computer technology. Controls and meters are digital, and selection of technical factors is by touch screen. Numerical technical-factor selection is sometimes replaced by icons indicating body part, size, and shape. Many of the features on the control panel are automatic, but the radiographer must know their purposes and their proper uses. Each of the console controls requires detailed examination. Thus line-compensation control, autotransformers, kVp adjustment, mA controls and selection, and five types of timers are discussed next.

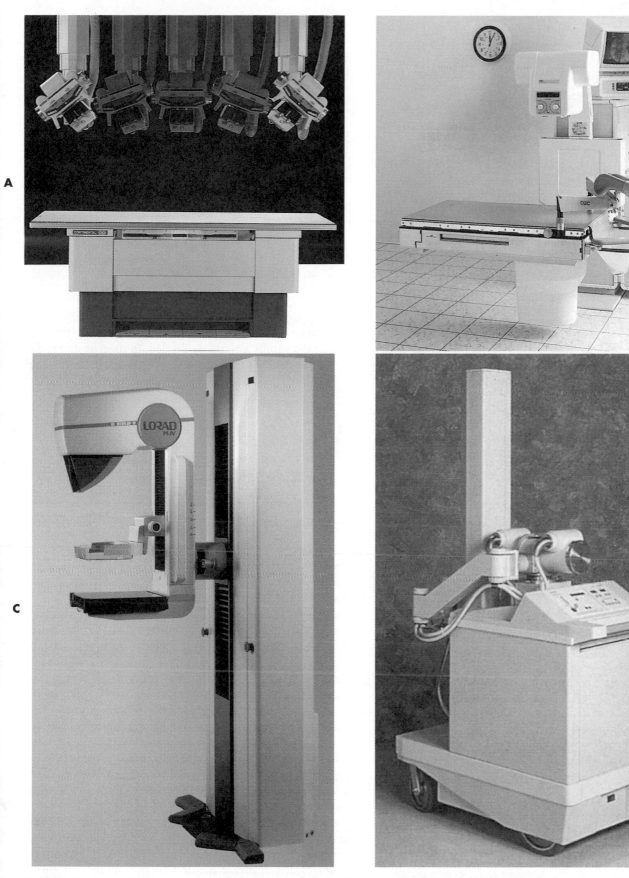

FIGURE 9-1 Types of diagnostic x-ray machines. **A,** Tomographic. **B,** Urologic. **C,** Mammographic. **D,** Portable. *(A, Courtesy Continental X-Ray Corporation; B, Courtesy OEC Medical Systems; C, Courtesy Lorad Medical Systems, Inc.; D, Courtesy Philips Medical Systems.)*

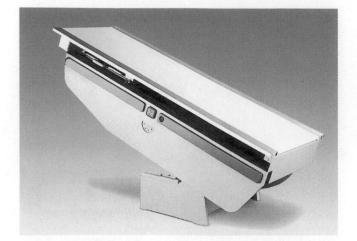

FIGURE 9-2 Tilting patient examination table. *(Courtesy Picker International.)*

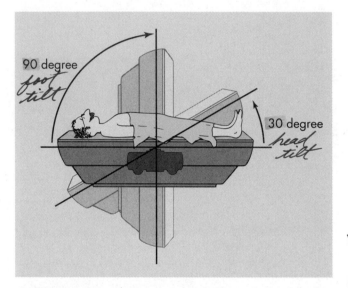

FIGURE 9-3 A fluoroscopic table is identified by its head and foot tilt.

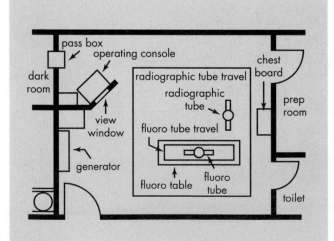

FIGURE 9-4 Drawing of a general purpose x-ray examination room showing location of the various x-ray apparatus.

Line Compensation. Most x-ray machines are designed to operate on 220 volts of power. Unfortunately, electric power companies are not capable of providing 220 volts accurately and continuously. Because of variations in power distribution and consumption by the various sections of the hospital, the voltage provided to an x-ray unit may easily vary by as much as 5%. Such variation in **supply voltage** results in a large variation in the x-ray beam. The x-ray beam cannot vary if high-quality radiographs are to be consistently produced.

Line Compensator

The line compensator incorporates a meter to measure the voltage provided to the x-ray machine and a control to adjust that voltage to precisely 220 volts.

The control is wired to the autotransformer. On some older units the radiographer must watch the meter and adjust the supply voltage as needed. In present-day radiographic units, line compensation is automatic. The power supplied to the x-ray machine is delivered to a special transformer called an *autotransformer.*

Autotransformer

The autotransformer is designed to supply a precise voltage to the filament circuit and to the high-voltage circuit of the x-ray machine.

The voltage supplied to the high-voltage transformer is controlled but variable. It is much safer and easier in terms of engineering to vary low voltage and then increase it than to increase low voltage to the kilovolt level and then vary its magnitude. The autotransformer works on the principle of electromagnetic induction but is very different from the conventional transformer. It has only one winding and one core. This single winding has a number of connections located along its length (Figure 9-7). Two of the connections, shown as A and A¹, conduct the input power to the autotransformer and are called *primary connections*. Some of the secondary connections, such as C, are located closer to one end of the winding than the primary connections. This allows the autotransformer to increase and decrease voltage. The autotransformer can be designed to increase voltage to approximately twice the input voltage value.

Because the autotransformer operates as an induction device, the voltage it receives (the primary voltage) and the voltage it provides (the secondary voltage) are in direct relation to the number of turns of the transformer enclosed by the respective connections.

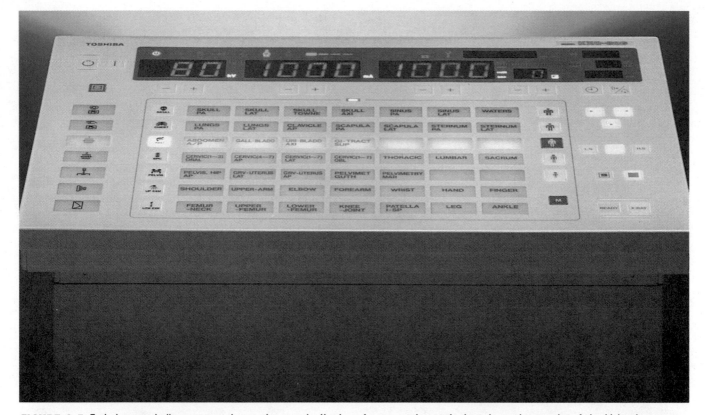

FIGURE 9-5 Typical anatomically programmed operating console. Number of meters and controls depends on the capacity of the high-voltage generator. *(Courtesy Toshiba American Medical Systems, Inc.)*

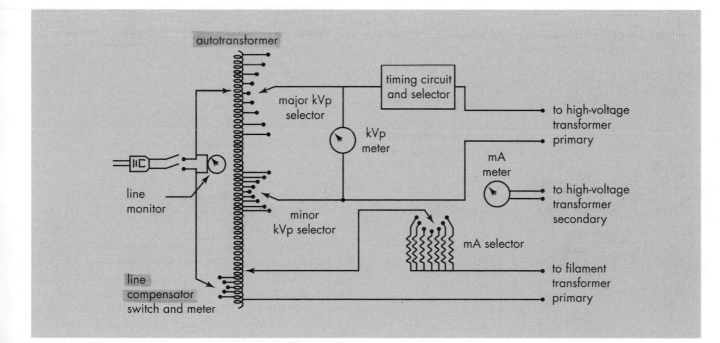

FIGURE 9-6 Circuit diagram of the operating console identifies the controls and meters.

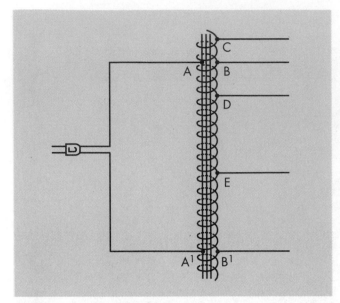

FIGURE 9-7 Autotransformer in simplified form.

(many connections on the single winding)

The **autotransformer** law is the same as the transformer law:

$$\frac{V_S \rightarrow N_S}{V_P \rightarrow N_P}$$ *directly proportional*

V_P = The primary voltage

V_S = The secondary voltage

N_P = The number of windings enclosed by primary connections

N_S = The number of windings enclosed by secondary connections

Question: If the autotransformer in Figure 9-7 is supplied with 220 volts to the primary connections AA^1, which enclose 500 windings, what will be the secondary voltage across BB^1 (500 windings), CB^1 (700 windings), and DE (200 windings)?

Answer: BB^1:$V_S = V_P\left(\dfrac{N_S}{N_P}\right)$ $\dfrac{V_S}{220V} = \dfrac{500}{500}$ $500 V_S = 110000$ $V_o = 220$

$\qquad = (220 \text{ V})\left(\dfrac{500}{500}\right) = 220$ volts is the secondary voltage across BB^1

$\qquad$ CB^1:$V_S = (220 \text{ V})\left(\dfrac{700}{500}\right)$

$\qquad = (220 \text{ V})(1.4) = 308$ volts is the secondary voltage across CB^1

$\qquad$ DE:$V_S = (220 \text{ V})\left(\dfrac{200}{500}\right)$

$\qquad = (220 \text{ V})(0.4) = 88$ volts is the secondary voltage across DE

kVp Adjustment. Some older x-ray operating consoles have adjustments labeled *major kVp* and *minor kVp*, and by selecting a combination of these controls the radiographer can provide precisely the required kVp.

> kVp determines the penetrating quality of the x-ray beam.

The major kVp adjustment and the minor kVp adjustment represent two separate series of connections on the autotransformer. If the primary voltage to the autotransformer is 220 volts, the output of the autotransformer can be controlled from about 100 to 400 volts, depending on the design of the autotransformer. This low voltage becomes the input to the high-voltage step-up transformer that increases the voltage to the kilovoltage required.

Question: An autotransformer, connected to a 440 volts supply, contains 4000 turns, all of which are enclosed by the primary connections. If 2300 turns are enclosed by secondary connections, what will be the voltage supplied to the high-voltage generator?

Answer: $V_S = V_P\left(\dfrac{N_S}{N_P}\right)$ $\dfrac{V_S}{V_P} = \dfrac{N_S}{N_P}$ $\dfrac{V_S}{440V} = \dfrac{2300}{4000}$

$\qquad = (440 \text{ V})\left(\dfrac{2300}{4000}\right)$ $4000 V_S = 1012000$

$\qquad = (440 \text{ V})(0.575)$ $V_S = \dfrac{1012000}{4000}$ $V_S = 253$

$\qquad = 253$ volts will be the voltage supplied to the high-voltage generator

The kVp meter is placed across the output terminals of the autotransformer and therefore actually reads the voltage and not the kilovoltage. However, the scale of the kVp meter on the control panel registers kilovolts. On most operating consoles the kVp meter registers even though an exposure is not being made and no current is flowing in the circuit. This type of meter is known as a *prereading voltmeter.* It allows the voltage to be monitored before an exposure.

> **mA**
> The x-ray tube current, the number of electrons crossing from cathode to anode per second, is measured in milliamperes (mA).

mA Control. The number of electrons emitted by the filament is determined by the temperature of the filament. The filament temperature is controlled by the filament current, which is measured in amperes (A). As filament current increases, the filament becomes hotter and more electrons are released by thermionic emission. Filaments normally operate at currents between 3 and 6 amperes. *3000 – 6000 milliamperes*

Question: A radiograph is made at 400 mA and an exposure time of 100 ms. Express this as mAs. *mAs = mA × time in seconds*

(.4 amperes)

Answer: 100 milliseconds = 0.1 seconds

(400 mA) (0.1 seconds) = 40 mAs

measured in amperes A

X-ray tube current is controlled through a separate circuit called the **filament circuit** (Figure 9-8). Voltage for the filament circuit is provided from connections on the autotransformer. This voltage is reduced by use of **precision resistors** to a value corresponding to the mA station provided. X-ray tube current normally is not continuously variable. Fixed-mA stations providing tube currents of 100, 200, and 300 mA and higher result from the precision resistors. In some units, mAs can be varied continuously during an exposure to the minimum exposure time. This is referred to as a **falling-load** mA. The voltage from the mA-selector switch is then delivered to the filament transformer. The filament transformer is a step-down transformer, therefore the voltage supplied to the filaments is lower, by a factor equal to the turns ratio, than the voltage supplied to the filament transformer. Similarly the current is increased across the filament transformer in proportion to the turns ratio. $= \dfrac{N_S}{N_P}$

Question: A filament transformer with a turns ratio of 1:10 provides 6.2 amperes to the filament. What is the current flowing through the primary coil of the filament transformer?

Answer: $\dfrac{I_P}{I_S} \bcancel{\times} \dfrac{N_S}{N_P}$

change in current across a transformer is in the opposite direction from the voltage change but in the same proportion.

$$I_P = I \left(\dfrac{N_S}{N_P} \right)$$

$$= (6.2) \left(\dfrac{1}{10} \right)$$

$$= 0.62 \text{ amperes}$$

Tube current is monitored with an mA meter that must be placed in the tube circuit. The mA meter is connected at the center of the secondary winding of the high-voltage step-up transformer. The secondary voltage alternates such that the center of this winding is always at zero volts. In this way, no part of the meter is in contact with the high voltage, and it may safely be put on the operating console. Variations of this meter are sometimes provided so that mAs can be monitored in addition to mA.

Exposure timers. For any given radiographic examination the number of x-rays reaching the image receptor is directly related to both the x-ray tube current and the time that the tube is energized.

mA

kVp

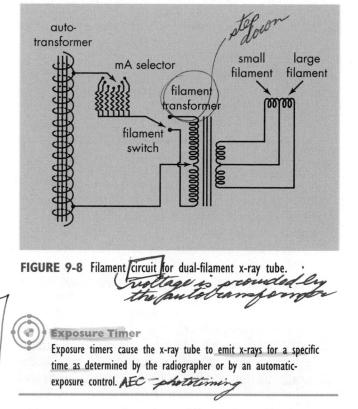

FIGURE 9-8 Filament circuit for dual-filament x-ray tube.

voltage is provided by the autotransformer

step down

Exposure Timer

Exposure timers cause the x-ray tube to emit x-rays for a specific time as determined by the radiographer or by an automatic-exposure control. *AEC — phototiming*

X-ray operating consoles provide a wide selection of x-ray beam-on times and, when used in conjunction with the appropriate mA station, provide an even wider selection of mAs values.

Question: A KUB examination (radiography of the *kid*neys, *u*reters, and *b*ladder) calls for 75 kVp and 80 mAs. If the radiographer selects the 200-mA station, what exposure time should be used?

Answer: $\dfrac{80 \text{ mAs}}{200 \text{ mA}}$ = 0.4 seconds, or $\frac{2}{5}$ seconds, or 400 ms is the exposure time

The timer circuit is separate from the other main circuits of the x-ray machine. It consists of mechanical or electronic devices whose action is to "make" and "break" the high voltage across the x-ray tube. This is nearly always done on the **primary side** of the high-voltage transformer. *5*

There are five types of timing circuits. Four can be controlled by the radiographer, and one is automatic. After studying this section, try to identify the types of timers on the equipment you use.

1. **Mechanical timers.** Mechanical timers are very simple devices used only in some portable and dental units. The mechanical timer operates by clockwork. A preset exposure time is dialed by turning a knob that winds a spring. When the exposure button is depressed, the spring is released and unwinds. The time required to unwind

corresponds to the exposure time. Mechanical timers are inexpensive but are not very accurate. They can be used only for exposure times greater than 250 milliseconds.

2. **Synchronous timers.** In the United States, electric current is supplied on a frequency of 60 Hz. In Europe, Latin America, and other parts of the world the frequency is 50 Hz. A special type of electric motor, known as a *synchronous motor,* is a precision device designed to drive a shaft at precisely 60 revolutions per second (rps). In some x-ray machines, synchronous motors are used as timing mechanisms. Machines with synchronous timers are recognizable because the minimum exposure time possible is $1/60$ second (17 milliseconds) and timing intervals increase by multiples thereof, for example $1/30$, $1/20$, and so on. Synchronous timers cannot be used for **serial exposures** because they must be reset after each exposure. Even when they are reset automatically they require too much time.

3. **Electronic timers.** Electronic timers are the most sophisticated, most complicated, and most accurate of the x-ray exposure timers. Electronic timers consist of rather complex circuitry based on the time required to charge a **capacitor** through a **variable resistance.** They allow a wide range of time intervals to be selected and are accurate to intervals as small as 1 millisecond. They can be used for **rapid serial exposures.** Today, most exposure timers are electronic.

4. **mAs timers.** Most x-ray apparatus is designed for accurate control of tube current and exposure time. The product of mA and time (mAs) determines the number of x-rays emitted. A special kind of electronic timer, called an *mAs timer,* monitors the product of mA and exposure time and terminates the exposure when the desired mAs is attained. The mAs timer is usually designed to provide the highest safe tube current for the shortest time of exposure for any mAs selected. Since the mAs timer must monitor the actual tube current, it is located on the secondary side of the high-voltage transformer.

5. **Automatic exposure controls.** Unlike the four previous timing devices, the phototimer does not require adjustment by the radiographer. A phototimer is a device that measures the quantity of radiation reaching the **image receptor.** It automatically terminates the exposure when sufficient radiation to provide the required **optical density** has reached the image receptor. Figure 9-9 shows the operation of two types of phototimers. The critical component of one type of phototimer is the **photomultiplier** sensing device. The photomultiplier views a fluorescent screen and converts the

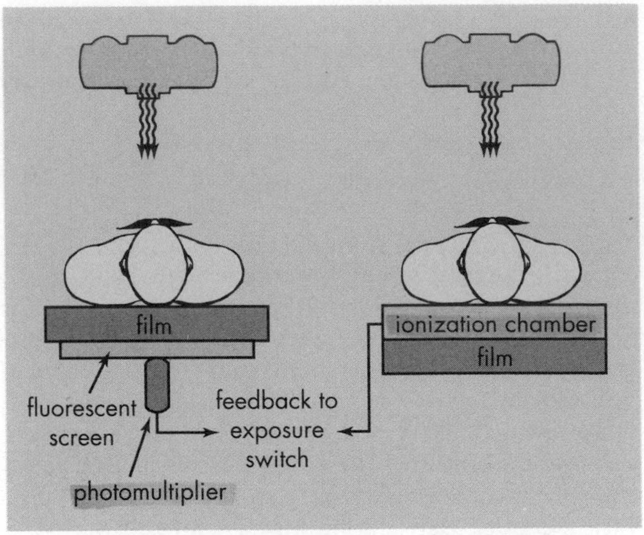

FIGURE 9-9 Phototimer automatically terminates the x-ray exposure at the desired film density. This is done with either a photomultiplier or an ionization chamber sensing device.

light from it into an electric charge. The intensity of the fluorescence is directly proportional to the intensity of **incident radiation.** The x-ray exposure is terminated when a preselected charge, corresponding to the desired optical density, has been reached by the photomultiplier. The type of phototimer used by most manufacturers incorporates a flat, parallel plate **ionization chamber** positioned between the patient and the image receptor. The chamber is made radiolucent so that it will not interfere with the radiographic image. Ionization within the chamber creates a charge proportional to optical density. When the appropriate charge has been reached, the exposure is terminated. The operation of a phototimer is simple. When a phototimed x-ray unit is installed, however, it must be **calibrated.** This calls for making exposures of a **phantom** and adjusting the phototimer for the range of optical densities required by the radiologist on the radiograph. Usually the service engineer takes care of this calibration. Once the phototimer has been placed in clinical operation, the radiographer simply selects the appropriate optical density and places the exposure timer in the phototime mode. When the electric charge from the ionization chamber reaches the preset level, a signal is returned to the operating console, and the exposure timer is turned off.

Phototimers are now widely used and often are provided on the console in addition to a **manual timer.** Care should be taken when using the phototime mode, especially in low-kVp examinations, such as in mammography. Because of the varying thickness and composition of breast tissue, the phototimer may not respond properly at low kVp, and the result is varying optical density. When radiographs are taken in the phototime mode, the manual timer should be set to 2 seconds as a backup timer in case the phototimer fails to terminate. This precaution should be followed for the safety of the patient and for the protection of the x-ray tube. There is an automatic backup timer on many units.

Checking the timer. The spinning top is a simple device that can be used to check the accuracy of x-ray timers in half-wave and full-wave–rectified units in which radiation output is pulsed (Figure 9-10). Solid-state radiation detectors are now used for exposure-timer checks (Figure 9-11). These devices operate with a very accurate internal clock based on a quartz-crystal oscillator. They are capable of measuring exposure times as short as 1 millisecond and, when used with an oscilloscope, can display the radiation waveform. These devices are usually used by medical physicists and service engineers to test x-ray equipment.

HIGH-VOLTAGE GENERATOR

High-Voltage Generator

The high-voltage generator of an x-ray machine is responsible for converting the low voltage from the electric power company into a kilovoltage of the proper waveform.

A cutaway view of a typical high-voltage generator is shown in Figure 9-12. The high-voltage generator contains the following three primary parts: (1) the **high-voltage transformer,** (2) the **filament transformer,** and (3) the **rectifiers** (all three are immersed in oil). Although some heat is generated in the high-voltage section, the oil is not used as a heat insulator but is used primarily for electrical insulation.

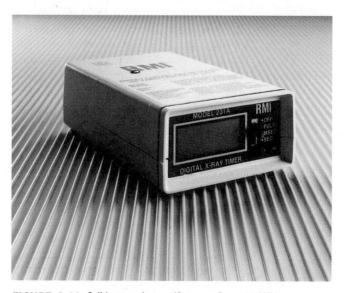

FIGURE 9-11 Solid state timers. *(Courtesy Gammex RMI.)*

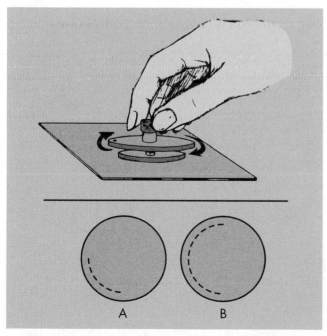

FIGURE 9-10 Spinning top tests can be used to check x-ray exposure timers. A 100 ms image of a spinning top test should result in 6 dashes for a half-wave rectified unit **(A)** and should result in 12 dashes for a full-wave rectified unit **(B).**

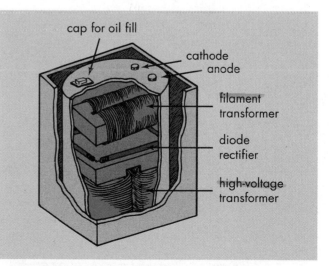

FIGURE 9-12 Cutaway view of typical high-voltage generator, showing oil-immersed diodes and transformers.

1) High-Voltage Transformer —

component of high-voltage generator 1 of 3
(Table 6-2 p64)

The high-voltage transformer is a **step-up** transformer. The secondary voltage is greater than the primary voltage because the number of secondary windings is greater than the number of primary windings. *2nd > 1st*

The ratio of the number of secondary windings to the number of primary windings is called the ***turns ratio*** $= \frac{N_s}{N_p}$ (see Chapter 8). The voltage increase is [proportional] to the turns ratio, according to the transformer law, and the current is reduced proportionately. The turns ratio of a high-voltage transformer is usually between 500:1 to 1000:1. Since transformers operate only on alternat(AC) ing current, the voltage waveform on both sides of a high-voltage transformer is sinusoidal (Figure 9-13). The only difference between the primary and secondary waveforms is the **amplitude**. The primary voltage is measured in volts, and the secondary voltage is measured in kilovolts.

Question: The turns ratio of a high-voltage transformer is 700:1, and the supply voltage is peaked at 120 volts. What is the secondary voltage supplied to the x-ray tube?

.12kV

Answer: (120 Vp) (700:1) = 84,000 Vp

= 84 kVp is the secondary voltage supplied to the x-ray tube

Voltage Rectification

Although transformers operate with alternating current, x-ray tubes must be provided with direct current. X-rays are produced by the acceleration of electrons from the cathode to the anode and cannot be produced by electrons flowing in the reverse direction from anode to cathode. The construction of the cathode assembly is such that it could not withstand the tremendous heat generated by such a process even if the anode could emit electrons thermionically. It would be disastrous to the x-ray tube for electron flow to be reversed. If the electron flow is to be only in the cathode-to-anode direction, the secondary voltage of the high-voltage transformer must be **rectified**. Rectification is the process of converting alternating voltage into direct voltage and therefore alternating current into direct current. Rectification is accomplished with **diodes**. A diode is an electronic device containing two electrodes. Originally, all diode rectifiers were vacuum tubes called ***valve tubes***. *electrical terminal connector* Anodes and cathodes of valve tubes are constructed much differently than those of an x-ray tube. As a result, x-rays are not emitted from valve tubes. The valve tube has been replaced in many x-ray units by **solid-state rectifiers** made of silicon (Figure 9-14).

Figure 9-15 shows the **unrectified voltage** at the secondary side of the high-voltage transformer. This voltage waveform appears as the voltage waveform sup-

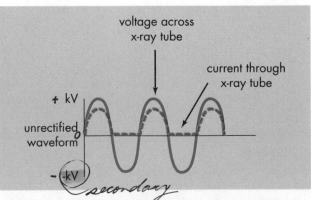

FIGURE 9-14 Rectifiers in most modern x-ray generators are the silicon, semiconductor type. *(Courtesy The Machlett Laboratories, Inc.)*

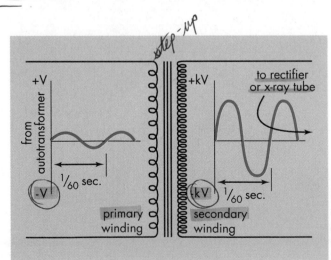

step-up

FIGURE 9-13 Voltage induced in the secondary winding of a high-voltage step-up transformer is alternating like the primary voltage but has a higher value. *2nd V > 1st V*

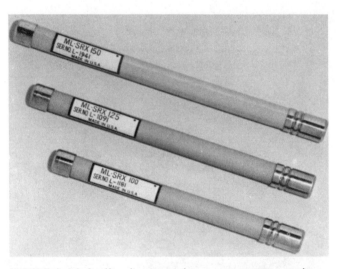

FIGURE 9-15 Unrectified voltage waveform on the secondary side.

plied to the primary side of the high-voltage transformer except its amplitude is much greater. The current passing through the x-ray tube, however, exists only during the positive half of the cycle, when the anode is positive and the cathode negative. During the negative half of the cycle, current can flow only from anode to cathode, but this does not occur because the anode is not constructed to emit electrons. The voltage across the x-ray tube during the negative half cycle is called *inverse voltage* and can cause failure of the x-ray tube. The inverse voltage is removed from the supply to the x-ray tube by rectification.

Half-wave Rectification

Half-wave rectification (Figure 9-16) represents a condition in which the voltage is not allowed to swing negatively during the negative half of its cycle.

Rectifying devices, either vacuum-tube or solid-state, can be assembled into electronic circuits capable of converting alternating current into the direct current necessary for the operation of an x-ray tube (Figure 9-17). During the positive portion of the AC waveform, the rectifier conducts freely and allows electric current to pass through the x-ray tube. During the negative portion of the AC waveform, however, the rectifier will not

conduct, and thus no electric current is allowed. The resulting current is a series of positive pulses separated by gaps where the negative current is not conducted. This output electric current is a rectified current, since electrons flow in only one direction. This form of rectification is called *half-wave rectification* because only one half of the AC waveform appears in the output. The negative portion of the AC waveform has been removed.

In some dental x-ray units the x-ray tube serves as the vacuum-tube rectifier. Such a system is said to be **self-rectified,** and the resulting waveform is the same as that of half-wave rectification. Self-rectification is not used in medical x-ray units because the x-ray tube cannot handle the higher power levels. Half-wave rectified circuits can always be recognized because they contain either zero, one, or two diodes. The x-ray output from a half-wave unit is pulsating, with 60 x-ray pulses produced each second.

One shortcoming of half-wave rectification is that it wastes half the supply power. It is possible, however, to devise a circuit that will rectify the entire AC waveform. Full-wave–rectified x-ray machines contain at least four diodes in the high-voltage circuit, usually arranged as in Figure 9-18.

Full-wave Rectification

In a full-wave–rectified circuit the negative half cycle corresponding to the inverse voltage is reversed so that a positive voltage is always directed across the x-ray tube (Figure 9-19).

In Figure 9-19 the current through the circuit is shown during both the positive and negative phases of the input waveform. In both cases the output voltage across the x-ray tube is positive, and there are no gaps in the output waveform. All of the input waveform is

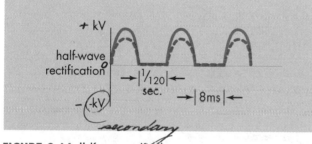

FIGURE 9-16 Half-wave rectification.

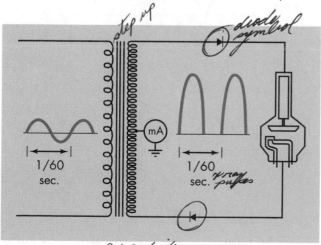

FIGURE 9-17 A half-wave–rectified circuit usually contains two diodes, although some contain one or more.

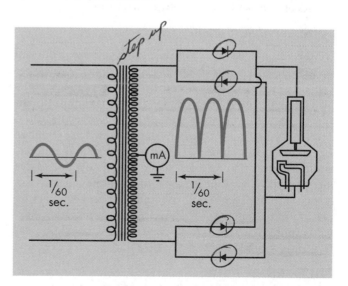

FIGURE 9-18 A full-wave–rectified circuit contains at least four diodes. Current is passed through the tube at 120 pulses per second.

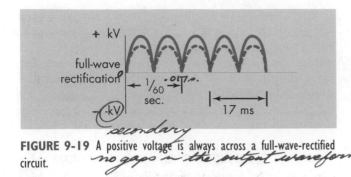

against the electron-flow

secondary

FIGURE 9-19 A positive voltage is always across a full-wave-rectified circuit. *no gaps in the output waveform*

rectified into usable output. This is the preferred circuit for use in x-ray devices, since it does not waste any of the input source.

Figure 9-20 helps explain how full-wave rectification works. During the positive half cycle of the secondary voltage waveform, electrons flow from the negative side to diodes C and D. Diode C is unable to conduct electrons in that direction, but diode D can. The electrons flow through diode D and the x-ray tube. The electrons then butt into diodes A and B. Only diode A is positioned to conduct them, and they flow to the positive side of the transformer, thus completing the circuit. During the negative half cycle, diodes B and C are pressed into service and diodes A and D block electron flow. Note that the polarity of the x-ray tube remains unchanged. The cathode is always negative and the anode always positive, even though the induced secondary voltage alternates between positive and negative. Full-wave rectification is used in nearly all stationary x-ray units. Its main advantage is that the exposure time for any given technique is cut in half. The half-wave–rectified x-ray tube emits x-rays only half the time it is on. The pulsed x-ray output of a full-wave–rectified machine occurs 120 times each second instead of 60 times per second as with half-wave rectification.

SINGLE-PHASE POWER

All the voltage waveforms discussed so far are produced by single-phase electric power. Single-phase power results in a pulsating x-ray beam. This is caused by the alternate swing in voltage from zero to maximum potential 120 times each second under full-wave rectification. The x-rays produced when the single-phase voltage waveform has a value near zero are of little diagnostic value because they are low energy and therefore have low penetrability. One method of overcoming this deficiency is to use some sophisticated electrical engineering principles to generate three simultaneous voltage waveforms out of step with one another. Such a manipulation results in three-phase electric power.

THREE-PHASE POWER

The engineering required to produce three-phase power involves the manner in which the high-voltage step-up transformer is wired into the circuit. Figure 9-21 shows

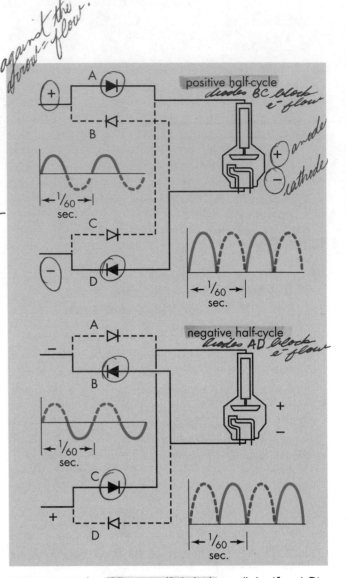

diodes BC block e⁻ flow

anode

cathode

positive half-cycle

diodes AD block e⁻ flow

negative half-cycle

FIGURE 9-20 In a full-wave-rectified circuit two diodes (**A** and **D**) conduct during the positive half-cycle and two (**B** and **C**) during the negative half-cycle.

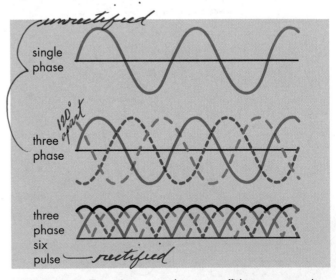

unrectified

120° apart

rectified

FIGURE 9-21 Three-phase power is a more efficient way to produce x-rays than is single-phase power. Shown are the voltage waveforms for unrectified, single-phase, three-phase, and associated rectified three-phase power.

the voltage waveforms for single-phase power, three-phase power, and three-phase power when full-wave rectified. With three-phase power, multiple voltage waveforms are superimposed on one another, which results in a waveform that maintains a nearly constant high voltage. There can be either six pulses per one sixtieth of a second or 12 pulses per one sixtieth of a second compared with the two pulses characteristic of single-phase power. With three-phase power, the voltage across the x-ray tube is nearly constant and never drops to zero during exposure. There are limitations to the speed of starting an exposure (**initiation time**) and ending an exposure (**extinction time**) because of how the iron in the transformer responds. Additional electronic circuits and hardware are necessary to correct this deficiency, which adds to additional size and cost of the three-phase generator.

High-Frequency Generator

The newest development in high-voltage generator design uses a **high-frequency circuit.** Full-wave–rectified power at 60 Hz is converted to a higher frequency, usually 500 to 25,000 Hz. One advantage of the high-frequency generator is size. Such generators can be placed within the **x-ray tube housing** and produce a nearly constant potential voltage waveform (Figure 9-22), which results in improved image quality at lower patient dose. Portable x-ray machines were the first to benefit from

this technology. High-frequency voltage generation uses **inverter** circuits (Figure 9-23). Inverter circuits are high-speed switches that convert DC into a series of **square pulses.** Many portable x-ray generators use storage batteries and silicon-controlled rectifiers (SCRs) to generate square waves at 500 Hz, which becomes the input to the anode transformer. The anode transformer operating at 500 Hz is about one tenth the size of a 60-Hz transformer, which is still rather large and heavy. At 500 Hz, one can sometimes hear the transformer "sing" during exposure. The small time gap between square wave pulses, unlike 60-Hz sine waves, is easy to filter, which produces a constant voltage of the anode. Such portable x-ray generators perform as well as the best three-phase generators.

High-frequency x-ray generators are sometimes grouped by frequency (Table 9-1). The principal differences are in the electrical components designed as the **inverter module.** The real advantage to such circuits is that they are much smaller, less costly, and more efficient than the older circuits.

Some portable units still use a high-voltage generator that operates by charging a bank of SCRs from the DC voltage of a nickel-cadmium (NiCd) battery. This is called a *capacitor discharge generator.* By stacking (in an electrical sense) the SCRs, the charge is stored at very high electrical potential or high voltage. During exposure the charge is released to form the x-ray tube current to produce x-rays. During capacitor discharge the voltage

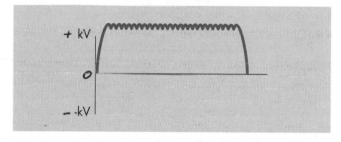

FIGURE 9-22 High frequency generator circuit voltage waveform.

TABLE 9-1	
Characteristics of High-Frequency X-ray Generators	
Frequency Range	**Inverter Features**
Up to 1 kHz	Thyristers
1 kHz to 10 kHz	Large SCRs (silicon-controlled rectifiers)
10 kHz to 100 kHz	Power field effect transistors

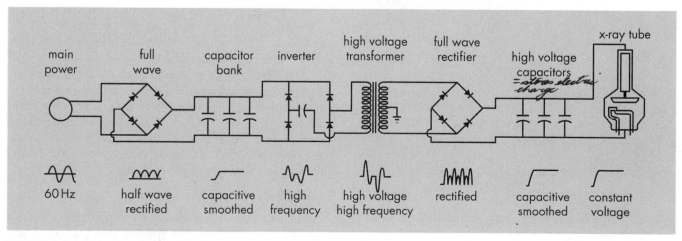

FIGURE 9-23 An inverter circuit.

falls by approximately 1 kV/mAs (Figure 9-24). This limits the available x-ray tube current and results in a falling kVp during exposure. As a result precise **radiographic technique charts** are needed.

Voltage Ripple

Another way to characterize these voltage waveforms is by **voltage ripple**.

Voltage ripple is the variation in peak voltage waveform.

O to the peak (repeated)

Single-phase power has **100% voltage ripple**. The voltage varies from zero to its maximum value. Three-phase, six-pulse power produces voltage with only approximately **13% ripple**, consequently the voltage supplied to the x-ray tube never falls below 87% of the maximum value. A further improvement in three-phase power results in 12 pulses per cycle rather than six. Three-phase, 12-pulse power results in a voltage supply of only **4% ripple**, and therefore the voltage supplied to the x-ray tube does not fall below 96% of the maximum value. High-frequency generators have less than **3% ripple** and therefore higher x-ray quantity and quality. It is even more efficient than three-phase power. Claims that higher frequency is better should be taken lightly. When the voltage ripple is less than approximately 3%, little is gained by even less ripple. Figure 9-25 shows the resulting voltage waveform provided to the x-ray tube by these various power sources. The approximate voltage ripple is also shown. The most efficient method of x-ray production also has the waveform with the lowest voltage ripple. There are many advantages to x-ray tube voltage generated with less ripple. The principal advantage is the higher radiation quantity and quality, which results from the more constant voltage supplied to the x-ray tube. The radiation quantity is higher because the efficiency of x-ray pro-

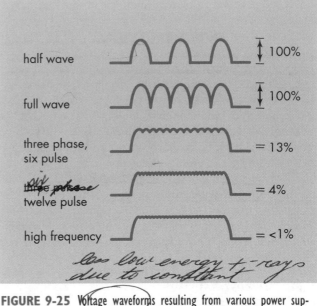

FIGURE 9-25 Voltage waveforms resulting from various power supplies.

provided (to the x-ray tube by)

duction is higher when x-ray tube voltage is high. Stated differently, for any projectile electron emitted by the x-ray tube cathode, more x-rays are produced when the electron energy (kVp) is high than when it is low. The radiation quality is increased with low-ripple power because there are fewer low-energy projectile electrons passing from cathode to anode to produce low-energy x-rays. Consequently the average x-ray energy is increased over single-phase operation.

Because the x-ray output intensity and penetrability are greater for low-ripple power than for single-phase power, technique charts developed for one cannot be used on the other. It is necessary to develop new technique charts when using three-phase or high-frequency equipment. Three-phase operation may require as much as a 10 kVp reduction to produce the same radiographic optical density when operated at the same mAs as single phase. A 12-kVp reduction may be necessary when using a high-frequency generator. Three-phase radiographic equipment is manufactured with tube currents as high as 1200 mA; therefore exceedingly short, high-intensity exposures are possible.

The principal disadvantage of three-phase x-ray apparatus is its initial cost. The cost of installation and operation, however, can be lower than those associated with single-phase equipment. High-frequency generators have a moderate cost. The overall capacity and flexibility provided by low-ripple generators are greater than those for single-phase equipment.

POWER RATING

Transformers and indeed high-voltage generators are usually identified by their **power rating** in kilowatts

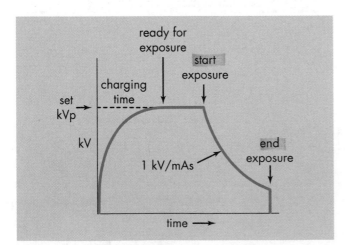

FIGURE 9-24 Tube voltage falls during exposure using a capacitor discharge generator.

(kW). Electrical power for any device is specified in watts as was shown in an equation in Chapter 6.

$$\begin{array}{l} \text{Power} = \text{Current} \times \text{Potential} \\ \text{Watts} = \text{Amperes} \times \text{Volts} \end{array}$$

A high-voltage generator for a basic radiographic unit would be rated at 30 to 50 kW.

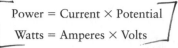

Maximum Available Power

When specifying high-voltage generators, the industry standard is to use the maximum tube current (mA) possible at 100 kVp for an exposure of 100 milliseconds. This combination generally results in the maximum available power.

The equation above shows that power is the product of amperes times volts. This assumes constant current and voltage, which does not exist in single-phase x-ray circuits. However, the low-ripple power of three phase and high frequency circuits is so close to constant current that the power equation above holds true.

Question: When a low-voltage ripple system is energized at 100 kVp, 100 milliseconds, the maximum tube current possible is 800 mA. What is the power rating?

Answer:
$$\begin{aligned} \text{Power rating} &= \text{amperes} \times \text{volts} \\ &= 800 \text{ mA} \times 100 \text{ kVp} \\ &= 80{,}000 \text{ mA} \times \text{kVp} \\ &= 80{,}000 \text{ watts} \\ &= 80 \text{ kW} \end{aligned}$$

Because the product of amperes × volts = watts, the product of milliampere × kilovolts = watts. However, power rating is expressed in kW, therefore the defining equation for three-phase and high-frequency power is as follows:

$$\text{Power rating (kW)} = \frac{\text{mA} \times \text{kVp}}{1000}$$

Single-phase generators have 100% voltage ripple and are less efficient x-ray generators. The single-phase expression of power rating is as follows:

$$\text{Power rating (kW)} = (0.7) \times \frac{\text{mA} \times \text{kVp}}{1000}$$

Question: A radiographic single-phase unit installed in a private office has a maximum capacity of 100 milliseconds of 120 kVp and 500 mA. What is its power rating?

Answer:
$$\text{Power rating} = (0.7) \frac{(500 \text{ mA}) (120 \text{ kVp})}{1000}$$
$$= 42 \text{ kW is the power rating}$$

X-ray Circuit

The three main sections of the x-ray machine—the x-ray tube, the operating console, and the high-voltage section—are represented in Figure 9-26 by a simplified schematic.

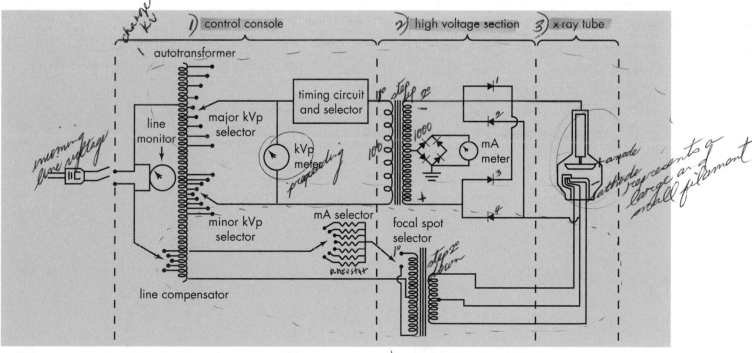

FIGURE 9-26 Simplified electric circuit diagram for the x-ray unit.

SUMMARY

There are three sections of the x-ray unit (1) the x-ray tube, (2) the operating console, and (3) the high-voltage generator. The design and operation of the x-ray tube is discussed in Chapter 10. The operating console and the high-voltage generator are presented in this chapter. The operating console consists of an on/off button, kVp selection control, mA and time or mAs selection control, and, in older units, a line-compensation switch or meter. Phototiming or automatic-exposure controls are also on the control panel. The high-voltage generator provides power to the x-ray tube in two different ways—single-phase power and three-phase power.

The difference between single- and three-phase power involves the manner in which the high-voltage step-up transformer is wired to the circuit. The waveforms for single-phase, three-phase, and three-phase fully rectified power are shown in Figure 9-21. With three-phase power the voltage across the x-ray tube is nearly constant during the exposure and never drops to zero, as does the voltage for single-phase power.

The parts of an x-ray unit are identified by their power rating in kW (kilowatts). Maximum available power for high-voltage generators equals the maximum tube current (mA) at 100 kVp for an exposure of 100 milliseconds.

REVIEW QUESTIONS

1. The general-purpose x-ray room contains a _____ and _____ with an _____. *p92*

2. The radiographic table must be radiolucent. Define *radiolucent.* *p92*

3. The Bucky tray is designed to hold a(n) _____ and _____. *p92*

4. When performing x-ray examinations in your clinical assignments, which examinations would not use the Bucky tray? *table top, portable, surgery,*

5. Describe the movements of a $^{80}/_{20}$ table. *80° tilt ft side; 20° tilt head side*

6. List the five major controls on the operator's console. *p92*

7. The line compensator adjusts voltage to the x-ray unit to precisely _____ *220* _____ volts.

8. What is the purpose of the autotransformer? Why is an autotransformer safer than a high-voltage transformer? *p94*

9. What is the relationship between the primary voltage and the secondary voltage in an autotransformer?

10. What does the prereading voltmeter allow? *p96*

11. Radiographic console controls are set at 200 mA with an exposure time of $\frac{1}{60}$ second. What is the mAs? *p97*

12. In an examination of a pediatric patient the controls are set at 600 mA at 30 milliseconds. What is the mAs? *.030.*

13. The mA stations in the filament circuit are not continuously variable. Instead, these values are fixed to specific current outputs because of the use of _____. *p.97*

14. The exposure timer circuit is located on the _____ of the high-voltage transformer.

15. Timers that have a minimum possible exposure time of one sixtieth of a second are _____.

16. Define *phototimer*.

17. Contrast the definitions of high-voltage generator and high-voltage transformer.

18. Why is rectification necessary in the x-ray circuit?

19. Match the power sources with the percent voltage ripple.

POWER	% VOLTAGE RIPPLE
single-phase	4%
three-phase, 12-pulse	100%
three-phase, six-pulse	13%
high-frequency	3%

Additional Reading

Pirtle OL: X-ray machine calibration: a study of failure rates, *Radiol Technol* 65(5):291, May-June, 1994.

10

The X-ray Tube

OBJECTIVES

At the completion of this chapter the student will be able to:

1. Describe the six support designs for the x-ray tube
2. List the parts of the housing that protect the x-ray tube
3. Identify the components of the glass or metal envelope that make up the x-ray tube
4. Discuss the cathode and filament current
5. Describe the parts of the anode and the induction motor that spins the rotating anode
6. Define the line-focus principle and the heel effect
7. Identify the three causes of x-ray tube failure
8. Explain the use of tube rating charts to prevent tube failure

OUTLINE

External Structure
   Support structures
   Protective housing
   Glass envelope
Internal Structure
   Cathode
   Anode

Tube Failure
   Causes
   Prevention of tube failure with tube
     rating charts

The external structure of the x-ray tube consists of three parts—(1) the support structure, (2) the protective housing, and (3) the glass or metal envelope. The internal structure of the tube is made up of a cathode and an anode enclosed in a vacuum. X-ray tubes should last many years with proper use.

An explanation of the external components of the x-ray tube and the internal structure of the x-ray tube is included in this chapter. At the end of the chapter, the causes and prevention of x-ray tube failure are discussed.

EXTERNAL STRUCTURE
Support Structures

The x-ray tube is very heavy and requires a sturdy structure to support its weight. Mechanisms are required so that the radiographer can move the weight of the tube easily. Figure 10-1 illustrates three of the six main methods to support the x-ray tube.

1. The **ceiling support** (Figure 10-1, *A*) is the most frequently used system. It consists of two sets of rails mounted to the ceiling directly over the radiographic table. The two sets of two rails are mounted perpendicular to each other so that the tube can move longitudinally along the length of the table and transversely in a perpendicular direction to the length of the table. A telescoping column attaches from the ceiling rails to the x-ray tube **housing,** and when the tube is manipulated by the radiographer, the column can change the distance to the table. The distance from the tube to the x-ray film or **cassette** is called the *source-to-image receptor distance (SID).* SID was formerly expressed as focal-film distance (FFD). When the tube is centered above the table at a standard SID, the tube is said to be in a **detent** or locked-in position. Positions other than detent also can be chosen by the operator.

2. The **floor-to-ceiling support** system has a single column with rollers attached to each end—one on a ceiling mounted rail and the other end on a floor mounted rail. The x-ray tube moves along the rails longitudinally, as well as up, down, and sideways on the column.

3. An alternative to the column mount is an x-ray tube mounted on a **floor-mount system** (Figure 10-1, *B*).

4. The **fluoroscopy** x-ray tube is mounted underneath the radiographic table and is energized only during fluoroscopy when the **image intensifier tower** is locked into place.

5. X-ray tubes can also be mounted on a support shaped like a C. These are called *C-arm* units (Figure 10-1, *C*) and are used as **portable fluoroscopy** units or in **special procedures** suites.

6. X-ray tubes also can be mounted on **portable** or **mobile machines** for use at the patient's bedside.

Protective Housing

When x-rays are produced, they are emitted **isotropically** with equal intensity in all directions. The **useful beam** is only those x-rays emitted through the special section of the x-ray tube called the *window* (Figure 10-2). Other x-rays that escape through the protective housing are termed *leakage radiation.* They contribute nothing in the way of diagnostic information and result in unnecessary exposure to the patient and to the radiographer. A properly designed protective housing reduces the level of leakage radiation when operated at maximum conditions. Manufacturers of x-ray tubes have standards for leakage radiation set by the federal government. That standard is less than 100 mR per hour at 1 meter. The protective housing also incorporates specially designed high-voltage receptacles to protect against accidental **electric shock.** Death by electrocution was a very real hazard to early operators. The protective housing also provides **mechanical support** for the x-ray tube and protects the tube from damage caused by handling. The protective housing around some x-ray tubes **contains oil that serves as both an electrical insulator and a thermal cushion.** Some protective housings have a cooling fan to air cool the tube or the oil in which the x-ray tube is immersed and a bellows like device to allow the oil to expand when heated. If the expansion is too great, a microswitch is activated so that the tube cannot be used until it cools down.

> **Remember:** The protective housing should *never* be held during an x-ray examination. In addition, patients' limbs should not rest on the tube or housing during an x-ray examination. The high-voltage cables and terminals should *never* be used as handles for positioning the tube.

Glass Envelope

An x-ray tube is a vacuum tube or **diode** with two electrodes: the **cathode** (filament) and the **anode** (target) (Figure 10-3). The components are contained within an evacuated **glass envelope.** The x-ray tube, however, is a special kind of vacuum tube. It is relatively large, perhaps 30 to 50 centimeters long and 20 centimeters in diameter. The glass envelope is made of Pyrex glass to enable it to withstand the tremendous heat generated. It maintains a **vacuum** or empty space inside the tube. This vacuum allows for more efficient x-ray production and longer tube life. If the tube were filled with gas, the electron flow from cathode to anode would be reduced, fewer x-rays would be produced, and more heat would be created. Early x-ray tubes, modifications of the Crookes tube, were not vacuum tubes but rather contained controlled quantities of gas within the glass en-

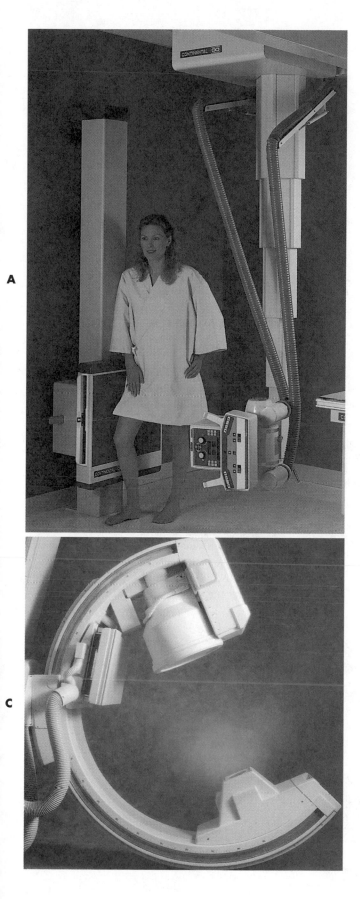

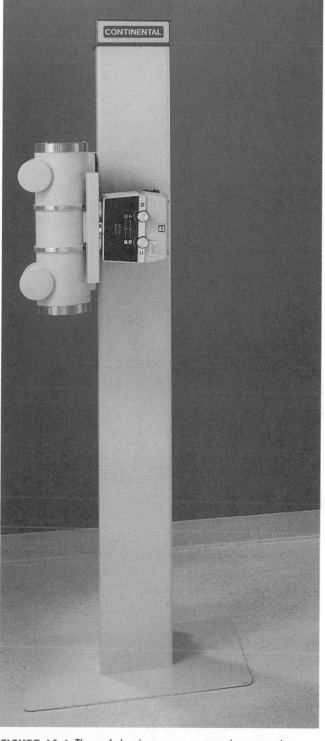

FIGURE 10-1 Three of the six ways to support the x-ray tube. **A,** Ceiling mount; **B,** floor stand; **C,** C-arm. *(Courtesy **A** and **B,** Continental X-ray Corp. **C,** Philips Medical Systems.)*

velope and were designed more like fluorescent lights. The modern x-ray tube, the Coolidge tube, is a vacuum tube. If it becomes gassy, that is, filled with gas molecules, x-ray production falls and the tube fails.

A recent improvement in tube design incorporates metal rather than glass as part or all of the envelope. As the glass envelope ages, some tungsten vaporizes and coats the inside. This alters the electric potential of the tube, which allows tube current to stray and interact with the glass envelope. The result is arcing and tube failure. Metal envelope tubes maintain a constant electric potential between the electrons of the tube current and the envelope. Therefore they have a longer life and are less likely to fail. Virtually all high-output x-ray tubes now use metal envelopes. The tube window is an area in the glass or metal envelope, approximately 5 centimeters square, that is thin and through which the useful x-ray beam is emitted. The thin window allows maximum emission of x-rays with minimum absorption from the glass or metal.

INTERNAL STRUCTURE
Cathode

Cathode →

The cathode is the negative side of the x-ray tube and has two primary parts—(1) a **filament** and (2) a **focusing cup**.

Figure 10-4 shows a photograph of a dual-filament cathode and a schematic drawing of its electrical supply.

Filament. The filament is a coil of wire similar to that in a kitchen toaster except much smaller. The filament is usually about 2 millimeters in diameter and 1 or 2 centimeters long. In the kitchen toaster an electric current is conducted through the coil, which causes it to glow and emit a large quantity of heat. An x-ray filament emits electrons when it is heated. When the current through the filament is sufficiently high, approximately 4 amperes and above, the outer-shell electrons of the filament atoms are literally boiled off and ejected from the filament. This phenomenon is known as *thermionic emission.* Filaments are usually made of **thoriated tungsten.** Tungsten provides for higher thermionic emission than other metals because its melting point is 3410° C, and therefore it is not likely to burn out. In addition, tungsten does not vaporize easily. If it did, the tube would quickly become gassy and its internal parts coated with tungsten. Ultimately, over long use, tungsten does vaporize and is deposited on internal components. This upsets some of the electrical characteristics

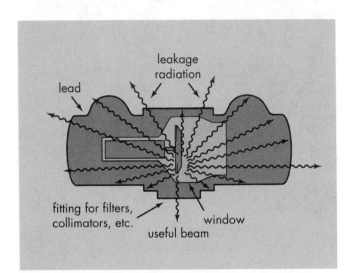

FIGURE 10-2 Protective housing reduces the intensity of leakage radiation to less than 100 mR/hr at 1 meter.

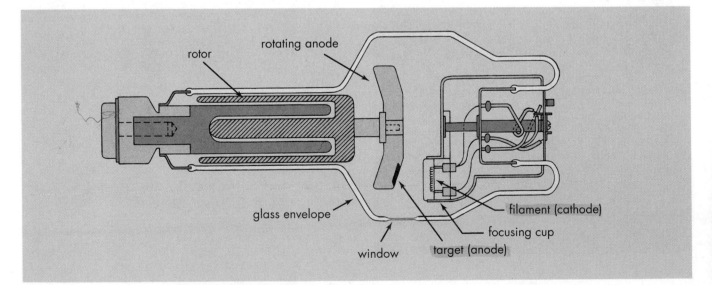

FIGURE 10-3 Principal parts of a modern rotating anode x-ray tube.

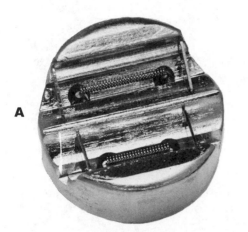

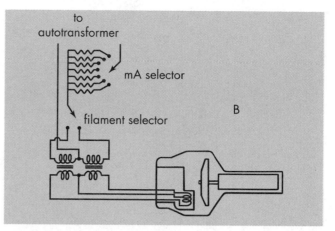

FIGURE 10-4 A, Dual-filament cathode designed to provide focal spots of 0.5 and 1.5 millimeters. **B,** Schematic for dual-filament cathode. (**A,** *Courtesy The Machlett Laboratories.*)

of the tube and can lead to tube failure. Although not spectacular or sudden, this is the most common cause of tube failure. The addition of 1% to 2% thorium to the tungsten filament increases efficiency of thermionic emission and prolongs tube life.

Focusing cup. The filament is embedded in a metal cup called the *focusing cup* (Figure 10-5). Because all the accelerating electrons coming from the cathode to the anode are electrically negative, the electron beam tends to spread out because of electrostatic repulsion. Some electrons can even miss the anode completely. The focusing cup is negatively charged so that it condenses the electron beam to a small area of the anode (Figure 10-6). The effectiveness of the focusing cup is determined by its size and shape, its charge, the filament size and shape, and the position of the filament within the focusing cup. Certain types of x-ray tubes called **grid-controlled** tubes are designed to be turned on and off very rapidly. Grid-controlled tubes are used in **portable capacitor discharge units** and in **digital subtraction angiography, digital radiography,** and **cineradiography,** all of which require multiple exposures at precise exposure times. The term *grid* is borrowed from vacuum-tube electronics and refers to an element in the tube that acts as the switch. In a **grid-controlled x-ray tube** the focusing cup is the grid and therefore the exposure switch.

Filament current. When the x-ray unit is first turned on, a low current flows through the filament to warm it and prepare it for the thermal jolt necessary for x-ray production. At low filament current, no tube current flows because the filament does not get hot enough for thermionic emission. Once the filament current is high enough for thermionic emission, a small rise in filament current results in a large rise in tube current. This relationship between filament current and tube current depends on the tube voltage (Figure 10-7).

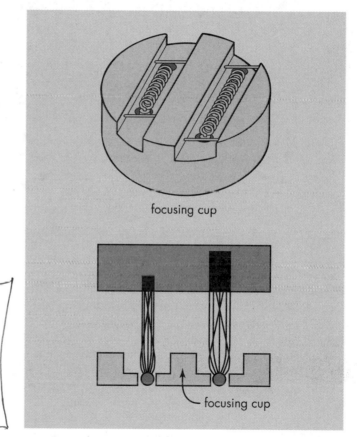

FIGURE 10-5 The focusing cup is a metal shroud surrounding the filament.

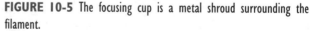

Filament Current

The x-ray tube current is adjusted by controlling the filament current.

Fixed stations of 100, 200, and 300 mA and so on correspond to discrete connections on the **filament transformer** or to **precision resistors.**

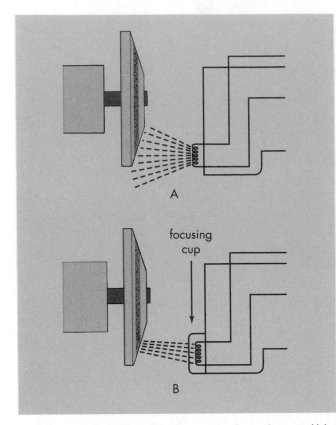

FIGURE 10-6 A, Without a focusing cup, the electron beam would be spread beyond the anode because of mutual electrostatic repulsion among the electrons. **B,** With a focusing cup, which is negatively charged, the beam is condensed and directed to the desired area of the anode.

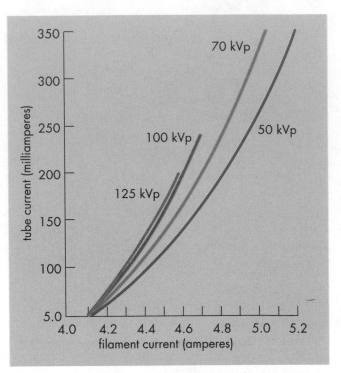

FIGURE 10-7 X-ray tube current is actually controlled by changing the filament current. Because of **thermionic emission,** a small change in filament current results in a large change in tube current.

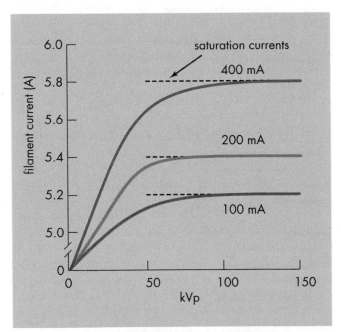

FIGURE 10-8 X-ray tube current reaches a maximum level called *saturation current.*

When emitted from the filament, electrons remain in the vicinity of the filament momentarily before being accelerated to the anode. Because these electrons carry negative charges, they repel one another and tend to form a cloud around the filament. This cloud of electrons, called a *space charge,* makes it difficult for subsequent electrons to be emitted by the filament because of the electrostatic repulsion. This phenomenon is called the *space-charge effect.* X-ray tubes under certain conditions of low kVp and high mA are said to be *space-charge limited.* A major obstacle in producing x-ray tubes with currents exceeding 1000 mA is the design of adequate space-charge compensating devices.

At any given filament current, for example, 5.2 amperes (Figure 10-8), the x-ray tube current will rise with increasing kVp to a maximum value. A further increase in kVp will not result in a higher mA because all of the available electrons are used. This is the **saturation current.** Saturation current is not reached at lower kVp because of space-charge limitation.

Dual-focus tube. Most diagnostic x-ray tubes have two **focal spots,** one large and the other small. The **small focal spot** is used when better **spatial resolution** is required. The **large focal spot** is used when technical factors that produce high heat are required. The selection of the large or small focal spot is generally made with the mA station selector on the operating console or with a focal-spot selection switch.

focal spot = size of the area the e⁻ hit

Large or Small Focal Spot

Normally either filament can be used with the lower mA stations (approximately 300 mA or less).

Large Focal Spot Only

At approximately 400 mA and up, only the large focal spot is recommended for use because the heat capacity of the anode could be exceeded if the small focal spot were used.

Small focal spots range from 0.1 to 0.5 millimeters; large focal spots usually range from 0.4 to 1.2 millimeters. Each filament of a modern dual-filament cathode assembly is embedded in the focusing cup (Figure 10-9). The small focal-spot size is associated with the small filament and the large focal-spot size with the large filament. The electric current flows through the appropriate filament.

Anode

Anode +

The anode is the positive side of the x-ray tube. There are two types of anodes—(1) **stationary** and (2) **rotating** (Figure 10-10). Both types have a support structure and a target (see below for an explanation of target).

Stationary-anode x-ray tubes are used in dental x-ray machines, some portable machines, and other special-purpose units in which high tube current and power are not required. General-purpose x-ray tubes use the rotating anode because they must be capable of producing high-intensity x-ray beams in a short time.

The anode serves three functions in an x-ray tube.
1. The anode is an **electrical conductor**. It receives electrons emitted by the cathode and conducts them through the tube to the connecting cables and back to the high-voltage generator.
2. The anode also provides **mechanical support** for the target.
3. The anode must also be a good **thermal conductor**. When the electrons slam into the anode, more than 99% of their kinetic energy is converted into heat. This heat must be conducted away quickly before it melts the anode. Adequate heat dissipation is the major engineering hurdle in the design of higher-capacity x-ray tubes.

Anode Materials

Copper, molybdenum, and graphite are the most common anode materials.

Target. In stationary-anode tubes the target consists of a **tungsten-alloy** metal embedded in the **copper anode** (Figure 10-11, *A*).

Target

The **target** is the area of the anode struck by the electrons from the cathode.

In rotating-anode tubes a tract around the face of the entire rotating disk is the target (Figure 10-11, *B*). This disk is usually made of a tungsten alloy. Alloying the **tungsten** (usually with **rhenium**) gives it added mechanical strength to withstand the stresses of high-speed rotation. High-capacity x-ray tubes have **molybdenum** and/or **graphite** layered under the **tungsten** target (Figure 10-12). Both molybdenum and graphite have lower mass density than tungsten, which makes the anode easier to rotate.

Target Material (reasons for choice)

Tungsten is the material of choice for the target for general radiography for three main reasons:
1. **Atomic number**—tungsten's high atomic number, 74, results in high-efficiency x-ray production and in high-energy x-rays.
2. **Thermal conductivity**—tungsten has a thermal conductivity nearly equal to that of copper. Therefore it is an efficient metal for dissipating the heat produced.
3. **High melting point**—any material, if heated sufficiently, will melt and become liquid. Tungsten has a high melting point (approximately 3400° C compared with about 1100° C for copper) and therefore can stand up under high tube current without **pitting** or **bubbling**.

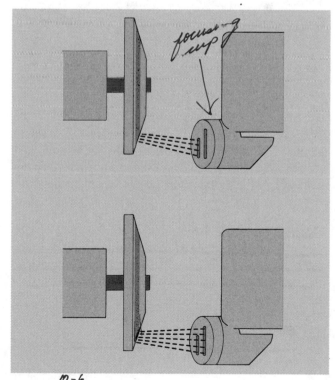

FIGURE 10-9 In a dual-focus x-ray tube, focal-spot size is controlled by heating one of the two filaments.

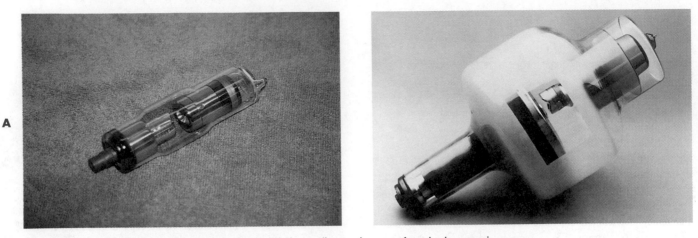

FIGURE 10-10 All diagnostic x-ray tubes can be classified according to the type of anode they contain. **A,** Stationary anode. **B,** Rotating anode. *(Courtesy Philips Medical Systems.)*

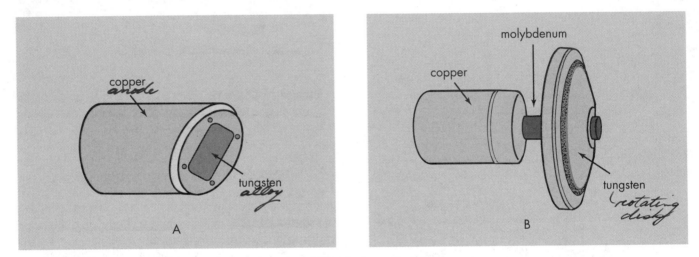

FIGURE 10-11 A, In a stationary-anode tube the target is embedded in the anode. **B,** In a rotating-anode tube the target is the rotating disk.

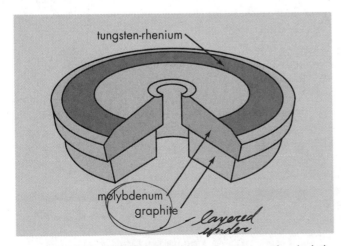

FIGURE 10-12 A layered anode consists of a target surface backed by one or more layers to increase capacity.

Speciality x-ray tubes for **mammography** have **molybdenum** or **rhodium** targets principally because of their low atomic number and low **K-characteristic** x-ray energy. Table 10-1 summarizes the properties of these target materials, all of which have excellent heat conduction.

Rotating anode. The rotating-anode x-ray tube allows the electron beam to interact with a much larger target area because the heating of the anode is not confined to one small spot as in a stationary-anode tube.

Rotating Anode

Higher tube currents and shorter exposure times are possible with the rotating anode.

Figure 10-13 compares the target areas of typical stationary-anode and rotating-anode x-ray tubes with

TABLE 10-1

Characteristics of X-ray Targets

Element	Chemical Symbol	Atomic Number	K X-ray Energy	Melting Temperature
1 Tungsten	W	74	69 keV	3400° C
2 Molybdenum	Mo	42	20 keV	2600° C
3 Rhodium	Rh	45	23 keV	3200° C

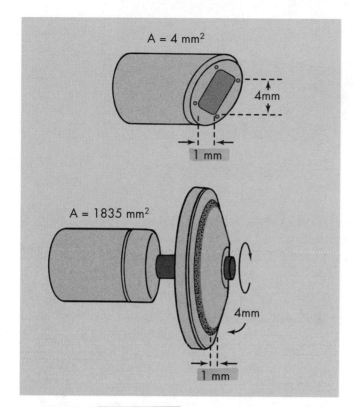

FIGURE 10-13 Stationary-anode tube with a 1-millimeter focal spot may have a target area of 4 millimeter². A comparable 4-centimeter rotating-anode target area has approximately 1835 mm² of area, which increases the heat capacity of the tube by a factor of nearly 500.

1-millimeter focal spots. The actual target area for the stationary tube is 1 mm × 4 mm = 4 mm². The actual target area for the 4 mm-wide rotating anode tract is 1835 mm², thus the rotating-anode tube provides approximately 500 times more area for the electron beam to interact than a stationary-anode tube. Heating capacity can be further improved by increasing the speed of rotation of the anode.

RPM of Anodes

Most rotating anodes revolve at 3400 revolutions per minute (rpm).

The anodes of high-capacity tubes rotate at 10,000 rpm. The neck of the anode is the shaft between the anode and the rotor. This shaft is usually molybdenum

because of its heat-conducting properties. Occasionally the rotor mechanism of a rotating-anode tube fails. When this happens, the anode becomes overheated and **pits** or **cracks**, which causes tube failure (Figure 10-14).

Induction motor. The anode rotates inside a glass envelope with no mechanical connection to the outside.

Rotating Anode

The anode is driven by an electromagnetic **induction motor** (Figure 10-15).

The induction motor consists of two principal parts that are separated from each other by a glass envelope. The part outside the glass envelope, called the *stator,* consists of a series of electromagnets equally spaced around the neck of the tube. Inside the glass envelope is a shaft made of bars of copper and soft iron fabricated into one mass. This mechanism is called the *rotor.* The induction motor works on electromagnetic induction similar to that for a transformer and on Lenz' law of induced currents. Current flowing in each stator winding induces a magnetic field that surrounds the rotor. The stator windings are energized sequentially so that the induced magnetic field rotates on the axis of the stator. This magnetic field interacts with the ferromagnetic rotor, which causes it to rotate synchronously with the activated stator windings. When the operator pushes the exposure button of a radiographic unit, there is a 1-second wait before taking the exposure. This allows the rotor to accelerate to its designed revolutions per minute. During this time, filament current is increased to provide the correct x-ray tube current. When using a **two-position exposure switch,** it is important for the radiographer to push the switch to its final position in one motion. That minimizes the time that the filament is heated, which prevents excessive space charge and thus prolongs tube life. When the exposure is completed on units equipped with **high-speed rotors,** the operator can hear the rotor slow down and stop because the induction motor is put into reverse. The rotor is a precisely balanced, low-friction device that if left alone might take many minutes to coast to a stop after use. In a new x-ray tube the **coast time** or anode stop time will be about 60 seconds. With age the coast time is reduced because of wear of the rotor bearings.

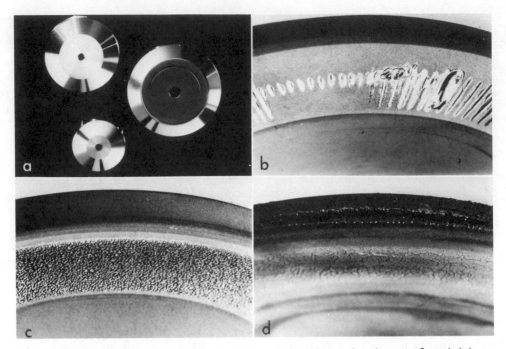

FIGURE 10-14 Comparison of smooth, shiny appearances of rotating anodes when new, **A,** and their appearance after failure, **B** to **D.** Examples of anode separation and surface melting shown were caused by slow rotation caused by bearing damage **(B),** repeated overload **(C),** and exceeding of maximum heat storage capacity **(D).** *(Courtesy The Machlett Laboratories.)*

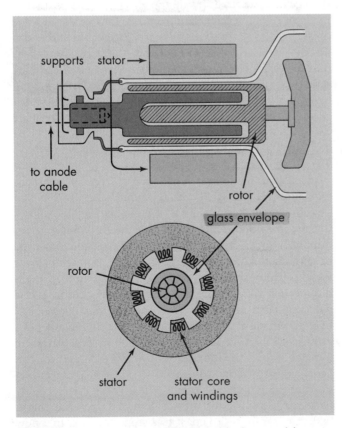

FIGURE 10-15 Target of a rotating-anode tube is powered by an induction motor, the principal components of which are the stator and the rotor.

Line-focus principle. X-ray units have small focal spots because the smaller the focal spot, the better the spatial resolution of the image.

> **Focal Spot**
> The **focal spot** is the area of the target actually being hit with electrons from which x-rays are emitted. The focal spot is the actual source of radiation.

Unfortunately, as the size of the focal spot decreases, the heating of the target is concentrated in a smaller area. This is the limiting factor to focal-spot size. Before the development of the rotating anode, another design was incorporated into x-ray tube targets to allow a large area for heating while maintaining a small focal spot. This design exhibits what is known as the *line-focus principle.* By angling the target, the **effective area** of the target is much smaller than the actual area of electron interaction (Figure 10-16).

> **Effective Focal Spot**
> The effective target area or **effective focal spot** is the focal spot projected onto the patient and the **image receptor.**

The effective focal-spot size is the value given when identifying large or small focal spots. When the **target angle** is made smaller, the effective focal-spot size will also be smaller. Diagnostic x-ray tubes have target angles varying from about 5 to 15 degrees. The advantage

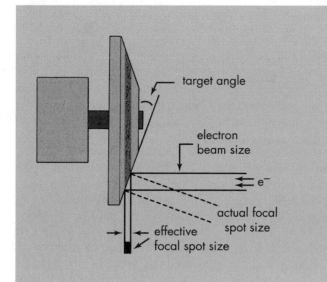

FIGURE 10-16 The line-focus principle allows high anode heating with small effective focal spots. As the target angle decreases, so does the effective focal-spot size.

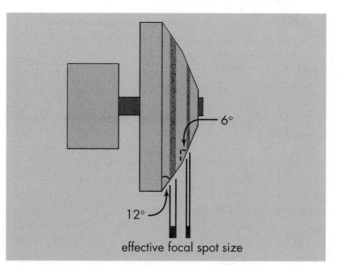

FIGURE 10-17 Some targets have two angles to produce two focal spots.

of the line-focus principle is that it simultaneously improves spatial resolution of the x-ray beam as well as the heat capacity of the anode.

Biangle targets are manufactured with two target angles on the same anode and two focal-spot sizes (Figure 10-17). Combining biangle targets with different length filaments results in a flexible combination. The National Electrical Manufacturers Association (NEMA) has established standards and variances for focal-spot sizes. When a manufacturer states that a focal spot is "nominal size," it means the focal spot on the equipment is within the acceptable standard.

Heel effect. One unfortunate consequence of the line-focus principle is the heel effect.

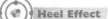
Heel Effect
The heel effect causes radiation intensity on the cathode side of the x-ray beam to be higher than on the anode side.

Electrons interact with target atoms at various depths into the target. The x-rays that constitute the useful beam are emitted from a depth in the target toward the anode side and must traverse a greater thickness of target material than the x-rays emitted in the cathode direction of the target (Figure 10-18). The intensity of x-rays emitted through the heel of the target is reduced because they have a longer path through the target to escape, and therefore there is increased absorption of those rays. This is the **heel effect.** Generally the smaller the anode angle, the larger the heel effect. The difference in radiation intensity across the useful beam of an x-ray field can vary as much as 45%.

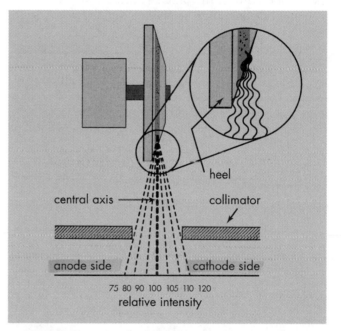

FIGURE 10-18 Heel effect results in reduced x-ray intensity on the anode side of the useful beam because of absorption in the heel of the target.

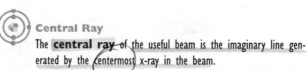
Central Ray
The **central ray** of the useful beam is the imaginary line generated by the centermost x-ray in the beam.

If the radiation intensity along the central ray is designated as 100%, then the intensity on the cathode side of the target may be as high as 120% and that on the anode side of the target may be as low as 75%. The heel effect is important when radiographing anatomic structures of different thicknesses or densities. (abdomen)

Remember: In general, positioning the cathode side of the x-ray tube over the thicker part of the anatomy provides more uniform optical density on the film.

The cathode and anode directions are usually indicated on the protective housing, sometimes near the cable connectors. The cathode is indicated as (−) and the anode is (+).

In chest radiography, for example, the cathode should be toward the feet. The lower thorax, in the region of the diaphragm, is considerably thicker than the upper thorax and therefore requires higher radiation intensity if there is to be uniform exposure of the image receptor. Abdominal imaging, on the other hand, should be taken so that the cathode is toward the head of the patient. The upper abdomen is thicker than the lower abdomen and pelvis and requires higher x-ray intensity for uniform optical density. Figure 10-19 shows two posteroanterior (PA) chest radiographs, one taken with the cathode down, the other with the cathode up. Try to figure out the difference before looking at the figure legend.

Another consequence of the heel effect is the changing focal-spot size. The effective focal spot is smaller on the anode side of the beam than on the cathode side (Figure 10-20). Manufacturers of mammography equipment take advantage of this property by angling the x-ray tube so that the smaller focal spot coincides with the thick tissue of the chest wall.

Extrafocal Radiation. X-ray tubes are designed so that projectile electrons from the cathode interact with the target only at the focal spot. Up to 15% of these electrons bounce off the focal spot and land on other areas of the target, which causes x-rays to be produced from outside of the focal spot (Figure 10-21). These x-rays are called *extrafocal* or *off-focus radiation*.

Extrafocal radiation is like squirting a water pistol at a concrete pavement. Some of the water splashes off and lands in a larger area. Extrafocal radiation is undesirable because it extends the size of the focal spot (Figure 10-22). The extrafocal radiation can significantly reduce **image contrast** and can expose patient tissue that was not intended to be imaged. Examples of such undesirable images are the ears in a skull examination, soft tissue beyond the cervical spine, and lung beyond the borders of the thoracic spine. Figure 10-23 is a postoperative radiograph of a cervical spine **fixation screw.** The area of interest is well collimated; however, the halo securing the patient's head into position has been exposed as well. This is an example of extrafocal radiation exposing areas outside the anatomy of interest. Extrafocal radiation is reduced by designing a fixed diaphragm in the tube housing near the window of the x-ray tube (Figure 10-24). Another effective solution is the metal envelope x-ray tube. Electrons reflected from the focal spot are extracted by the metal envelope and conducted away.

TUBE FAILURE
Causes

With careful use, x-ray tubes can provide many years of service. With unknowledgeable radiographers, tube life

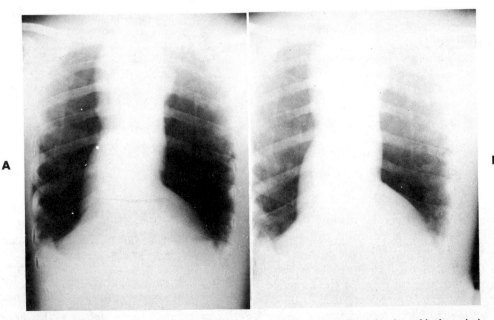

FIGURE 10-19 PA chest radiographs demonstrating the heel effect. **A,** Radiograph taken with the cathode up (superior). **B,** Radiograph with cathode down (inferior). More uniform radiographic density is obtained with the cathode positioned to the thicker side of the anatomy **(B).**

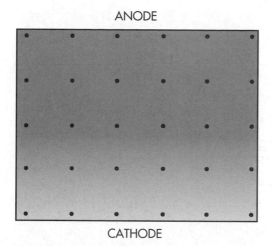

ANODE

CATHODE

FIGURE 10-20 The effective focal spot changes size and shape across the projected x-ray field.

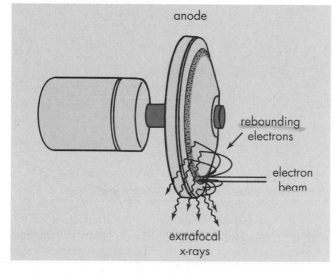

anode

rebounding electrons

electron beam

extrafocal x-rays

FIGURE 10-21 Extrafocal x-rays result from electrons interacting outside the focal spot.

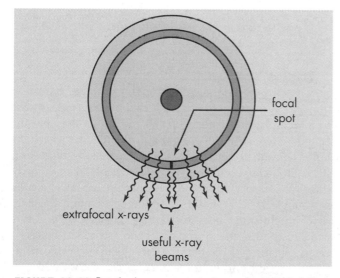

focal spot

extrafocal x-rays

useful x-ray beams

FIGURE 10-22 Extrafocal x-rays create a larger than intended focal spot. *(Courtesy Don Jacobson.)*

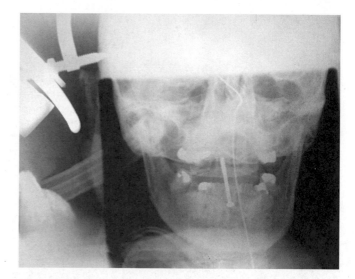

FIGURE 10-23
Extrafocal radiation exposes areas outside the anatomy of interest.

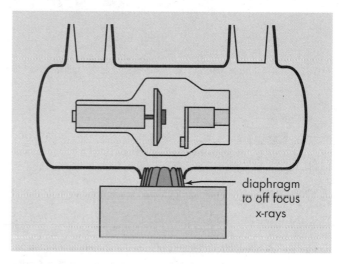

diaphragm to off focus x-rays

FIGURE 10-24 An additional diaphragm is positioned close to the focal spot to reduce extrafocal radiation.

may be shortened substantially and the tube may even fail abruptly. X-ray tube life is under the control of the radiographer. Tube life is extended by using the radiographic factors of mA, kVp, and exposure time that are appropriate for each examination. In recent years the use of faster image receptors and shorter exposure times has resulted in longer tube life. There are several causes of tube failure, all of which are related to the thermal characteristics of the x-ray tube. Enormous heat is generated in the anode of the x-ray tube during x-ray exposure. This heat must be dissipated in order for the x-ray tube to continue to function. Heat can be dissipated in three ways—(1) radiation, (2) conduction, and (3) convection (Figure 10-25). **Radiation** is the transfer of heat by the emission of infrared radiation. Heat lamps emit not only visible light but also infrared

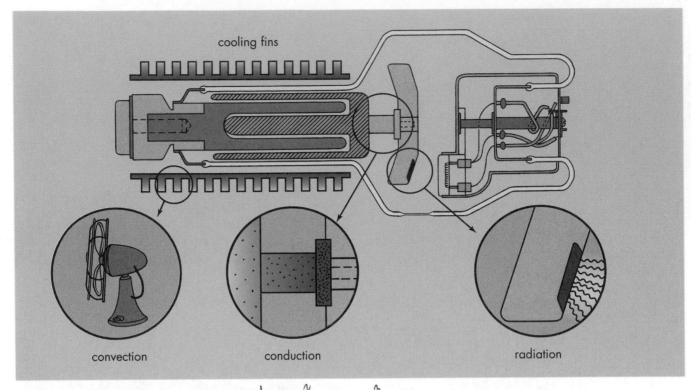

FIGURE 10-25 Heat from an anode is dissipated by radiation, conduction, and convection.

energy. **Conduction** is the transfer of energy from one area of an object to another. The handle of a heated skillet becomes hot because of conduction. **Convection** is the transfer of heat by the movement of a heated object such as air, water, or oil from one place to another. Convection can only occur in a gravity field. Many homes and offices are heated by the convection of hot air. All three modes of heat transfer occur in an x-ray tube. Most of the heat is dissipated by radiation during exposure. The anode may glow red hot. It will always emit infrared energy. Some heat is conducted through the neck of the anode to the rotor and glass envelope. The heated glass envelope raises the temperature of the oil bath, which convects the heat to the tube housing and then to room air.

Single excessive exposure. When the temperature of the anode is excessive during a single exposure, localized surface melting and pitting of the anode can occur. These surface irregularities result in variable and reduced radiation output. If the surface melting is sufficiently severe, the tungsten can be vaporized. The vaporized tungsten plates the inside of the glass envelope, which causes filtering of the x-ray beam and interference with electron flow from cathode to anode. If the temperature of the anode increases too rapidly, the anode may crack, become unstable in rotation, and render the tube useless.

Remember: To prevent pitting and cracking, maximum radiographic technical factors should never be applied to a cold anode.

If maximum technical factors are required for a particular examination, the anode should first be warmed with low-technique operation. The **warm-up procedure** is performed after 45 minutes of non-use of the x-ray unit. The procedure is as follows or as specified by the equipment manufacturer.

Warm-up procedure = three exposures 3 seconds apart at 200 mA, 1 second, 80 kVp.

Long exposure times. A second type of tube failure results from maintaining the anode at elevated temperatures for prolonged periods. During exposures lasting 1 to 3 seconds, the temperature of the anode may be sufficient to cause it to glow like an incandescent light bulb. During exposure, heat is dissipated by radiation. Between exposures, this heat is dissipated, primarily through conduction into the oil bath in which the tube is immersed. Some heat is conducted through the narrow molybdenum neck to the **rotor assembly,** and this can cause subsequent heating of the rotor bearings. Excessive heating of the bearings results in increased rotational friction and an imbalance of the rotor-anode assembly. Bearing damage is another cause of tube failure.

If the **thermal stress** on the x-ray tube anode is maintained for prolonged periods, such as during fluoroscopy, the **thermal capacity** of the total anode system and of the x-ray tube housing suffers. During fluoroscopy, the x-ray tube current is generally less than 5 mA, rather than hundreds of mA as in radiography. Under such conditions the rate of heat dissipation from the rotating target attains equilibrium with the rate of heat input, and this rate rarely is sufficient to cause surface defects in the target. The tube can fail, however, because of the continuous heat delivered to the rotor assembly, the oil bath, and the x-ray tube housing. Bearings can fail, the glass envelope can crack, and the tube housing protection can fail.

Filament vaporization. A final cause of tube failure involves the filament. Because of the high temperature of the filament, tungsten atoms are slowly vaporized even with normal use and cover the inside of the glass or metal envelope. This tungsten, along with that vaporized from the anode, can disturb the electrical balance of the x-ray tube, which causes abrupt, intermittent changes in tube current or can lead to arcing and tube failure.

Tube Failure
Vaporization of the filament and plating of the glass or metal envelope is the most frequent cause of tube failure.

Excessive heating of the filament caused by high mA operation for prolonged periods vaporizes the filament. The filament wire becomes thinner and eventually breaks, causing an **open filament**. This is the same type of failure that occurs when an incandescent light bulb burns out. In the same way that the life of a light bulb is measured in hours (2000 hours is standard) that of an x-ray tube is measured in tens of thousands of exposures. Some CT tubes are now guaranteed for 50,000 exposures.

Question: A CT x-ray tube is guaranteed for 25,000 scans. Each scan is limited to a 1-second exposure. What is the x-ray tube life in hours?

Answer: Guaranteed tube life = (25,000 scans)
(1 second/scan)

= 25,000 seconds

= 6.9 hours is the tube life for the CT tube

Prevention of Failure with Tube Rating Charts

The radiographer is guided in the use of x-ray tubes by **x-ray tube rating charts.** It is absolutely essential that the radiographer be able to read and understand these charts. Three types of x-ray tube rating charts are particularly significant to the radiographer—(1) the **radiographic rating chart,** (2) the **anode cooling chart,** and (3) the **housing cooling chart.**

Radiographic rating chart. Of the three rating charts, the radiographer rating chart is the most important.

Remember: The **radiographic rating chart** is the most important because it states which radiographic technical factors are safe and which factors are unsafe for tube operation.

Each chart in Figure 10-26 contains a family of curves representing the various tube currents in mA. The x-axis and y-axis show scales of the two other radiographic parameters—time and kVp. For a given mA, any combination of kVp and time that lies below the mA curve is safe. Any combination of kVp and time that lies above the curve is unsafe. If an unsafe exposure was made, the tube might fail abruptly.

Safe Operating Exposures
X-ray units have a built-in safety feature that will not allow an exposure to be made when the technique selected would cause the tube to exceed the safe conditions of the radiographic rating chart.

A series of radiographic rating charts accompanies every x-ray tube. These charts cover the various modes of operation possible with that tube. There are different charts for each filament (large or small focal spot), the speed of anode rotation (3400 rpm or 10,000 rpm), the target angle, and the voltage rectification (half wave, full wave, or three phase). Be sure to use the proper radiographic rating chart with each tube. This is particularly important after the replacement of x-ray tubes. An appropriate radiographic rating chart is supplied with each replacement x-ray tube and can be different from that of the original tube. The application of radiographic rating charts is not difficult.

Question: With reference to Figure 10-26, which of the following exposure factors are safe and which are unsafe?
a. 95 kVp, 150 mA, 1 second; 3400 rpm; 0.6-millimeter focal spot
b. 80 kVp, 400 mA, 0.5 second; 3400 rpm; 1-millimeter focal spot
c. 125 kVp, 500 mA, 0.1 second; 10,000 rpm; 1-millimeter focal spot
d. 75 kVp, 700 mA, 0.3 second; 10,000 rpm; 1-millimeter focal spot
e. 88 kVp, 400 mA, 0.1 second; 10,000 rpm; 0.6-millimeter focal spot

Answer: a. Unsafe   c. Safe e. Unsafe
b. Unsafe   d. Safe

Question: Radiographic examination of the abdomen with a tube that has a 0.6-mm focal spot and anode rotation of 10,000 rpm requires tech-

Small focal spot

large focal spot

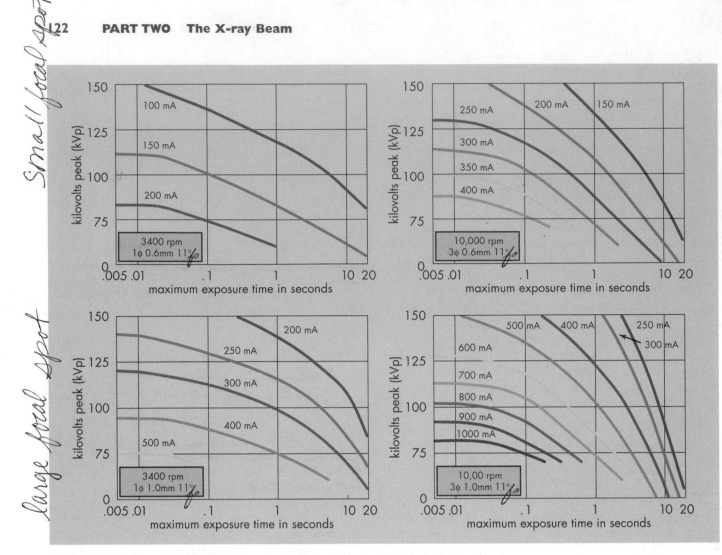

FIGURE 10-26 Representative radiographic rating charts for given x-ray tube. Each chart specifies the conditions of operation to which it applies. *(Courtesy General Electric Company.)*

nique factors of 95 kVp, 150 mAs. What is the shortest possible exposure time for this examination?

Answer: Locate the proper radiographic rating chart (upper right in Figure 10-26) and the 95 kVp line (horizontal line near middle of chart). Beginning from the left (shorter exposure time) determine the mAs for the intersection of each mA curve with the 95 kVp level.
1. The first intersection is approximately 350 mA at 0.03 second, which equals 10.5 mAs. This is not enough.
2. The next intersection is approximately 300 mA at 0.2 second, which equals 60 mAs. This is not enough.
3. The next intersection is approximately 250 mA at 0.6 second, which equals 150 mAs. This is sufficient.

Consequently, 0.6 second is the minimum possible exposure time.

Anode Cooling Chart. The anode has a limited capacity for storing heat. Although heat is dissipated to the oil bath and tube housing, it is possible through prolonged use or multiple exposures to exceed the heat storage capacity of the anode. Thermal energy is conventionally measured in units of calories, British thermal units (BTU), or joules. In x-ray applications, thermal energy is measured in **heat units (HU)**. The capacity of the anode and the housing to store heat is measured in heat units.

Heat Units for Single-phase Units

One heat unit is equal to the product of 1 kVp, 1 mA, and 1 second.

$$HU = kVp \times mA \times seconds$$

mAs

Question: Radiographic examination of the lateral lumbar spine requires 98 kVp at 120 mAs. How many heat units are generated by this exposure?

Answer: Number of heat units = 98 kVp × 120 mAs

= 11,760 HU is generated by the lateral lumbar spine exposure

Question: A fluoroscopic examination is performed at 76 kVp and 1.5 mA for 3½ minutes. How many heat units are generated?

Answer: Number of heat units = 76 kVp × 1.5 mA × 3½ minutes × 60 seconds/minute

= 23,940 HU are generated during the fluoroscopic examination

More heat is generated when three-phase equipment is used than when single-phase and high-frequency equipment is used. A modification factor is necessary for calculating three-phase heat units, so the previous equation becomes:

Heat Units for Three-phase Units

Heat Units for Three-phase 6-pulse Units

$$HU = 1.35 \times kVp \times mA \times seconds$$

Heat Units for Three-phase 12-pulse Units

$$HU = 1.41 \times kVp \times mA \times seconds$$

Question: Six sequential skull films are exposed with a three-phase generator operated at 82 kVp and 120 mAs. What is the total heat generated?

Answer: Number of heat units/film = 1.35 × 82 kVp × 120 mAs

= 13,284 HU

Total HU = 6 × 13,284 HU

= 79,704 HU for six skull films

The thermal capacity of an anode and its heat-dissipation characteristics are contained in a rating chart called an *anode cooling chart* (Figure 10-27). Unlike the radiographic rating chart, the anode cooling chart is not dependent on the filament size or the speed of rotation. The tube represented in Figure 10-27 has a maximum anode heat capacity of 350,000 HU. The chart shows that if the maximum heat load were attained, it would take 15 minutes for the anode to completely cool. The rate of cooling is rapid at first and slows as the anode cools. In addition to determining the maximum heat capacity of the anode, the anode cooling chart is used to determine the length of time required for complete cooling after any level of heat input.

Question: A particular examination results in 50,000 HU being delivered to the anode in a matter of seconds. How long will it take the anode to cool completely?

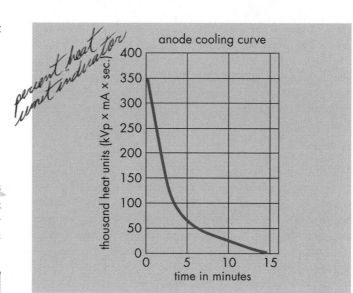

FIGURE 10-27 Anode cooling chart, which shows the time required for heated anode to cool. *(Courtesy General Electric Company.)*

Answer: The 50,000 HU level intersects the anode cooling curve at approximately 6 minutes. From that point on the curve to complete cooling requires an additional 9 minutes (15 − 6 = 9). Therefore 9 minutes are required for complete cooling.

Although the heat generated in producing x-rays is expressed in heat units, joules are the equivalent.

1 watt = 1 volt × 1 amp

= 1 kV × 1 mA

One watt of electric power is also equal to 1 joule per second.

1 watt = 1 volt × 1 amp

= 1 joule/coulomb × 1 coulomb/second

= 1 joule/second

Therefore:

1 watt = 1 joule/second = 1 kV × 1 mA

= 1 kV × 1 mA × 1 second

= 1 HU

Question: How much heat energy (in joules) is produced during a single high-frequency mammographic exposure of 25 kVp at 200 mAs?

Answer: 25 kVp × 200 mAs = 5000 joule

= 5 kJ of heat is produced during a mammographic exposure

Housing Cooling Chart

The cooling chart for the housing of the x-ray tube has a shape similar to that of the anode cooling chart and is used in precisely the same way. X-ray tube housings generally have maximum heat capacities in the range of 1 to 1.5 million HU. Complete cooling after maximum heat capacity requires from 1 to 2 hours. About twice that amount of time is required without auxiliary fan-powered air circulation.

SUMMARY

The primary support structure for the x-ray tube, which allows the greatest ease of movement and range of position, is the ceiling support system. The protective housing covers the x-ray tube and provides the following three functions: (1) it reduces leakage radiation to 100 mR per hour at 1 meter, (2) it provides mechanical support protecting the tube from damage, and (3) it serves as a way to conduct heat away from the x-ray target. The glass or metal envelope surrounds the cathode ($-$) and anode ($+$), which are the electrodes at the ends of the vacuum tube. The cathode contains the tungsten filament, which is the source of space charge of electrons. The rotating anode is the tungsten-rhenium disk, which serves as a target for the accelerating electrons streaming from the cathode. To prevent wear of the target, most tubes have a target that is powered by an induction motor. Anode designs that exhibit the line-focus principle have angled targets. The heel effect is defined as the variation in x-ray intensity across the beam because of absorption of the x-rays in the heel of the target.

Tube failure can be prevented, and safe operation of the x-ray tube is the responsibility of the radiographer. The causes of tube failure are threefold:

1. A single excessive exposure causes pitting or cracking of the anode.
2. Long exposure times cause excessive heating of the anode components, resulting in damage to the bearings in the rotor assembly. Bearing damage causes warping and rotational friction of the anode eventually causing tube failure.
3. Even with normal use, vaporization of the filament causes tungsten atoms to coat the glass or metal envelope, which eventually causes arcing and tube failure. Tube rating charts printed by manufacturers of x-ray tubes aid the radiographer in using acceptable exposure levels to maintain x-ray tube life.

REVIEW QUESTIONS

1. List the six main methods used to support the x-ray tube and briefly describe each method.
2. Define SID.
3. _____ _____ contributes nothing in the way of diagnostic information and results in unnecessary exposure to the patient and radiographer.
4. What is the length and diameter of an x-ray tube?
5. Why are arcing and tube failure no longer a problem in modern x-ray tube design?
6. Explain the phenomenon of thermionic emission.
7. Describe the principal cause of x-ray tube failure. What addition to the filament material prolongs tube life?
8. What is the reason for the filament to be embedded in a focusing cup?
9. The cloud of electrons surrounding the filament is called the _____ _____ .
10. Why are x-ray tubes manufactured with two focal spots?
11. Match the following:
    Anode   Negative charge
    Cathode   Positive charge
12. List and describe the two types of anodes.
13. What are the three functions the anode serves in an x-ray tube? List the three common anode materials.
14. How does atomic number, thermal conductivity, and melting point affect the anode target material?
15. Draw diagrams of the stationary and the rotating anodes.
16. The revolutions per minute of the rotating anode equal _____ .
17. How does the anode rotate inside a glass envelope with no mechanical connection to the outside?
18. Use a drawing to show the difference between the actual and effective focal spot.
19. Define the heel effect and describe how it can be used advantageously.
20. List the x-ray tube warm-up procedure and explain the three causes of x-ray tube failure.

TUBE RATING CHART QUESTIONS

1. Using a single-phase radiographic unit, a shoulder x-ray examination is performed using 70 kVp at 12 mAs. How many heat units are generated using this exposure?
2. A series of x-rays were completed in rapid succession on a multitrauma case from a motor vehicle accident. Using the following list and technical factors, determine the heat units generated from this case on a three-phase 6 pulse unit.
   Pelvis (anterior position) 80 kVp at 40 mAs
   Hip (lateral cross-table) 80 kVp at 50 mAs

Thoracic spine (anterior position) 80 kVp at 20 mAs

Thoracic spine (lateral position) 70 kVp at 50 mA at 2.5 seconds

3. Refer to the radiographic rating charts in Figure 10-26 to complete the following question. The radiographer selects the high speed anode (10,000 rpm) on the three-phase unit and the large focal spot for a pediatric case. Because the radiographer wants to use the shortest possible exposure time to minimize patient motion, 1000 mA was selected. What is the highest possible kVp that can be used on this case?

Additional Reading

Pirtle OL: X-ray machine calibration: a study of failure rates, *Radiol Technol* 65(5):291, May-June 1994.

X-ray Production

OBJECTIVES

At the completion of this chapter the student will be able to:

1. Discuss the interactions between electrons and the x-ray target
2. Identify the graphs depicting the x-ray emission spectra for characteristic and bremsstrahlung radiation
3. Explain how mAs, kVp, added filtration, target material, and voltage ripple affect x-ray emission spectra

OUTLINE

Electron-Target Interactions
   Heat production
   Characteristic radiation
   Bremsstrahlung radiation
X-ray Emission Spectrum
   Characteristic x-ray spectrum
   Bremsstrahlung x-ray spectrum
   Minimum wavelength equals
    maximum x-ray energy

Factors Affecting X-ray Emission Spectrum
   Effect of mA
   Effect of kVp
   Effect of added filtration
   Effect of target material
   Influence of voltage waveform

I n Chapter 10 the internal components of the x-ray tube, the cathode and anode within the evacuated glass or metal envelope, are outlined. This chapter explains the interaction between the stream of electrons from the cathode and the tungsten target or anode.

. . . .

ELECTRON-TARGET INTERACTION
Heat Production

The primary function of the x-ray tube is to accelerate electrons from the cathode to the anode. The three principal parts of an x-ray unit are as follows: (1) the operating console, (2) the high-voltage generator, and (3) the x-ray tube. All the components are designed to provide a large number of electrons in the cathode to be accelerated and focused toward a small spot on the anode. When the electrons speed toward the anode, they have high kinetic energy. Remember that kinetic energy is the energy of motion. Stationary objects have no kinetic energy. Objects in motion have kinetic energy proportional to their masses and to the square of their velocities.

Kinetic Energy Review

The equation used to calculate kinetic energy is as follows:

$$KE = \tfrac{1}{2} m \times v^2$$

m is the mass in kilograms
v is the velocity in meters per second
KE is the kinetic energy in joules

For example, a 1000-kilogram automobile has four times the kinetic energy that a 250-kilogram motorcycle has when they are traveling at the same speed (Figure 11-1). If the motorcycle were to double its velocity, however, it would have the same kinetic energy as the automobile.

Kinetic Energy and Velocity
In determining the magnitude of the kinetic energy of a projectile, velocity is more important than mass.

In an x-ray tube the projectile is the electron. All electrons have the same mass; therefore, electron kinetic energy is increased by raising kVp. As electron kinetic energy is increased, both the intensity (mAs) and the energy (kVp) of the x-ray beam increases.

The modern x-ray machine is remarkable. It conveys to the target an enormous number of electrons at a precisely controlled kinetic energy. At 100 mA, for example, 6×10^{17} electrons travel from the cathode to the anode of the x-ray tube every second. In an x-ray unit

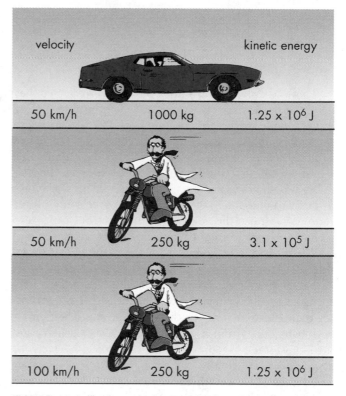

velocity		kinetic energy
50 km/h	1000 kg	1.25×10^6 J
50 km/h	250 kg	3.1×10^5 J
100 km/h	250 kg	1.25×10^6 J

FIGURE 11-1 Kinetic energy is proportional to the product of mass and velocity squared. If the weight of a motorcycle is one fourth that of an automobile and the motorcycle is traveling twice as fast as the automobile, then the motorcycle and the automobile have equal kinetic energies.

operating at 70 kVp, each electron arrives at the target with a maximum kinetic energy of 70 keV. Since there are 1.6×10^{-16} J per keV, this energy is equivalent to the following:

$$(70 \text{ keV}) (1.6 \times 10^{-16} \text{ J/keV}) = 1.12 \times 10^{-14} \text{J}$$

is the energy of electrons arriving at the target at 70 keV

Inserting this energy into the kinetic energy equation and solving for the velocity of the electrons, we find the following:

$$KE = \tfrac{1}{2} m \times v^2$$

$$v^2 = 2\,\frac{KE}{m}$$

$$1.12 \times 10^{-14} \text{ J} = \tfrac{1}{2}(9.1 \times 10^{-31} \text{ kg})v^2$$

$$v^2 = \frac{(2)\,(1.12 \times 10^{-14} \text{ J})}{(9.1 \times 10^{-31} \text{ kg})}$$

$$= 0.25 \times 10^{17} \text{ m}^2/\text{s}^2$$

$v = 1.6 \times 10^8$ m/s is the velocity of electrons arriving at the target at 70 keV

Question: At what fraction of the velocity of light do 70 keV electrons travel?

127

Answer: $\dfrac{v}{c} = \dfrac{1.6 \times 10^8 \text{ m/s}}{3.0 \times 10^8 \text{ m/s}} = 0.53$

70 keV electrons travel at 0.53 times the velocity of light

These calculations are not precisely correct, but they do serve to illustrate the point and demonstrate the use of the kinetic energy equation on page 127. According to the theory of relativity, the mass of the electron increases as it approaches the speed of light, thus the actual value of v/c is 0.47 at 70 keV. The distance between the filament and the target is only 1 to 3 centimeters. It is not difficult to imagine the intensity of the accelerating force required to raise the velocity of the electrons from zero to half the speed of light in so short a distance.

The electrons traveling from the cathode to the anode comprise the x-ray-tube current and are sometimes called *projectile electrons*. When these projectile electrons hit the heavy metal atoms of the target, they transfer their kinetic energy to the target atoms. These interactions occur within a very small depth of penetration into the target. As they occur, the projectile electrons slow down and finally come nearly to rest. Then they are conducted through the x-ray anode assembly and out into the associated electronic circuitry. The projectile electron interacts with either the orbital electrons or the nuclei of target atoms. The interactions result in the conversion of kinetic energy into thermal energy (heat) and electromagnetic energy in the form of **infrared radiation** and x-rays.

The projectile electrons interact with the outer-shell electrons of the target atoms but do not transfer sufficient energy to these outer-shell electrons to ionize them. Instead, the outer-shell electrons are simply raised to an excited, or higher, energy level. The outer-shell electrons immediately drop back to their normal energy level with the emission of infrared radiation or heat. The constant **excitation** and return of outer-shell electrons are responsible for the heat generated in the anodes of x-ray tubes.

Heat Production

Generally, more than 99% of the kinetic energy of projectile electrons is converted to heat, which leaves less than 1% available for the production of radiation (Figure 11-2).

Sophisticated as the x-ray tube is, it is really very inefficient. The production of heat in the anode increases directly with increasing tube current. Doubling the tube current doubles the quantity of heat produced. Heat production also increases directly with increasing kVp, at least in the diagnostic range. Although the relationship between varying kVp and varying heat production is approximate, it is sufficiently exact to allow the computation of heat units for use with anode cooling charts. The efficiency of x-ray production is independent of the

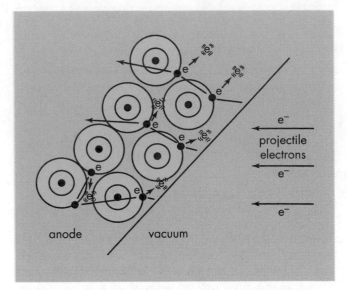

FIGURE 11-2 Most of the kinetic energy of projectile electrons is transformed into heat by interactions with outer-shell electrons of target atoms. These interactions are primarily excitations rather than ionizations.

tube current. Consequently, regardless of what mA station is selected, the efficiency of x-ray production remains constant. The efficiency of x-ray production increases with increasing kVp. At 60 kVp, only 0.5% of the electron kinetic energy is converted to x-rays. At 100 kVp, approximately 1% is converted to x-rays, and at 20 MV, 70% of the kinetic energy is converted into x-rays.

Characteristic Radiation

Characteristic Radiation

If the projectile electron interacts with an inner-shell electron of the target atom rather than with an outer-shell electron, **characteristic x-rays** can be produced. Characteristic x-rays result when the interaction is sufficiently violent to ionize the target atom by totally removing an inner-shell electron.

The inner-shell electron is tightly bound to the nucleus (see Chapter 4). Thus, K-shell electrons or inner-shell electrons have a higher binding energy than outer-shell electrons. Tungsten is a large atom with 74 orbiting electrons. As atomic complexity increases, the electrons in any given shell are more tightly bound than in a less complex atom.

Figure 11-3 illustrates how these characteristic x-rays are produced. When the projectile electron ionizes a target atom by removing a K-shell electron, a temporary electron void is produced in the K shell. This is a highly unnatural state for the target atom and is corrected by an outer-shell electron falling into the void in the K shell. Tungsten, for example, has electrons in shells out to the P shell, and when a K-shell electron is ionized, its

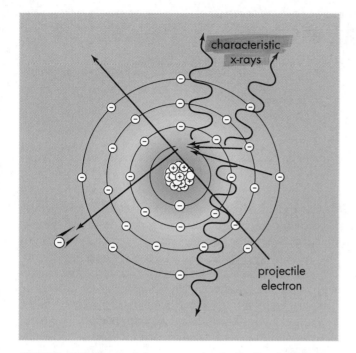

FIGURE 11-3 Characteristic x-rays are produced after the ionization of a K-shell electron. When an outer-shell electron fills the vacancy in the K shell, an x-ray is emitted.

position can be filled with electrons from any of the outer shells. The transition of an orbital electron from an outer shell to an inner shell is accompanied by the emission of an x-ray.

Characteristic Radiation

The x-ray has energy equal to the difference in the **binding energies** of the orbital electrons involved.

Question: A K-shell electron is removed from a tungsten atom and is replaced by an L-shell electron. What is the energy of the characteristic x-ray that is emitted?

Answer: Refer to Figure 11-4, which shows that for tungsten, K electrons have binding energies of 69.5 keV and L electrons are bound by 12.1 keV. Therefore the characteristic x-ray emitted has an energy of

69.5 − 12.1 = 57.4 keV

By the same procedure, the energy of x-rays resulting from M-to-K, N-to-K, O-to-K, and P-to-K transitions can be calculated. All these x-rays are called *K x-rays* because they result from ionization of K-shell electrons. Similar characteristic x-rays are produced when the target atom is ionized by removal of electrons from shells other than the K shell. A diagram of this would show the removal of an L-shell electron by the projectile electron. The vacancy in the L shell would be filled by an

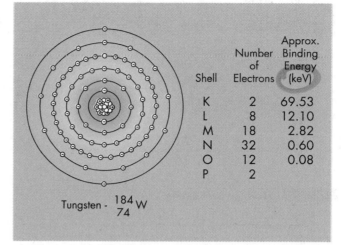

FIGURE 11-4 Atomic configuration and electron-binding energies for tungsten.

electron from any of the outer shells. X-rays resulting from electron transitions to the L shell are called *L x-rays* and are much less energetic than K x-rays, since the binding energy of an L-shell electron is much lower than that of a K-shell electron.

Similarly, M-characteristic x-rays, N-characteristic x-rays, and even O-characteristic x-rays can be produced in a tungsten target. Table 11-1 summarizes the production of characteristic x-rays in tungsten. Although many characteristic x-rays can be produced, it should be emphasized that they can be produced only at specific energies, equal to the differences in the electron-binding energies for the various electron transitions.

K X-rays   *diagnostic significance*

Except for K x-rays, all the characteristic x-rays have very low energy. Only the K-characteristic x-rays with an effective energy of 69 keV are useful for making a diagnostic radiograph.

The L x-rays, with approximately 12 keV of energy, penetrate only a few centimeters into soft tissue. Consequently, they are totally useless as diagnostic x-rays, as are all the other low-energy characteristic x-rays. The last column in Table 11-1 shows the effective energy for each of the characteristic x-rays of tungsten. These effective values will be referred to later.

In summary, characteristic x-rays are produced by transitions of orbital electrons from outer to inner shells. Because the electron binding energy for every element is different, the energy of characteristic x-rays produced in the various elements is also different. This type of radiation is called *characteristic radiation* because it is a characteristic of the target element. The effective energy of characteristic x-rays increases with the increasing atomic number of the target element.

TABLE 11-1

Characteristic X-rays of Tungsten and Their Effective Energies (keV)

Character	Electron Transistion From					Effective Energy
	L Shell	M Shell	N Shell	O Shell	P Shell	
K	57.4	66.7	68.9	69.4	69.5	69 keV
L		9.3	11.5	12.0	12.1	12 keV
M			2.2	2.7	2.8	2 keV
N				0.52	0.6	0.6 keV
O					0.08	0.08 keV

Bremsstrahlung Radiation

The production of heat and characteristic x-rays involves interactions between the projectile electrons and the electrons of target atoms. Another type of interaction in which the projectile electron can lose its kinetic energy is an interaction with the nucleus of a target atom. In this type of interaction the kinetic energy of the projectile electron is converted into electromagnetic energy.   *kinetic → electromagnetic*

A projectile electron that completely avoids the orbital electrons as it passes through a target atom may come sufficiently close to the nucleus of the atom to come under its influence (Figure 11-5). Because the electron is negatively charged and the nucleus is positively charged, there is an electrostatic force of attraction between them. The closer the projectile electron gets to the nucleus, the more it is influenced by the elec-

trostatic field of the nucleus. This field is very strong because the nucleus contains many protons and the distance between the nucleus and projectile electron is very small. As the projectile electron passes by the nucleus, it slows down, changes its course, and leaves with reduced kinetic energy in a different direction. This loss in kinetic energy reappears as an x-ray. These types of x-rays are called *bremsstrahlung x-rays*. Bremsstrahlung is a German word for slowing down or braking.

> **Bremsstrahlung Radiation**
> Bremsstrahlung radiation can be considered radiation resulting from the braking of projectile electrons by the nucleus.

A projectile electron can lose any amount of its kinetic energy in an interaction with the nucleus of a target atom, and the bremsstrahlung radiation associated with the loss can take on a corresponding range of values. For example, when an x-ray unit is operated at 70 kVp, projectile electrons have kinetic energies up to 70 keV. An electron with kinetic energy of 70 keV can lose any level of kinetic energy in a bremsstrahlung interaction. Therefore the bremsstrahlung x-ray produced can have any energy in the range of 0 to 70 keV.

This is different from the production of characteristic x-rays, which have specified energies. Bremsstrahlung x-rays are randomly emitted from the target. A low-energy bremsstrahlung x-ray results when the projectile electron is barely influenced by the nucleus. A maximum-energy x-ray occurs when the projectile electron loses all its kinetic energy and simply drifts away from the nucleus. Bremsstrahlung x-rays can be produced at any projectile electron energy. However, K-characteristic x-rays require a tube potential of at least 70 kVp because of the K-shell binding energy of tungsten.

> **Bremsstrahlung Radiation**
> In the **diagnostic range,** most x-rays are of bremsstrahlung origin.

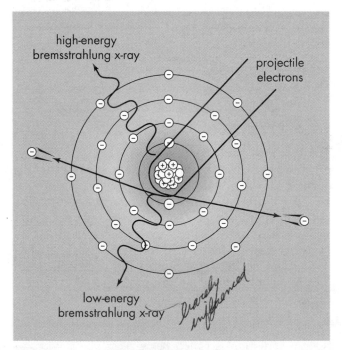

FIGURE 11-5 Bremsstrahlung x-rays result from an interaction between a projectile electron and a target nucleus. The electron is slowed down and its direction is changed.

At 100 kVp, for example, only approximately 15% of the x-ray beam results from characteristic radiation.

X-RAY EMISSION SPECTRUM

Most people have seen or heard of pitching machines (the devices used by baseball teams for batting practice so that the pitchers do not get worn out). There are similar machines for automatically ejecting bowling balls, tennis balls, and even ping-pong balls. Suppose there was a device that could eject all these types of balls at random at a rate of one per second. The most straightforward way to determine how often each type of ball is ejected on the average would be to catch each ball as it was ejected, identify it, and drop it into a basket, so that at the end of the observation period the total number of each type of ball could be counted. Suppose that the results obtained for a 10-minute period are those shown in Figure 11-6. A total of 600 balls were ejected. Perhaps the easiest way to represent these results graphically would be to plot the total number of each type of ball emitted during the 10-minute observation period and represent each total by a bar (Figure 11-7). Such a bar graph can be described as a <u>discrete ball-ejection spectrum</u> that is representative of the automatic pitching machine. It is a plot of the number of balls ejected per unit of time based on the type of ball. Only five distinct types of balls are involved. Connecting the bars with a curved line as shown would indicate a large number of different balls. Such a curve is called a *continuous ejection spectrum*. The word *spectrum* refers to the range of types. The total number of balls ejected is represented by the sum of the areas under the bars, in the case of the discrete spectrum, and the area under the curve, in the case of the continuous spectrum. Without regard to the absolute number of balls emitted, Figure 11-7 could also be identified as a <u>relative</u> ball-ejection

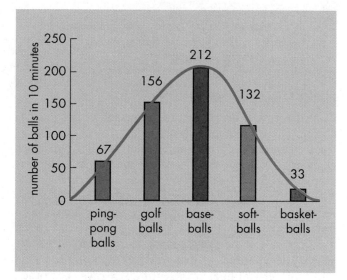

FIGURE 11-7 Bar graph representing results of 10-minute observation of balls ejected by the automatic pitching machine in Figure 11-6.

spectrum since at a glance one can tell the relative frequency of ejection of each type of ball. Relatively speaking, baseballs are ejected most frequently and basketballs least frequently. If the ball-ejection machine operated randomly, the results of this 10-minute observation would be characteristic of any time of observation.

This type of relationship is fundamental to describing the output of an x-ray unit. If one could stand in the middle of the useful x-ray beam and could catch each individual x-ray and measure its energy, one could describe what is known as the *x-ray emission spectrum* (Figure 11-8). Here the relative number of x-rays emitted is plotted as a function of the energy of each individual x-ray. Although a person cannot catch and identify each individual x-ray, there are instruments available that can do just that. X-ray emission spectra have been measured for all types of x-ray machines.

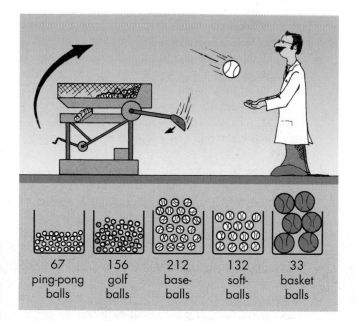

FIGURE 11-6 In a 10-minute period an automatic ball-throwing machine might eject 600 balls that are distributed as shown.

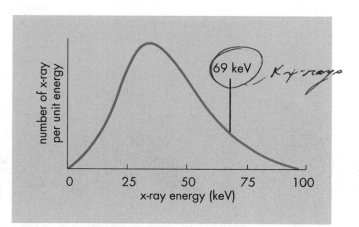

FIGURE 11-8 General form of an x-ray emission spectrum.

X-ray Emission Spectra

Understanding x-ray emission spectra is a key to understanding how changes in kVp, mA, time, and filtration affect the optical density and contrast of a radiograph.

Characteristic X-ray Spectrum

Characteristic x-rays have precisely fixed or discrete energies. These energies are characteristic of the differences between electron-binding energies of a particular element. A characteristic x-ray from tungsten, for example, can have 1 of 15 energies and no others (Table 11-1). A plot of the frequency with which characteristic x-rays are emitted as a function of their energy would look like that shown for tungsten in Figure 11-9. Such a plot is called the *characteristic x-ray emission spectrum.* There are five vertical lines representing K x-rays and four vertical lines representing L x-rays. The other, lower-energy lines represent characteristic emissions from the outer electron shells. The relative intensity of the K x-rays is greater than that of the lower-energy characteristic x-rays because of the nature of the interaction process. K x-rays are the only characteristic x-rays of tungsten with sufficient energy to be of value in diagnostic radiology. Although there are five K x-rays, it is customary to represent them as one, as has been done with a single vertical line at 69 keV in Figure 11-9. Only this line will be shown in later graphs.

Bremsstrahlung X-ray Spectrum

If it were possible to measure the energy contained in each bremsstrahlung photon emitted from an x-ray tube, one would find that these energies range from the peak electron energy all the way down to zero. In other words, when an x-ray tube is operated at 70 kVp, bremsstrahlung photons with energies ranging from 0 to 70 keV are emitted. A typical **bremsstrahlung x-ray emission spectrum** is shown in Figure 11-10. The gen-

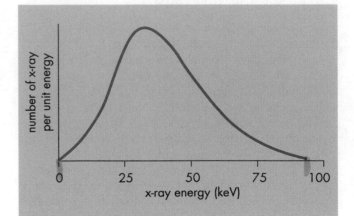

FIGURE 11-10 Bremsstrahlung x-ray emission spectrum extends from zero to maximum projectile electron energy, with the highest number of x-rays having approximately one third the maximum energy.

kVp = max. energy

eral shape of the bremsstrahlung x-ray spectrum is the same for all x-ray machines. The maximum energy that an x-ray can have is numerically equal to the kVp of operation. This is why it is called *kVp* (peak kilovoltage). However, the greatest number of x-rays emitted have energies approximately one third of the maximum energy. The number of x-rays emitted decreases at very low energies and below 5 keV nearly reaches zero.

Question: At what kVp was the x-ray machine represented in Figure 11-10 operated?

Answer: Because the bremsstrahlung spectrum intersects the energy axis at approximately 90 keV, the machine must have been operated at approximately 90 kVp.

There are four principal factors influencing the shape of an x-ray emission spectrum:

1. The electrons accelerated from cathode to anode do not all have the peak kinetic energy. Depending on the type of rectification and high-voltage generator, many of these electrons may have very low energies when they strike the target. Such electrons can produce only low-energy x-rays.
2. The target of a diagnostic x-ray tube is relatively thick. Consequently, many of the bremsstrahlung x-rays emitted result from multiple interactions of the projectile electrons. For each successive interaction, the projectile electron has less and less energy.
3. Low-energy x-rays are more likely to be absorbed in the target.
4. **External filtration** is nearly always added to the x-ray tube assembly. This added filtration serves to selectively remove low-energy x-rays from the beam.

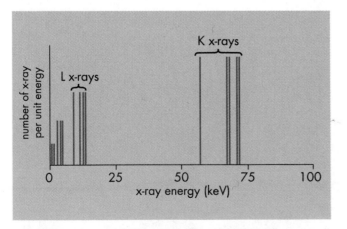

FIGURE 11-9 Characteristic x-ray emission spectrum for tungsten contains 15 different x-ray energies.

Question: Construct the expected emission spectrum for an x-ray machine with a pure molybdenum target (effective energy of K x-ray equals 19 keV) operated at 95 kVp.

Answer: The spectrum should look similar to the figure below. The curve intersects the energy axis at 0 and 95 keV and has the general shape shown in Figure 11-8, except the bremsstrahlung spectrum is much lower. A line extends above the curve at 19 keV to represent the characteristic x-rays.

Minimum Wavelength Equals Maximum X-ray Energy

As described in Chapter 5 the energy of an x-ray photon is equal to the product of the photon frequency and Planck's constant (h). X-ray energy is also inversely proportional to the photon wavelength (the equation in which $E = h \times c/\lambda$). As photon wavelength increases, photon energy decreases.

> **Minimum Wavelength**
>
> Maximum x-ray energy is associated with minimum x-ray wavelength (λ_{min}).

To solve for the minimum wavelength of x-ray emission, follow the next calculation.

To calculate λ_{min}, one must solve the following equation for λ:

$$\lambda = \frac{h \times c}{E}$$

Planck's constant

Both h and c are constant (h − 4.15×10^{-15} eV-s, $c = 3 \times 10^8$ m/s) and therefore:

$$\lambda - \frac{12.4 \times 10^{-7}\ \text{eV-m}}{E}$$

Because the minimum wavelength of x-ray emission corresponds to the maximum x-ray energy and the max-

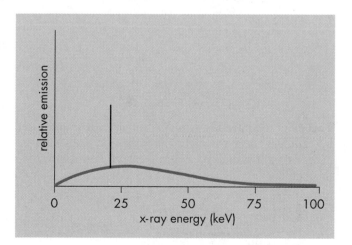

Graph of relative emission versus x-ray energy in keV.

imum x-ray energy is numerically equal to the kVp (or kVp = keV), the previous equation can be expressed as follows:

$$\lambda_{min} = \frac{12.4 \times 10^{-10}}{kVp}$$

kVp = keV

where λ_{min} is in meters.

To express λ_{min} in nanometers (nm) apply the following conversion factor:

$$1\ \text{nm} = 10^{-9}\ \text{meters}$$

Question: What is the minimum wavelength associated with the x-rays emitted from an x-ray machine operated at 100 kVp?

Answer: At 100 kVp, the maximum photon energy will be 100 keV.

$$\lambda_{min} = \frac{12.4 \times 10^{-10}}{100\ \text{kVp}}$$

$$= 0.124 \times 10^{-10}\ \text{m}$$

$$= 0.0124\ \text{nm is the minimum wavelength associated with 100 kVp.}$$

FACTORS AFFECTING THE X-RAY EMISSION SPECTRUM

The total number of x-rays emitted from an x-ray tube could be determined by adding the number of x-rays emitted at each energy over the entire spectrum through a process called *integration*. Graphically, the total number of x-rays emitted is equivalent to the area under the curve. The general shape of an emission spectrum is always the same, but its relative position along the energy axis can change. The farther to the right a spectrum is, the higher the effective energy or quality of the x-ray beam. The greater the area under the curve, the higher the x-ray intensity or quantity of photons in the beam. Factors that are controlled by the radiographer influence the size and shape of the x-ray emission spectrum.

Effect of mA = *quantity*

Changing the mA station from 200 to 400 mA while all other conditions remain constant results in twice as many electrons flowing from cathode to anode. This operating change produces twice as many x-rays of every energy. In other words the x-ray emission spectrum will be changed in amplitude but not in shape (Figure 11-11). Each point on the curve labeled 400 mA is precisely two times higher than the associated point on the 200-mA curve.

> **Effect of mA**
>
> A change in mA results in a directly proportional change in the amplitude of the x-ray emission spectrum at all energies.

greater area under the curve.

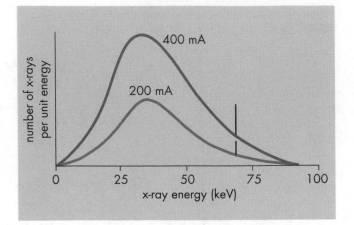

FIGURE 11-11 Change in tube mA results in a proportionate change in the amplitude of the x-ray emission spectrum at all energies.

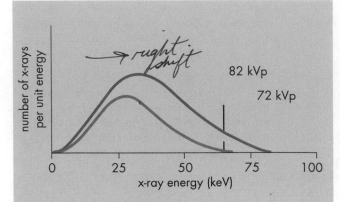

FIGURE 11-12 Change in kVp results in an increase in the amplitude of the emission spectrum at all energies but a greater increase at high energies than at low energies. Therefore the spectrum is shifted to the right, or high-energy, side.

This relationship also is true for changes in mAs. Thus the area under the x-ray emission curve varies directly in proportion to changes in mA or mAs, as does the x-ray quantity.

Question: Suppose the area under the 200-mA curve in Figure 11-11 totals 4.2 cm², and the x-ray quantity is 325 mR (84 μC/kg). What would the area under the curve and the x-ray quantity be if the tube current were increased to 400 mA while other operating factors remained constant?

Answer: In going from 200 to 400 mA, the tube current has been increased by a factor of two. The area under the curve and the x-ray quantity are increased proportionately:

$$\text{Area} = 4.2 \text{ cm}^2 \times 2 = 8.4 \text{ cm}^2$$

$$\text{Intensity} = 325 \text{ mR} \times 2 = 650 \text{ mR}$$

Effect of kVp

> **Effect of kVp**
> A change in kVp affects both the amplitude and the position of the x-ray emission spectrum. When kVp is increased, the relative distribution of emitted x-rays shifts to the right to higher x-ray energies.

As kVp is raised, the area under the curve increases to an area approximating the square of the factor by which kVp was increased. Accordingly, the x-ray quantity increases with the square of this factor as well. Figure 11-12 demonstrates the effect of increasing the kVp while other factors remain constant. The lower spectrum represents x-ray operation at 72 kVp, and the upper spectrum represents operation at 82 kVp, which is a

10-kVp increase. It can be seen that the area under the curve has approximately doubled, and the relative position of the curve has been shifted to the right to the high-energy side. More x-rays are emitted at all energies during operation at 82 kVp than during operation at 72 kVp. The increase, however, is relatively greater for high-energy x-rays than for low-energy x-rays. A change in kVp does not shift the position of the discrete x-ray emission spectrum.

Question: Suppose the curve labeled 72 kVp in Figure 11-12 covers a total area of 3.6 cm² and represents an x-ray quantity of 125 mR (32 μC/kg). What area under the curve and what x-ray quantity would be expected for operation at 82 kVp?

Answer: The area under the curve and the output intensity are proportional to the **square** of the ratio of the kVp. A ratio can be established.

$$\left(\frac{82}{72}\right)^2 (3.6 \text{ cm}^2) = (1.3)(3.6 \text{ cm}^2)$$

$$= 4.7 \text{ cm}^2$$

and

$$(1.3)(125 \text{ mR}) = 163 \text{ mR}$$

This example partially explains the rule of thumb used by radiographers to relate the kVp and mAs changes necessary to produce a constant optical density on a radiograph.

> **15% kVp Rule**
> The rule states that a 15% increase in kVp is equivalent to doubling the mAs.

At low kVp levels (e.g., 50 to 60 kVp), a 7-kVp increase is equivalent to doubling the mAs. At tube potentials above about 100 kVp, a 15-kVp change may be necessary. A 15% increase in kVp does not double the output intensity from an x-ray machine, but a 15% increase is equivalent to doubling the mAs to obtain a given optical density on the radiograph. To double the output intensity by increasing kVp, one would have to raise the kVp by as much as 40%. Radiographically, only a 15% increase in kVp is necessary because with increased kVp, the penetrability of the beam is increased and less radiation is absorbed by the patient, leaving proportionately more to expose the film.

Effect of Added Filtration

Adding filtration to an x-ray tube has an effect on the relative shape of the spectrum similar to that of increasing the kVp. This effect is shown in Figure 11-13 in which a tube is operated at 95 kVp with 2 millimeters aluminum (Al) added filtration compared with the same operation with 4 millimeters Al added filtration. Added filtration effectively absorbs low-energy x-rays and allows high-energy x-rays to pass through. Therefore the bremsstrahlung x-ray emission spectrum is reduced more on the left than on the right.

> **Added Filtration**
> The overall result of added filtration is an increase in the effective energy of the x-ray beam (higher quality) with an accompanying reduction in x-ray quantity.

Adding filtration is sometimes called *hardening* the x-ray beam. The characteristic spectrum is not affected nor is the maximum energy of x-ray emission. Furthermore, there is no simple method to calculate the changes in x-ray quality and quantity with a change in filtration.

Effect of Target Material

The atomic number of the target material affects both the number (quantity) and the effective energy (quality) of x-rays.

> **Target Material**
> As the atomic number of the target material increases, the efficiency of the production of bremsstrahlung radiation increases and the high-energy x-rays increase in number more than the low-energy x-rays.

The change in the bremsstrahlung x-ray spectrum is not nearly so pronounced as the change in the characteristic spectrum. After an increase in the atomic number of the target material, the characteristic spectrum is shifted to the right, representing the higher-energy characteristic radiation. This phenomenon is a direct result of the higher electron-binding energies associated with increasing atomic numbers. These changes are shown schematically in Figure 11-14. Tungsten is the primary component of x-ray targets, but some specialty tubes use gold as target material. The atomic numbers for tungsten and gold are 74 and 79, respectively. Molybdenum (Z = 42) and rhodium (Z = 45) are target elements used for mammography. Most dedicated mammography machines have molybdenum targets. The x-ray quantity from such targets is low due to the inefficiency of x-ray production (Figure 11-14). This occurs as a result of molybdenum's low atomic number. Low atomic numbers also produce low-energy characteristic x-rays, but low-energy x-rays are required for imaging at low kVp (23 to 32) levels for the soft tissue detail in mammography.

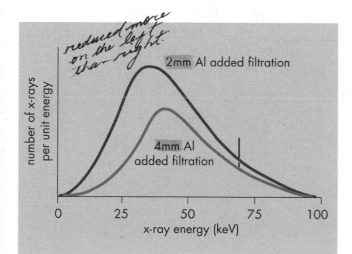

FIGURE 11-13 Adding filtration to an x-ray tube results in reduced x-ray intensity but increased effective energy. The emission spectra represented here result from operation at the same mAs and kVp but with different filtration.

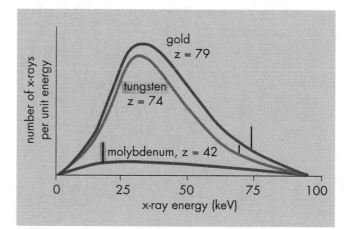

FIGURE 11-14 Discrete emission spectrum shifts to the right with an increase in the atomic number of the target material. The continuous spectrum increases slightly in amplitude, particularly to the high-energy side, with an increase in target atomic number.

Influence of Voltage Waveform

In Chapter 9 the various types of voltage waveforms produced by modern x-ray generators are discussed. There are principally five voltage waveforms: (1) half-wave rectification; (2) full-wave rectification; (3) three-phase, six-pulse power; (4) three-phase, 12-pulse power; and (5) high frequency.

Half-wave and full-wave–rectified voltage waveforms are the same except for the frequency of x-ray pulse repetition. There are twice as many x-ray pulses per cycle with full wave rectification as with half-wave rectification.

The difference between three-phase, six-pulse and three-phase, 12-pulse power is simply the reduced ripple obtained with 12-pulse generation compared with six-pulse generation. High-frequency generators are based on fundamentally different electrical engineering principles. They produce the lowest voltage ripple of all generators.

Figure 11-15 shows an exploded view of a full-wave–rectified voltage waveform for an x-ray unit operated at 100 kVp. Recall that the amplitude of the waveform corresponds to the applied voltage and that the horizontal axis represents time. At t = 0, the voltage across the x-ray tube is 0 volts, indicating that at this instant no electrons are flowing and no x-rays are being produced. At t = 1 millisecond, the voltage across the x-ray tube has increased from 0 to approximately 10,000 volts. The x-rays produced at this instant are of relatively low intensity and energy; none exceeds 10 keV. At t = 2.1 milliseconds, the tube voltage has increased to approximately 25,000 volts and is rapidly approaching its peak value. At t = 4.2 millisecond, the maximum tube voltage is obtained and the maximum energy and intensity of x-ray emission are produced. For the following one-quarter cycle between 4.2 and 8.3 milliseconds, the x-ray quantity and quality decrease again to zero.

The number of x-rays emitted at each instant through a cycle is not proportional to the voltage. The number increases slowly at lower voltages and more rapidly at higher voltages. The quantity of x-rays is much higher at peak voltages than at lower voltages. Consequently, voltage waveforms of three-phase or high-frequency operation result in considerably more intense x-ray emission than those of single-phase operation. This relationship between x-ray quantity and type of high-voltage generator is the basis for another rule of thumb used by radiographers.

> **Three-Phase Power versus Single-Phase Power**
> Operation with three-phase power is equivalent to a 12% increase in kVp or almost a doubling of mAs over single-phase power.

For example, if a lateral skull technique calls for 72 kVp on single-phase equipment, on three-phase equipment approximately 64 kVp produces similar results. High-frequency generators result in an approximate equivalent of a 16% increase in kVp.

This discussion is summarized in Figure 11-16. An x-ray emission spectrum from a full-wave–rectified unit is compared with that from a 12-pulse, three-phase generator and a high-frequency generator, all operated at 92 kVp and the same mAs. The x-ray emission spectrum resulting from high-frequency operation is more efficient than either single-phase or three-phase. The area under the curve is considerably greater and the

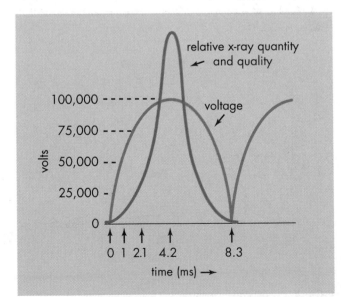

FIGURE 11-15 As the voltage across the x-ray tube increases from zero to its peak value, the x-ray intensity and energy increase, slowly at first and then rapidly as peak voltage is obtained.

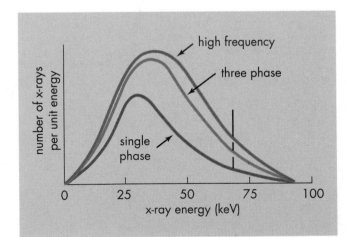

FIGURE 11-16 Three-phase and high-frequency operation are considerably more efficient than single-phase operation. Both the x-ray intensity (area under the curve) and the effective energy (relative shift of amplitude) are increased. Shown are representative spectra for 92-kVp operation.

x-ray emission spectrum is shifted to the high-energy side.

The characteristic x-ray emission spectrum remains fixed in its position along the energy axis but increases slightly in magnitude because of the increased number of projectile electrons available for K-shell electron interaction. There is no simple way to calculate the differences in x-ray quantity between single-phase and three-phase operation.

Question: What would be the difference in the x-ray emission spectra between a full-wave–rectified operation compared with a half-wave-rectified operation if the kVp and mAs are held constant?

Answer: Under constant conditions of kVp and mAs there should be no difference in the x-ray emission spectra. The x-ray quantity and quality will remain constant for each x-ray pulse.

Table 11-2 presents a summary of the effect on x-ray quantity and quality from each of the factors that affect the x-ray emission spectrum. Although five factors are listed, only the first two, mAs and kVp, are routinely controlled by the radiographer. Occasionally the added filtration will be changed if the collimator design permits.

■ ■ ■ ■ ■ ■ ■ ■ ■ ■ ■ ■ ■ ■ ■ ■ ■ ■ ■

SUMMARY

When electrons stream from the space charge at the cathode and bombard the target or anode, three effects take place. There is the production of heat, the formation of characteristic radiation, and the formation of bremsstrahlung radiation. Characteristic radiation occurs when an electron interacts with an inner-shell electron of the target atom. As the inner-shell void is filled, an x-ray is emitted. Bremsstrahlung radiation is produced by the sudden stopping, breaking, or slowing down of an electron by the target-atom nucleus. Most x-rays in the diagnostic range (50 to 150 kVp) are the result of bremsstrahlung radiation.

X-ray emission spectra can be graphed as the number of x-rays in relation to the energy level in keV, as shown

TABLE 11-2

Changes in X-ray Beam Quality and Quantity by Factors that Influence the Emission Spectrum

Increased	Results
mAs	An increase in quantity. No change in quality.
kVp	An increase in quantity and quality.
Added mm Al	A decrease in quantity. An increase in quality.
Target material	An increase in quantity and quality.
Voltage ripple	A decrease in quantity and quality.

TABLE 11-3

Factors Affecting the Size and Position of X-ray Emission Spectra

Factor	Effect
Tube current	Amplitude of spectrum
Tube voltage	Amplitude and position of spectrum
Added filtration	Amplitude at low energy
Target material (Z)	Amplitude and position of line spectrum
Voltage waveform	Amplitude at high energy

in Figure 11-8. Characteristic x-rays of tungsten, also shown in Figure 11-8, have a discrete energy level of 69 keV. Bremsstrahlung x-rays contain a range of energies from 0 to 70 keV.

The following are four factors that influence the x-ray emission spectrum: (1) low-energy electrons interact to produce low-energy x-rays, (2) successive interactions of electrons result in the production of x-rays with lower and lower energy x-rays, (3) low-energy x-rays are most likely to be absorbed by the target material, (4) added filtration (2 millimeters aluminum) removes low-energy x-rays from the useful beam.

Factors that affect the size and relative position of x-ray emission spectra are summarized in Table 11-3.

■ ■ ■ ■ ■ ■ ■ ■ ■ ■ ■ ■ ■ ■ ■ ■ ■ ■ ■

REVIEW QUESTIONS

1. The space-charge electrons all have the same mass and, therefore, the same kinetic energy. How is the kinetic energy of the electrons streaming across the x-ray tube increased to increase the intensity and energy level of the x-ray beam?

2. At 80 kVp, what is the energy in joules of the electrons arriving at the target?

3. Calculate the following: 80 keV electrons travel at what fraction of the velocity of light?

4. What is the distance between the filament and the target in the x-ray tube? At 80 keV, what is the range of acceleration from filament to target?

5. Why is the x-ray tube considered an inefficient machine?

6. Draw the diagram and write the description of the formation of characteristic radiation.

7. Using Figure 11-4, calculate the energy of the characteristic x-ray if the K-shell electron is replaced by a M-shell electron.

8. What is the importance of K-characteristic x-rays in forming a diagnostic radiograph?

9. Draw the diagram and write the description of the formation of bremsstrahlung radiation.

10. What is the range of energies of bremsstrahlung radiation?

11. In the diagnostic range, most x-rays are of _____ origin.

12. What is the importance of studying the x-ray emission spectrum?

13. Maximum x-ray energy is associated with _____ x-ray wavelength.

14. What is the minimum wavelength associated with x-rays emitted from an x-ray tube operated at 90 kVp?

15. Define integration as it refers to the x-ray emission spectrum.

16. List the factors that affect the x-ray emission spectrum and briefly describe how the spectrum is affected by each factor.

17. Define and explain the 15% kVp rule.

18. What is considered the diagnostic range of x-ray kVp values?

19. What is considered the range of mammographic kVp values? What type of radiation is useful for mammography and not useful for general diagnostic exposures?

20. In your clinical setting, observe or ask what filtration is used on the x-ray tubes. Why is filtration important?

Additional Reading

Mosby's radiographic instructional series: radiologic physics [slide set], St Louis, 1996, Mosby.

12

X-ray Emission

OBJECTIVES

At the completion of this chapter the student will be able to:

1. Define radiation quantity in relation to intensity in roentgens
2. Define radiation quantity in relation to mAs
3. List and discuss the factors affecting the quantity of x-rays in the beam
4. Explain x-ray quality or penetrability
5. List and discuss the factors affecting the quality of the x-ray beam

OUTLINE

X-ray Quantity
  Output intensity
  Factors affecting x-ray quantity
    review

X-ray Quality
  Penetrability
  Half-value layer
  Factors affecting x-ray quality
    review

X-rays are emitted through a window in the glass or metal envelope to form a beam of varied energies. The tube output is characterized by **quantity** (the number of x-rays) and **quality** (the penetrability of the beam.)

X-RAY QUANTITY
Output Intensity

The output intensity of an x-ray unit is measured in roentgens (R) or milliroentgens (mR) and is termed the *x-ray quantity* or *radiation exposure*. Both quantity and radiation exposure have the same meaning. The roentgen is a measure of the number of ion pairs produced in air by a quantity of x-rays. The ionization of air is measured in coulombs of charge per kilogram of air (1 R = 2.58×10^{-4} C/kg) and increases as the number of x-rays in the beam increases. The relationship between the x-ray quantity as measured in roentgens and the number of x-rays in the beam is not always one to one. There are some small variations related to the effective x-ray energy, but these variations are unimportant over the x-ray energy range used in radiography.

Radiation Quantity

The number of x-rays in the useful beam, which is the beam forming the radiographic image, is the radiation quantity. The radiation quantity can also be defined as the intensity of radiation, usually measured in mR.

When operated at approximately 70 kVp, general-purpose radiographic tubes produce x-ray intensities of approximately 5 mR/mAs (75 to 150 µC/kg/mAs) at the 100-centimeter source-to-image receptor distance (SID). Figure 12-1 is a **nomogram,** a graph made up of parallel curves for estimating x-ray intensity for a wide range of techniques. These curves apply only for single-phase, full-wave–rectified apparatus. As the legend under the nomogram explains, the quantity, mR/mAs, can be easily estimated by first knowing the filtration level of the x-ray tube and the kVp in use, then drawing a vertical line from the filtration level and finding the curved kVp line of the appropriate value. The horizontal line drawn from the kVp value to the y-axis indicates the mR/mAs radiation exposure value for that x-ray tube. Nomograms are also available for three-phase apparatus.

Factors Affecting X-ray Quantity

The following four factors affect x-ray quantity: (1) mAs, (2) kVp, (3) SID, and (4) filtration. This section may serve primarily as a review because the factors affecting x-ray quantity are nearly the same as those controlling **optical density** on a radiograph (Table 12-1).

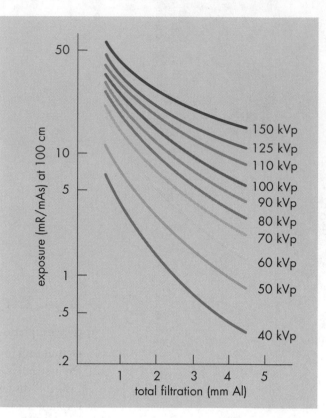

FIGURE 12-1 Nomogram for estimating intensity of x-ray beams. From the position on the x-axis corresponding to the filtration of the machine, draw a vertical line until it intersects with the appropriate kVp. A horizontal line from that point will intersect the y-axis at the appropriate x-ray quantity for the machine. *(Modified from E. McCullough, and J. Cameron, University of Wisconsin.)*

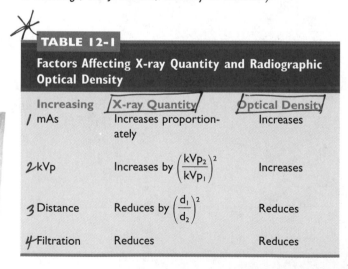

TABLE 12-1

Factors Affecting X-ray Quantity and Radiographic Optical Density

Increasing	X-ray Quantity	Optical Density
mAs	Increases proportionately	Increases
kVp	Increases by $\left(\dfrac{kVp_2}{kVp_1}\right)^2$	Increases
Distance	Reduces by $\left(\dfrac{d_1}{d_2}\right)^2$	Reduces
Filtration	Reduces	Reduces

Milliampere-seconds (mAs). X-ray quantity is directly proportional to the mAs. When the mAs is doubled, the number of electrons striking the tube target is doubled and therefore the number of x-rays emitted is doubled. The following equation represents the relationship between intensity in R or mR and mAs:

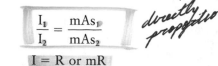

$$\frac{I_1}{I_2} = \frac{mAs_1}{mAs_2}$$

directly proportional

$$I = R \text{ or } mR$$

$$mAs = milliamps \times seconds$$

Question: Lateral chest radiographic technical factors call for 110 kVp at 10 mAs, which results in an x-ray intensity of 32 mR (8.3 µC/kg) at the patient. If the mAs is increased to 20 mAs, what will the x-ray intensity be?

Answer:

$$\frac{x}{32 \text{ mR}} = \frac{20 \text{ mAs}}{10 \text{ mAs}}$$

$$x = \frac{(32 \text{ mAs})(20 \text{ mR})}{10 \text{ mAs}}$$

$$= 64 \text{ mR is the increased x-ray intensity}$$

Question: The radiographic technical factor for a KUB examination (kidneys, ureter, and bladder) is 74 kVp at 60 mAs. The result is a patient exposure of 248 mR. What will be the potential exposure if the mAs can be reduced to 45 mAs?

Answer:

$$\frac{x}{248 \text{ mR}} = \frac{45 \text{ mAs}}{60 \text{ mAs}}$$

$$x = \frac{(248 \text{ mR})(45 \text{ mAs})}{60 \text{ mAs}}$$

$$= 186 \text{ mR is the reduced x-ray intensity}$$

Remember that mAs is just a measure of the total number of electrons that travel from cathode to anode to produce x-rays.

$$mAs = mA \times seconds$$

$$= mC/s \times seconds$$

$$mAs = mC$$

C (coulomb) is a measure of electrostatic charge, and $1 \text{ C} = 6.25 \times 10^{18}$ electrons.

Question: A radiograph is made at 74 kVp at 100 mAs. How many electrons interact with the target?

Answer: 100 mAs = 100 mC

$$= 6.25 \times 10^{17} \text{ electrons will interact with the target}$$

Question: If the radiographic output intensity is 6.2 mR/mAs, how many electrons are required to produce 1.0 mR?

Answer: 6.2 mR/mAs = $6.2 \text{ mR}/6.25 \times 10^{15}$ electrons will be required to produce 1.0 mR; stated inversely: 6.25×10^{15} electrons/6.2 mR = 1×10^{15} electrons/mR

 kVp

kVp

The change in x-ray quantity is proportional to the square of the ratio of the kVp. If kVp were doubled, the x-ray intensity would increase by a factor of four. Mathematically this is expressed as follows:

$$\frac{I_1}{I_2} = \left(\frac{kVp_1}{kVp_2}\right)^2$$

I_1 and I_2 are the x-ray intensities at kVp_1 and kVp_2, respectively

Question: Lateral chest radiographic technical factors call for 110 kVp at 10 mAs and results in an x-ray intensity of 32 mR (8.3 µC/kg). What will the intensity be if the kVp is increased to 125 and the mAs remains fixed?

Answer:

$$\frac{I}{32 \text{ mR}} = \left(\frac{125 \text{ kVp}}{110 \text{ kVp}}\right)^2$$

$$I = (32 \text{ mR})\left(\frac{125 \text{ kVp}}{110 \text{ kVp}}\right)^2$$

$$= (32 \text{ mR})(1.14)^2$$

$$= (32 \text{ mR})(1.29)$$

$$= 41.3 \text{ mR is the increased intensity}$$

Question: An extremity is examined with a technique of 58 kVp at 8 mAs, which results in an x-ray intensity of 24 mR. If the technical factor is changed to 54 kVp, at 8 mAs what will be the x-ray intensity?

Answer:

$$\frac{I}{24 \text{ mR}} = \left(\frac{54 \text{ kVp}}{58 \text{ kVp}}\right)^2$$

$$I = 24 \text{ mR} \left(\frac{54 \text{ kVp}}{58 \text{ kVp}}\right)^2$$

$$= (24 \text{ mR})(0.93)^2$$

$$= (24 \text{ mR})(0.867)$$

$$= 20.8 \text{ mR is the reduced x-ray intensity}$$

In practice, radiographic technical factors are selected from a narrow range of values, usually between 40 to 150 kVp. In theory, to double the x-ray intensity by kVp manipulation alone, the kVp must be increased by 41%. However, a 41% increase in kVp to double the intensity does not work in practice. As kVp is increased, the penetrability of the x-ray beam is increased as well, which results in fewer x-rays absorbed in the patient. More x-rays go through the patient, do not interact with tissue, and are recorded on the image. To maintain a constant exposure of the film, an increase of 15% in kVp should be accompanied by a one half reduction in mAs.

Question: Radiographic technical factors call for 80 kVp at 30 mAs and results in an intensity of 135 mR. What is the expected intensity if the kVp is increased to 92 kVp (+15%) and the mAs reduced by one half to 15 mAs?

Answer:
$$\frac{I}{135 \text{ mR}} = \left(\frac{15 \text{ mAs}}{30 \text{ mAs}}\right)\left(\frac{92 \text{ kVp}}{80 \text{ kVp}}\right)^2$$

$$I = 135 \text{ mR} \left(\frac{15 \text{ mAs}}{30 \text{ mAs}}\right)\left(\frac{92 \text{ kVp}}{80 \text{ kVp}}\right)^2$$

$$= 135 \text{ mR} \ (0.5) \ (1.32)$$

= 89 mR is the intensity resulting from the change in mAs and kVp

4) Distance

Inverse Square Law

Radiation intensity from an x-ray tube varies inversely with the square of the distance from the target. This relationship is known as the *inverse square law* (see Chapter 5). This relationship can be calculated by the following formula:

$$\frac{I_1}{I_2} = \frac{(d_2)^2}{(d_1)^2}$$

Question: An examination with a portable x-ray unit is normally conducted at 100 centimeters SID and results in an intensity of 12.5 mR (3.2 μC/kg) at the film. If 91 centimeters is the maximum SID that can be obtained for a particular situation, what will be the radiation intensity at the film?

Answer:
$$\frac{I}{12.5 \text{ mR}} = \left(\frac{100 \text{ cm}}{91 \text{ cm}}\right)^2$$

$$I = (12.5 \text{ mR}) \left(\frac{100 \text{ cm}}{91 \text{ cm}}\right)^2$$

$$= (12.5 \text{ mR}) \ (1.1)^2$$

$$= (12.5 \text{ mR}) \ (1.21)$$

= 15.1 mR is the increased intensity at the reduced distance

Question: A posterior-anterior (PA) chest examination (120 kVp at 3 mAs) with a chest radiographic unit is taken at an SID of 300 centimeters (10 feet). The intensity at the image receptor is 12 mR. If the same technique is used at an SID of 100 centimeters, what will be the x-ray intensity?

Answer:
$$\frac{I}{12 \text{ mR}} = \left(\frac{300 \text{ cm}}{100 \text{ cm}}\right)^2$$

$$I = 12 \text{ mR} \left(\frac{300 \text{ cm}}{100 \text{ cm}}\right)^2$$

$$= (12 \text{ mR}) \ (3)^2$$

$$= (12 \text{ mR}) \ (9)$$

= 108 mR is the increased intensity at the decreased distance

3) Filtration

Filtration

X-ray units have metal filters, usually 1- to 3-mm aluminum (Al), positioned in the useful beam. The primary purpose of these filters is to reduce the number of low-energy x-rays that reach the patient.

Low-energy x-rays contribute nothing to the diagnostic quality of the radiograph. Low-energy x-rays increase the patient dose unnecessarily because they are absorbed in superficial tissues and do not penetrate the body part to reach the film. When filtration is inserted in the x-ray beam, the patient dose is reduced because there are fewer low-energy x-rays to reach the patient. Calculation of the amount of reduction in exposure requires a knowledge of **half-value layer (HVL),** which is discussed in the following section. An estimate of exposure reduction can be made from the **nomogram** in Figure 12-1, where it is shown that the reduction is not proportional to the thickness of added filter but is related in a complex way.

X-RAY QUALITY
Penetrability

As the energy of an x-ray beam is increased, the **penetrability** is also increased.

Penetrability

Penetrability refers to the attenuation of x-rays in tissue. Higher-energy x-rays are able to penetrate through tissue farther than low-energy x-rays.

The penetrability or penetrating power of an x-ray beam is called the *x-ray quality*. X-rays with high penetrability are termed *high-quality* or *hard x-rays*. Those with low penetrability are of low quality and are called *soft x-rays*. X-ray quality is identified numerically by **HVL (half-value layer).** The half-value layer is affected by the kVp and the amount of filtration in the useful beam, and therefore x-ray quality is influenced by kVp and filtration. Factors that affect beam quality also influence radiographic contrast. Distance and mAs do not affect radiation quality, but they do affect radiation quantity as explained in the next section.

Half-Value Layer

High-energy x-rays are considerably more penetrating than low-energy x-rays. 100 keV x-rays are attenuated or absorbed at the rate of only 3% per centimeter of soft tissue, but 10 keV x-rays are absorbed at the rate of 15% per centimeter of soft tissue. X-rays of any given energy are more penetrating in low atomic number tissue such as skin or muscle than in high atomic number tissue such as bone.

In radiography the quality of x-rays is characterized by the half-value layer.

> ⊙ **Half-value Layer**
>
> The half-value layer of an x-ray beam refers to the thickness of absorbing material necessary to reduce the x-ray intensity to half of its original value.

The half-value layer characterizes the x-ray beam. A diagnostic x-ray beam usually has a half-value layer in the range of 3 to 5 millimeters of aluminum or 4 to 8 centimeters of soft tissue.

Half-value layers are determined by using experimental devices similar to those shown in Figure 12-2. The following three principal parts of the experimental arrangement detect the half-value layer: (1) the x-ray tube (with collimation), (2) graded thicknesses of aluminum used as a filter, and (3) a radiation detector. First a radiation measurement is made with no filter between the x-ray tube and the detector. Then measurements of radiation intensity are made for successively thicker sections of filter. The thickness of filtration that reduces the x-ray intensity to half of its original value is the half-value layer.

A number of methods can be used to determine the half-value layer of an x-ray beam. Perhaps the most straightforward is to graph the measurements made with the devices in Figure 12-2. The graph in Figure

12-3 shows how this can be done when the following steps are completed. Sample numerical values are shown in Table 12-2.

1. Determine the x-ray quantity with no absorbing material in the beam and with a known thickness of absorber.
2. Plot the ordered pairs of data (thickness of absorber and x-ray quantity).
3. Determine the x-ray quantity equal to half the original quantity and locate this value on the y, or vertical, axis of the graph (A).
4. Draw a horizontal line parallel with the x-axis from the point A in step 3 until it intersects the curve (B).
5. From point B of the intersection, drop a vertical line to the x-axis.

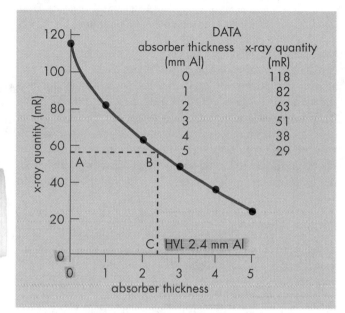

DATA	
absorber thickness (mm Al)	x-ray quantity (mR)
0	118
1	82
2	63
3	51
4	38
5	29

FIGURE 12-3 Data in table are typical for half-value layer determination. The plot of these data shows a half-value layer of 2.4 millimeter aluminum.

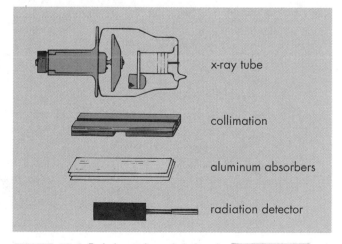

FIGURE 12-2 Typical experimental devices for determination of half-value layer.

- x-ray tube
- collimation
- aluminum absorbers
- radiation detector

TABLE 12-2

Experimental Data Obtained to Determine Half-Value Layer

Added mm Al	mR
None	94
0.5	79
1.0	67
1.5	57
2.0	49
2.5	42
3.0	38
3.5	33

This data is plotted in Figure 12-3.

6. On the x-axis, read the thickness of absorber required to reduce the x-ray intensity to half of its original value point (C). This is the half-value layer.

Question: The list of data on Table 12-2 is obtained with the radiographic tube operated at 70 kVp while the detector is positioned 100 centimeters from the target with 0.5-millimeter aluminum filters inserted halfway between the target and the detector. Estimate the half-value layer from a simple observation of this data, then plot the data to see how close you were.

Answer: One half of 94 is 47, therefore the half-value layer must be between 2 and 2.5 millimeters of aluminum. A plot of the data shows the half-value layer to be 2.4 millimeters aluminum.

Different combinations of added filtration and kVp can result in the same x-ray beam half-value layer. For example, measurements may show that a single unit has the same half-value layer when operated at 90 kVp with 2 millimeters aluminum total filtration as when operated at 70 kVp with 5 millimeters aluminum total filtration. In this case, x-ray penetrability remains constant, as does the half-value layer. It would be erroneous to specify beam quality by either kVp or filtration alone.

Factors Affecting X-ray Quality

Kilovoltage. As kVp is increased, so is x-ray beam quality and therefore the half-value layer. An increase in kVp results in a shift of the x-ray emission spectrum toward the high-energy side, which causes an increase in the energy of the beam. The result is a more penetrating x-ray beam. Table 12-3 shows the measured change in the half-value layer as kVp is increased from 50 to 150 kVp for a representative x-ray unit. The total filtration of the beam is 2.5 millimeters aluminum equivalent.

TABLE 12-3	
Relationship Between kVp and Half-value Layer for Fixed Radiographic Units Having Total Filtration of 2.5 Millimeters Aluminum Equivalent	
kVp	**HVL (2.5 mm Al equivalent)**
50	1.9
75	2.8
100	3.7
125	4.6
150	5.4

Filtration. The primary purpose of adding filtration to an x-ray beam is to selectively remove low-energy x-rays that have no chance of getting to the film. Figure 12-4 shows x-ray emission spectra representing unfiltered, normally filtered, and ideally filtered x-ray beams. The ideally filtered x-ray beam would have nearly all the same energy or be **monoenergetic**. It is desirable to totally remove all x-rays with energies below a certain level. This level is determined by the type of x-ray examination, and the goal is to reduce patient dose. It is also desirable to remove x-rays with energies above a certain level to improve image contrast. Unfortunately, total removal of regions of an x-ray beam is not possible.

Almost any material could serve as an x-ray filter. Aluminum is chosen because it is efficient in removing low-energy x-rays and because it is available, inexpensive, and easily shaped into filters. Copper (Z = 29), tin (Z = 50), **gadolinium** (Z = 64), and **holmium** (Z = 67) have been used occasionally.

Effect of Filtration
As filtration is increased, so is beam quality, but quantity is decreased.

Filtration of diagnostic x-ray beams has the following two components: (1) **inherent filtration** and (2) **added filtration**. The glass envelope of an x-ray tube

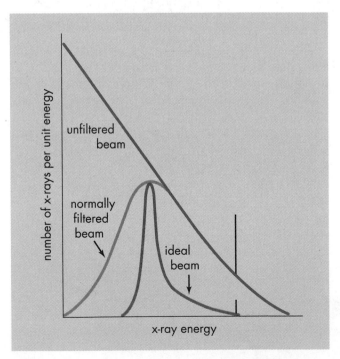

FIGURE 12-4 Filtration is used to selectively remove low-energy x-rays from the useful beam. Ideal filtration would remove all low-energy x-rays.

filters the emerging x-ray beam, which is **inherent filtration.** Inspection of an x-ray tube will reveal that the part of the glass envelope, or window through which x-rays are emitted, is thin. This is to provide for low inherent filtration. The inherent filtration of a general-purpose x-ray tube is approximately 0.5 millimeter aluminum equivalent. With age, inherent filtration tends to increase as some of the tungsten metal of both target and filament is vaporized and deposited on the inside of the glass envelope. Special-purpose tubes, such as those used in mammography, have very thin x-ray tube windows. They are sometimes made of **beryllium** (Z = 4) rather than glass and have inherent filtration of approximately 0.1 millimeter aluminum.

Added filtration consists of sheets of aluminum placed between the protective tube housing and the external housing or **collimator.** The addition of a filter to an x-ray beam attenuates x-rays of all energies emitted by the x-ray tube, but it attenuates more low-energy x-rays than high-energy x-rays. This shifts the x-ray emission spectrum to the high-energy side, which results in an x-ray beam with higher energy, greater penetrability, and higher quality. The addition of filtration results in an increased half-value layer. The extent of increase in the half-value layer cannot be predicted even when the thickness of added filtration is known.

Because added filtration attenuates the x-ray beam, it affects x-ray quantity. This value can be predicted if one knows the half-value layer of the beam. The addition of filtration equal to the beam half-value layer reduces the beam quantity to half its prefiltered value and results in a **harder** x-ray beam.

Question: A general-purpose x-ray tube has a half-value layer of 2.2 millimeters of aluminum. The exposure from this machine is 2 mR/mAs (0.5 µC/kg/mAs) at 100 centimeters SID. If 2.2 millimeters of aluminum is added to the beam, what will be the x-ray intensity or quantity?

Answer: This is an addition of one half-value layer. Therefore the x-ray quantity will be 1 mR/mAs (0.25 µC/kg/mAs).

Added filtration usually has two sources and totals 2 and 3 millimeters of aluminum equivalent. First, 1- or 2-millimeter sheets of aluminum will be permanently installed in the port of the x-ray tube housing, between the housing and the collimator. If the collimator is a conventional **light-localizing variable-aperture collimator,** the collimator will contribute an additional 1 millimeter aluminum equivalent added filtration. This filtration results from the silver surface of the mirror in the collimator (Figure 12-5). One of the most difficult tasks facing the radiographer is producing an image of uniform optical density when examining a body part

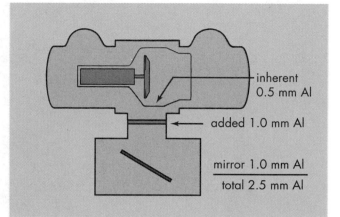

FIGURE 12-5 Total filtration consists of the inherent filtration of the x-ray tube, an added filter, and filtration by the mirror of the light-localizing collimator.

that varies greatly in thickness or tissue composition. During PA chest radiography, for instance, if the left chest is radiopaque because of fluid and the right chest is normal and filled with air, then the image would have very low optical density on the left side of the chest and very high optical density on the right. Compensation for this density variation is made using a filter so that the thinner part of the filter is positioned over the left side of the chest. When a filter is used in this fashion, it is called a *compensating filter* because it compensates for differences in **subject radiopacity.** Compensating filters can be fabricated for many procedures and therefore come in various sizes and shapes. They are nearly always constructed of aluminum, but plastic materials can also be used. Figure 12-6 shows some commonly used compensating filters.

A **wedge filter** is principally used when radiographing a body part, such as the foot, that varies considerably in thickness from the toes to the heel (Figure 12-7). During an AP projection of the foot, the wedge would be positioned with its thick portion shadowing the toes and the thin portion toward the heel.

A **bilateral wedge filter** or a **trough filter** is sometimes used in chest radiography (Figure 12-8). The thin central region of the wedge is positioned over the **mediastinum** (includes heart and great vessels), whereas the lateral thick portion shadows the lung fields (filled with air). The result is a radiograph with more uniform optical density. Special compensating wedges of this type are used for chest radiography.

Special **bow-tie–shaped filters** are used with some CT scanners to compensate for the shape of the head or body. **Conic filters,** either concave or convex, find application in **digital fluoroscopy,** where the image receptor and the image-intensifier tube are round.

A **step-wedge filter** is an adaptation of the wedge filter (Figure 12-9). It is used in some special procedures,

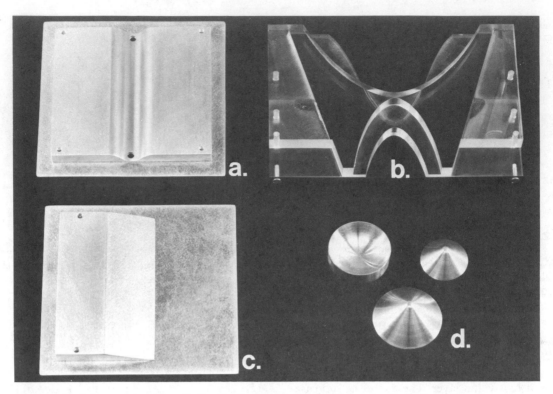

FIGURE 12-6 Compensating filters. **A,** Trough filter. **B,** Bow-tie filter for use in CT. **C,** Wedge filter. **D,** Conic filters for use in digital fluoroscopy.

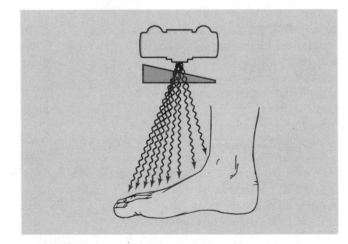

FIGURE 12-7 Use of a wedge filter for examination of a foot.

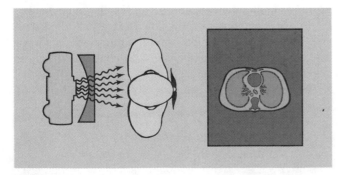

FIGURE 12-8 Use of a trough filter for examination of the chest.

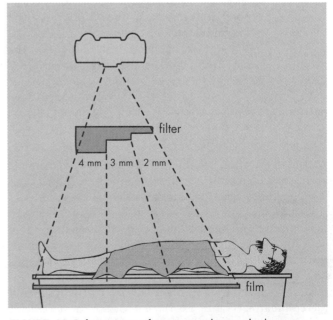

FIGURE 12-9 Arrangement of apparatus using an aluminum step wedge for serial radiography of the abdomen and lower extremities.

TABLE 12-4

Factors Affecting X-ray Quality and Radiographic Optical Density

An Increase in	Effect on X-ray Quality	Effect on Radiographic Optical Density
1 mAs	None	Increase
2 kVp	Increase	Increase
3 Distance	None	Reduce
4 Filtration	Increase	Reduce

usually where long sections of the anatomy are radiographed and imaged with two or three separate films. A common application of this technique uses a three-step aluminum wedge and three 14 × 17 inch (30 × 36 centimeters) films in a **rapid change** for **translumbar** and **femoral arteriography** and **venography**.

A summary of the factors affecting x-ray quality and radiographic optical density are listed in Table 12-4.

SUMMARY

Radiation quantity is the number of x-rays in the useful beam. The factors affecting the number of x-rays in the beam are as follows:
1. mAs, which is directly proportional to radiation quantity
2. kVp, which if doubled would increase radiation quantity by a factor of four
3. Distance squared, which varies inversely with radiation quantity
4. Filtration, which reduces quantity by eliminating the low-energy x-rays reaching the patient
To summarize, refer to Table 12-1.
Radiation quality is the penetrating power of the x-ray beam. *Penetrability* refers to the attenuation or absorption of x-rays in tissue. The penetrability is quantified by measuring the half-value layer, which is the thickness of filtration that reduces x-ray intensity in roentgens (R) to half its original value. The factors affecting beam penetrability or radiation quality are as follows:
1. kVp, which increases penetrability as it is increased
2. Filtration when added to the beam reduces low-energy x-rays and thus increases radiation quality
The following are the three types of filtration: (1) inherent filtration built into the glass or metal envelope, (2) added filtration in the form of aluminum sheets, and (3) compensating filters, which provide variation in beam quality, depending on tissue thickness. The factors affecting quality of the x-ray beam are summarized in Table 12-4.

In this chapter the x-ray beam has been characterized as having quantity (the number of x-rays) and quality (penetrability). Chapter 13 describes the interactions between the x-ray beam and matter.

REVIEW QUESTIONS

1. MATCH   Tube output   Quality of the beam
   Penetrability   Quantity of x-rays
2. Tube output is measured in _____ and is the measure of _____ _____.
3. A radiographic exposure is 80 kVp at 50 mAs. How many electrons will interact with the target?
4. The radiation intensity of an exposure is 2 mR. How many electrons will interact with the target?
5. An extremity is radiographed using factors of 60 kVp at 10 mAs with an x-ray intensity of 28 mR. If the technique is changed to 55 kVp with the mAs constant, what is the resulting x-ray intensity?
6. A chest film taken at 180 centimeters results in an exposure of 12 mR. What would be the radiation exposure if the same factors were used at (a) 90 centimeters SID and (b) 100 centimeters SID?
7. An increase of _____ in kVp is accompanied by a _____ in one half the mAs to maintain constant exposure.
8. State the inverse square law.
9. What is the primary purpose of x-ray filters?
10. Fill in the following chart:

Increasing	Effect on Quantity of the X-ray Beam	Effect on Optical Density
mAs		
kVp		
Distance		
Filtration		

11. What is the relationship between x-ray quantity and mAs?
12. What are hard x-rays? What are soft x-rays?
13. Define half-value layer.
14. List the two ways an x-ray beam emission spectrum can be shifted to higher energy levels.
15. Why is aluminum used for x-ray beam filtration?
16. Define the term light-localizing variable-aperture collimator.
17. Describe the use of a wedge filter when x-raying a foot.

18. Does adding filtration to the x-ray beam affect the quantity of x-rays reaching the film?

19. Fill in the following chart:

Increasing	Effect on X-ray Quality	Effect on Optical Density
mAs		
kVp		
Distance		
Filtration		

Additional Reading

Mosby's radiographic instructional series: radiologic physics [slide set], St Louis, 1996, Mosby.

13

X-ray Interaction with Matter

OBJECTIVES

At the completion of this chapter the student will be able to:

1. Describe each of the five x-ray interactions with matter
2. Define and compare differential absorption and attenuation
3. Explain the effect of atomic number and mass density of tissue on the differential absorption of the x-ray beam
4. Discuss why radiologic contrast agents are used to highlight soft tissue structures and organs in the human body

OUTLINE

X-ray Interactions with Matter
    Classical scattering
    Compton effect
    Photoelectric effect
    Pair production
    Photodisintegration

Differential Absorption
    Dependence on the density of matter
Attenuation
    Absorption
Radiologic Contrast Agents

X-ray beam photons interact with matter in the following five ways: (1) by classical scattering, (2) through the Compton effect, (3) through the photoelectric effect, (4) by pair production, and (5) by photodisintegration.

. . . .

X-RAY INTERACTIONS WITH MATTER

In Chapter 5 the interaction between electromagnetic radiation and matter is described. The interaction has wavelike and particle-like properties, and electromagnetic radiation interacts with structures similar in size to its wavelength. X-rays have very short wavelengths, no larger than 10^{-8} to 10^{-9} meters. The higher the energy of an x-ray, the shorter its wavelength. Consequently, low-energy x-rays tend to interact with whole atoms, which have diameters of approximately 10^{-9} to 10^{-10} meters. Moderate-energy x-rays generally interact with electrons, and high-energy x-rays generally interact with nuclei.

In this chapter the interaction between x-rays and matter is presented. In radiography, matter is defined as human tissue. The interaction between x-rays and human tissue is important for the radiographer to study because specific technical factors (kVp and mAs) are required to image certain tissue and, if chosen appropriately, may actually decrease the radiation exposure to the patient.

This chapter introduces the fundamental interactions between x-rays and all matter, which includes human tissue. The following are five basic ways x-rays interact with matter: (1) classical scattering, (2) Compton effect, (3) photoelectric effect, (4) pair production, and (5) photodisintegration. Two of these, the Compton effect and the photoelectric effect, are particularly important to radiography.

Classical Scattering

Low-energy x-rays, those with energies below about 10 keV, interact with matter by **classical scattering**, sometimes called *coherent scattering* (Figure 13-1). JJ Thomson described the classical scattering of an x-ray with an electron, and that interaction is named after him. When the interaction is with the entire atom, it is **Rayleigh scattering.** In classical scattering the incident x-ray interacts with a target atom, which causes it to become excited. The target atom immediately releases this excess energy as a scattered x-ray with a wavelength equal to that of the incident x-ray ($\lambda = \lambda'$) and therefore of equal energy. The direction of the scattered x-ray, however, is different from that of the incident x-ray. The net result of classical scattering is a change in direction of the x-ray without a change in its energy. There is no energy transfer and therefore no ionization. Most classically scattered x-rays are scattered forward.

Classical scattering is of little importance to diagnostic radiology because it primarily involves low-energy

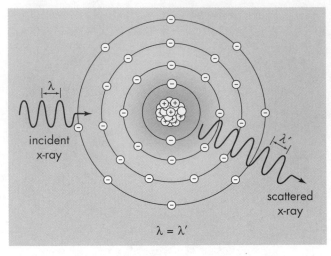

FIGURE 13-1 Classical scattering is an interaction between low-energy x-rays and atoms. The x-ray loses no energy but changes direction slightly. The wavelength of the incident x-ray is equal to the wavelength of the scattered x-ray.

x-rays, which contribute little to the radiograph. Classical scattering occurs throughout the diagnostic range but is more prevalent at lower (<10 keV) energies. At 70 kVp, 3% of x-rays undergo classical scattering, which contributes a small amount to **film fog** (general graying of the radiograph).

Compton Effect

Moderate-energy x-rays throughout the diagnostic range can undergo an interaction with outer-shell electrons. This interaction not only scatters the x-ray but reduces its energy and ionizes the atom as well. This interaction is called the *Compton effect* or *Compton scattering* (Figure 13-2). With the Compton effect, the

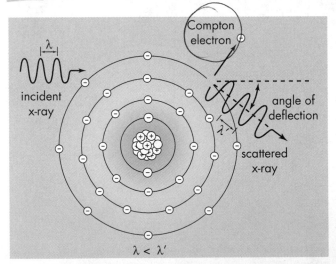

FIGURE 13-2 Compton effect occurs between moderate-energy x-rays and outer-shell electrons. It results in ionization of the target atom, change in photon direction, and reduction of photon energy. The wavelength of the scattered x-ray is greater than that of the incident x-ray.

incident x-ray interacts with an outer-shell electron, ejects it from the atom, and ionizes the atom. The x-ray continues in a different direction with less energy. The energy of the Compton-scattered x-ray is equal to the difference between the energy of the incident x-ray and the energy of the ejected electron. The energy of the ejected electron is equal to its binding energy plus the kinetic energy it has when it leaves the atom. Mathematically this energy transfer is represented as the following:

Compton Effect-Energy Transfer

$$E_i = E_s + (E_b + E_{KE})$$

In the Compton effect, E_i is the energy of the incident x-ray; E_s is the energy of the scattered x-ray; E_b is the electron binding energy; and E_{KE} is the kinetic energy of the electron.

Question: A 30-keV x-ray ionizes an atom of barium by ejecting an O-shell electron with 12 keV of kinetic energy. What is the energy of the scattered x-ray?

Answer: The binding energy of an O-shell electron of barium is 0.04 keV; therefore

$$30 \text{ keV} = E_s + (0.04 \text{ keV} + 12 \text{ keV})$$

$$E_s = 30 \text{ keV} - (0.04 \text{ keV} + 12 \text{ keV})$$

$$= 30 \text{ keV} - (12.04 \text{ keV})$$

$$= 17.96 \text{ keV is the energy of the scattered x-ray}$$

During a Compton interaction, most of the energy is divided between the following: (1) the **scattered x-ray** and (2) the **Compton electron**, which is also called the *secondary electron*. Usually the scattered x-ray retains most of the energy, but both the scattered x-ray and the secondary electron may have sufficient energy to undergo more ionizing interactions before losing all their energy. Ultimately, the scattered x-ray is absorbed. The secondary electron loses all of its kinetic energy by ionization and excitation. It then drops into a vacancy in an electron shell previously created by some other ionizing event.

Compton-scattered x-rays can be deflected in any direction, including 180 degrees from the incident x-ray. At a deflection of 0 degrees, no energy is transferred. As the angle of deflection increases to 180 degrees, more energy is transferred to the secondary electron. Even at a 180-degree deflection the scattered x-ray retains about two thirds of its original energy. X-rays scattered back in the direction of the incident x-ray beam are called *backscatter radiation.* In radiography, backscatter from tissue or objects immediately behind the cassette can cause artifacts such as the cassette-strap image

seen in Figure 13-3. The probability that a given x-ray will undergo Compton effect is a complex function of the energy of the incident x-ray. Generally the probability of Compton effect decreases as x-ray energy increases.

The probability of Compton effect does not depend on the atomic number of the atom involved. Any given x-ray is just as likely to undergo Compton effect with an atom of soft tissue as with an atom of bone (Figure 13-4). Table 13-1 summarizes Compton scattering.

Compton scattering can occur with all x-rays. Therefore it is of considerable importance in radiography but in a negative sense. Scattered x-rays provide no useful information on the radiograph. Compton-scattered x-rays produce a uniform optical density on the radiograph (fog), which results in reduced image contrast. There are ways of reducing scattered radiation, which are discussed later, but none is totally effective. Radiographs always appear duller and flatter because of Compton-scattered x-rays.

The scattered x-rays from Compton interactions can create a serious radiation exposure hazard in radiography, particularly in fluoroscopy. A large amount of radiation can be scattered from the patient during fluoroscopy. Such radiation is the source of most of the occupational radiation exposure that radiographers receive. During film radiography, the hazard is less severe because no one other than the patient is in the examining room. Nevertheless, scattered-radiation levels are high enough to have federal requirements for protective shielding in the x-ray examining room.

3 Photoelectric Effect

X-rays in the diagnosis range also undergo ionizing interactions with inner-shell electrons. The x-ray is not scattered but is totally absorbed. This process is called the *photoelectric effect* (Figure 13-5).

Photoelectric Effect

The photoelectric effect is an x-ray absorption interaction in which the x-ray is not scattered but is totally absorbed. The electron or photoelectron is removed from the atom and escapes with kinetic energy equal to the difference between the energy of the incident x-ray and the binding energy of the electron. Mathematically this is shown as follows:

$$E_i = E_b + E_{KE}$$

The symbols are the same as in the previous equation.

For low atomic number atoms, such as those found in soft tissue, the binding energy of even K-shell electrons

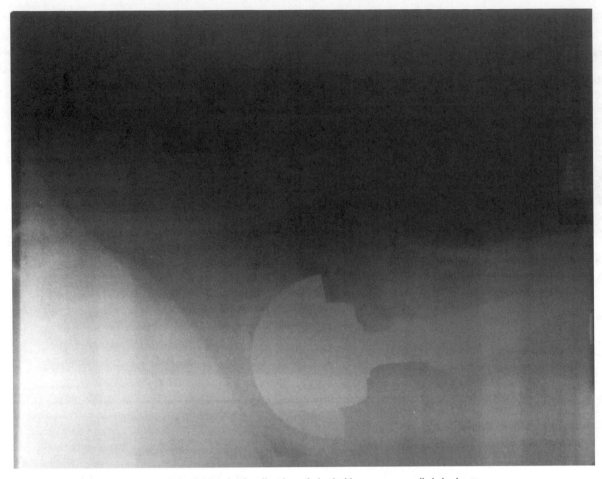

FIGURE 13-3 Compton x-rays scattered back in the direction of the incident rays are called *backscatter radiation*. Backscatter is responsible for the cassette-strap image sometimes seen on a radiograph, even though the strap is on the back of the cassette. *(Courtesy Napoleon Martin.)*

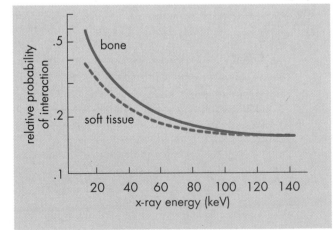

FIGURE 13-4 The probability that an x-ray will interact by Compton effect is about the same for target atoms of soft tissue and bone. This probability decreases with increasing photon energy.

TABLE 13-1	
Characteristics of Compton Scattering	
Most likely to occur	• With outer shell electrons
	• With loosely bound electrons
As x-ray energy increases	• Increased probability of penetration through tissue without interaction
	• Increased probability of Compton scattering relative to photoelectric effect
	• Reduced probability of Compton scattering
As atomic number of matter increases	• No effect on probability of Compton scattering
As mass density of matter increases	• Proportional increase in x-ray attenuation
	• More Compton scattering

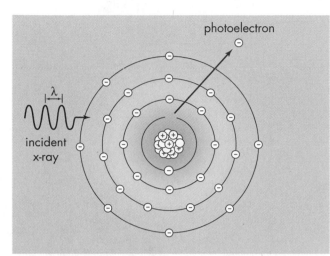

FIGURE 13-5 Photoelectric effect occurs when an incident x-ray is totally absorbed during the ionization of an inner-shell electron. The incident photon disappears, and the K-shell electron, now called a photoelectron, is ejected from the atom.

is low (e.g., 0.284 keV for carbon). Therefore the photoelectron is released with kinetic energy nearly equal to the energy of the incident x-ray. For higher atomic number target atoms, the electron binding energies are higher (37.4 keV for barium K-shell electrons). Therefore the kinetic energy of the photoelectron from barium is proportionately lower. Table 13-2 shows the approximate K-shell binding energy for some elements.

Characteristic x-rays are produced after a photoelectric interaction in a manner similar to what is described in Chapter 11. The ejection of a K-shell photoelectron by the incident x-ray results in a vacancy in the K shell. This is an unnatural state that is immediately corrected

TABLE 13-2

Atomic Number and K-shell Electron Binding Energy

Element	Atomic Number	Rounded K-shell Electron Binding Energy
Hydrogen	1	0.02 keV
Carbon	6	0.3 keV
Nitrogen	7	0.4 keV
Oxygen	8	0.5 keV
Aluminum	13	1.6 keV
Calcium	20	4.1 keV
Molybdenum	42	20 keV
Rhenium	45	24 keV
Iodine	53	33 keV
Barium	56	37 keV
Tungsten	74	69 keV
Lead	82	88 keV

by an outer-shell electron, usually from the L shell, which drops into the vacancy. This electron transition is accompanied by the emission of an x-ray with energy that is equal to the difference in the binding energies of the shells involved. This transition does not occur often. The characteristic x-rays are **secondary radiation** and behave in the same manner as scattered radiation. Secondary radiation contributes nothing of diagnostic value to the radiographic image.

Question: A 50 keV x-ray interacts photoelectrically with (a) a carbon atom and (b) a barium atom. What is the kinetic energy of each photoelectron and the energy of each characteristic x-ray if an L-to-K transition occurs?

Answer: a. Carbon atom binding energies: K shell = 0.284 keV; L shell = 0.01 keV

$$E_{KE} = E_i - E_b$$

$$= 50 \text{ keV} - 0.284 \text{ keV}$$

$$= 49.72 \text{ keV is the kinetic energy of the photoelectron displaced in a carbon atom}$$

$$E_x = 0.284 \text{ keV} - 0.01 \text{ keV}$$

$$= 0.274 \text{ keV is the energy of the characteristic x-ray emitted from the carbon atom}$$

b. Barium atom binding energies: K shell = 37.4 keV; L shell = 5.989 keV

$$E_{KE} = E_i - E_b$$

$$= 50 \text{ keV} - 37.4 \text{ keV}$$

$$= 12.6 \text{ keV is the kinetic energy of the photoelectron displaced in a barium atom}$$

$$E_x = 37.441 \text{ keV} - 5.989 \text{ keV}$$

$$= 31.452 \text{ keV is the energy of the characteristic x-ray emitted from the barium atom}$$

The probability that a given x-ray will undergo a photoelectric interaction is a function of both the x-ray energy and the atomic number of the atom with which it interacts. A photoelectric interaction cannot occur unless the incident x-ray has energy equal to or greater than the electron binding energy. A barium K-shell electron bound to the nucleus by 37.441 keV cannot be removed by a 25 keV x-ray. If the incident x-ray has sufficient energy, the probability that it will undergo a photoelectric effect decreases with the third power of the photon energy ($1/E^3$). The probability of photoelectric effect is inversely proportional to the third power of the x-ray energy. This relationship is shown graphically in Figure 13-6 for soft tissue and bone.

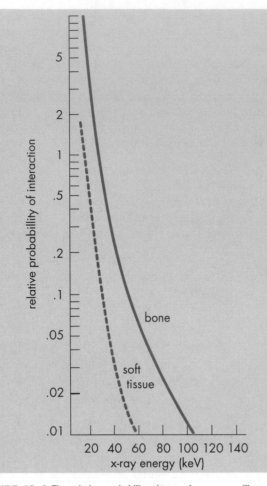

FIGURE 13-6 The relative probability that a given x-ray will undergo a photoelectric interaction is inversely proportional to the third power of the photon energy and directly proportional to the third power of the atomic number of the absorber. **A,** Relationship for soft tissue. **B,** Relationship for bone.

As the relative vertical displacement between the graphs of soft tissue and bone demonstrates, a photoelectric interaction is much more likely to occur with high-Z atoms than with low-Z atoms (Figure 13-7). In fact the probability of photoelectric interaction is directly proportional to the third power of the atomic number of the absorbing material. Table 13-3 presents the effective atomic numbers of atoms.

Question: If an 80-keV x-ray enters the first centimeter of soft tissue, what is its relative probability of interacting with the following:

    a. Fat (Z = 6.3)
    b. Barium (Z = 56)
    Probability = $\left(\frac{1}{E^3}\right)$ (refer to Table 13-3)

Answer:

    a. $\left(\dfrac{6.3}{7.4}\right)^3 = 0.62$ or 62% chance of interacting with fat

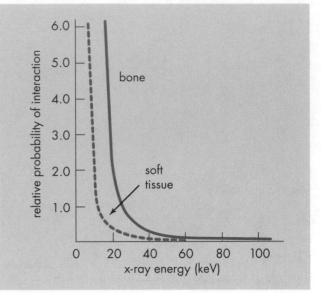

FIGURE 13-7 Relative probability for photoelectric interaction ranges over several orders of magnitude. If it is plotted in the conventional arithmetic fashion, one cannot estimate its value above an energy of about 20 keV.

TABLE 13-3	
Effective Atomic Numbers of Various Materials Important to Diagnostic Radiology	
Type of Substance	**Effective Atomic Number**
Human tissue	
Fat	6.3
Muscle	7.4
Lung	7.4
Bone	13.8
Contrast agent	
Air	7.6
Iodine	53
Barium	56
Other	
Concrete	17
Molybdenum	42
Tungsten	74
Lead	82

    b. $\left(\dfrac{56}{7.4}\right)^3 = 433$ or 43,300% chance of interacting with barium

Cubic relationships. The probability of interaction proportional to the third power changes rapidly. For the photoelectric effect, this means that a small variation in atomic number of the tissue atom or a small variation in x-ray energy results in a large change in the chance of photoelectric interaction. This is unlike the situation that exists for the Compton interaction.

Question: If the relative probability of photoelectric interaction with soft tissue for a 20 keV x-ray is 1, how much less likely will an interaction be for a 50 keV x-ray? How much more likely is interaction with iodine than with soft tissue for a 70 keV x-ray?

Answer:

$$\left(\frac{20 \text{ keV}}{50 \text{ keV}}\right)^3 = \left(\frac{2}{5}\right)^3$$

$= 0.064$ or 6.4% is the probability of 50 keV interaction compared with 20 keV interaction

Atomic number of iodine $= 53$

Atomic number of soft tissue $= 7.4$

$$\left(\frac{53}{7.4}\right)^3 = 368 \text{ or } 36{,}800\% \text{ is the}$$

probability of interaction with iodine compared with soft tissue

Table 13-4 summarizes the photoelectric effect.

Pair Production
takes energy and creates matter

If an incident x-ray has sufficient energy, it may escape interaction with the electron shells and come close enough to the nucleus of the atom to be influenced by the strong electrostatic field of the nucleus. The interaction between the x-ray and the nuclear electrostatic field causes the x-ray to disappear. In its place appear two electrons, one positively charged **positron** and one negatively charged **electron**. This process is called *pair production* (Figure 13-8).

In Chapter 5, the energy equivalence of the mass of an electron is calculated to equal 0.51 MeV. Since two

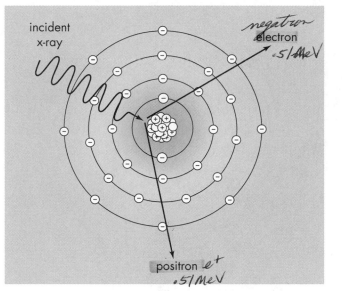

FIGURE 13-8 Pair production occurs with x-rays that have energies greater than 1.02 MeV. The photon interacts with the nuclear force field, and two electrons that have opposite electrostatic charges are created.

electrons are formed in a pair-production interaction, the incident photon must have at least 1.02 MeV of energy. An x-ray with less than 1.02 MeV cannot undergo pair-production. Any of the energy in excess of 1.02 MeV is distributed equally between the two electrons as kinetic energy. Because pair production involves only x-rays with energies greater than 1.02 MeV, it rarely occurs in the diagnostic x-ray range.
= pair annihilation

Photodisintegration

Very high-energy x-rays, those with energy above 10 MeV, can escape interaction with electrons and the nuclear electrostatic field and be absorbed directly by the nucleus. When this happens, the nucleus is raised to an excited state and instantaneously emits a nucleon or other nuclear fragment. This process is called *photodisintegration* (Figure 13-9). Because it involves only x-rays with energies greater than approximately 10 MeV, photodisintegration, like pair production, rarely occurs in the diagnostic x-ray range.

DIFFERENTIAL ABSORPTION

Of the five ways an x-ray can interact with tissue, only the following two occur in the diagnostic range: (1) the Compton effect and (2) the photoelectric effect. The Compton effect results in no diagnostic information reaching the image. The photoelectric effect results in x-rays that are completely absorbed. Those x-ray photons that pass through the body without interacting produce the x-ray image. Figure 13-10 shows schematically how each of these three types of x-ray contributes

TABLE 13-4	
Features of Photoelectric Effect	
Most likely to occur	• With inner-shell electrons • With tightly bound electrons • When x-ray energy is just higher than electron binding energy
As x-ray energy increases	• Increased probability of penetration through tissue without interaction • Less probability of photoelectric effect relative to Compton scattering • Reduced absolute photoelectric effect
As atomic number of absorber increases	• Probability increases proportionally with the cube of the atomic number (Z^3)
As mass density of absorber increases	• Proportional increase in x-ray absorption • More photoelectric effect

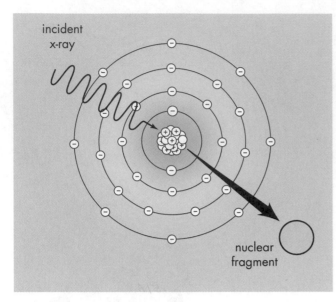

FIGURE 13-9 Photo disintegration is an interaction between high-energy photons and the nucleus. The photon is absorbed by the nucleus, and a nuclear fragment is emitted.

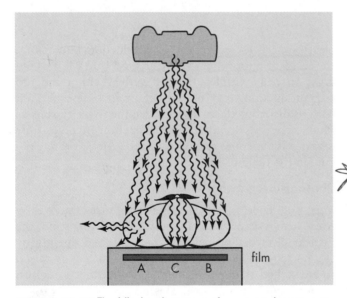

FIGURE 13-10 The following three types of x-rays are important to the making of a radiograph; **A,** those scattered by Compton interaction; **B,** those absorbed photoelectrically, and **C,** those transmitted through the patient without interaction.

to a radiograph. It should be clear that the Compton-scattered x-ray contributes no useful information to the radiograph. When a Compton-scattered x-ray interacts with the **film emulsion,** it carries no information about the tissue through which it passed (Figure 13-11). These scattered x-rays result in **film fog,** a generalized dulling of the image on the radiograph by optical densities that do not represent diagnostic information. To reduce fog, there are techniques and devices that reduce the number of scattered x-rays reaching the film.

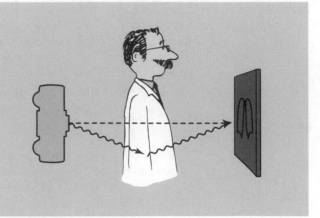

FIGURE 13-11 When an x-ray is Compton scattered, the image receptor responds as if it came straight from the target.

X-rays that undergo photoelectric interaction provide diagnostic information to the image receptor or film. They do not reach the film, but these x-rays represent anatomic structures with high x-ray absorption. Such structures are **radiopaque.** The photoelectric absorption of x-rays results in the bright areas of a radiograph, which correspond to bone or other dense tissue. Other x-rays penetrate the body with no interaction whatsoever. They result in the dark (high optical density) areas of a radiograph. The anatomic structures through which these x-rays pass are **radiolucent.**

Basically, an x-ray image results from the difference between those x-rays absorbed photoelectrically and those not absorbed at all. This characteristic is called ***differential absorption.*** Except at very low kVp, most x-rays that interact do so by the Compton effect. This is one reason that radiographs are not as sharp and clear as photographs. Generally less than 5% of the incident x-rays passing through a patient reach the film. Less than half of those that reach the film interact to form an image. The radiographic image results from only 1% of the x-rays emitted by the x-ray unit. Consequently, careful control and selection of the x-ray beam is necessary to produce high-quality radiographs. Producing a high-quality radiograph requires the proper selection of kVp so that the effective x-ray energy results in **maximum differential absorption.** Because absorption increases as the kVp is reduced, reduced kVp results in increased patient dose. An optimum kVp is used to provide a compromise between absorption and penetration based on the atomic number(z) of the tissue.

Consider the radiograph of an extremity (Figure 13-12). An image of the bone is produced because many more x-rays are absorbed photoelectrically in bone than in soft tissue. Recall that the probability of an x-ray undergoing photoelectric absorption is pro-

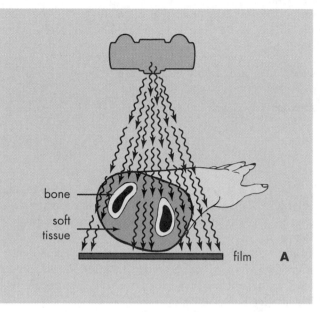

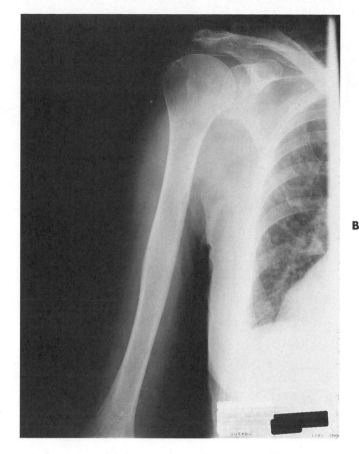

B

FIGURE 13-12 Radiograph of bony structures results from the differential absorption between bone and soft tissue as shown in **A,** a drawing of a forearm, and **B,** a radiograph of an upper arm and shoulder. (**B,** *Courtesy John Lampign.*)

portional to the third power of the atomic number of the tissue. According to Table 13-3, bone has an atomic number of 13.8; soft tissue has an atomic number of 7.4. Consequently, the probability that an x-ray will undergo a photoelectric interaction is approximately seven times greater in bone than in soft tissue.

Question: How much more likely is an x-ray to interact with bone than muscle?

Answer:

$$\frac{(13.8)^3}{(7.4)^3} = \frac{2628}{405} = 6.5 \text{ times more likely to interact with bone than muscle}$$

These relative values of interaction are apparent in Figure 13-6 when one pays particular attention to the logarithmic scale of the vertical axis (see Chapter 2). Notice that the relative probability of interaction between bone and soft tissue (differential absorption) remains constant, whereas the absolute probability of each decreases with increasing energy. With higher x-ray energy, fewer interactions occur; thus more x-rays are transmitted without interaction.

Question: What is the relative probability that a 20-keV x-ray will undergo photoelectric interaction in bone compared with fat?

Answer:

$$Z_{bone} = 13.8, Z_{fat} = 6.8$$

$$\left(\frac{13.8}{6.8}\right)^3 = 8.36 \text{ times more probable an interaction will occur in bone than in fat}$$

Compton scattering of x-rays is independent of the atomic number (Z) of different tissue (Figure 13-4). The probability of Compton scattering for bone atoms and for soft tissue atoms is about equal and decreases with increasing x-ray energy. This decrease in scattering, however, is not as rapid as that occurring with photoelectric absorption.

Probability of Interaction Formulas

The probability of Compton scattering is inversely proportional to x-ray energy ($1/E$). The probability of photoelectric effect is approximately inversely proportional to the third power of energy ($1/E^3$).

At low energies the majority of x-ray interactions are photoelectric. At high energies, Compton scattering predominates. Of course, as x-ray energy is increased, the chance of any interaction at all decreases, more x-rays get to the film, and therefore a lower x-ray quantity (lower mAs) is required. Figure 13-13 combines all these factors into one graph. At 20 keV the probability of photoelectric effect equals the probability of Comp-

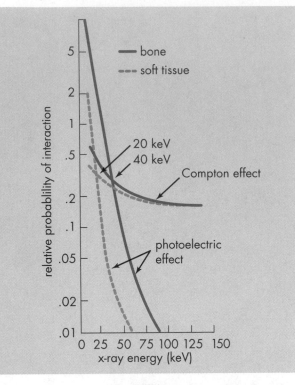

FIGURE 13-13 Graph showing probabilities of photoelectric and Compton interaction with soft tissue and bone. The intersections of these curves indicate those x-ray energies at which the chance of photoelectric absorption equals the chance of Compton scattering.

ton scattering in soft tissue. Below this energy most x-rays interact with soft tissue photoelectrically. Above this energy the predominate interaction with soft tissue is Compton scattering. To image small differences in soft tissue, as in mammography, low kVp results in maximum differential absorption.

In summary, photoelectric interactions in bone and soft tissue depend on the atomic number (Z) of tissue. Maximum differential absorption forms the highest quality radiograph. The loss of radiographic contrast is due to fog caused by Compton scattering. When the amount of scattered radiation becomes too high, **grids** are used. Grids do not affect differential absorption; they simply reduce the scattered radiation reaching the film.

The following two other factors are also important in making an image: (1) the x-ray emission spectrum and (2) the mass density of patient tissue.

Dependence on the Density of Matter

Bone could be imaged even if differential absorption were not related to atomic number because bone has higher mass density than soft tissue. **Mass density** is not to be confused with optical density. Mass density is the quantity of matter per unit volume, usually specified in

units of kilograms per cubic meter (kg/m³). Sometimes mass density is reported in grams per cubic centimeter (gm/cm³).

Question: How many gm/cm³ are there in 1 kg/m³?

Answer: $gm/cm^3 = (1 \ gm/cm^3) \left(\frac{kg}{10^3 \ gm}\right)\left(\frac{100 \ cm}{m}\right)^3$

$= (1 \ gm/cm^3) \ (10^{-3} \ kg/gm) \ (10^6 \ cm^3/m^3)$

$gm/cm^3 = 10^3 \ kg/m^3$

Table 13-5 gives the mass densities of several materials. Mass density is related to the mass of each atom and tells how tightly the atoms of a substance are packed. Water and ice are composed of precisely the same atoms, but ice occupies more volume. The mass density of ice is 917 kg/m³ compared with 1000 kg/m³ for water. Ice floats in water because of this difference in mass density. Ice is lighter than water.

Mass Density

The interaction between x-rays and tissue is proportional to the mass density of the tissue.

When the mass density is doubled, the chance for x-ray interaction is doubled because there are twice as many electrons available for interaction. Therefore, even without the Z-related photoelectric effect, nearly twice as many x-rays would be absorbed and scattered in bone as in soft tissue.

TABLE 13-5	
Mass Density of Various Materials Important to Diagnostic Radiology	
Type of Substance	**Mass Density (kg/m³)**
Human tissue	
Lung	320
Fat	910
Muscle	1000
Bone	1850
Contrast material	
Air	1.3
Barium	3500
Iodine	4930
Other	
Calcium	1550
Concrete	2350
Molybdenum	10200
Rhenium	12500
Tungsten	19300
Lead	11350

Question: What is the relative probability that 60 keV x-rays will undergo Compton scattering in bone compared with soft tissue?

Answer: Mass density of bone = 1.85 kg/m³

Mass density of soft tissue = 1.0 kg/m³

$$\frac{1.85}{1.00} = 1.85 \text{ more probable that Compton scattering will occur in bone than in soft tissue}$$

Lungs are imaged on a chest radiograph primarily because of differences in mass density. According to Table 13-5, the mass density of soft tissue is 773 times that of air. For the same thickness, 773 times as many x-rays interact with soft tissue than with air. The atomic numbers of air and soft tissue are about the same (7.4 for soft tissue and 7.6 for air). Thus differential absorption in air-filled soft tissue cavities is primarily due to mass-density differences. Figure 13-14 demonstrates differential absorption in air, soft tissue, and bone caused by mass-density differences. Table 13-6 summarizes the various relationships of differential absorption.

Question: Assume that all x-ray interactions during mammography are photoelectric. What is the differential absorption of x-rays in **microcalcifications** (bone) relative to fatty tissue? (See Tables 13-3 and 13-5).

Answer: Differential absorption due to atomic number:

$$\frac{(13.8)^3}{(6.3)^3} = \frac{2628}{250} = 10.5$$

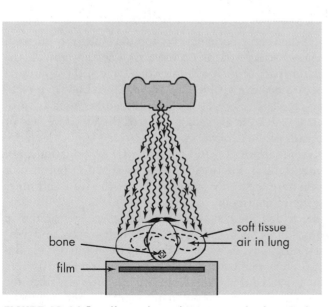

FIGURE 13-14 Even if x-ray interaction was not related to atomic number (Z), differential absorption would occur because of differences in mass density.

TABLE 13-6
Characteristics of Differential Absorption

As x-ray energy increases	• Fewer Compton interactions occur • Much fewer photoelectric interactions occur • More photons are transmitted through tissue
As tissue atomic number increases	• No change in the number of Compton interactions occurs • Many more photoelectric interactions occur • Less x-ray transmission
As tissue mass density increases	• Proportional increase in Compton interactions • Proportional increase in photoelectric interactions • Proportional reduction in x-ray transmission

Differential absorption due to mass density:

$$\frac{1850}{910} = 2.0$$

Total differential absorption:

$$(10.5)(2.0) = 21$$

ATTENUATION
Absorption

When x-rays penetrate any type of tissue, they interact with the atoms of that tissue by any of the five mechanisms discussed previously. The relative frequency of interaction by each mechanism depends primarily on the atomic number of the tissue atoms and the x-ray energy. The photoelectric effect is called **absorption** because the x-ray disappears. Interactions in which the x-ray is only partially absorbed, such as the Compton effect, are **scattering** processes. Classical scattering, pair production, and photodisintegration also represent scattering events because the x-rays emerging from the interaction travel in a direction different from that of the incident x-rays.

Attenuation

The total reduction in the number of x-rays remaining in an x-ray beam after penetration through a given thickness of tissue is called **attenuation.**

When a broad beam of x-rays penetrates any tissue, some of the x-rays are absorbed and some are scattered. The result is a reduction in the number of x-rays, thus attenuation equals absorption plus scattering.

X-rays are **attenuated exponentially,** which means that they do have a fixed range in tissue. They are reduced in number by a given percentage for each incremental thickness of tissue they go through.

Consider the situation diagrammed in Figure 13-15. One thousand x-rays are incident on tissue 5 centimeters thick. The x-ray energy and the atomic number of the tissue are such that 50% of the x-rays are removed per centimeter. Therefore in the first centimeter 500 x-rays are removed, leaving 500 available to enter the second centimeter. By the end of the second centimeter, 50% of the 500 x-rays have been removed, which leaves 250 x-rays to enter the third centimeter of thickness. Similarly, 125 x-rays enter the fourth centimeter of thickness and 63 enter the fifth centimeter. Half of the 63 x-rays are attenuated in the last centimeter of tissue and, therefore only 32 emerge. The total effect of these interactions is 3% transmission and 97% attenuation of the x-ray beam. A plot of this hypothetical beam attenuation, which closely resembles the actual situation, appears in Figure 13-16. It should be clear that, theoretically at least, the number of x-rays emerging from any thickness of absorber never reaches zero. Each succeeding thickness can attenuate the x-ray beam only by a fractional amount, and a fraction of any positive number is always greater than zero. The beam exiting from tissue and hitting the x-ray film emulsion is called *remnant radiation*. Remnant radiation remains after attenuation by matter.

RADIOLOGIC CONTRAST AGENTS

Barium and iodine compounds are used as an aid for imaging internal organs. The atomic number (Z) of barium is 56 and the atomic number (Z) of iodine is 53. Each has a much higher atomic number and mass density than soft tissue. When used to help see organs by filling them in, they are called *contrast agents*.

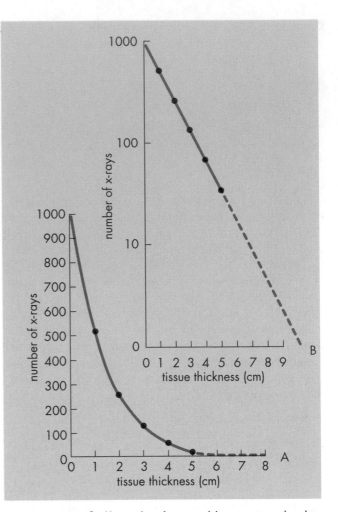

FIGURE 13-16 A, Linear plot of exponential x-ray attenuation data in Figure 13-15. **B,** Semilog plot of same data.

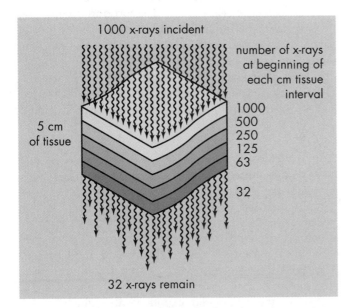

FIGURE 13-15 Interaction of x-rays by absorption and scatter is called *attenuation*. In this example the x-ray beam has been attenuated 97%; 3% have been transmitted.

When an iodinated compound fills the **internal carotid artery** or a blood vessel or when barium fills the colon (part of the gastrointestinal tract), these internal organs become visible on a radiograph. Low-kVp technique (e.g., below 80 kVp) is sometimes used to produce high-contrast radiographs of the blood vessels or organs of the genitourinary (GU) tract. Higher kVp operation (above 90 kVp) is used in GI examinations, not only to fill in the organ under investigation but also to penetrate the contrast media to see the wall and inner space of the organ.

Air was used at one time as a contrast medium in procedures such as **pneumoencephalography** and **ventriculography**. In these procedures the normal body fluids filling these internal cavities were replaced by air. Such procedures have disappeared, however, since the introduction of computed tomography and magnetic resonance imaging. However, air is still used as a contrast agent in a gastrointestinal examination, called a *double-contrast examination*.

SUMMARY

The following are five fundamental interactions between x-rays and matter:

1. Classical scattering is a change in the direction of an incident x-ray without a loss of energy.
2. The Compton effect occurs when incident x-rays ionize atoms and the x-ray then changes direction with a loss of energy.
3. The photoelectric effect occurs when the incident x-ray is absorbed in one of the inner electron shells and emits a photoelectron with energy nearly equal to the energy of the incident x-ray.
4. Pair production occurs when the incident x-ray interacts with the electrostatic field of the nucleus. The x-ray disappears and two electrons appear, one positively charged (positron) and one negatively charged (electron).
5. Photodisintegration occurs when the incident x-ray is directly absorbed by the nucleus. The x-ray disappears and nuclear fragments are released.

The interactions that occur most frequently in the diagnostic x-ray range (23 to 150 kVp) are the Compton effect and the photoelectric effect.

Differential absorption is used to make a radiograph. The x-ray image results from the difference between those x-rays absorbed by photoelectric interaction and those x-rays that pass through the body and form remnant radiation. Attenuation is the reduction of the x-ray beam intensity as it penetrates through a thickness of tissue. Differential absorption and attenuation of the x-ray beam depends on the following two factors: (1) the atomic number (Z) of the atoms in tissue and (2) the mass density of the atoms in tissue.

Radiologic contrast agents, such as iodine and barium, use the principles of differential absorption and attenuation to image soft tissue organs within the body. Iodine is used in vascular, renal, and biliary imaging. Barium is used for gastrointestinal imaging. Both elements have high atomic (Z) numbers (iodine is 53, barium is 56) and mass densities greater than soft tissue.

REVIEW QUESTIONS

1. Electromagnetic radiation interacts with structures similar in size to _____.
2. _____ _____ is a change of direction of an x-ray without a change in its energy.
3. The energy of the Compton-scattered x-ray is equal to the difference of what two energies?
4. The secondary electron is associated with _____ interaction.
5. The probability of the Compton effect depends on the atomic number of the target atom. True or False? Defend your answer.
6. When x-ray energy is increased, is there an increase or a reduction of Compton scattering?
7. Describe the photoelectric effect.
8. X-ray interaction with the nucleus results in _____ _____.
9. When x-ray energy is increased, what is the relationship between x-ray production from the photoelectric effect versus Compton scattering?
10. Photodisintegration involves x-ray energies greater than _____.
11. Define differential absorption.
12. How much more likely is it that an x-ray will interact with bone than muscle?
13. What is the relationship between the atomic number (Z) of tissue and differential absorption?
14. What is the relationship between the mass density of tissue and differential absorption?
15. Define mass density.
16. Attenuation is _____.
17. Attenuation equals _____ plus _____.
18. The x-rays remaining after attenuation by matter are _____ _____.
19. In a contrast radiographic examination using iodine, what is the probability that the x-ray beam will interact with iodine rather than tissue?
20. What kVp level is used to penetrate barium in a contrast examination?

Additional Reading

Magalhaes SD, Eichler J, Goncalves OD, Rizzo P: Scattering of photons and influence in diagnostic radiology, *Appl Radiat Isot* 46(6-7):647, June-July 1995.

Mosby's radiographic instructional series: radiologic physics [slide set], St. Louis, 1996, Mosby.

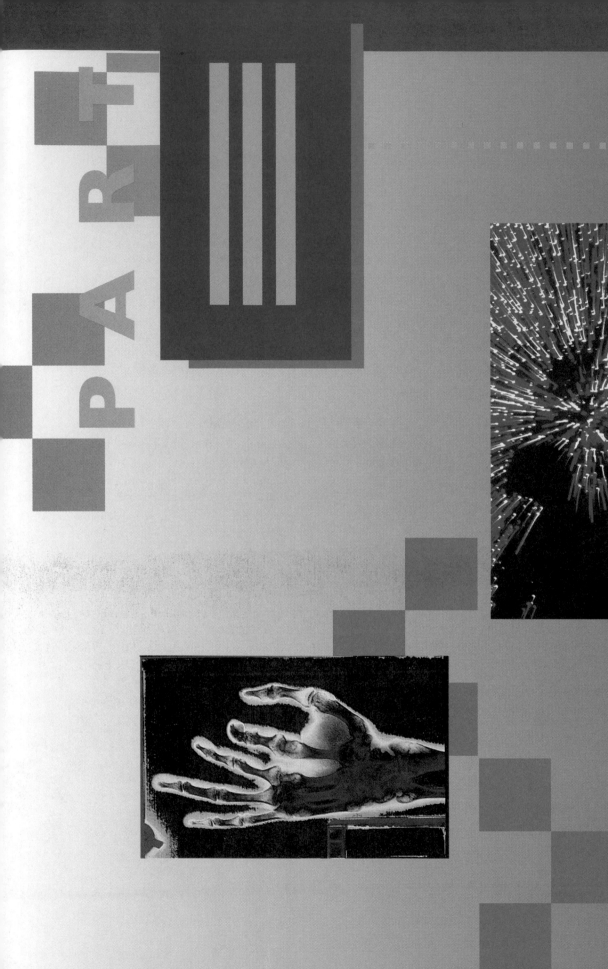

PART III

THE RADIOGRAPHIC IMAGE

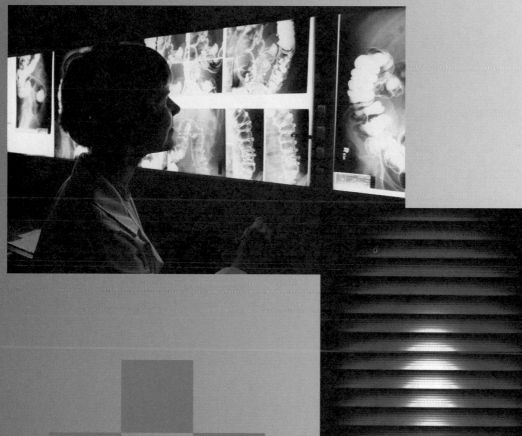

14 Radiographic Film

OBJECTIVES

At the completion of this chapter the student will be able to:

1. Discuss the construction of radiographic film
2. Describe the formation of the latent image
3. List and define the characteristics of x-ray film
4. Identify the types of film used in diagnostic imaging departments
5. Explain proper film storage and handling procedures

OUTLINE

Remnant Radiation
Radiographic Film
  Film construction
  Formation of latent image

Radiographic film characteristics
Types of film
Handling and storage of films

R emnant radiation exits the **anatomic part** and exposes the radiographic screens placed in the protective radiographic **cassette**. The **intensifying screens** emit light energy to expose the radiographic film placed between the two screens.

REMNANT RADIATION

The useful beam is transmitted from the target of the x-ray tube. Although the beam is composed of x-ray photons of varied energy, the photons are nearly uniformly distributed throughout the beam. After interaction with the patient, the beam is attenuated. The attenuation of the beam depends on the atomic number and mass density of the tissue through which it passes. What was once a nearly uniform beam before interaction with the patient becomes a **remnant beam** of varied intensity.

Remnant Radiation
Remnant radiation remains in the beam after attenuation by matter.

The remnant beam then interacts with the **image receptor**, the **x-ray film**, and the **x-ray screen** combination mounted in a protective **cassette**. The remnant beam activates the material within the screens, which changes x-ray energy to **visible light**. Visible light is then emitted from the screens, exposing the radiographic film within the cassette. Because visible light exposes the x-ray film, the characteristics of x-ray film is similar to the characteristics of photographic film. X-ray film is manufactured with high quality control and has a **spectral response** different from that of photographic film, but otherwise it is the same.

RADIOGRAPHIC FILM

Film Construction

Radiographic film basically has two parts: (1) **base** and (2) **emulsion** (Figure 14-1). Most x-ray film has the emulsion coated on both sides and therefore is called *duplitized* or *double-emulsion film.* Between the emulsion and the base is a thin coating of material called the *adhesive layer,* which ensures a uniform adhesion of the emulsion to the base. This adhesive layer allows the emulsion and base to maintain proper contact during use and processing. The emulsion is encased by a protective covering of gelatin called the *supercoating.* This supercoating protects the emulsion from scratching, pressure, and contamination during handling, processing, and storage and allows for relatively rough manipulation of x-ray film before exposure. **Processed film** may be handled with even less regard for damage.

Base. The base is the support for the radiographic film emulsion. Its primary purpose is to provide a rigid

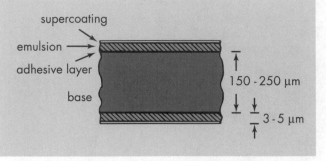

FIGURE 14-1 Cross-sectional view of radiographic film. The bulk of the film is the base. The emulsion contains the diagnostic information.

structure onto which the emulsion can be coated. The base is flexible and unbreakable to allow easy handling, but it is sufficiently rigid to be snapped into a view box. Conventional photographic film has a much thinner base than radiographic film and therefore is not as rigid. Imagine attempting to snap a 14×17 inch conventional photographic negative into a view box. The base of radiographic film maintains its size and shape during use and processing. The rigidity of the base prevents distortion of the radiographic image. This rigid property of the base is known as *dimensional stability.* The base is of uniform **lucency**, nearly transparent to light, so that there is no unwanted pattern on the film caused by the base. During manufacture, however, dye is added to the base to tint the film blue. This coloring results in less eyestrain and fatigue for the radiologist and therefore is conducive to more efficient and accurate diagnoses.

The original radiographic film base was a glass plate. Radiologists used to refer to radiographs as x-ray plates. During World War I, the availability of the high-quality glass used as the radiographic film base became severely limited (see Chapter 1). At the same time, medical applications of x-rays, particularly by the military, were increasing rapidly. A substitute material, **cellulose nitrate,** soon became the standard base. Cellulose nitrate, however, had one serious deficiency. It was inflammable. The improper storage and handling of some x-ray film files resulted in severe hospital fires during the 1920s and early 1930s. By the mid-1920s, film using a safety base, **cellulose triacetate,** was introduced. Cellulose triacetate has properties similar to those of cellulose nitrate but is not as inflammable. In the early 1960s a **polyester** base was introduced. Polyester has taken the place of cellulose triacetate as the film base of choice. Polyester is more resistant to warping from age and is stronger than cellulose triacetate, permitting easier transport through automatic processors. Its dimensional stability is superior. Polyester bases at 175 μm are thinner than triacetate bases at 200 μm but are just as strong. The polyester base is similar in composition to the polyester fibers in clothing. Principally two chemicals, ethylene glycol and dimethyl terephthalate, are formed into a molten polymer (a very large molecule made from two or more smaller ones) by mixing at high temperature and low pressure. For clothing, the polyester is produced in thin strands like thread. For film, it is formed into thin sheets of appropriate size.

2) **Emulsion.** The emulsion is the most important part of the x-ray film. It is the material with which x-rays or light photons from screens interact and transfer information. The emulsion consists of a homogeneous mixture of **gelatin** and **silver-halide crystals.** It is coated evenly with a 3 to 5 μm thick layer. The gelatin is similar to that used in gelatin salads and desserts but is of much higher quality. It is clear, so that it transmits light, and is sufficiently porous for the processing chemicals to penetrate to the crystals of silver halide. Its principal function is to provide mechanical support for the silver-halide crystals by holding them uniformly in place. The silver-halide crystal is the active ingredient of the radiographic emulsion. In the typical emulsion, 95% of the silver halide is **silver bromide.** The remainder is usually **silver iodide.** These atoms have relatively high atomic numbers ($Z_I = 53$, $Z_{Br} = 35$, $Z_{Ag} = 47$) compared with the gelatin and base (for both, $Z = 7$). The interaction of x-ray and light photons with these high-Z atoms ultimately results in the formation of an image on the radiograph. The silver-halide crystals are flat and trigonal, approximately 1 μm on a side. The arrangement of atoms in the crystals is cubic, as shown in Figure 14-2. The crystals are made by dissolving metallic **silver (Ag)** in **nitric acid (HNO₃)** to form **silver nitrate (AgNO₃).** The light-sensitive **silver-bromide (AgBr)** crystals are formed by mixing the **silver nitrate** with **potassium bromide (KBr)** in the following reaction:

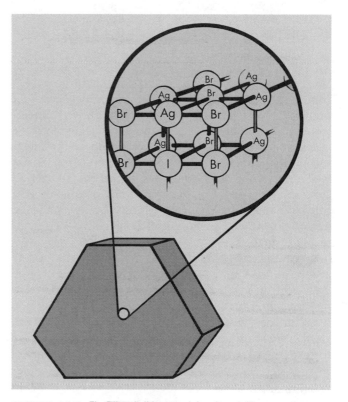

FIGURE 14-2 The silver-halide crystal is trigonal. The arrangement of atoms in the crystal is cubic.

Silver-Halide Crystal Reaction

$$AgNO_3 + KBr \rightarrow AgBr \downarrow + KNO_3$$

The arrow ↓ indicates that the silver bromide is precipitated, whereas the potassium nitrate, which is water-soluble, is washed away.

At the manufacturing plant, the entire process of forming silver-halide crystals takes place in a vat of gelatin, with the temperature, the pressure, and the rate at which ingredients are mixed precisely controlled. The emulsion is then ready to spread onto the polyester base.

The shape and lattice structure of the silver-halide crystals are not perfect, and some of the imperfections result in the imaging property of the crystals. An imperfection thought to be a chemical contaminant, usually silver sulfide (AgS), intrudes into the crystal lattice or resides on the crystal surface. This contaminant has been given the name *sensitivity speck.* It has been shown that during the processing of the radiographic image the silver atoms are attracted to and concentrate at the location of the sensitivity speck.

The differences in **speed, contrast,** and **resolution** among various radiographic films are determined by how the silver-halide crystals are manufactured and by how the crystals are mixed into the gelatin. The number of sensitivity specks per crystal, the concentration of crystals in the emulsion, and the size and distribution of the crystals also affect the performance characteristic of radiographic film. The concentration of silver-halide crystals determines film characteristics. The composition of the radiographic emulsion is a **proprietary secret** closely guarded by each manufacturer. The making of radiographic film is conducted in total darkness. From the moment of emulsion, ingredients are brought together until final packaging, no light is present.

Formation of Latent Image

The remnant radiation exiting the patient and hitting the radiographic film deposits energy (primarily by photoelectric interaction) into the atoms of the silver-halide crystal. This energy is deposited in a pattern representative of the object or part of the anatomy being radiographed. If one observed the film immediately after exposure, no image would be seen. There is, however, an image present, which is called a *latent image.*

Latent Image

The latent image is the invisible change induced in the silver-halide crystals.

With proper chemical processing, the latent image becomes a **manifest image**. The interaction between light photons and silver-halide crystals is fairly well understood, as is the processing of the latent image into the manifest image. However, the formation of the latent image, sometimes called the *photographic effect,* is not well understood and continues to be the subject of considerable research. The following discussion is a brief summary of the Gurney-Mott theory, which is the accepted, although incomplete, explanation of latent-image formation.

Silver-Halide Crystal. The silver, bromide, and iodine atoms are fixed in the **crystal lattice in ion form** (Figure 14-3). Silver is a positive ion. Bromine and iodine are negative ions. An ion is an atom that has either too many or too few electrons and therefore, as a whole, is electrically charged. When a silver-halide crystal is formed, the silver atoms each release an outer-shell electron, which becomes attached to a halide atom (either bromine or iodine). Thus the silver atom is missing an electron and is a positively charged ion, identified as **Ag$^+$**. The bromine and iodine atoms each have one extra electron, are negatively charged ions, and are identified as **Br$^-$** and **I$^-$**. The silver halide crystal is not rigid. Diamond crystals, for example, are very rigid. Under certain conditions both atoms and electrons are free to migrate within the crystal. The halide ions, bromine and iodine, are generally in greatest concentration along the surface of the crystal. Therefore the crystal takes on a negative surface charge, which is matched by the positive charge of the **interstitial** silver ions or the silver ions inside the crystal. The sensitivity speck is believed to be located on or near the surface. A model of the silver-halide crystal is shown in Figure 14-4.

Photon Interaction with Silver-Halide Crystal. When light interacts with film, most photon energy is trans-

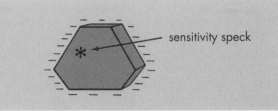

FIGURE 14-4 Model of a silver-halide crystal, emphasizing sensitivity speck and concentration of negative ions on surface.

ferred to the gelatin. It is the interaction with the silver and halide atoms (Ag, Br, and I) that responds to form the latent image. If the light photon is totally absorbed (Figure 14-5, *A*), its interaction is photoelectric. If the light photon is partially absorbed, its interaction is Compton. In both cases a **secondary electron**, either a photoelectron or Compton electron, is released with sufficient energy to travel a large distance in the crystal. While crossing the crystal, the secondary electron may have sufficient energy to dislodge additional electrons from the crystal lattice. Consequently, as a result of one interaction, a number of electrons are released and travel through the crystal lattice. The release of these secondary electrons is represented as follows:

$$Br^- + photon \rightarrow Br + e^-$$

The result is the same if the interaction involves x-rays using **direct-exposure film,** but because x-ray photons have higher energy, fewer are needed to produce an

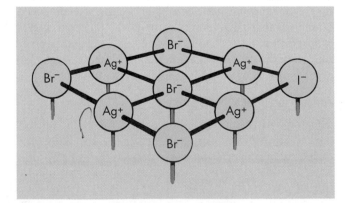

FIGURE 14-3 Silver-halide crystal lattice contains ions. Electrons from Ag atoms are attached to Br and I atoms.

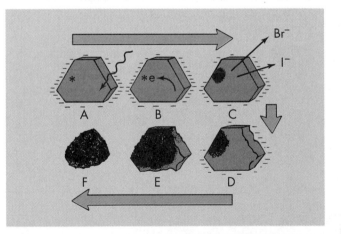

FIGURE 14-5 Production of the latent image and the conversion of the latent image into a manifest image follow several simultaneous steps. **A,** Light or radiation interaction releases electrons. **B,** These electrons migrate to the sensitivity speck. **C,** At the sensitivity speck, atomic silver is formed. **D,** This process is repeated many times, which results in the disappearance of the negative surface electrification and the buildup of silver atoms. **E,** The remaining silver halide is converted with processing. **F,** The resulting silver grain.

equal number of migrating secondary electrons. Some of these migrating electrons pass near or through the sensitivity speck (Figure 14-5, *B*). Here many of them are trapped by the positively charged silver ion. This reaction is represented as follows (Figure 14-5, *C*):

$$e^- + Ag^+ \rightarrow Ag$$

Most of these electrons come from the bromine and iodine ions, since these negative ions have one extra electron. These negative ions therefore are converted to neutral atoms, and the loss of ionic charge results in a disruption of the crystal lattice. The bromine and iodine atoms are now free to migrate, since they are no longer bound by ionic forces. They migrate out of the crystal into the gelatin portion of the emulsion . The deterioration of crystalline structure also makes it easier for remaining silver ions to migrate.

Latent Image. The concentration of electrons at the sensitivity speck produces a region of negative electrification. As the halide atoms are removed from the crystal, the positive silver ions are electrostatically attracted to the sensitivity speck. After migrating to the sensitivity speck, the silver ions are neutralized by electrons and converted to atomic silver (Figure 14-5, *D*). In each crystal, less than ten silver atoms are deposited at the sensitivity speck in this fashion. Consequently, this silver deposition is not observable, even microscopically. This group of silver atoms is called a *latent-image center.* It is here that visible quantities of silver form during processing to create the radiographic image. Crystals with silver deposited at the sensitivity speck develop into black grains. Crystals that have not been irradiated remain crystalline and inactive. The unobservable information contained in light-activated and inactivated silver halide crystals constitutes the latent image. *Processing* is the term applied to the chemical reactions that transform the latent image into a manifest radiographic image (Figure 14-5, *E* and *F*). Because of its importance, this subject is dealt with separately in Chapter 15.

Radiographic Film Characteristics

Medical imaging, especially radiography, is becoming extremely technical and sophisticated. This is reflected in the number and variety of the radiographic films used. The major film manufacturers each produce over 25 different films for medical imaging. When combined with the various film sizes produced, over 500 selections are possible. Table 14-1 shows the standard film sizes in English and metric (SI units).

In most cases the sizes are not exactly equivalent, but they are usually interchangeable. By far the most commonly used film is that customarily referred to as *screen film.* Even screen film, however, comes in a variety of types. In addition to screen film, there is **direct-exposure film,** which is sometimes called *nonscreen film.* There is also special application films such as film used in mam-

TABLE 14-1	
Standard Film Sizes	
English Units	**Metric Units**
	18 × 43 centimeters
8 × 10 inches	20 × 25 centimeters
	24 × 30 centimeters
10 × 12 inches	
	28 × 35 centimeters
14 × 14 inches	35 × 35 centimeters
14 × 17 inches	35 × 43 centimeters

mography, **video recording, duplication, subtraction, cineradiography,** and dental radiography. Each has particular reasons for use. The following is a brief description of the characteristics of radiographic film.

Spectral Matching. Perhaps the most important consideration in selecting modern **screen film** is its **spectral absorption characteristics.** Since the introduction of **rare-earth screens** in the early 1970s, one must be particularly cautious to use a film whose sensitivity to various colors of light, its **spectral response,** is properly matched to the spectrum of light emitted by the screen. Calcium tungstate screens, used before the development of rare-earth screens, emit blue and blue-violet light and therefore must be exposed only with standard silver-halide film. These films respond to violet and blue light but not to green, yellow, or red. They are called *blue-sensitive films.* If rare-earth screens are used, they should be matched with a film that is sensitive not only to blue light but also to green light. Such film is **orthochromatic** and is called *green-sensitive film.* This is distinct from **panchromatic film,** which is used in photography and is sensitive to the entire visible-light spectrum. Figure 14-6 shows the spectral response of blue- and green-sensitive

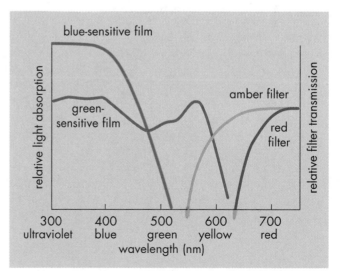

FIGURE 14-6 Radiographic films are either blue sensitive or green sensitive, and they require amber- and red-filtered safelights, respectively.

film. Blue-sensitive film should be used with calcium-tungstate screens. Green-sensitive film is usually exposed with rare-earth screens, although several phosphors, notably **lanthanum oxybromide** and **barium strontium sulfate**, emit in the blue-violet region of the spectrum. If there is an improper match of the spectral emission of a screen with the spectral sensitivity of film, the image-receptor speed will be greatly reduced, and patient dose will be increased. Proper **spectral matching** results in the correct **film-screen combination**.

Speed. Film is also available with different sensitivity to light photons or speed. Usually a manufacturer offers two or three different films having different speeds and different emulsions. In general, the thicker the emulsion, the more sensitive is the film to light and therefore the higher the speed. To optimize speed, screen films are almost always double emulsion, that is, emulsion is layered on either side of the base. This provides for twice the speed that could be obtained with a single-emulsion film, even if the single emulsion were made twice as thick. There is a limit to film speed, however, because the light from the **intensifying screen** is absorbed very rapidly in the superficial layers of the emulsion. If the emulsion thickness is too great, the portion next to the film base remains largely unexposed. In general, large-grain emulsions are more sensitive than small-grain emulsions. Current emulsions contain less silver yet produce the same optical density per unit exposure. This more efficient use of silver in the emulsion is termed the **covering power** of the emulsion. The reported speed of a film is nearly always that for the total image receptor, that is, the film and two screens in combination. When screens and film are properly matched, the speed re-ported by the manufacturer will be accurate. Mismatch can result in significant error in exposure of the radiograph.

Contrast. Most manufacturers offer screen films with multiple **contrast** levels. **High-contrast film** produces a black-and-white image, whereas a **low-contrast film** image is gray. Contrast is dealt with in more detail in Chapter 19.

Latitude. The contrast of an image receptor is inversely proportional to its exposure **latitude,** that is, the range of exposure techniques that produces an acceptable image. Consequently, screen films are available in multiple latitudes. Usually the manufacturer identifies these as medium-, high-, or higher-contrast films. The difference is basically one of **silver-halide crystal size** and **distribution**. A high-contrast emulsion contains smaller silver-halide grains with a relatively uniform grain size. Lower-contrast films, on the other hand, contain larger grains that have a wider range of sizes. Wide-latitude film forms an acceptable image with as much as 15% technique error by the operator. The use of wide-latitude film minimizes repeats and reduces patient radiation exposure.

Crossover. Until recently, silver-halide crystals were fat and three dimensional (Figure 14-7, *B*). New emulsions (Figure 14-7, *A*) are called *tabular grain* because the silver-halide crystals are flat, a shape that results in a large surface area to volume ratio. The result is not only improved covering power but significantly lower **crossover**. When light is emitted by an intensifying screen, it not only exposes the adjacent emulsion but also the emulsion on the other side of the base. The light **crosses over** the base and causes increased blur on the

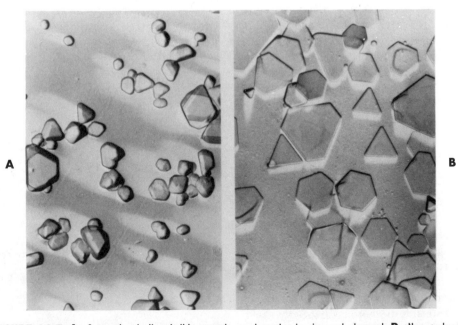

FIGURE 14-7 A, Conventional silver-halide crystals are irregular in size and clumped. **B,** New technology produces flat, tabletlike grains that are more evenly dispersed. *(Courtesy Eastman Kodak.)*

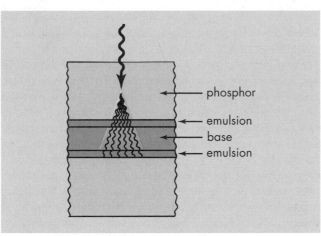

FIGURE 14-8 Crossover occurs when screen light crosses the film base and exposes the film emulsion on the other side.

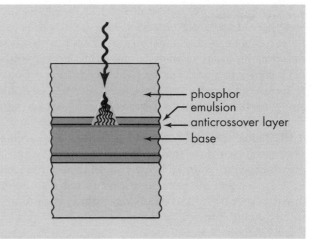

FIGURE 14-9 Crossover is reduced by adding a dye to the base.

other emulsion (Figure 14-8). Crossover is reduced with the use of tabular grain emulsions. The increased covering power produces increased light absorption from the screen and increased light transmitted through the emulsion. The addition of a light-absorbing dye in an anticrossover layer reduces crossover to near zero (Figure 14-9). The anticrossover layer has the following three critical characteristics: (1) it absorbs most of the crossover light; (2) it does not diffuse into the emulsion but remains as a separate layer; (3) it is completely removed during processing.

Reciprocity Law. The reciprocity law states that the exposure of radiographic film depends on the intensity of x-rays of the remnant beam and the time the film is exposed to those x-rays.

$$\text{Exposure} = \text{Intensity} \times \text{Time}$$

The reciprocity law holds for direct-exposure film, but the reciprocity law fails when film is exposed to light from intensifying screens. Radiographers must be aware of this. **Reciprocity law failure** is important when long exposure times are used, as in mammography or when short exposure times are used, as in pediatric examinations. The result is reduced response or speed. An increase in technique may be required to compensate for the reduced speed of the film-screen combination. Table 14-2 shows percent speed of film-screen combinations at different exposure times.

Safelights. The use of radiographic film requires precautions in the **darkroom. Safelights** are lamps with color filters that provide sufficient illumination in the darkroom but ensure that the film remains unexposed. Proper darkroom illumination depends not only on the color of the filter but also on the wattage of the bulb and the distance between the lamp and the work surface. A 15-watt bulb should be no closer than 5 feet

TABLE 14-2
Approximate Reciprocity Law Failure

Exposure Time	Relative Speed (%)
1 millisecond	95
10 milliseconds	100
100 milliseconds	100
1 second	90
10 seconds	60

from the work surface. With blue-sensitive film, or film used with calcium-tungstate screens, an **amber filter** is used. The amber filter transmits light that has wavelengths longer than about 550 nm, which is above the spectral response of blue-sensitive film. The use of an amber filter would fog green-sensitive film (used with rare-earth screens); therefore a **red filter,** which transmits light above about 600 nm, must be used. A red filter is suitable with both green- and blue-sensitive film. Figure 14-6 shows the approximate transmission characteristics for amber and red safelight filters.

Types of Film

Direct-Exposure Film. In the past, x-ray film was manufactured for use without intensifying screens. Direct-exposure film was used for radiographing thin body parts that present low radiation risk, such as hands and feet. Until the early 1970s, it was also used for mammography; however, patient dose was much too high. This film typically requires 10 to 100 times more radiation than intensifying screen film. Today, it is used only when the benefits outweigh the risks of exposure. The emulsion of a direct-exposure film is thicker than that of screen film, and it contains a higher concentration of silver-halide crystals to enhance direct x-ray interaction. Direct-exposure film is not sensitive to light and therefore should not be used with screens. Direct-exposure film is usually used with a cardboard cassette, although some are available in individually packaged paper wrappings. Most extremity examinations now use fine-grain, high-detail screens and double-emulsion film as the image receptor rather than the antiquated direct-exposure film.

2) **Mammography Film.** Mammography was originally performed with an **industrial-grade,** double-emulsion direct-exposure film. The radiation doses associated with such a technique were much too high, and consequently specialty films were developed, including Lo Dose by EI duPont de Nemours and Company and Min-R by Eastman Kodak Company. These mammography films are **fine-grain,** single-emulsion films designed to be exposed with a single intensifying screen. Lo Dose uses a calcium-tungstate screen and Min-R uses a rare-earth screen. The spectral response of each emulsion is adjusted accordingly. The surface of the base opposite the screen is coated with a special light-absorbing dye to reduce reflection of screen-light that is transmitted through the emulsion and base. This effect is called *halation* and the absorbing dye is an **antihalation coating.** Such antihalation coating is used on all single-emulsion screen films, not just mammography film. The antihalation coating is removed during processing.

3) **Video Film.** The use of video film is growing rapidly because of the introduction and increasing use of computed tomography, digital radiography, ultrasound, and magnetic resonance imaging. In each of these imaging processes the image receptor is not film but rather some type of radiation detector. The image is formed by computer-assisted analysis of the detected radiation. The image is then displayed on a video monitor. To provide the radiologist with a permanent image, a negative photograph of the video image is made. This is called *video imaging* or *CRT imaging.* The television picture tube is a **cathode-ray tube (CRT).** When used in office equipment, the CRT is a principal component of a **video display terminal (VDT).** Patient dose is not a consideration in video imaging because it is totally independent of the manner in which the video image is obtained. What is important is that the video film be sensitive so that images can be obtained in a short time and the film can be properly matched to the spectral emission of the CRT. Images are obtained with what is known as a *blue-dot* or *green-dot CRT phosphor.* CRT phosphor images must be recorded with blue- or green-sensitive film. Although some video-imaging films are spectrally matched for either blue or green CRT emission, most are orthochromatic films and therefore can be used with any type CRT. Panchromatic films are not used because they would become fogged with existing darkroom safelights. Video-imaging films incorporate a single emulsion that is relatively thin. They are usually exposed in

a device called a *multiformat camera* (Figure 14-10). These devices allow multiple images to be placed on a single sheet of film. The best cameras can accommodate many different film sizes and provide either a single image on the film or up to 16 images per film. This multi-imaging capacity uses a **film mask** and lens system on the multiformat camera.

4) **Laser Film.** A **laser printer** uses the digital electronic signal from an imaging unit like an MRI or CT computer. The intensity of the laser beam is varied in direct proportion to the strength of the image signal. This process is called *laser-beam modulation.* While being modulated, the laser beam writes in **raster fashion** over the entire film. Laser printers provide exceptionally consistent image quality for multiple-size films and multiple-image formats per film. They can be electronically interfaced with multiple digital imaging modalities such as CT, MRI, and computed radiography. For even greater productivity, laser printers can be linked to an automatic film processor (Figure 14-11). Laser film is silver-halide film sensitized to the red light emitted by the laser in much the same way blue- and green-sensitive screen film is sensitized. Different types of lasers are used in laser printers, and laser film is particularly light sensitive, therefore laser film must be handled in total darkness. Figure 14-12 illustrates in cross section a representative sample of single-emulsion film such as that used for mammography, video imaging, and laser imaging.

5) **Speciality film.** Occasionally a radiographer will be requested to use **speciality film.** To duplicate an existing radiography, **duplicating film** is used. Duplicating film is designed for same-size use; that is, the size of duplicating film is equal to the size of the film being duplicated. Duplicating film is a single-emulsion film that is exposed to ultraviolet light through the existing radiograph to produce a copy.

a) **Subtraction film** is sometimes used in angiography, although with the increasing application of digital fluoroscopy, its use is declining. Subtraction film is single emulsion with generally two types. One type is designed to prepare the **subtraction mask,** and the other type accommodates the superimposed image of the original radiograph and subtraction mask. Subtraction film has a high contrast to enhance the existing subject contrast.

b) **Cinefluorography** is a special examination reserved almost exclusively for the **cardiac catheterization** laboratory. The radiographer who assists in cardiac catheterization uses **cine film.** Cine film comes in two sizes, 16 and 35 millimeter, and is supplied in 100- and 500-foot rolls. Most cine film is, in fact, the same 35 millimeter movie type of film that is seen in the theater. Some gastrointestinal studies in fluoroscopy that require rapid-sequence filming, such as swallowing studies, use 16-millimeter cine film. Although both have the same

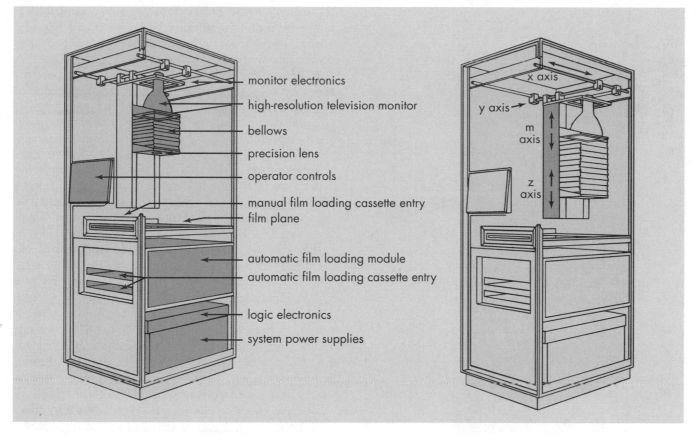

FIGURE 14-10 A multiformat camera. *(Courtesy Matrix Instruments.)*

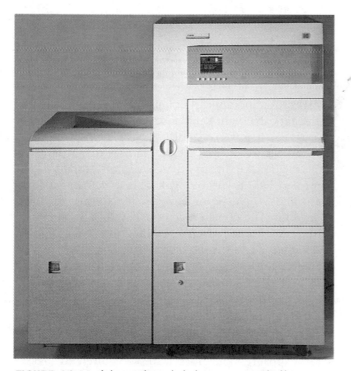

FIGURE 14-11 A laser printer docked to an automatic film processor. *(Courtesy Eastman Kodak.)*

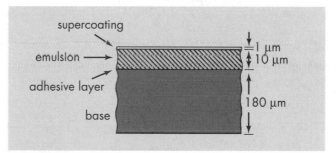

FIGURE 14-12 Cross section of single-emulsion mammography film.

resolution when viewed with the proper projector, the perceived image obtained on 35-millimeter film will be better than that obtained on 16-millimeter film. Since the area of the 35-millimeter film is nearly four times that of a 16-millimeter film, the patient dose is increased proportionately.

Spot Films. Roll films from 70 to 105 millimeter in width are used in a number of different types of **spot-film cameras.** These films are similar to cine film but are called *spot films.* Spot film is larger than cine film and therefore can be viewed directly on a conventional view box without resorting to a projector. Figure 14-13

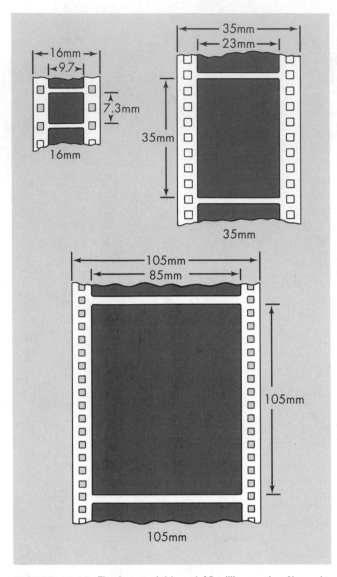

FIGURE 14-13 The format of 16- and 35-millimeter cine film and 105-millimeter spot film.

shows the format of the more popular sizes of cine and roll type of spot films. **Quality control** in processing of cine film and spot film is critical. The roll type of spot film usually can be adequately processed in the automatic processor used for conventional radiographs. Cine film, on the other hand, should be processed with specially designed movie film-processing equipment because when the image is magnified during projection, artifacts are likewise magnified.

Handling and Storage of Films

Radiographic film is sensitive. Improper handling and storage will result in poor radiographic images with artifacts that can interfere with diagnosis. For this reason, when handling radiographic film, do not bend, crease, or otherwise subject film to rough handling. Hands

should be cleaned before handling film. Hand lotions and hand creams should not be used in the darkroom. Creams or oils from the hands cause fingerprint artifacts on the film emulsion.

Artifacts. Any type of improper handling causes **artifacts.** Artifacts are marks that sometimes appear on the processed radiograph. Radiographic film is pressure sensitive, so rough handling or the imprint of any sharp object is reproduced on the processed radiograph. Creasing the film before processing produces a fingernail-appearing artifact. Dirt on the hands or on intensifying screens results in spot artifacts. In a dry environment, static electricity can cause tree-like artifacts. Identifying artifacts and their causes is covered in Chapter 32.

Heat and Humidity. Radiographic film is sensitive to the effects of elevated temperature and humidity, especially if stored for long periods. Heat increases fog and reduces visualization of the image on a radiograph. Consequently, radiographic film should not be stored at temperatures in excess of about 20° C (68° F). Ideally, radiographic films should be stored under refrigeration. Storage for a year or longer is acceptable if the film is maintained at 10° C (50° F). Film should never be stored near steam pipes or other sources of heat.

Storage under conditions of elevated humidity (over 60%) also reduces contrast and increases fog. Consequently, radiographic film should be stored in a cool, dry place before use, ideally in a climate-controlled environment. Storage under dry conditions can be equally objectionable. If the relative humidity dips below about 40%, static artifacts are possible.

Film Storage

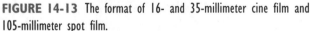

Radiographic film should be stored at temperatures <68° F (20° C) and at a humidity between 40% and 60%.

Light. Radiographic film must be stored and handled in the dark. No light should expose the emulsion before processing. If low-level, diffuse light exposes the film, film fog occurs. If bright light exposes or partially exposes the film, an obvious dark artifact is produced. The control of light is ensured by having a well-sealed darkroom and a light-proof **film bin** for storage of unexposed film. The film storage bin should have an electrical interlock that prevents the bin from being opened when the door to the darkroom is ajar.

Radiation. Ionizing radiation, other than the useful beam, creates an image artifact by increasing fog and reducing visualization of the image. Darkrooms located next to x-ray rooms need to be lead lined. It is usually acceptable to lead line only the storage shelf and film bin. Radiographic film is sensitive to any unwanted x-ray exposure. Therefore lead is required to protect film. The fog level for unprocessed film is only 0.2 mR

(52 pC/kg), and therefore the thickness of the lead barrier should be designed to keep the total exposure of unexposed film below this level. This requires some assumptions about the storage time of the film. If the turnover of film is monthly, then the required lead shielding would be four times more than weekly exposure requirements.

Care should be taken to ensure that the receiving area for radiographic film is not the same as that for the radioactive material used in nuclear medicine. Even though the packaging of radioactive material ensures the safety of those who handle it, the low-level radiation can fog film if the radioactive material and film are stored together for even a short period of time.

Shelf Life. Most radiographic film is supplied in boxes of 100 sheets. Some film is packaged in an **interleaved** fashion with chemically treated protective paper between each sheet of film. Each box contains an expiration date, which indicates the maximum shelf life of the film. Under no circumstances should film be stored for longer periods. It must be used before its expiration date, which is usually a year after purchase. The aging film results in loss of speed and contrast and an increase in fog. It is always wise to store boxes of film on edge rather than lying flat. When stored on edge, warping of the sheets of film is minimized. The storage of film should be sequenced so that the oldest film is used first. Rotation of film, much like the rotation of perishables in a supermarket, is appropriate. Most hospitals receive film on a monthly basis and purchase enough film for 5 weeks of use. The extra few days above monthly use are necessary to cover civil emergencies when an unexpectedly large number of x-ray examinations would be necessary. The maximum storage time for radiographic film is 45 days.

SUMMARY

Remnant radiation is the part of the x-ray beam that exits a patient and exposes the image receptor. X-ray film is made up of a polyester base covered on both sides or duplitized with a radiographic emulsion. The x-ray film emulsion contains light sensitive silver-bromide crystals, which are made from the mixture of silver nitrate and potassium bromide. The following is the silver halide crystal reaction: $AgNO_3 + KBr \rightarrow AgBr \downarrow + KNO_3$. At the manufacturing plant the emulsion is spread onto the base in darkness or under red lights because the AgBr molecule is light sensitive. The latent image is formed in the film emulsion when light photons interact with the silver-halide crystals. The unobservable information contained in the silver halide crystals that have been activated by light photons is the latent image. Processing of the radiographic film makes the image manifest.

The following is a list of the characteristics of x-ray film:

1. **Spectral matching.** The x-ray beam does not directly expose the x-ray film. Intensifying screens are contained in the cassette, which are activated when the x-ray beam is on. The intensify screens release light energy, which then exposes the radiographic film. The light energy emitted is a particular energy or color and each manufacturer has its own proprietary spectral make-up for the screens. In any case the response of the film must match the emissions of the screen. This is called *spectral matching*. If the screens emit blue-green light, the film must be designed to respond to blue-green light to get an image. Use of safelights in the darkroom prevents film exposure. With blue-sensitive film an amber filter is used on the safelight, and a red filter is required for green-sensitive film.

Spectral Matching	
Screens	**Emitted Light**
Calcium tungstate ———→	Blue *amber*
Rare earth ——————→	Green *red*

2. **Speed.** Speed is the sensitivity of the film-screen combination to x-rays and light. Fast film-screen combinations need fewer x-rays to activate the screens and less light to expose the film. Slow film-screen combinations, although producing sharper radiographs with more detail, require more x-rays to activate the screens and more light from the screens to expose the film.
3. **Contrast.** High-contrast film produces black-and-white images. Low-contrast film produces images with shades of gray.
4. **Latitude.** Latitude is the range of exposure techniques (kVp and mAs) that will produce an acceptable image.
5. **Crossover.** When light is emitted from an intensifying screen, it exposes not only the adjacent film emulsion but also the emulsion on the other side of the base. The light crosses over the base and causes blur on the radiographic image.
6. **Reciprocity law.** Intensify screens and radiographic film speed vary if very short or very long exposures are used.

Table 14-3 summarizes the types of film available in diagnostic imaging departments.

Film should be handled carefully and stored at specific temperatures and humidities. Artifacts on radiographic film are caused by rough handling, which results in increased marks, or low humidity in the darkroom, which causes static artifacts.

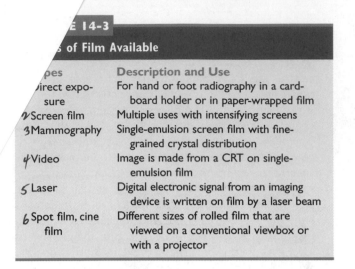

TABLE 14-3

Types of Film Available

Types	Description and Use
1 Direct exposure	For hand or foot radiography in a cardboard holder or in paper-wrapped film
2 Screen film	Multiple uses with intensifying screens
3 Mammography	Single-emulsion screen film with fine-grained crystal distribution
4 Video	Image is made from a CRT on single-emulsion film
5 Laser	Digital electronic signal from an imaging device is written on film by a laser beam
6 Spot film, cine film	Different sizes of rolled film that are viewed on a conventional viewbox or with a projector

REVIEW QUESTIONS

1. X-ray film that has emulsion on both sides is _____.

2. Diagram the cross-sectional view of radiographic intensifying screen film. Identify the base emulsion, the adhesive layer, and supercoating. Label the composition and thicknesses of each.

3. Define dimensional stability and explain why this is an important property of x-ray film.

4. Briefly discuss the history of the development of x-ray film.

5. List the ingredients in the radiographic emulsion and indicate their atomic numbers.

6. Write the silver-halide crystal reaction. What does the arrow pointing down represent?

7. What determines the speed of an x-ray film?

8. What is the term for closely guarded information held by film manufacturers?

9. Explain the Gurney-Mott theory of latent-image formation.

10. Explain how Compton and photoelectric reactions relate to latent-image formation.

11. Refer to Table 14-1 of standard film sizes. 8 × 10 inch film size in English units is equivalent to what film size in metric units?

12. Nonscreen film is also known as _____ _____ _____.

13. When were rare-earth screens developed?

14. What is the difference between panchromatic film and orthochromatic film?

15. Name two rare-earth phosphors.

16. What is the importance in spectral matching in choosing film-screen combinations?

17. Why do radiographers need to be aware of reciprocity law failure?

18. An amber filter on a safelight is used under what conditions? A red filter on a safelight is used under what conditions?

19. Discuss the difference between regular screen film and mammography screen film?

20. List the proper film storage conditions: (a) temperature, (b) humidity, and (c) shelf-life.

Additional Reading

Bohland RJ; Film/cassette size: time for a change? *Radiol Technol* 65(5):287, May-June 1994.

Eastman Kodak Company: *Introduction to medical radiographic imaging,* Rochester, NY, 1993, Eastman Kodak.

Haus AG: *Screen-film image receptors and film processing,* Rochester, NY, 1994, Eastman Kodak.

Haus AG, Dickerson RE: *Characteristics of screen-film combinations for conventional medical radiography,* Rochester, NY, 1995, Eastman Kodak.

Mosby's radiographic instructional series: radiographic imaging [slide set] St Louis, 1996, Mosby.

15

Processing the Latent Image

OBJECTIVES

At the completion of this chapter the student will be able to:

1. Discuss the historical development from hand processing to automatic processing
2. List the processing chemicals used in each processing step
3. Discuss the use of each chemical
4. Explain the systems of the automatic processor, including the transport system, the temperature-control system, the circulation system, the replenishment system, the dryer system, and the electrical system
5. Describe the three alternative processing methods, including daylight processing

OUTLINE

The Development of Radiographic Film Processing
  Hand processing
  Automatic processing
  Sequence of processing steps
Processing Chemistry
  Wetting
  Development
  Fixing
  Washing
  Drying

Components of the Automatic Processor
  Transport system
  Temperature-control system
  Circulation system
  Replenishment system
  Dryer system
  Electrical system
Alternative Processing Methods
  Rapid processing
  Extended processing
  Daylight processing

Processing of the latent image causes all the silver ions in the silver-halide crystal that have been exposed to light to be converted into the microscopic black grain of silver. The processing sequence has the following six steps: (1) wetting, (2) developing, (3) stop bath, (4) fixing, (5) washing, and (6) drying.

THE DEVELOPMENT OF RADIOGRAPHIC FILM PROCESSING

Hand Processing

Before the introduction of automatic film processing in radiography, x-ray films were **hand processed.** In hand processing the exposed radiographic film is first immersed in developing chemicals for approximately 5 minutes at 20° C. Films are then put in a **stop bath,** which is followed by immersion in a **fixer solution.** The film is **washed** in running water and hung to drip **dry.** These hand-processing steps take 1 hour to obtain a completely dry and ready-to-read radiograph.

Automatic Processing

The first automatic x-ray film processor was introduced by Pako in 1942 (Figure 15-1). The first commercially

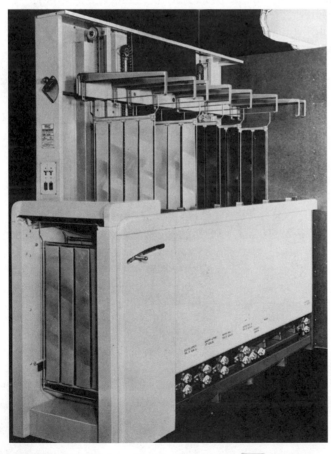

FIGURE 15-1 The first automatic processor, circa 1942. *(Courtesy Art Haus.)*

available model could process 120 films per hour by using special film hangers. These film hangers were dunked from one tank to another. The total cycle time for processing one film was approximately 40 minutes.

A significant improvement in automatic x-ray film processing came in 1956 when the first roller transport system for processing medical radiographs was introduced by the Eastman Kodak Company. This processor accommodated all medical x-ray films that were designed for exposure with intensifying screens, even films from surgery or the emergency department. The roller transport automatic processor shown in Figure 15-2 is about 10 feet long and weighs nearly three quarters of a ton. Automatic processing revolutionized busy departments. Finished radiographs became available in 6 minutes, and the variability in results caused by dunking and drying by hand was eliminated. Automatic processing enabled radiologists and radiographers to standardize techniques (kVp and mAs) so that fewer retakes were needed. Departmental efficiency, work flow, and radiographic quality all improved.

Another significant breakthrough in the production of radiographs was the introduction of 90-second rapid processing in 1965 by the Eastman Kodak Company. Rapid processing was possible because of the development of new chemistry, new emulsions, and the faster drying permitted by polyester film base. With rapid processing, 215 sheets of film per hour can be processed, which remains the standard of the industry today.

In 1987, Konica introduced an automatic film processor that has a processing cycle of approximately 45 seconds. This processor, however, requires special films and chemicals. In the future, 20- to 45-second processing may become the standard.

Sequence of Processing Steps

A number of steps are involved in the processing of radiographic film, and these are presented on Table 15-1.

Most radiographic processing is done automatically today. The chemicals involved in automatic and manual processing are basically the same. In automatic processing the times for each step are shorter and the chemical concentrations and temperature are higher than in manual processing.

1. **Wetting.** The first step in the processing sequence is to wet the film to loosen the emulsion so that subsequent chemical baths can reach all parts of the emulsion uniformly. This step is often omitted, and the **wetting agent** then is incorporated into the second step—development.
2. **Development.** The development step is the stage of processing in which the latent image is converted to a manifest image.
3. **Stop bath.** After development the film is rinsed in an acid solution that is designed to stop the development process and remove excess developer chemi-

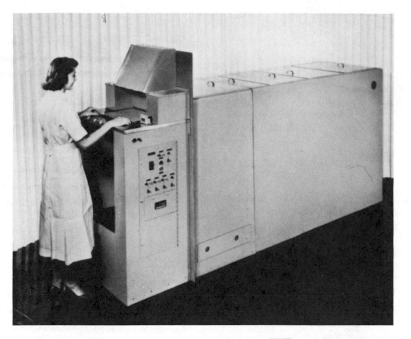

FIGURE 15-2 The first roller transport automatic processor, circa 1956. *(Courtesy Eastman Kodak Company.)*

cals from the emulsion. Photographers call this step the *stop bath*, and in processing radiographs the stop bath is sometimes included in the next step—fixation.

4. **Fixing.** During **fixation,** the silver halide that was not exposed to radiation or light is dissolved and removed from the emulsion. The gelatin portion of the emulsion is **hardened** at the same time to make it structurally more sound.
5. **Washing.** Fixation is followed by a vigorous washing of the film to remove any remaining chemicals from the previous processing steps.
6. **Drying.** Finally the film is **dried** to remove the water used to wash it and to make the film acceptable for handling and viewing.

The steps of development and fixation are the most important in the processing of radiographic film. An explanation of each step follows because of the importance **processing** plays in producing a high-quality radiograph.

PROCESSING CHEMISTRY
Wetting

A **solvent** is a liquid into which various solids and powders can be dissolved. The universal solvent is water. Water is the solvent for all the chemicals used in processing a radiograph. For these chemicals to penetrate through the emulsion, the radiograph must first be treated by a wetting agent. The wetting agent is water, and it penetrates through the gelatin of the emulsion, which swells it and causes it to expand. In automatic processing the wetting agent or water is in the developer.

TABLE 15-1

Sequence in Processing a Radiograph

Step	Purpose	Approximate Time	
		Manual	*Automatic*
1 Wetting	Swelling of the emulsion to permit subsequent chemical penetration	15 seconds	—
2 Development	Production of a manifest image from the latent image	5 minutes	22 seconds
3 Stop bath	Termination of development and removal of excess chemical from emulsion	30 seconds	—
4 Fixing	Removal of remaining silver halide from emulsion and hardening of gelatin	15 minutes	22 seconds
5 Washing	Removal of excess chemicals	20 minutes	20 seconds
6 Drying	Removal of water and preparation of radiograph for viewing	30 minutes	26 seconds

Development

> ### Development
> The principal action of development is to change silver ions of the exposed crystals into metallic silver and to concentrate this metallic silver in the region of the sensitivity speck.

The developer is the chemical solution that performs this task. In addition to the solvent water, it contains a number of other ingredients. This composition of the developer and the function of each ingredient are outlined in Table 15-2. For the ionic silver to be changed to metallic silver, an electron must be supplied to the silver ion. Chemically the reaction is described as follows:

$$Ag^+ + e^- \rightarrow Ag$$

When an electron is given up by a chemical, the **developing agent** in this case, to neutralize a positive ion, the process is called *reduction*. The silver ion is said to be **reduced** to metallic silver, and the chemical responsible for this is called a *reducing agent.* The opposite of reduction is **oxidation,** which is a reaction that produces an electron. Oxidation and reduction occur simultaneously and are called *redox* reactions. To help recall the proper association, think of EUR/OPE—electrons are used in reduction/oxidation produces electrons.

The precise chemical compositions of film developers are closely guarded as proprietary secrets by manufacturers. The principal component, however, is a compound called *hydroquinone.* Secondary constituents of the developing agent are **phenidone** and **metol.** Usually, hydroquinone and metol are combined for manual pro-

cessing, and hydroquinone and phenidone are combined for rapid processing. As reducing agents, each of these molecules has an abundance of electrons that can be easily released to neutralize positive silver ions. These molecules are not ions but are constructed in such a way that many of their electrons are concentrated on their outside surfaces.

The **optical density** of a processed radiograph comes from the **synergistic** action of hydroquinone and phenidone. **Synergism** means that the action of two agents working together is greater than the sum of the action of each agent working independently. Hydroquinone is rather slow acting but is responsible for the very blackest shades. Phenidone acts rapidly and influences the lighter shades of gray.

An unexposed silver-halide crystal has a negative electrostatic charge distributed over its entire surface. An exposed silver-halide crystal, on the other hand, has a negative electrostatic charge distributed over its surface except in the region of the sensitivity speck. The similar electrostatic charges on the developing agent and the silver-halide crystal make it difficult for the developing agent to penetrate the crystal surface except in the region of the sensitivity speck in an **exposed crystal.** In such a crystal the developing agent penetrates the crystal through the sensitivity speck and reduces the remaining silver ions to atomic silver. The difference between the development of unexposed and exposed crystals is illustrated in Figure 15-3.

Development occurs over a period of time and depends on factors such as crystal size, developer concentration, and temperature. If one could observe the process in action, one would see a slow buildup of metallic silver at the site of the sensitivity speck. After complete development, exposed crystals have been destroyed and a grain of black metallic silver is all that remains. Unexposed crystals remain unaffected. The reduction of a silver ion is accompanied by the release of

TABLE 15-2		
The Components of the Developer and Their Functions		
Component	**Chemical**	**Function**
Developing agent	Phenidone	Reducing agent; produces shades of gray rapidly
Developing agent	Hydroquinone	Reducing agent; produces black tones slowly
Buffering agent	Sodium carbonate	Helps swell gelatin; produces alkalinity; controls pH
Restrainer	Potassium bromide	Antifog agent; keeps unexposed crystals from being chemically attacked
Preservative	Sodium sulfite	Controls oxidation; maintains balance among developer components
Hardener	Glutaraldehyde	Controls emulsion swelling; aids archival quality
Sequestering agent	Chelates	Removes metallic impurities; stabilizes developing agent
Solvent	Water	Dissolves chemicals for use

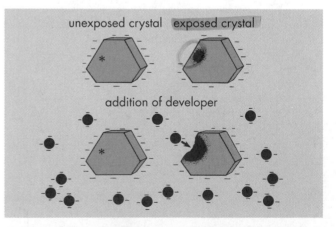

unexposed crystal   exposed crystal

addition of developer

FIGURE 15-3 Development is the chemical process that amplifies the latent image. Only crystals that contain a latent image are reduced to metallic silver by the addition of developer.

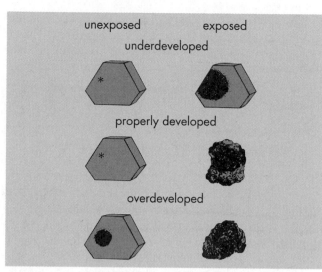

unexposed   exposed
underdeveloped

properly developed

overdeveloped

FIGURE 15-4 Underdevelopment results in a dull radiograph because the crystals that contain a latent image have not been completely reduced. Overdevelopment produces a similar radiograph because of the partial reduction of unexposed crystals. Proper development results in maximum contrast.

a bromine ion. The bromine ion migrates through the remnant of the crystal into the gelatin portion of the emulsion. From there it is dissolved into the developer and removed from the film.

The developer contains **alkali compounds** such as **sodium carbonate** and **sodium hydroxide**. These **buffering agents** enhance the action of the developing agent by controlling the **concentration** of **hydrogen ions,** which is called the *pH.* These alkali compounds are caustic, that is, they are very corrosive and can eat away at your skin. Sodium hydroxide is the strongest alkali and is commonly called *lye.*

Remember: Be very cautious if you mix a developer solution containing sodium hydroxide. You must wear gloves and goggles.

Potassium bromide and **potassium iodide** are added to the developer as **restrainers.** These compounds restrict the action of the developing agent to react with only those silver-halide crystals that have been irradiated. Without the restrainer, even those crystals that had not been exposed would be reduced to metallic silver. This results in an increased fog that is termed *development fog.*

A **preservative** is also included in the developer to control the oxidation of the developing agent by air. Air is introduced into the chemistry when it is mixed, handled, and stored. When oxidation occurs, it is called *aerial oxidation.* By controlling aerial oxidation, the preservative helps maintain proper development rate. Mixed chemistry lasts only a couple of weeks. Close-fitting lids on replenishment tanks are needed to control aerial oxidation. Hydroquinone is particularly sensitive

to aerial oxidation. Premixed chemistry, when stored at room temperature, lasts a year. It is easy to tell when the developing agent has been oxidized because it turns a brownish color. The addition of a preservative causes the developer to remain clear. **Sodium sulfite** is the usual preservative.

All developers used in automatic processors contain a **hardener,** usually **glutaraldehyde.** If the emulsion swells too much or becomes too soft, the film will not be transported properly through the system because of the very close tolerances of the transport system rollers. The hardener controls the swelling and softening of the emulsion. Sometimes when films drop from the processor and are damp, the cause is depletion of the hardener. Lack of sufficient glutaraldehyde may be the biggest cause of problems with automatic processing.

Metal impurities and soluble salts may exist in the developer. When these impurities are present, they can accelerate the oxidation of hydroquinane, which renders the developer unstable. **Chelates,** compounds having metal ions, are introduced as **sequestering agents** to form stable complexes with these metallic ions and salts.

Proper development implies that all exposed crystals containing a latent image are reduced to metallic silver, whereas those crystals unexposed are unaffected. The development process, however, is not perfect. Some crystals containing a latent image remain undeveloped (unreduced), whereas other crystals that are unexposed may be developed. Both of these actions reduce the quality of the radiograph.

Film development is basically a chemical reaction. Like all chemical reactions, it is governed by three physical characteristics: (1) time, (2) temperature, and (3) concentration of the developer. Long development time leads to increased reduction of the silver in each grain and increased development of the total number of grains. High developer temperature has the same effect. Similarly, silver reduction is controlled by the concentration of the developing chemicals. With increased developer concentration, the reducing agent becomes more powerful and can more readily penetrate both exposed and unexposed silver-halide crystals.

Manufacturers of x-ray film and developer chemicals have very carefully determined the optimal conditions of time, temperature, and concentration for proper development. Optimal images with proper contrast and density can be expected if the manufacturer's recommendations for development are followed. Deviation from the manufacturer's recommendations can result in loss of image quality. Refer to Figure 15-4 again, which illustrates the three degrees of development for unexposed and exposed crystals. A fogged film is dull and washed-out and lacks proper contrast. There are many causes of fog. An increase in the time, temperature, or developer concentration above manufacturer recom-

Causes of fog...

mendations will result in increased fog. Fog can also be produced by chemical contamination of the developer (**chemical fog**), by unintentional exposure to radiation, (**radiation fog**), or by improper storage at elevated temperature and humidity.

Fixing

Once development is complete, the film must be treated so that the image will be permanent. This stage of processing is termed *fixing*. The image is said to be fixed on the film and this produces film of archival quality. Archival quality refers to the permanence of the radiograph. The archival quality image does not deteriorate with age but remains in its original state.

When the film is removed from the developer, some developer is trapped in the emulsion and continues its reducing action. If developing is not stopped, development fog will result. In manual processing the step after development is called stop bath, and its function is to neutralize the residual developer in the emulsion and stop its action. The chemical used in the stop bath is **acetic acid.**

In automatic processing a stop bath is not used because the **rollers** of the **transport system** squeeze the film clean. Furthermore, the fixer contains acetic acid, which behaves as a stop bath. This acetic acid, however, is called an *activator.* It neutralizes the pH of the emulsion and stops developer action. Table 15-3 lists the chemical components of the fixer.

When referring to the fixing agent, the terms *clearing agent, hypo,* and *thiosulfate* can be used interchangeably. Fixing agents remove unexposed and undeveloped silver-halide crystals from the emulsion. It is sodium thiosulfate that has been classically referred to as *hypo.* Ammonium thiosulfate, however, is the fixing agent used in most fixer chemistries. Sodium thiosulfate is seldom used.

Hypo retention is a term used to describe the undesirable retention of the fixer in the emulsion. Excess hypo slowly oxidizes and causes the image to discolor to brown over a long period of time. Fixing agents retained in the emulsion combine with silver to form silver sulfide.

Hypo Retention in Fixing

Silver-sulfide stain is the most common cause of poor archival quality radiographs.

The fixer also contains a chemical called a hardener. As the developed and unreduced silver bromide is removed from the emulsion during fixation, the emulsion shrinks. The hardener accelerates this shrinking process and causes the emulsion to become more rigid or hardened. The purpose of hardeners is to ensure that the film is transported properly through the wash-and-dry section and also to ensure rapid and complete drying. The chemicals commonly used as hardeners are either **potassium alum, aluminum chloride,** or **chromium alum.**

The fixer also contains a **preservative** that is of the same composition and that serves the same purpose as the preservative in the developer. The preservative is **sodium sulfite,** and it is necessary to maintain the chemical balance because of the carryover of developer and fixer from one tank to another.

The alkalinity or acidity (pH) of the fixer must remain constant. This is achieved by adding a **buffer,** usually acetate, to the fixer.

In the same manner that metallic ions were sequestered in the developer, so must they be in the fixer. Aluminum ions are the principal impurity at this stage. Boric acids and boric salts are used to form stable complexes of these metallic ions.

Finally the fixer contains filtered water as the solvent. Other chemicals might be applicable as a solvent, but they would be thicker and more apt to gum up the transport mechanism of the automatic processor.

Washing

The next stage in processing is to wash away any residual chemicals remaining in the emulsion, particularly hypo clinging to the surface of the film. Water is used as the wash agent. Inadequate washing leads to excess hypo retention and the production of an image that will fade, turn brown with time, and be of generally poor archival quality.

Drying

The final step in processing is to dry the radiograph. This is done by blowing warm dry air over both surfaces of the film as it is transported through the drying chamber.

TABLE 15-3		
The Components of the Fixer and Their Functions		
Component	**Chemical**	**Function**
Activator	Acetic acid	Neutralizes the developer and stops its action
Fixing agent	Ammonium thiosulfate	Removes undeveloped silver bromide from emulsion
Hardener	Potassium alum	Stiffens and shrinks emulsion
Preservative	Sodium sulfite	Maintains chemical balance
Buffer	Acetate	Maintains proper pH
Sequestering agent	Boric acid/ salts	Removes aluminum ions
Solvent	Water	Dissolves other components

The total sequence of events involved in **manual processing** requires over 1 hour. Most **automatic processors** are 90-second processors.

The process of converting the latent image to a manifest image can be summarized as a three-step process (Figure 15-5). First the latent image is formed by exposure of silver-halide grains. Next the exposed grains and only the exposed grains are made visible by development. Finally, fixing removes the unexposed grains from the emulsion and makes the image permanent.

COMPONENTS OF THE AUTOMATIC PROCESSOR

The efficiency of radiology services increased considerably with the introduction of roller transport automatic processing in 1956. The time between exposure and the finished radiograph was shortened from an hour to matter of minutes. The requirement for darkroom personnel diminished proportionately. In addition to increased efficiency, automatic processing has resulted in better image quality because each radiograph is processed exactly the same way.

Figure 15-6 is a cutaway view of an automatic processor. The principal components of an automatic processor are as follows: (1) the transport system, (2) the temperature-control system, (3) the circulation system, (4) the replenishment system, (5) the dryer system, and (6) the electrical system. Table 15-4 briefly describes each of these component systems of automatic processing.

Transport System

The transport system begins at the feed tray. In the darkroom the film to be processed is placed on the feed tray and inserted into the automatic processor. Here, entrance rollers grip the film as it begins its trip through the processor. Here also is a microswitch that controls the replenishment rate of the processing chemicals. Always feed the film evenly using the side rails of the feed tray and alternate sides from film to film. This ensures even wear of the transport system components.

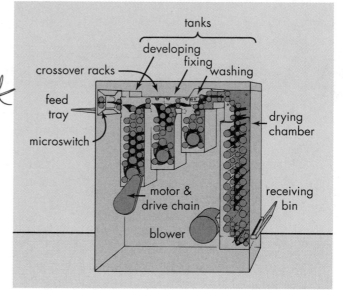

FIGURE 15-6 A cutaway view of an automatic processor with the major components identified.

TABLE 15-4		
The Principal Components of an Automatic Processor		
System	Subsystem	Purpose
Transport		Transport film through various stages at precise time intervals
	Roller	Steer film movement
	Transport rack	Rollers and guide shoes to move and change direction of film
	Drive	Provide power to turn rollers at a precise rate
Temperature control		Monitor and adjust temperature of each stage
Circulation		Agitate fluids
	Developer	Continuously mix, filter
	Fixer	Continuously mix
	Wash	Single pass at constant flow rate
Replenishment	Developer	Meter film and replace solutions
	Fixer	Meter and replace
Dryer		Remove moisture, vent exhaust
Electrical		Distribute fused power to above systems

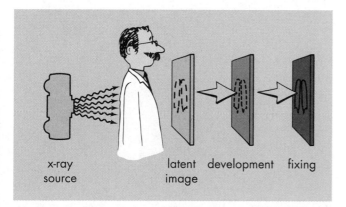

FIGURE 15-5 Converting the latent image to a manifest image is a three-step process.

x-ray source — latent image — development — fixing

Remember: The shorter dimension of the film should always be against the side rail to maintain the proper **replenishment rate** (Figure 15-7).

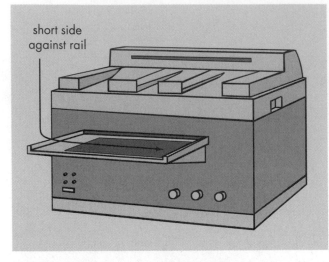

FIGURE 15-7 Place the short side of the film against the guide rail to maintain proper replenishment rate.

From the entrance rollers, the film is transported by rollers and racks through the wet chemistry tanks and drying chamber and finally is dropped in the receiving bin. The transport system not only transports the film but also controls processing by controlling the time the film is immersed in each of the wet chemistries. The sequence of times for each step in processing is accomplished by moving the film through each stage at a carefully controlled rate. The transport system consists of the following three principal subsystems: (1) **rollers,** (2) **transport racks,** and (3) **drive motor.**

Roller subassembly. There are basically three types of rollers used in the transport system. **Transport rollers** are 1-inch diameter rollers that convey the film along its path. They are positioned opposite one another in pairs or are offset from one another (Figure 15-8). When the film makes a turn in the processor, and most of the turns are designed to reverse the direction of the film, a 3-inch

diameter **master roller,** or solar roller, is used (Figure 15-9). The master roller usually has positioned around it a number of **planetary rollers** and metal or plastic **guide shoes.**

Transport-rack subassembly. Except for the entering rollers at the feed tray, most of the rollers in the transport system are positioned on a rack assembly (Figure 15-10). These racks are easily removable and provide for convenient maintenance and efficient cleaning of the processor.

When the film is transported in one direction along the rack assembly, only the 1-inch diameter rollers are required to guide and propel it. At each bend, however, there is a curved metal lip with smooth grooves to guide the film around the bend. These are called *guide shoes.* For a 180-degree bend, the film would be positioned for the turn by the leading guide shoe, propelled around the curve by the master roller and its planetary rollers, and leave the curve by entering the next straight run of rollers through the trailing guide shoe.

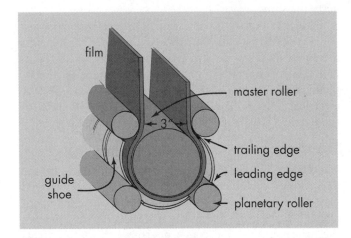

FIGURE 15-9 A master roller with planetary rollers and guide shoes is used to reverse the direction of film in a processor.

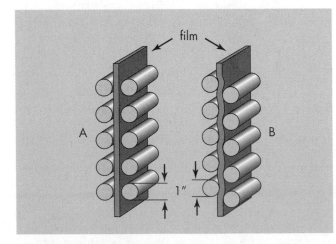

FIGURE 15-8 A, Transport rollers positioned opposite each other. **B,** Transport rollers positioned offset from one another.

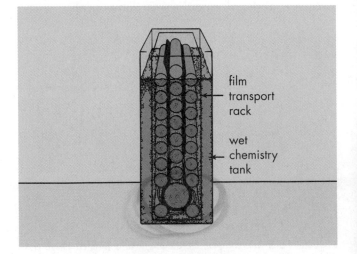

FIGURE 15-10 A transport-rack subassembly.

Such a system of a master roller, planetary rollers, and guide shoes is called a *turnaround assembly*. The turnaround assembly is located at the bottom of the transport-rack assembly. Each wet-chemistry cycle has a transport-rack assembly positioned in the tank. When the film exits the top of the rack assembly, it is guided to the adjacent rack assembly through a **crossover rack.** The crossover rack is a smaller rack assembly than the turnaround assembly, but it is also composed of rollers and guide shoes.

Drive subsystem. Power for the transport system is provided by a fractional horsepower drive motor. The shaft of the drive motor is usually reduced to 10 to 20 rpm through a **gear-reduction assembly.** A chain, pulley, or gear assembly transfers power to the transport rack and drives the rollers. Figure 15-11 illustrates the three principal mechanical devices—a belt and pulley, a chain and sprocket, and gears—used to connect the mechanical energy of the drive motor to the drive mechanism of the rack assembly.

The speed of the transport system is controlled by both the speed of the motor and the gear-reduction system used. The tolerance on this mechanical assembly is quite rigid. Film transport time should not vary by more than ±2% of the time specified by the manufacturer.

Temperature-Control System

The developer requires precise temperature control.

> **Temperature Control**
> The developer temperature is critical, and it is usually maintained within plus or minus 5° F of the optimal temperature.

The optimal temperature has been determined experimentally and is 95° F (35° C).

Temperature is monitored by a **thermocouple** or **thermistor.** A thermostatically controlled heating element is in the developer tank.

Circulation System

Anyone who has manually processed a radiograph knows how important it is to agitate the film during

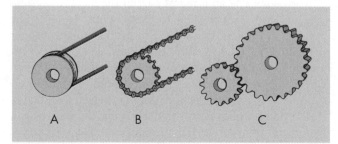

FIGURE 15-11 A, Belt and pulley. **B,** Chain and sprocket. **C,** Gears. These are the three means by which transfer of power to the transport rack can be accomplished.

processing. Agitation is necessary to continually mix the processing chemistry, to maintain a constant temperature throughout the processing tank, and to aid in the exposure of the emulsion to the chemistry.

In automatic processing, agitation is provided by a circulation system that continuously keeps the developer and fixer tanks in constant agitation. A filter that traps particles down to approximately 100 μm in size is required in the developer-circulation system to trap flecks of gelatin that are dislodged from the emulsion. Thus the particles have less chance of becoming attached to the rollers, where they can produce artifacts on the film during transport. These filters are not 100% efficient, and sludge can build up on the rollers. Consequently, cleaning the tanks and the transport system should be a part of the routine maintenance of any processor.

Filtration in the fixer-circulation system is normally unnecessary, since the fixer hardens and shrinks the gelatin so that coating of the rollers does not occur. Furthermore, the fixer neutralizes the developer, and the products of this reaction will not affect the final radiograph.

Circulation of water through the wash tank is necessary to remove all of the processing chemicals from the surface of the film before drying to ensure archival quality. Rather than using a **closed-circulation system,** this is usually done with an **open system.** Fresh tap water is piped into the tank at the bottom and overflows out the top, where it is collected and discharged directly to the outflow system. The minimum flow rate for the wash tank in most processors is 12 liters per minute (3 gallons per minute).

Replenishment System

Each time a film makes its way through the processor, it uses some of the processing chemistry. Some developer is absorbed into the emulsion and is neutralized during fixing. The fixer, likewise, is absorbed during processing, and some is carried over into the wash tank. If neither the developer nor the fixer were replenished, they would quickly lose chemical balance, the level of solution in each tank would drop, and short contact times with the chemistry would result.

The replenishment system puts into each tank the proper amount of chemistry to maintain volume and chemical activity. Although the replenishment of the developer is more important, the fixer also has to be replenished. Wash water is not recirculated. It is continuously replenished with fresh tap water.

Replenishment rates are based on the amount of film processed. Usually the rate is established for every 14 inches of film travel. When a film is inserted into the feed tray with its widest dimension gripped by the leading rollers and its narrow side against the guide fence, a microswitch is activated that turns on the replenishment for as long as film travels through the microswitch. Replenishment rates are approximately 60 to 70 milliliters of developer and 100 to 110 milliliters of fixer for every 14 inches of film. If the replenishment rate is increased, a slightly increased radiographic contrast results. If the rate is too low, a significant decrease in contrast occurs.

5 Dryer System

If a finished radiograph is wet or damp, it picks up dust particles in the air, which results in artifacts on the film. Additionally, a wet or damp film is difficult to handle on a view box. When stored, a damp film can become sticky and the emulsion will be destroyed. The dryer system consists of a blower, ventilation ducts, drying tubes, and an exhaust system. It completely extracts all residual moisture from the processed radiograph so that it drops into the receiving bin dry.

The blower sucks in room air and blows it across heating coils through duct work to the drying tubes. The room air therefore should be at low humidity and dust free. Sometimes as many as three heating coils, each approximately 2500-watt capacity, are used. The temperature of the air entering the drying chamber is thermostatically regulated.

The drying tubes are long hollow cylinders with slit-like openings that extend the length of the cylinder and face the film. They are positioned on both sides of the film as the film is transported through the drying chamber. The hot moist air is exhausted from the drying chamber and vented to the outside, much like the air in a clothes dryer. Some fraction of the exhaust air may be recirculated in the dryer system.

When damp films drop into the receiving bin, there is immediate suspicion that a malfunction of the dryer system has occurred. It seems, however, that most processing faults that lead to damp film occur because of a depletion of glutaraldehyde, the hardener in the developer.

6 Electrical System

Electrical power must be provided to the thermal and mechanical components of each of the previously mentioned systems. This is done, of course, through proper wiring of the automatic processor. Normally, each major electrical component is fused. The fuse box is the only part of the electrical system that is of importance to the radiographer.

ALTERNATIVE PROCESSING METHODS

There is a tendency to think that most of the recent advances in medical x-ray imaging are associated with imaging equipment, but excellent developments have been made by the radiographic film manufacturers that have improved image quality and the efficiency of radiology departments. Rapid processing, extended processing, and daylight processing are fast becoming standard in medical imaging.

Rapid Processing

No matter what the task, today people want to do it faster. Medical imaging is no exception, and the manufacturers of radiographic film have developed microprocessor-controlled equipment and specially formulated processing chemicals for this task. Processing as rapidly as 30 seconds is now available.

These rapid processors prove to be useful in angiography, special procedures, surgery, and emergency rooms where time is critical. Here, it is important to have radiographic images available for physicians as soon as possible. When used with proper chemistry, rapid processing produces images similar to 90-second processing.

For rapid processing, the chemicals are more concentrated and developer and fixer temperatures are higher.

Extended Processing

Extended processing has particular application in mammography. Whereas the standard processing time is 90 seconds, extended processing may be as long as 3 minutes. Developer immersion time is nearly doubled, but it is not necessary to alter developer temperature. Furthermore, standard chemicals may be used. The only significant disadvantage is the longer time.

There are two principal advantages with extended processing—greater image contrast and lower patient dose. Contrast is increased approximately 15%. Image-receptor sensitivity is increased by at least 30%. Thus patient radiation dose is reduced.

The improvements in contrast and patient dose with extended processing occur only with single-emulsion film. Extended processing is not recommended for double-emulsion films, since it does not significantly influence contrast or dose with such films.

Daylight Processing

Daylight systems are being adopted as the standard in emergency department x-ray rooms. In a daylight system the radiographer only needs to position a cassette with an exposed film into the appropriate slot of the system (Figure 15-12). The film is automatically extracted from the cassette and sent to the processor. The processor may be an integral part of the daylight system or a separate unit docked to the daylight system. The cassette is reloaded with unexposed film of the proper size before it is released by the system for the next exposure. The daylight system allows the radiographer to watch over the patient in the x-ray room without interruption. It takes only seconds for a patient to need help. If the radiographer is in the darkroom, the patient can be left unassisted. Daylight processing also can reduce cassette handling time. It takes only about 15 seconds for the radiographer to insert the exposed cassette into the daylight loader and retrieve a fresh cassette. Total load, unload, and process time is about 2 minutes, and

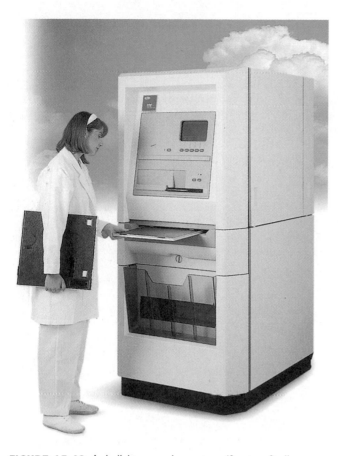

FIGURE 15-12 A daylight processing system. *(Courtesy Sterling Diagnostic Imaging.)*

multiple film sizes are automatically accommodated. Microprocessor technology makes daylight systems possible. The microprocessor monitors the unloading and reloading of the cassette automatically by sensing the cassette size and film consumption rate. Most can accommodate up to 1000 sheets of radiographic film of various sizes. Some units can also annotate data on the radiograph, including the date, time, and other examination characteristics. System status is continuously indicated with light-emitting diodes (LED) or liquid-crystal displays (LCD).

SUMMARY

The process of converting the latent image to a manifest image in the emulsion is a three-step process. First the latent image is formed when silver-halide grains are exposed to light or x-ray energy. Next, only the grains exposed to photon energy are made visible by development. Finally, fixing removes the unexposed grains from the emulsion and makes the image permanent.

In 1965 the Eastman Kodak Company developed a 90-second radiographic film rapid processor, which is still the standard of the industry. The steps for manual and automatic processing are the same but because

manual processing takes up to an hour, it is rarely used in modern departments. The sequence of processing steps are as follows: (1) wetting, (2) development, (3) stop bath, (4) fixing, (5) washing, and (6) drying. Tables 15-2 and 15-3 list the chemicals and their functions in the developing and fixing processes.

The components of the automatic processor are (1) the transport system, (2) the temperature-control system, (3) the circulation system, (4) the replenishment system, (5) the dryer system, and (6) the electrical system. Most diagnostic imaging departments have 90-second rapid processors and at least one alternative processing system as well. The extended processing method is used to develop speciality films such as single-emulsion mammography screen film. The daylight processing system allows radiographers to maintain uninterrupted patient care. The daylight system commonly is used in critical care areas such as the emergency department.

REVIEW QUESTIONS

1. When was automatic processing first introduced?
2. Which company invented the first roller transport processing system?
3. What type of processors are used in the clinical sites you visit?
4. List the steps of automatic processing and the times of each step in a 90-second processor.
5. Name the universal wetting agent.
6. What is the principal action of development?
7. Give an example of a redox reaction.
8. _____ means that the action of two agents working together is greater than the sum of the action of each agent working independently.
9. Name the principal component in developer solutions.
10. Why is it recommended to wear gloves and goggles when mixing or handling developer solutions?
11. Why is a preservative added to the developer? What happens over time if the preservative is not added?
12. If a film drops into the receiving bin damp or wet, this could indicate a problem with the developer solution. What is wrong?
13. Define what archival quality of radiographic film means.
14. Why does the film need to go through the fixer tank?
15. If a radiographic film turns brown once it has been stored in the file room, what may be the problem?
16. What changes took place in the processing chemistries to reduce the time of processing from

the 1 hour of hand processing to 90 seconds of automatic processing?

17. List and explain the components of the automatic processor transport system.

18. How should each size of x-ray film be fed onto the feed tray of the automatic processor to maintain a proper replenishment rate in the processing tanks?

19. At what temperature should the developer be maintained?

20. Explain the use of the extended processing system.

Additional Readings

Eastman Kodak Company: *Introduction to medical radiographic imaging,* Rochester, NY, 1993, Eastman Kodak.

Fitterman AS, Brayer FC, Cumbo PE: *Processing chemistry for medical imaging,* Rochester, NY, 1995, Eastman Kodak.

Haus AG: *Film processing in medical imaging,* Rochester, NY, 1993, Eastman Kodak.

Haus AG: *Screen-film image receptors and film processing,* Rochester, NY, 1994, Eastman Kodak.

Haus AG et al: *Automatic film processing in medical imaging: system design considerations,* Rochester, NY, 1992, Eastman Kodak.

Hewitt P: Reducing the risks in x-ray processing, *Occup Health (Lond)* 46(7):244, July 1994.

Ketchum LE: Dry-process film eliminates need for darkroom and chemicals, *Appl Radiol* 23(5):39, May 1994.

Mosby's radiographic instructional series: radiographic imaging [slide set], St Louis, 1996, Mosby.

Pirtle OL: Study shows inconsistency in film processing quality, *Radiol Technol* 64(3):154, January-February 1993.

Utt D: Solving your darkroom problem, *Radiol Technol* 66(1):65, September-October 1994.

16 Intensifying Screens

OBJECTIVES

At the completion of this chapter the student will be able to:

1. List and describe the layers that make up an intensifying screen
2. Discuss luminescence
3. Compare the characteristics of screen versus nonscreen imaging regarding intensification factor
4. Identify the screen characteristics of x-ray absorption, the x-ray to light conversion efficiency, and the speed of screens
5. Define noise
6. Explain image blur
7. Discuss film-screen combinations, including calcium-tungstate and rare-earth systems
8. Describe the handling and cleaning of intensifying screens

OUTLINE

Screen Construction
  Protective coating
  Phosphor layer
  Reflective layer
  Base
Luminescence
Screen Characteristics
  Screen designs
  X-ray absorption
  Conversion efficiency
  Image noise
  Spatial resolution or image blur

Screen-Film Combinations
  Compatibility
  Cassette
  Direct-exposure film, calcium-tungstate screens, and rare-earth systems
  Rare earth elements
Care of Intensifying Screens

Intensifying screens are part of the radiographic cassette. The cassette is the protective holder for the intensifying screens and the radiographic film.

Even though some x-rays reach the film emulsion, it is actually visible light from the intensifying screens that exposes the radiographic film. Visible light is emitted from the phosphor layer of the intensifying screens, which is activated by the remnant radiation exiting the patient.

SCREEN CONSTRUCTION

Less than 1% of the x-ray beam exposing radiographic film contributes to the latent image. To increase efficiency, radiographic film is placed in contact with intensifying screens within the radiographic cassette. Intensifying screens convert the energy of the x-ray beam into visible light. This visible light then interacts with the radiographic film to form the latent image. Approximately 30% of the x-rays striking an intensifying screen will interact with the screen. For each interaction a large number of visible-light photons are emitted.

Intensifying Screens
The intensifying screen acts as an amplifier of the remnant radiation reaching the film.

Use of an intensifying screen results in considerably lower patient dose and increased subject contrast. Compared with direct-exposure film, using intensifying screens causes a slight blurring of the image. However, modern intensifying-screen technology minimizes blur and, as a result, image detail is improved.

Intensifying screens resemble flexible sheets of plastic or cardboard and are manufactured in sizes corresponding to the sizes of film. Radiographic film called *double-emulsion film* is placed between the two intensifying screens in the cassette.

Most screens are composed of the four distinct layers shown in cross section in Figure 16-1. The intensifying screen contains a protective coating, the phosphor, reflective layers, and the base.

Protective Coating

The layer of the intensifying screen closest to the x-ray film is the **protective coating.** It is 10 to 20 μm thick and is applied to the face of the screen to make the screen resistant to abrasion caused by handling. It also helps eliminate the buildup of static electricity and provides a surface for routine cleaning without disturbing the active phosphor. Naturally, the protective layer is transparent to light.

Phosphor Layer

The active layer of the intensifying screen is the **phosphor layer.** In the phosphor layer the phosphor emits

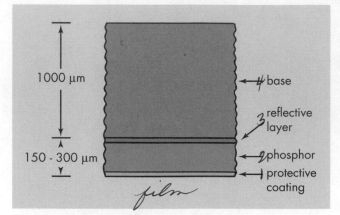

FIGURE 16-1 Cross-sectional view of an intensifying screen, showing its four principal layers.

light during stimulation by x-rays. Phosphor layers vary in thickness from 150 to 300 μm, depending on the type of screen. The phosphor has one purpose—to convert the energy of the x-ray beam into visible light. The action of the phosphor can be demonstrated by viewing an opened cassette in a darkened x-ray room through the protective barrier of the control booth. The intensifying screen will glow brightly when exposed to x-rays. There are many materials satisfactory for use in radiography, but they must possess the characteristics given in the box below. Through the years, materials have been used as phosphors because they exhibit these characteristics. These materials are **calcium tungstate, zinc sulfide,** and **barium lead sulfate,** and since 1972 the rare-earth phosphors are **gadolinium, lanthanum,** and **yttrium.**

Roentgen discovered x-rays quite by accident. He observed the luminescence of **barium platinocyanide,** a phosphor that has never been applied to diagnostic imaging with success. Within a year of Roentgen's discovery of x-rays, calcium tungstate was developed as a phosphor by the American inventor, Thomas A. Edison.

Properties of an Intensifying Screen Phosphor

The phosphor should have a **high atomic number** so that x-ray absorption is high.
The phosphor should emit a large amount of light per absorption of x-ray photons. This is called the *x-ray conversion efficiency.*
The spectral emission of the screen must match the sensitivity of the x-ray film. This is called *spectral matching.*
Phosphor **afterglow,** the continuing emission of light after exposure of the phosphor to x-rays, should be minimal.
The phosphor should not be affected by heat, humidity, or other environmental agents.

Edison demonstrated the use of screens before the beginning of the twentieth century, but screen-film imaging did not come into general use until about the time of World War I with the renewed use of calcium tungstate.

For a time, barium-lead sulfate screens were used, particularly with high-kVp techniques. Zinc sulfide was once used for low-kVp techniques but never gained wide acceptance. Calcium tungstate, because of improved manufacturing techniques and quality-control procedures, was used until the 1970s. Since then, rare-earth screens have been used in diagnostic imaging departments. These screens are faster than those made of calcium tungstate, rendering them more useful for most types of radiographic imaging. Use of rare-earth screens results in lower patient dose, less thermal stress on the x-ray tube, and reduced radiation shielding requirements for x-ray rooms.

Differences in screen imaging characteristics are basically caused by differences in the composition of the phosphor. The thickness of the phosphor layer and the concentration and size of the phosphor crystals also influence the action of intensifying screens. The thickness of the phosphor layer ranges from approximately 50 to 250 μm, with individual phosphor crystals ranging from 5 to 15 μm.

Reflective Layer

In a calcium-tungstate screen there is a reflective layer between the phosphor and the base (Figure 16-2) that is approximately 25 μm thick and is made of a shiny substance such as **magnesium oxide** or **titanium dioxide.** When x-rays interact with the phosphor, light is emitted **isotropically,** that is, with equal intensity in all directions. Less than half the light is emitted in the direction of the film. The reflective layer intercepts light headed in other directions and redirects it to the film. The reflec-

tive layer increases the efficiency of the intensifying screen, nearly doubling the number of light photons reaching the film. Some screens incorporate special dyes in the phosphor layer to selectively absorb those diverging light photons that increase image blur. Because they must travel a longer distance in the phosphor than those emitted perpendicularly to the film, these photons are more easily absorbed by the dye, but this process does result in a reduction in screen efficiency.

Rare-earth screens do not need this reflective layer because of the efficiency of the x-ray absorption and emission of light photons to expose the film.

Base

The layer farthest from the film is called the *base.* The base is 1 millimeter thick and serves principally as a mechanical support for the active phosphor layer. It is made of high-grade cardboard or polyester. Polyester is the popular base material in screen construction just as it is for radiographic film. The requirements for high-quality base material are given in the box below.

LUMINESCENCE

Any material that emits light in response to some outside stimulation is called a **luminescent material,** or a **phosphor,** and the visible light emitted is called **luminescence.** Materials can be caused to luminesce by a number of different energy sources, such as electric current (the fluorescent light), biochemical reactions (the lightning bug), visible light (a watch dial), and x-rays (an intensifying screen). Luminescence is a process similar to characteristic x-ray emission. However, luminescence involves **outer-shell electrons** (Figure 16-3). In an intensifying screen a single x-ray absorption causes thousands of light photons to be emitted. When a luminescent material is stimulated, the outer shell electrons far from the nucleus are raised to an excited energy state. This effectively creates a hole in the outer electron shell, which is an unstable condition for the atom. The hole is filled when the excited electron returns to its normal state, and this transition is accompanied by the emission of electromagnetic energy as visible-light photons. Energy is required to raise the outer-shell electron

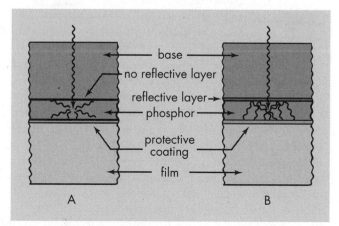

FIGURE 16-2 A, Screen without reflective layer. **B,** Screen with reflective layer. Screens without reflective layers are not as efficient as those with reflective layers because fewer light photons reach the film.

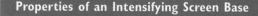

Properties of an Intensifying Screen Base
It must be **sturdy** and moisture resistant.
It must not suffer radiation damage nor **discolor** with age.
It must be **chemically inert** and not interact with the phosphor layer.
It must be **flexible.**
It must not contain **impurities** that would be imaged by x-rays.

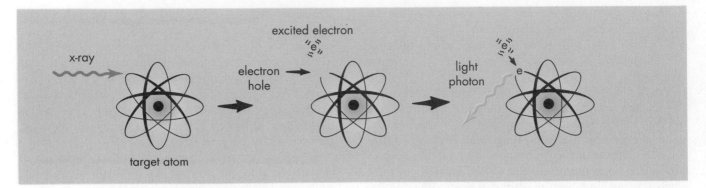

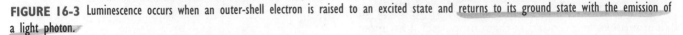

FIGURE 16-3 Luminescence occurs when an outer-shell electron is raised to an excited state and returns to its ground state with the emission of a light photon.

to an excited state, and this energy is released when the electron returns to its normal state. Only a narrow range of excited energy states for an outer-shell electron is possible, and these states depend on the structure of the luminescent material. The wavelength of the emitted light is determined by the level of excitation to which the electron was raised and is characteristic of a given luminescent material. Consequently, luminescent materials emit light of a characteristic color.

There are two types of luminescence: (1) If visible light is emitted only during the stimulation of the phosphor, the process is called *fluorescence*. (2) If the phosphor continues to emit light after stimulation, then the process is called *phosphorescence*. Some materials can phosphoresce for long periods after stimulation. For example, a light-stimulated watch dial fades slowly in the dark. X-ray intensifying screens mainly fluoresce. Phosphorescence in an intensifying screen is called *screen lag*, or *afterglow*, and is objectionable. There is a precise distinction between fluorescence and phosphorescence related to the motion of the excited electron around the nucleus. If the electron returns to its normal state with the emission of light within one revolution after stimulation, then fluorescence has occurred. If more than one revolution is required, then the process is phosphorescence. The time required for an electron to make one revolution about the nucleus is 10 nanoseconds. To perceive this with the human eye, ask a radiographer or the radiography instructor to x-ray an intensifying screen in a darkened x-ray room. The luminescence, as well as the characteristic color of the

phosphor, is visible. The luminescence is visible because there are many light photons released with each x-ray interaction.

SCREEN CHARACTERISTICS

The primary characteristics of x-ray intensifying screens that are important to the radiographer are (1) x-ray absorption, (2) screen conversion efficiency, (3) image noise, and (4) spatial resolution or image blur.

The property used to compare nonscreen exposures with screen-film exposures and may be considered a screen characteristic. Since intensifying screens have always been used to reduce patient dose, it is important to know the magnitude of dose reduction compared with nonscreen exposures. This property is called the *intensification factor*.

Screen speed is often used in reference to intensifying screens, however, *image receptor speed* is a more accurate term. The speed of a film-screen system depends on the whole imaging chain from x-ray exposure intensity to the processing of the x-ray film.

Image receptor speed is determined by manufacturers, often in inconsistent ways. Generally, image receptor speed is characterized by a relative number that relates to the amount of radiation used to produce the radiograph. The numbers commonly used by manufacturers to differentiate image receptor speed are 100, 200, 400, 800, and 1000. The systems may be identified as a particular speed by the manufacturer, but factors in the imaging department, for example developer temperature in the processor, may cause inconsistency of the stated image receptor speed.

Par-speed calcium-tungstate screens are assigned a value of 100 and through the years have been the basis for comparison of all other screens, even though calcium-tungstate screens are not in modern use. There are two factors that theoretically contribute to screen speed even though there are actually many contributing factors. Screen speed is determined by the number of x-rays interacting with the screen phosphor layer and

Luminescence	
Fluorescence	**Phosphorescence**
No lag	Afterglow
$<10^{-8}$ seconds	$>10^{-8}$ seconds
(less than)	(greater than)

the efficiency of conversion of x-ray energy into visible light that interacts with the film.

Screen Designs

The design characteristics of intensifying screens that affect x-ray absorption and x-ray-to-light conversion efficiency are given in the box below. These characteristics are the manufacturer's proprietary design.

Remember the speed of an image receptor is a number compared with that of calcium-tungstate screens. This speed number does not convey information concerning dose reduction to the patient. The information of dose reduction from nonscreen radiography to intensifying screen radiography is conveyed by the **intensification factor (IF)**. The intensification factor is defined as the ratio of the exposures required to produce the same optical density with and without the use of screens as follows:

$$IF = \frac{\text{Exposure required without screens}}{\text{Exposure required with screens}}$$

The optical density chosen for comparing one screen with another is usually 1. The value of the intensification factor can be used to determine the dose reduction accompanying the use of an intensifying screen.

Question: A pelvic examination using 100-speed screens is taken at 75 kVp, 100 mAs and results in an exposure to the patient of 200 mR (52 μC/kg). A similar examination taken without screens would result in a patient exposure of 6400 mR (1.7 mC/kg). What is the approximate intensification factor of the 100-speed screen-film combination?

Manufacturer's Design of Intensifying Screens

Phosphor composition. Rare-earth elements efficiently convert x-rays into usable light.

Phosphor thickness. The thicker the phosphor layer, the higher is the relative number of x-rays converted into light.

Reflective layer. The presence of a reflective layer increases x-ray to light conversion efficiency but also increases image blur.

Dye. Light-absorbing dyes are added to some phosphors to control the spread of light. These dyes improve spatial resolution.

Crystal size. Larger individual phosphor crystals produce more light emission per x-ray interaction. The phosphor crystals range from approximately 4 to 8 μm.

Concentration of phosphor crystals. Higher crystal concentration results in higher x-ray to light conversion efficiency.

Answer:

$$IF = \frac{6400}{200} = 32 \text{ is the intensification factor}$$

X-ray Absorption

Absorption efficiency is a concept describing the percent absorption of x-rays in the phosphor layer of intensifying screens. Figure 16-4, A illustrates 1000 x-rays incident on the intensifying screen and 800 x-rays exiting through the screen that have not interacted with the screen's phosphor layer. The difference, 200 x-rays, has been absorbed in the phosphor layer. With a simple calculation, this becomes a 20% absorption efficiency of the intensifying screen under investigation.

Conversion Efficiency

Intensifying screens are also characterized by the efficiency of converting x-ray energy into light energy. This is called **conversion efficiency**. The x-ray energy in ergs (joules) is measured at input, and the light energy exiting the intensifying screen is measured also. With a fixed x-ray absorption efficiency, changes in conversion efficiency are the greatest contributor to the change in image receptor speed. Figure 16-4, B shows how an increase in conversion efficiency can make a screen brighter and thus directly influence the image receptor speed. There are laboratories, one at Eastman Kodak Company, Rochester, NY, that investigate x-ray to light conversion efficiency. Even with research, new designs, and new phosphors, it is difficult to achieve a conversion efficiency of more than approximately 15% to 20%.

Image Noise

Noise is the term used to describe the deterioration of the radiographic image. Deterioration of the image is caused by many factors. Noise, for the most part, is caused by (1) the number of x-rays used to expose the patient or mAs, (2) the limited absorption efficiency of x-rays in the intensifying screen, and (3) the randomness of the x-ray to light-conversion process.

The number of x-rays used to expose the patient, or mAs, is a predominant cause of image noise on a radiograph. The fewer x-rays used to expose the patient, the greater the image noise. **Quantum mottle** is the term used to describe the mottled or noisy appearance of an image that has been exposed by a limited number of x-ray photons. An example of quantum mottle is often seen in the fluoroscopy image. Very low exposure rate is used in fluoroscopy, and image graininess is often evident on the fluoroscopy monitor. Raising the kVp often degrades the subject contrast; however, raising the exposure rate and increasing the number of x-rays used generally improve the fluoroscopic image.

Absorption efficiency also contributes to image noise. Because absorption efficiency is a random process, the

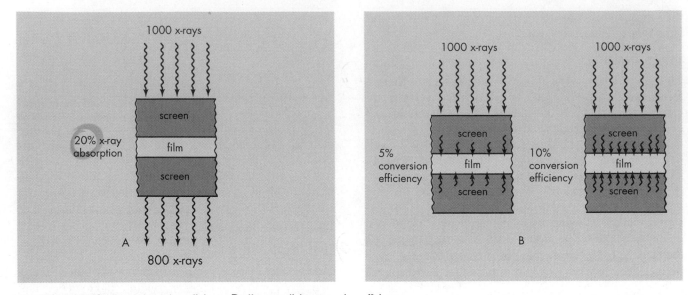

FIGURE 16-4 A, X-ray absorption efficiency. **B,** X-ray to light conversion efficiency.

fluctuations can cause radiographic image deterioration. Noise also occurs from the random flux of the intensity of light emitted from the phosphor layer. The noise resulting from random fluctuation of conversion efficiency can be as much as 30%.

Dectective quantum efficiency (DQE) is the term commonly used by manufacturers of imaging receptors to define the noise efficiency of an imaging system. DQE calculations include noise from all aspects of the imaging chain, a few of which are as follow: some types of processing nonuniformities, the random placement size of the phosphor grains in the phosphor layer, and random placement and size of the silver-halide crystals in the film emulsion.

Spatial Resolution or Image Blur

Spatial resolution or **image blur** of the screen is its ability to produce an accurate and clear image. Resolution is usually measured by the **minimum line spacing** or **line pairs per millimeter (lp/mm)** that can be detected on the radiograph.

The use of intensifying screens adds one more step to the process of imaging the human body with x-rays. Although screens are used everywhere, they have the disadvantage of lower spatial resolution compared with direct-exposure radiographs. When calcium-tungstate screens were in use, extremity examinations were performed on direct-exposure film. Figure 16-5 compares the spatial resolution between screen-film and direct-exposure film. The direct-exposure film has clearer detail throughout; however, the increased patient exposure outweighs the benefit of increase in image detail. Direct-exposure film requires 10 to 40 times more exposure than using screen-film for extremity radiographs.

Spatial resolution or image blur is measured in a number of ways and can be given a numerical value. Resolution is related to the ability of a system to image an object exactly. A photograph in focus shows good spatial resolution; one out of focus shows poor spatial resolution and therefore much image blur. Figure 16-5 shows the differences in spatial resolution between a direct-exposure film and a par-speed screen-film combination obtained when imaging an x-ray test pattern. Such a test pattern is called a *line-pair test pattern.* It has lead lines separated by equal size interspaces. As discussed more completely in Chapter 29, spatial resolution may be expressed by the number of line pairs per millimeter (lp/mm). The higher the number, the better the detail of the object to be imaged. The 800 to 1000 class image receptors can resolve approximately 6 lp/mm, and 100 class image receptors can resolve 10 lp/mm (see Table 16-4). Direct-exposure film can resolve 50 lp/mm. The unaided eye can resolve about 10 lp/mm.

Generally, those conditions that increase the intensification factor between nonscreen film and screen-film combinations also reduce spatial resolution. Resolution improves with smaller phosphor crystals and thinner phosphor layers. Figure 16-6 shows how these factors affect image resolution.

In mammography the screens and the film are specially positioned to improve detail. The screen is positioned in contact with the emulsion on the side of the cassette away from the x-ray source to reduce screen blur and improve spatial resolution (Figure 16-7).

SCREEN-FILM COMBINATIONS
Compatibility

Screens and films are manufactured for compatibility. The best results will be obtained if they are selected with this in mind.

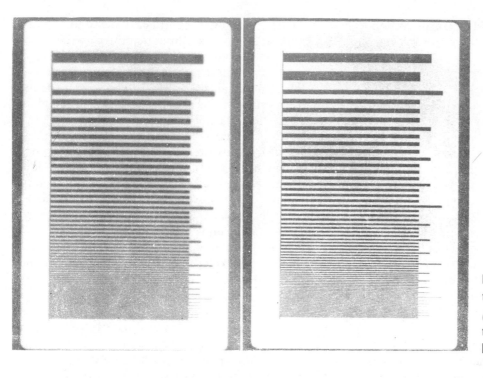

FIGURE 16-5 Radiographs of an x-ray test pattern made with direct-exposure film *(right)* and a par-speed screen-film combination *(left)*. Note the difference in image blur.

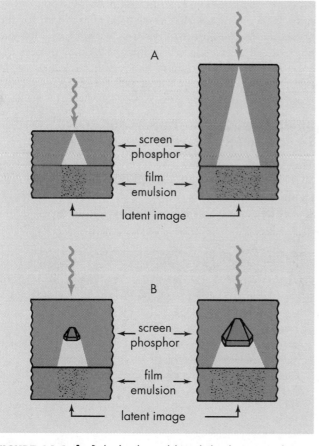

FIGURE 16-6 **A,** Reduction in spatial resolution is greater when phosphor layers are thick. **B,** Reduction is also greater when crystal size is large. These same conditions increase screen speed by producing more light photons per incident x-ray.

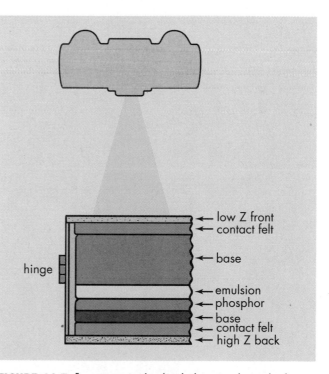

FIGURE 16-7 For mammography the single screen is on the far side of the emulsion to reduce screen blur.

Remember: Screens and film are selected for compatability. The film has to match the screen. Check with the film and screen manufacturers for proper selection and use.

Intensifying screens are nearly always used in pairs. Figure 16-8 is a cross section of a properly loaded radiographic cassette containing front and back screens with a double-emulsion film. Production of the latent image will be nearly evenly divided between front and back screens with less than 1% being contributed directly by x-ray interaction. Each screen exposes the emulsion with which it is in contact.

Cassette

The **cassette** is the rigid holder that contains the screens and film. The front surface, the side facing the x-ray source, should be made of material with a low atomic number that will not attenuate the x-ray beam, such as plastic or cardboard. It should be as thin as practical yet sturdy.

Attached to the inside of the front cover of the cassette is the front screen, and attached to the back cover is the back screen. The radiographic film is sandwiched between the two screens. Between each screen and the cassette cover will be some sort of **compression device**, such as felt or rubber, that maintains close **film-screen contact** when the cassette is closed and latched. The

back cover is usually made of heavy metal to minimize *backscatter*. The x-rays transmitted through the screen-film combination to the back cover will be absorbed photoelectrically more readily in a high-Z material than in a low-Z material. If the back cover were made of a low-Z material, x-rays could be transmitted through the entire cassette and some might be scattered back to the film by the cassette holding device or a nearby wall. This is called backscatter radiation and results in image blur. Sometimes the cassette hinges or hold-down clamps on the back cover are seen on the radiograph (see Figure 13-3). This is due to backscatter radiation and normally occurs only during high-kVp radiography when the x-ray beam is sufficiently penetrating.

One of the materials the United States developed early in its space exploration program was **carbon fiber.** This material was developed for the nose cone of the space capsule because of its exceedingly high strength and heat resistance. It consists principally of graphite fibers ($Z_C = 6$) in a plastic matrix that can be formed to any shape or thickness. This material is now used widely in radiographic devices that are designed to reduce patient exposure. A cassette with a front consisting of carbon fiber material will absorb only half the x-rays that are absorbed in an aluminum or cardboard cassette. Carbon fiber is also being used as material for fluoroscopic examination tables and computed tomography couches. Use of carbon fiber not only reduces the patient exposure but may also result in longer x-ray tube life because of the lower radiographic techniques required.

Direct-Exposure Film, Calcium-Tungstate Screens, and Rare-Earth Systems

The principal advantage of intensifying screens is that fewer x-ray photons are needed than in direct-exposure techniques. The box below lists the advantages of screen-film use over direct-exposure film use.

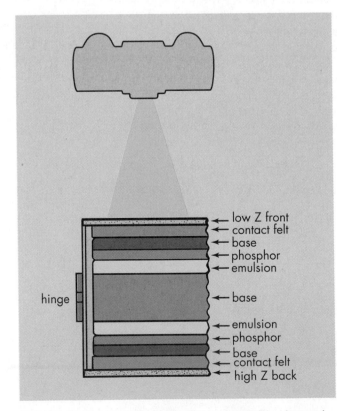

FIGURE 16-8 Cross-sectional view of cassette containing front and back screens and loaded with double-emulsion film.

Advantages of Screen-Film over Direct-Exposure Film Use
INCREASED
Flexibility of kVp selection
Adjustment of radiographic contrast
Spatial resolution when using smaller focal spots
Ability for magnification radiography
X-ray tube life
DECREASED
Patient dose
Occupational exposure
X-ray tube heat production
X-ray exposure time
X-ray tube mA
Possible focal-spot size

Table 16-1 shows the relative number of x-ray and light photons at various stages of the imaging process for radiographs taken with direct exposure film and with a calcium tungstate screen-film. The steps where major differences occur are due to the interaction of x-rays with the screen phosphor and to the large number of visible-light photons produced by each of these interactions. Unfortunately the number of latent images formed is less than 1% of the number of visible photons produced.

Calcium-tungstate phosphors emit visible light in the violet-to-blue region. A stimulated calcium-tungstate screen observed through a protective window appears dark blue. The sensitivity of radiographic film matching calcium-tungstate screens is highest in the blue-violet region of the spectrum. Consequently the light emitted by calcium-tungstate screens is readily absorbed if the radiographic film is **spectrally matched** (Figure 16-9). If the screen phosphor emitted green or red light, its conversion efficiency would be greatly reduced because it would not be spectrally matched with the radiographic film. From its introduction in 1896 by Thomas Edison until the 1970s, calcium tungstate ($CaWO_4$) was used almost exclusively as the phosphor for radiographic intensifying screens.

As newer phosphor materials have been developed, they have become the material of choice in modern imaging departments. Except for barium fluorochloride, the other new phosphors are identified as rare earth, and therefore all these screens have come to be known as *rare-earth screens.*

To be fully effective, rare-earth screens must be used only in conjunction with film emulsions with proper spectral matching. Table 16-2 lists the composition and color emission of rare-earth phosphors. The spectral emissions of rare-earth phosphors are specific, as indicated by the many peaks in the spectrum (Figure 16-10).

TABLE 16-1

Comparison of Relative Number of X-ray Photons and Light Photons at Various Stages for Direct and Screen-Film Exposures*

Stage	Type of Exposure	
	Direct	Screen-film
Incident x-ray photons	1000	20
X-rays absorbed by film	10	<1
X-rays absorbed by screens	—	5
Light photons produced	—	5000
Light photons incident on film	—	3000
Light photons absorbed on film	—	1000
Latent images formed	10	10

*Intensification factor = 1000/20 = 50

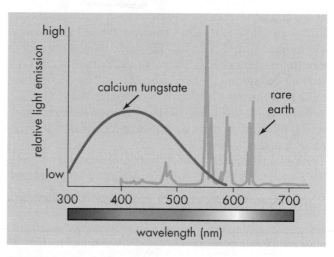

FIGURE 16-10 Calcium tungstate emits a broad spectrum of light centered in the blue region. Rare-earth screens have discrete emissions centered near the green-yellow region.

TABLE 16-2

Composition and Emission of Rare-Earth Intensifying Screens

Phosphor	Activator	Color
Barium strontium sulphate	Europium	Ultraviolet
Barium sulphate	Lead	Ultraviolet
Yttrium tantalate	Thuliuim	Ultraviolet/blue
Zinc sulfide	Silver	Ultraviolet/blue
Calcium tungstate	Lead	Blue
Lanthanum oxybromide	Thulium	Blue
Yttrium oxysulfide	Terbium	Blue
Gadolinium oxysulfide	Terbium	Green
Lanthanum oxysulfide	Terbium	Green
Zinc cadmium sulphide	Silver	Yellow-green

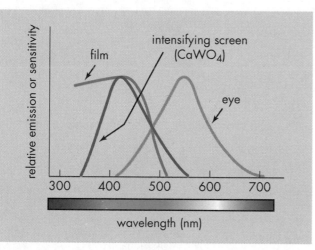

FIGURE 16-9 Importance of spectral matching is demonstrated by showing the relative emission spectrum for an intensifying screen and the relative sensitivity of radiograph film to the light from the screen.

Terbium activation is the element responsible for the shape and intensity of this emission spectrum, which is centered in the green region at 540 nanometers. Specially designed green-sensitive film must be used with rare-earth screens (Figure 16-11). If a green-emitting screen was used with blue-sensitive film, the emissions in the green region would go undetected and the system response would be greatly reduced. To obtain maximum advantage from rare-earth screens, the film used must be spectrally matched to the emissions of the screen. Also, safelights in the darkroom must be of the appropriate tint to prevent film fog. Red safelight lenses are required when developing rare-earth screen film.

Rare Earth Elements

The term *rare earth* describes those elements of group IIIa in the periodic table (see Figure 3-3) that have atomic numbers of 57 to 71. These elements are transitional metals found in low abundance in nature. Those used in rare-earth screens are **gadolinium, lanthanum,** and **yttrium.** The compositions of the five principal rare-earth phosphors are (1) terbium-activated **gadolinium oxysulfide** (Gd$_2$O$_2$S: Tb), (2) terbium-activated lanthanum oxysulfide (La$_2$O$_2$S: Tb), (3) terbium-activated **yttrium oxysulfide** (Y$_2$O$_2$S: Tb), (4) **lanthanum oxybromide** (LaOBr), and (5) **yttrium tantalate** (YTaO$_4$).

Table 16-2 is a list of the rare-earth intensifying screen phosphors, their activator, and the color of phosphor emission.

Rare-earth screens have a single, principal advantage over calcium-tungstate screens—**conversion efficiency.** Rare-earth screens are manufactured to perform at several speed levels, but each is at least twice as fast as the calcium-tungstate screen counterpart. This increase in conversion efficiency is obtained without loss of resolu-

tion. However, with the fastest rare-earth screens the effects of **quantum mottle** (radiographic noise) can be noticeable (see Chapter 19). Since rare-earth screens are faster, lower radiographic technique can be used, which results in lower patient dose. Rare-earth screens provide a general reduction of radiation in the controlled radiation environment. The lower radiographic technique also results in increased x-ray tube life. Rare-earth screens obtain their increased sensitivity through higher x-ray absorption and more efficient conversion of x-ray energy into light.

X-ray absorption. When diagnostic x-rays interact with a calcium-tungstate screen, approximately 30% of the x-rays are absorbed. The mechanism of absorption is almost entirely the photoelectric effect. Recall that photoelectric absorption occurs readily with the inner electrons of high atomic number atoms. In a calcium-tungstate screen, it is the tungstate atom that determines its absorption properties. Tungsten has an atomic number of 74 and a K-shell electron binding energy of 70 keV. In the diagnostic range, x-ray absorption in tungsten follows the relationship shown in Figure 16-12.

At very low energies photoelectric absorption is very high, but as the x-ray energy increases, the probability of absorption decreases rapidly until the x-ray energy is equal to the binding energy of the K-shell electrons. At x-ray energies below the K-shell electron binding energy, the incident photon does not have sufficient energy to ionize K-shell electrons.

When the x-ray energy equals the K-shell electron binding energy, the two K-shell electrons become available for photoelectric interaction. Consequently, at this energy, there is an abrupt increase in the probability of photoelectric absorption. This abrupt increase is followed by another rapid reduction in photoelectric absorption with increasing x-ray energy.

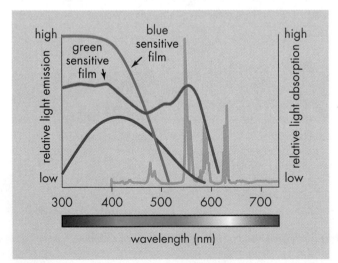

FIGURE 16-11 It is essential that blue-sensitive film be used with blue-emitting screens and green-sensitive film with green-emitting screens.

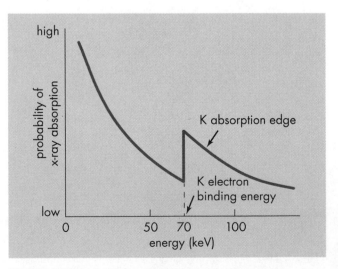

FIGURE 16-12 Probability of x-ray absorption in a calcium-tungstate screen as a function of the incident x-ray energy.

When the incident x-ray has energy equal to the K-shell electron binding energy, photoelectric absorption is maximum for those electrons. The abrupt rise in absorption at this energy is called the *K-shell absorption edge.*

K-edge effect in rare-earth systems. The rare-earth materials used for radiographic intensifying screens all have atomic numbers less than that for tungsten. Consequently, they each have a lower K-shell electron binding energy. Table 16-3 lists the important physical characteristics of the high atomic number elements in intensifying screens. Elements with lower atomic numbers and lower K-shell electron binding energies have lower x-ray absorption probability over most of the x-ray absorption spectrum.

Figure 16-13 shows that the probability for x-ray absorption in rare-earth screens is lower than that for calcium-tungstate screens at all x-ray energies except those between the respective K-shell electron binding energies. Below the K-shell absorption edge for the rare-earth elements, x-ray absorption is higher in tungsten. At an x-ray energy equal to the K-shell electron binding energy of the rare-earth elements, however, the probability of photoelectric absorption is considerably higher than that for tungsten. The absorption probability of the rare earths decreases with increasing x-ray energy, as does calcium tungstate. At x-ray energies above the K-shell absorption edge for tungsten, the rare-earth elements again exhibit lower absorption than that for tungsten.

Each of the rare-earth screens has an absorption curve characteristic of the phosphor that determines the speed of the screen and how it changes with kVp. Figure 16-14 shows the x-ray absorption in two phosphors relative to calcium tungstate. For instance, barium strontium sulfate has higher x-ray photon absorption at lower kVp than gadolinium oxysulfide.

The result of this complex interaction process is that in the x-ray energy range between the K-shell absorption edge for the rare earths and tungsten shows that the rare-earth screens absorb approximately five times more x-rays than a calcium-tungstate screens. Furthermore, for each x-ray absorbed, more light is emitted by the rare-earth screens.

Rare-earth screens exhibit better absorption properties than calcium-tungstate screens only in the energy range between the respective **K-shell absorption edges.** This energy range extends from approximately 35 to 70 keV and corresponds to most of the useful x-rays emitted during routine x-ray examinations.

Conversion efficiency. An additional property of the rare-earth phosphors, the **conversion efficiency**, contributes to their extraordinary speed. The conversion efficiency is defined as the ratio of visible-light energy emitted to the x-ray energy absorbed.

When an x-ray photon interacts photoelectrically with a phosphor and is absorbed, its energy reappears

TABLE 16-3

Atomic Number and K-shell Electron Binding Energy of High-Z Elements in Intensifying Screen Phosphors

Element	Chemical Symbol	Atomic Number (Z)	K-shell Electron Binding Energy (keV)
Yttrium	Y	39	17
Barium	Ba	56	37
Lanthanum	La	57	39
Gadolinium	Gd	64	50
Tungsten	W	74	70

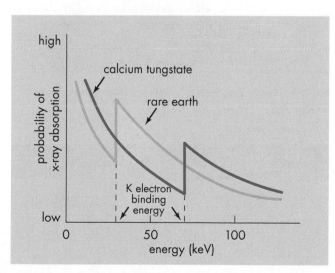

FIGURE 16-13 X-ray absorption probability in a rare-earth screen compared with that for a calcium-tungstate screen. In the energy interval between respective K-shell electron binding energies, absorption in a rare-earth screen is higher.

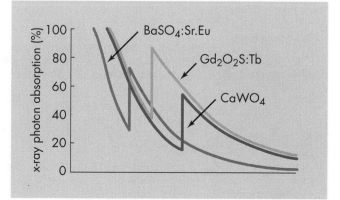

FIGURE 16-14 X-ray absorption for three intensifying screen phosphors.

as either heat or light through a rearrangement of electrons in the crystal lattice of the phosphor. If all the energy reappeared as heat, the phosphor would be worthless as a radiographic intensifying screen. In calcium tungstate, approximately 5% of the absorbed x-ray energy reappears as light. *Rare-earth phosphors exhibit conversion efficiencies of 15% to 20%.*

It is the combination of improved conversion efficiency and higher x-ray absorption that results in the increased sensitivity of rare-earth screens. When using rare-earth screen-film systems with relative speeds as high as 600, image quality may be degraded somewhat by increased quantum mottle, but this may be acceptable for some types of examination in view of the significantly reduced patient dose.

The following table compares and summarizes the characteristics of calcium tungstate and the various speed classes of rare-earth screens (Table 16-4).

Recent developments. Consider the double-emulsion screen-film combination in Figure 16-15. If each screen has an absorption efficiency of 50%, the back screen will have only the 50% of x-rays transmitted with which to work. Therefore the backscreen will absorb only 25% of the x-rays hitting the cassette which results in only one half of the exposure of the back emulsion as compared with the front emulsion. This difference in exposure can be remedied by making the back screen thicker. It can also be remedied by using a different screen and emulsion combination. Such screens and film emulsions are termed *asymmetric* and have been developed by the Eastman Kodak Company. Asymmetric film-screen systems are used to great advantage in applications such as chest, pediatric, and portable radiography. In chest radiography with the Kodak InSight system, for example, the front screen and film emulsion is a slower system, whereas the back screen and film emulsion is a faster system (Figure 16-16). The result is a more balanced image of wide latitude and high contrast over both the lung fields and the mediastinum (Figure 16-17).

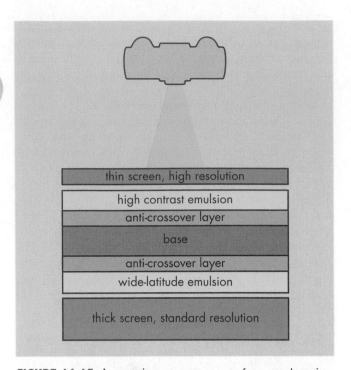

FIGURE 16-15 Asymmetric screens compensate for x-ray absorption in the front screen.

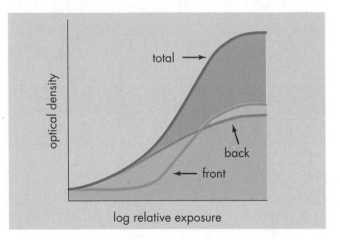

FIGURE 16-16 Characteristic curves from an asymmetric screen-emulsion image receptor.

TABLE 16-4					
Characteristics of Calcium-Tungstate and Modern Rare-Earth X-ray Intensifying Screens					
		Speed Classes Of Rare-Earth Screens			
	Ca Wo Par Speed	100 Class	200 Class	400 Class	800 to 1000 Class
Relative Exposure (OD)	1	1	0.5	0.25	0.1
Resolution lp/mm	Approximately 10 lp/mm	Approximately 10 lp/mm	Approximately 8 lp/mm	Approximately 7 lp/mm	Approximately 6 lp/mm
Radiographic Noise		Low	Medium low	Medium	High
Application	Not in use	Extremity, fine detail	Extremity, chest	General radiography	Special procedures

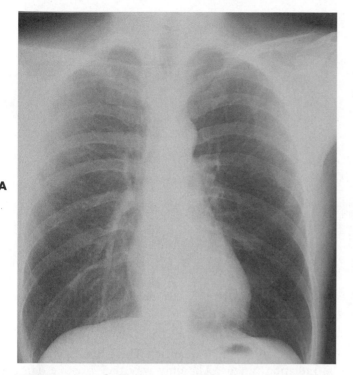

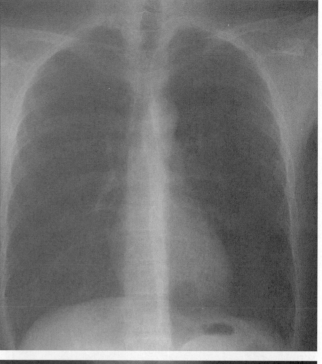

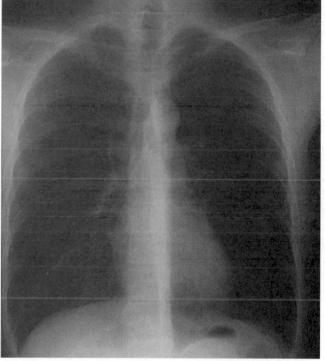

FIGURE 16-17 **A,** The front image of this asymmetric screen-emulsion image receptor shows high contrast. **B,** The back image shows wide latitude. **C,** The total image shows enhanced rendering of mediastinal and subdiaphramatic tissue and plural spaces.

CARE OF INTENSIFYING SCREENS

Screens must be properly cared for if high-quality radiographs are to be consistently produced. When handling screens, use utmost care. Even a small fingernail scratch can produce artifacts and degrade the radiographic image. When loading cassettes do not slide in the film. A sharp corner or the edge can scratch the screen. Place the film in the cassette carefully. Remove the film by rocking the cassette on the hinged edge and letting it fall to your fingers. Do not dig the film out of the cassette with your fingernails. Do not leave cassettes open, because the screens can be damaged by dust or darkroom chemical fumes. Screens should be handled only when they are new and when they are being cleaned. When screens are newly mounted in a cassette, the manufacturer's instructions must be followed carefully.

Screens must be cleaned periodically. The required frequency of cleaning is determined primarily by the following two factors: (1) the amount of use the screens receive and (2) dust in the environment. In a busy imaging department, it may be necessary to clean screens once a month. Under other circumstances, cleaning frequency may safely be extended to 2 to 3 months. Screens must only be cleaned with products recommended by the screen manufacturer, and the manufacturer's instructions should be followed carefully. One advantage to using these commercial preparations is that they often contain **antistatic** compounds, which can be quite helpful.

An equally important requirement in caring for screens is maintaining **screen-film contact.** Screen-film contact can be checked by radiographing a **wire-mesh device.** Figure 16-18, *A* is a radiograph showing good screen-film contact. If there are any areas of blurring, as in Figure 16-18, *B,* then poor screen-film contact

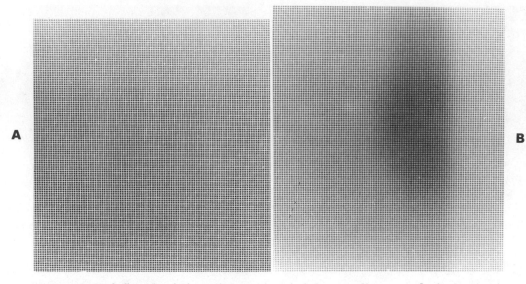

FIGURE 16-18 Radiographs of wire mesh are used to check for screen-film contact. **A,** Good contact is evident. **B,** Region of poor contact is present because of a warped cassette cover.

exists and should be corrected by replacing the cassette.

When new screens are installed in a cassette, this examination for screen-film contact should be made and the radiograph retained as a baseline evaluation. Additional wire-mesh radiographs for screen-film contact should be made once a year and compared with the baseline film.

To test for screen-film contact, expose the cassette through the wire mesh at 50 kVp at 5 mAs and an SID of 100 centimeters. To view the result optimally, back away 2 to 3 meters from the viewbox. Areas of poor screen-film contact will appear blurred and cloudy, indicating that the cassette should be repaired or replaced.

The box below summarizes the most common causes of poor screen-film contact. Observe that nearly all the causes listed can result from rough handling of cassettes. Rough handling is the principal cause of loss of good screen-film contact. Although the cassettes appear sturdy, they are precision pieces of equipment and should be handled carefully.

Properly maintained x-ray intensifying screens will last indefinitely. X-ray interaction with the phosphor

does not cause them to wear out. There is no such thing as radiation fatigue. The only way they become damaged enough to require replacement is through improper handling and maintenance.

SUMMARY

Intensifying screens are permanently placed within the radiographic cassette. The x-ray film used for each exposure is placed between them. The intensify screens are so named because they change the energy of the remnant radiation exiting the patient into light energy striking the radiographic film. As the remnant beam activates the screen phosphor, radiation is converted into light. It is light from the intensifying screens that actually exposes the radiographic film. Intensifying screens are composed of the following four distinct layers: (1) a protective coating, (2) the phosphor layer, (3) the reflective layer, and (4) the base. The phosphor layer has one purpose—to convert x-ray energy into visible light. This process is called *luminescence.* Intensifying screens display a particular kind of luminescence called *fluorescence,* which means the phosphor is stimulated to emit light only when struck by x-ray or light energy. Once the energy is terminated, the light presents no lag or afterglow.

Intensifying screens, like radiographic film, display characteristics in response to radiation. Screens display an x-ray absorption efficiency and an x-ray to light conversion efficiency. Intensifying screens also exhibit image deterioration called *noise* and display spatial resolution, which results in an accurate and clear image on the film.

Intensification factor is a characteristic that compares nonscreen film exposure with screen-film exposure. The intensification factor is defined as follows:

Most Common Causes of Poor Screen-Film Contact
Worn contact felt
Loose, bent, or broken hinges
Loose, bent, or broken latches
Warped screens caused by excessive moisture
Warped cassette front
Sprung or cracked cassette frame
Foreign matter under the screen

$$IF = \frac{\text{Exposure required without screens}}{\text{Exposure required with screens}}$$

Because of the efficiency of the conversion of x-rays to light energy, sometimes short exposure times are required, which limits the quantity of photons emitted by the tube. Fewer photons cause less information to reach the film, which causes deterioration of the image or quantum mottle. Spatial resolution is the accuracy with which the screen reproduces the image. Spatial resolution is measured in line pairs per millimeter of a test object.

When producing intensifying screens, manufacturers change components within the screen to exhibit changes in x-ray absorption, conversion efficiency, spatial resolution, and noise reduction. Manufacturers work with the parameters in their screen designs as listed in Table 16-3.

Calcium-tungstate screen phosphors were used almost exclusively until 1972, when rare-earth phosphors were developed for medical x-ray use. Calcium-tungstate par-speed intensifying screens are used as the standard for determining screen speed. Screen speed is a number determined by the amount of radiation used to expose the patient. Par-speed screens ($CaWO_4$) are assigned a value of 100. Table 16-4 summarizes optical density, resolution in lp/mm, image noise, and application of various intensifying screens.

Finally, intensifying screens must be properly cared for if high-quality radiographs are to be consistently produced. Avoid artifacts on the radiographic film by handling the screens and film carefully. Spots will show up on the radiograph if dust or other deposits cover the screen. Because of dust accumulation, screens need to be cleaned regularly. Clean screens only with products recommended by the screen manufacturer.

■ ■ ■ ■ ■ ■ ■ ■ ■ ■ ■ ■ ■ ■ ■ ■ ■ ■

REVIEW QUESTIONS

1. What percentage of the x-ray beam exposing the radiographic film contributes to the latent image?

2. What is the function of intensifying screens in the radiographic cassette?

3. Why are two intensifying screens placed in the radiographic cassette?

4. What is the purpose of the phosphor layer of the intensifying screen in the radiographic cassette?

5. Why would afterglow be objectionable as a characteristic of an intensifying screen?

6. Name six materials, three used before 1972 and three used after 1972, that are phosphors in intensifying screens.

7. List the four distinct layers that make up an intensifying screen.

8. The _____ of the intensifying screen intercepts light headed in other directions and redirects it to the film.

9. Name the five properties of an intensifying screen base.

10. Discuss the process of luminescence.

11. Define fluorescence and phosphorescence.

12. List the four primary characteristics of x-ray intensifying screens.

13. Explain intensification factor. Write the IF formula.

14. What are the six design characteristics of intensifying screens that are the manufacturer's proprietary information?

15. Draw an illustration showing a 20% x-ray absorption efficiency of the phosphor layer of the intensifying screen.

16. The efficiency of an intensifying screen in converting x-ray energy into light energy is called _____.

17. Define quantum mottle.

18. The higher the number in line pairs per millimeter visualized in the line-pair test pattern, the _____ the detail of the object to be imaged.

19. What is the importance of having radiographic film and intensifying screen phosphor spectrally matched? List five rare-earth phosphors and their emission colors.

20. Describe the factors involved in the care and handling of intensifying screens.

Additional Reading

Introduction to Medical Radiographic Imaging, Rochester, NY, 1993, Eastman Kodak.

Haus AG, Dickerson RE: *Characteristics of screen-film combinations for conventional medical radiography*, Rochester, NY, 1995, Eastman Kodak.

Haus AG: *Screen-film image receptors and film processing*, Rochester, NY, 1994, Eastman Kodak.

Scatter Radiation and Beam-Restricting Devices

OBJECTIVES

At the completion of this chapter the student will be able to:

1. Identify two kinds of x-rays that are responsible for remnant radiation
2. List three factors that contribute to scatter radiation
3. Discuss three devices developed to minimize scatter radiation

OUTLINE

Scatter Radiation
    Factors affecting scatter radiation
    Beam-restricting devices

Three factors contribute to an increase in scatter radiation: increased kVp, increased x-ray field size, and increased anatomic part thickness. Beam-restricting devices control and minimize scatter radiation.

. . . .

SCATTER RADIATION

The following two kinds of x-rays are responsible for the optical density on a radiograph: (1) those that pass through the patient without interacting and (2) those that are scattered in the patient through Compton interaction. Together these two types of x-rays are called *remnant x-rays* (Figure 17-1). As the number of scattered x-rays increases, the radiograph loses contrast and looks dull, fogged, and blurred. There are three primary factors that influence the intensity of scatter radiation reaching the film. They are kilovoltage, x-ray beam field size, and patient or anatomic part thickness.

Factors Affecting Scatter Radiation

Kilovoltage. As x-ray energy is increased, the number of x-rays that undergo Compton interaction increases. The absolute number of Compton interactions decreases with increasing x-ray energy, but the number of photoelectric interactions decreases much more rapidly.

Table 17-1 shows the percentage of x-rays incident on a 10-centimeter thickness of soft tissue that will undergo photoelectric interaction and Compton interaction at selected kVp levels from 50 to 120. Kilovoltage is one of the factors that affects the level of scatter radiation. Scatter radiation is controlled by keeping

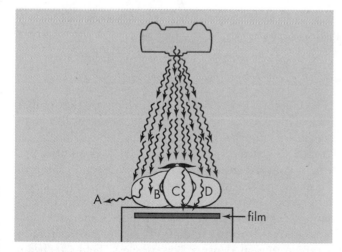

FIGURE 17-1 A, Some x-rays interact with the patient and are scattered away from the film. **B,** Others interact with the patient and are absorbed. X-rays that arrive at the film are those transmitted through the patient without interacting **(C),** and those scattered in the patient **(D).** X-rays of types **C** and **D** are called *remnant radiation.*

kVp at low levels, but to assume that all radiographs should be taken at the lowest reasonable kVp is not the best practice.

Table 17-1 shows that x-rays that interact photoelectrically increase greatly as kVp is lowered. Photoelectric interaction results in a considerable increase in patient dose. Also, fewer x-rays reach the film at low kVp, and thus the technical factors must be compensated for by increasing the mAs. The end result is a higher patient dose.

If the normal technique factors for an AP film of the abdomen are not sufficient to image the abdomen adequately, the radiographer has a choice of increasing mAs or kVp. Increasing the mAs usually generates enough x-rays to provide a satisfactory image on the film but may result in an unacceptably high patient dose. On the other hand, a much smaller increase in kVp is usually sufficient to provide enough x-rays, and kVp can be increased at a much lower patient dose. When kVp is increased, the total amount of scatter radiation decreases. Unfortunately, when kVp is increased, the level of scatter radiation making the film also increases. Because it has a higher energy level and more penetration, an increase in scatter radiation causes the radiographic contrast on the film to decrease.

To reduce the level of scatter radiation, beam-restricting devices called *collimators* and *grids* are used. Figure 17-2 shows a series of radiographs of a skull phantom taken at 70, 80, and 90 kVp using appropriate collimation and grids with the mAs adjusted to produce radiographs of nearly equal optical density. Notice that the patient dose at 90 kVp is approximately one third the patient dose at 70 kVp. In general, because of this reduction in patient dose, high-kVp technique is preferred to low-kVp technique.

X-ray beam field size. Another factor affecting the level of scatter radiation is x-ray beam field size. As field size is decreased, scatter radiation decreases (Figure 17-3). Also the relative intensity of scatter radiation increases with increasing field size as graphed in Figure

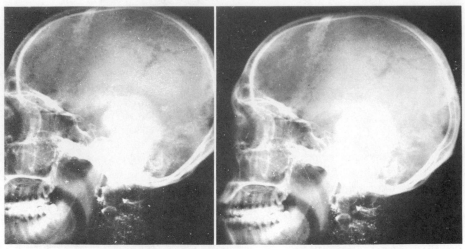

70 kVp / 120 mAs
665 mR

80 kVp / 60 mAs
545 mR

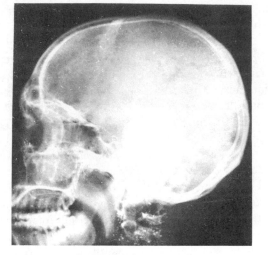

90 kVp / 30 mAs
230 mR

FIGURE 17-2 All these skull radiographs are of acceptable quality. The technique factors for each are shown, along with the resulting patient exposure.

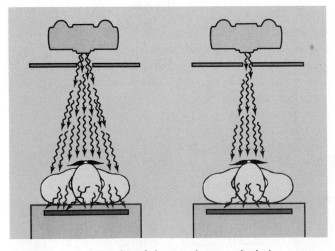

FIGURE 17-3 Collimation of the x-ray beam results in less scatter radiation.

17-4. Figure 17-5 shows two AP films of the lumbar spine. One was taken on a full 14 × 17 inches (35 × 43 centimeter) film, and the other film had a field size restricted to just the spinal column. There is a noticeable loss of contrast in the 14 × 17 radiograph because of the increased scatter radiation that accompanies larger field sizes. When the x-ray beam is collimated, radiographic exposure factors may have to be increased, because reduced scatter radiation results in lower radiographic optical density. Nevertheless, field-size beam restriction is recommended.

Restriction of field size to improve image quality is perhaps even more important during fluoroscopy than for general radiography. Figure 17-6 shows two spot films taken with a spatial resolution grid embedded in the middle of a tissue **phantom** that is 20 centimeters thick.

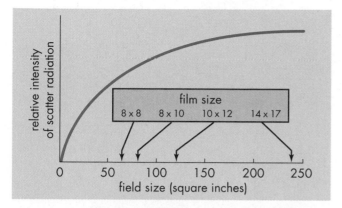

FIGURE 17-4 This graph is representative of operation at 70 kVp with a patient who is 20 centimeters thick. The relative intensity of scatter radiation increases with increasing field size.

The first image was taken with a full-field exposure, and the second with the field size restricted to the area of the grid. The difference in image contrast and spatial resolution is seen.

Patient or part thickness. More scatter radiation results from imaging thick parts of the body than from imaging thin parts of the body. Compare the bony structures in an extremity radiograph with the bony structures in a pelvis or chest radiograph. The extremity radiograph will be much sharper because of the reduced amount of scatter radiation (Figure 17-7).

Figure 17-8 shows the intensity of scattered x-rays in a thickness of soft tissue in an 8 × 10 inch (20 × 25 centimeter) field. Exposing a 3-centimeter thick extremity at 70 kVp results in about 45% scatter radiation. Exposing a 30-centimeter thick abdomen results in

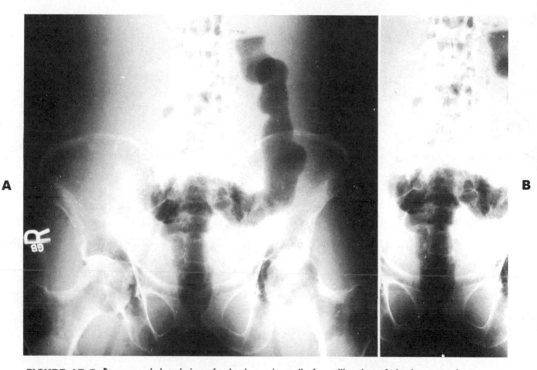

FIGURE 17-5 Recommended technique for lumbar spine calls for collimation of the beam to the vertebral column. The full-field technique results in reduced image contrast. **A,** Full-field technique. **B,** Preferred collimated technique.

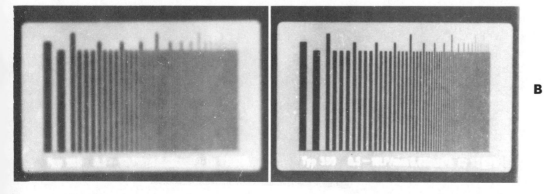

FIGURE 17-6 These spot films of a test pattern in the middle of 20 centimeters of tissue equivalent material were taken with, **A,** full-field exposure and, **B,** with the x-ray beam restricted to the area of the test pattern. The image in **B** is better because the smaller field size resulted in less scatter radiation.

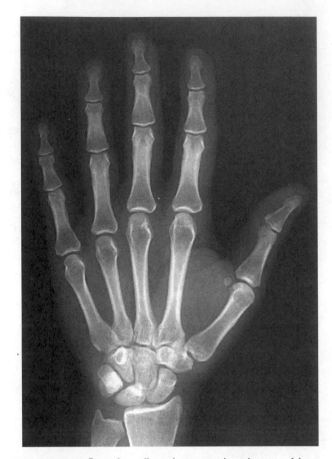

FIGURE 17-7 Extremity radiographs appear sharp because of less tissue and hence less scatter radiation. *(From Ballinger PW: Merrill's atlas of radiographic positions and radiologic procedures,* vol 1, ed 2, *St Louis, 1995, Mosby.)*

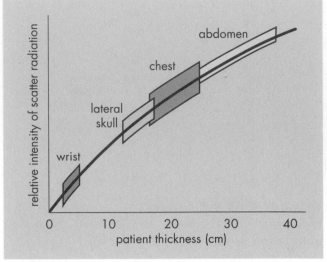

FIGURE 17-8 Relative intensity of scatter radiation increases with increasing thickness of the irradiated part.

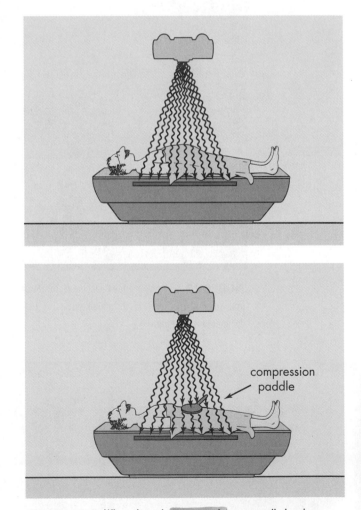

FIGURE 17-9 When tissue is compressed, scatter radiation is reduced, dose is lower, and contrast is higher.

nearly 100% of the x-rays exiting the patient as scattered x-rays. With increasing patient thickness, more x-rays undergo multiple scattering, so that the average angle of scatter in the remnant beam is greater.

Even though more x-rays are scattered with increasing patient thickness, the radiographer can produce high-quality radiographs by choosing the proper technique factors and by using devices designed to reduce the amount of scatter radiation reaching the film.

Compression devices, for example, improve spatial resolution by reducing patient thickness and bringing the tissue closer to the image receptor (Figure 17-9). Compression reduces patient dose and improves image contrast. Compression is particularly important during mammography.

Beam-Restricting Devices

The radiographer uses two types of devices to reduce the amount of scatter radiation reaching the film. They are **beam-restricting devices** and grids (discussed in Chapter 18). The aperture diaphragm, cones or cylinders, and the variable-aperture collimator are three types of beam-restricting devices. (Figure 17-10).

The x-ray beam is restricted for the following two reasons: (1) to reduce patient dose and (2) to improve image contrast. *By reducing scatter radiation*

Only the tissue being examined should be exposed. Large x-ray fields beyond the anatomy of interest result in unnecessary patient exposure. Proper collimation of the x-ray beam has the primary effect of reducing patient dose by restricting the volume of tissue irradiated.

Proper collimation has the secondary effect of improving image contrast by reducing the scatter radiation reaching the film. By reducing scatter radiation and thus reducing film fog, there is a corresponding increase in image contrast. Ideally, only those x-rays not interacting with tissue would reach the film.

Aperture diaphragm. An aperture diaphragm is the simplest of all beam-restricting devices. It is basically a lead or lead-lined metal plate attached to the x-ray tube head. The opening in the plate or diaphragm is designed to cover just less than the size of the image receptor used. Figure 17-11 shows the relationships among the x-ray tube, an aperture diaphragm, and the image receptor. A properly designed aperture diaphragm projects onto the image receptor an image 1 centimeter smaller on all sides than the size of the image receptor. Therefore, when a diaphragm is used, an unexposed border should be visible on each edge of the radiograph.

Question: If a 20-centimeter square film is to be imaged at 100 centimeters SID and the diaphragm is placed 10 centimeters from the target, what should the dimension of one side of the diaphragm opening be? A border of 1 centimeter is left on each side, which means a reduction in beam size to 18 centimeters.

Answer:
$$\frac{A}{10 \text{ centimeters}} = \frac{18 \text{ centimeters}}{100 \text{ centimeters}}$$

$$A = \frac{(10 \text{ centimeters})(18 \text{ centimeters})}{100 \text{ centimeters}}$$

= 1.8 centimeters is the dimension of one side of the diaphragm opening

X-ray head units present the most familiar example of the use of aperture diaphragms. The typical head unit has a fixed SID, and some are equipped with diaphragms to accommodate film sizes of 5 × 7 inches (13 × 18 centimeters), 8 × 10 inches (20 × 25 centimeters), and 10 × 12 inches (25 × 30 centimeters). Head units are being replaced by more flexible, general trauma radiography

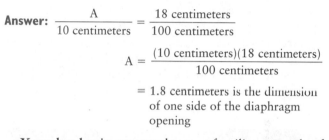

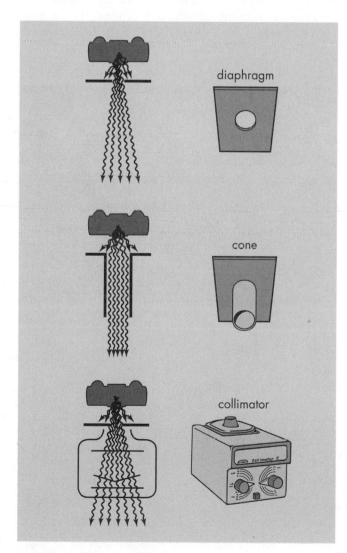

FIGURE 17-10 Beam-limiting devices.

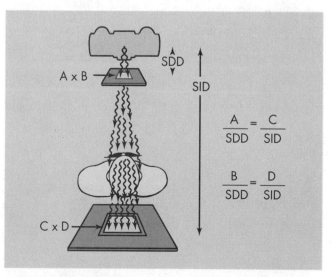

FIGURE 17-11 The aperture diaphragm is a fixed lead opening designed for a fixed image-receptor size and constant SID. SDD is the source-to-diaphragm distance.

units that can be positioned to image all parts of the body (Figure 17-12). When using an aperture diaphragm, the radiographer should ensure that it is inserted into the tube head so that the **long axis** of the diaphragm is parallel to the long axis of the image receptor. If it is not, diaphragm cutoff can result, which leaves large portions of the radiograph unexposed and causes unnecessary exposure to the patient because of repeat examinations.

X-ray units to be used specifically for chest examinations are supplied with aperture diaphragms. Usually these diaphragms are securely fastened to the radiographic head and are not easily removed. Aperture diaphragms for chest rooms are designed to leave a 1-centimeter border on a 14 × 17 inch (35 × 43 centimeters) film.

Dental radiography is another area where aperture diaphragms may be used. Dental radiographs are customarily obtained at 20- or 40-centimeters SID. The diaphragm used in these techniques must provide a circular x-ray beam not exceeding 7 centimeters in diameter at the skin level of the patient. Typically the diameter of an aperture diaphragm for 20-centimeters SID is 18 mil-

limeters, and the diameter of the aperture diaphragm for 40-centimeters SID is 9 millimeters.

Extension cones and cylinders. Radiographic extension cones and cylinders are considered modifications of the aperture diaphragm. Typical cones and cylinders are diagrammed in Figure 17-13. Both use an extended metal structure to restrict the useful beam to the required size. Unlike the beam produced by the aperture diaphragm, the useful beam produced by a cylinder or cone is usually circular. Both these beam restrictors are routinely called *cones,* even though the type used most widely is actually a cylinder.

One difficulty with using cones is alignment. If the x-ray tube, the extension cone, and the image receptor are not aligned on the same axis, the cone may interfere with the x-ray beam and one side of the image will be cut off. Such interference is called *cone cutting.*

The same limitations that apply to aperture diaphragms apply to cones and cylinders. Their openings are fixed so that they are appropriate for only specific types of examinations. At one time, cones were used extensively in diagnostic radiology. Today, they are reserved primarily for examinations of the head, sinuses,

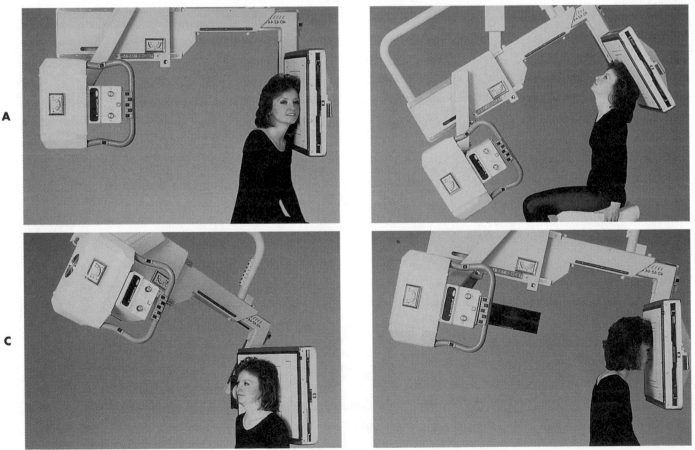

FIGURE 17-12 Trauma radiography unit as used for imaging the skull and its internal structures. Such units are flexible and adaptable for examination of all parts of the body. **A,** Lateral skull. **B,** Axial. **C,** Townes. **D,** Caldwell. *(Courtesy Fischer Imaging.)*

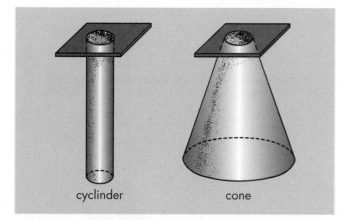

FIGURE 17-13 Radiographic cones and cylinders produce restricted useful x-ray beams of a circular shape.

cyclinder   cone

and **coned-down** views of the spine. Figure 17-14 shows the improvement in image contrast that results when an extension cone is used for the examination of the **sella turcica.** In modern radiography the **light-localizing variable-aperture collimator** has replaced the extension cone and aperture diaphragms in most examinations.

Beam-defining cones are used frequently in dental radiography. Figure 17-15 is a photograph of four typical dental cones. Dental cones are usually made of plastic. Some are lead lined. The long lead-lined dental cones result in slightly less exposure to the patient than the other types. The 20-centimeter plastic pointer cones used on dental x-ray units result in unnecessarily high patient exposure caused by scattering of the useful beam in the cone tip. Many dentists now use the lead-lined ex-

tension cone technique. Proper alignment is a little more difficult, but the images produced have less distortion, and the patient receives a lower dose. The dental cone and circular diaphragm are often made as one device. Together they provide excellent beam restriction for dental radiography.

Variable-aperture collimator. The light-localizing variable-aperture collimator is the most common beam-restricting device in diagnostic imaging departments. The photograph in Figure 17-16 is an example of a modern automatic variable-aperture collimator, and Figure 17-17 identifies the principal parts.

Not all x-rays are emitted precisely from the focal spot of the x-ray tube. Some x-rays are produced when projectile electrons stray and interact on the anode other than the focal spot. Such radiation is called *off-focus radiation* and results in an increase in image blur. To control off-focus radiation, a first-stage entrance shuttering device that has multiple collimator blades protrudes from the top of the collimator into the x-ray tube housing. The second-stage collimator shutters are usually a 3-millimeter thickness of lead. These two collimators work in pairs and are independently controlled, thereby allowing for both longitudinal and transverse field changes by the operator.

Light localization as part of a variable-aperture collimator is accomplished with a small lamp and mirror. The mirror must be far enough on the tube side of the collimator to project a sufficiently sharp light pattern through the collimator when the lamp is on. The lamp, mirror, and collimator must all be adjusted so that the projected light field coincides with the x-ray beam. If the light field and x-ray beam do not coincide, adjust-

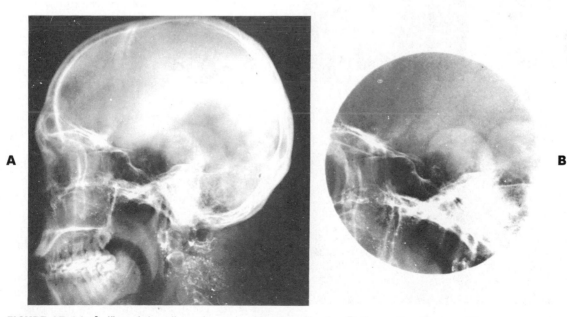

FIGURE 17-14 A, View of the sella turcica made with open collimation. **B,** View made with cone collimation. Use of a cone improves image contrast.

A

B

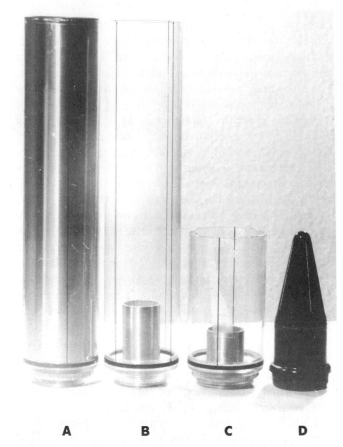

FIGURE 17-15 Four typical dental cones. **A,** Long, lead-lined, plastic, open-end cone. **B,** Long, plastic, open-end cone. **C,** Short, plastic, open-end cone. **D,** Plastic pointer cone.

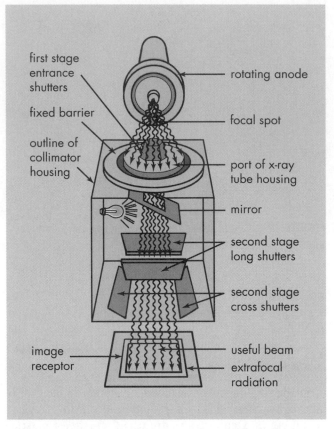

FIGURE 17-17 Simplified schematic of a light-localizing variable-aperture collimator.

(Labels in figure: first stage entrance shutters; fixed barrier; outline of collimator housing; image receptor; rotating anode; focal spot; port of x-ray tube housing; mirror; second stage long shutters; second stage cross shutters; useful beam; extrafocal radiation)

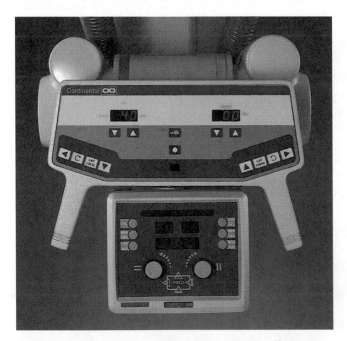

FIGURE 17-16 Automatic variable-aperture collimator. *(Courtesy Continental X-ray Corporation.)*

ment of the mirror or lamp is required. Radiation- and light-field testing is a critical part of a **quality control program** in diagnostic imaging departments.

There is always a scale marked on the collimator to indicate field size at fixed SIDs. In addition, the clear plastic exit surface of the collimator has two crossed lines marked to project the **central ray** of the x-ray beam onto the center of the tissue being radiographed. Often a bright slit of light will project onto the table to assist the centering of the image receptor in the table Bucky device.

Today, nearly all light-localizing collimators manufactured in the United States for fixed radiographic equipment are automatic. They are called *positive beam limiting (PBL)* devices. When a cassette is inserted in the Bucky tray and clamped into place, sensing devices in the tray identify the size and alignment of the cassette. An electric signal is transmitted to the collimator housing, which actuates the synchronous motors that drive the collimator leaves to a precalibrated position, so that the x-ray beam is restricted to the image receptor size in use. When properly adjusted, the automatic collimator provides an unexposed border on all sides of the finished radiograph. Even with PBL, if conditions warrant, the radiographer should manually collimate to reduce patient dose and improve image quality.

Remember: under no circumstances should the x-ray beam exceed the size of the image receptor.

Collimator filtration. Because prescribed thicknesses of filtration are needed to produce high-quality radiographs with minimum patient exposure, some collimator housings are designed to allow easy changing of the added filtration. Most commonly, filtration stations of 0, 1, 2, and 3 millimeters aluminum are provided.

Even in the zero position, however, the added filtration to the x-ray tube is not zero because collimator structures intercept the beam. The exit portal, usually plastic, and the reflecting mirror provide filtration in addition to the inherent filtration of the tube. The added filtration of the collimator assembly is usually equivalent to approximately 1 millimeter aluminum.

SUMMARY

The following are two types of x-rays that exit the patient: (1) remnant x-rays that pass through tissue without interacting and (2) x-rays that are scattered in tissue by Compton interaction. The three factors that contribute to an increase in scatter radiation and ultimately to film fog are increasing kVp, increasing x-ray field size, and increasing anatomic part thickness. Although an increase in kVp does increase scatter radiation, there is a trade-off with reduced patient exposure. The increase in scatter can be controlled and minimized by using beam-restricting devices such as the aperture diaphragm, extension cones and cylinders, and the variable aperture collimator, which is the most commonly used beam-restricting device in diagnostic imaging departments.

REVIEW QUESTIONS

1. List and describe the two types of remnant radiation.

2. At the 80-kVp level, what percentage of the x-ray beam is scattered through Compton interaction?

3. _____ is one of the factors that affects the level of scattered radiation.

4. Refer to Table 17-1 and compare the 70 kVp and 120kVp rows on the chart. Answer the following questions:
   a. What is the difference in scatter radiation resulting from these two kVp levels?
   b. Photoelectric interaction at 70 kVp is 60%. At 120 kVp, photoelectric interaction is 18%. How would contrast be affected on each of these radiographs?
   c. What is the trade-off when percent transmission of the remnant beam reaches 9% for 120 kVp?

5. Name the two types of devices used to reduce the level of scatter radiation.

6. As x-ray beam field size increases, _____ _____ increases also.

7. When collimating the x-ray beam, radiographic exposure factors must be _____.

8. Compression of tissue is particularly important during what examination?

9. List the two reasons for restricting the x-ray beam.

10. Describe the design of the aperture diaphragm.

11. What is the reason to show an unexposed 1-centimeter border on the edge of the radiograph?

12. Explain a difficulty that can come about when using extension cones.

13. In dental radiography, the 20-centimeter plastic pointer may result in unnecessary high patient exposure. Why?

14. X-rays produced when projectile electrons stray and do not interact with the focal spot are called _____ _____ _____.

15. Where do the two crossed lines to mark central ray location on the tissue to be radiographed originate?

16. What does the abbreviation PBL stand for?

17. If the light field and the radiation field do not coincide, what needs to be adjusted?

18. When should the x-ray field exceed the size of the image receptor?

18 The Grid

OBJECTIVES

At the completion of this chapter the student will be able to:

1. Recognize the relationship between scatter radiation and image contrast
2. Explain the components of grid construction
3. Calculate grid ratio, grid frequency, contrast improvement factor, Bucky factor, and selectivity
4. Describe eight different types of grids
5. Discuss the five common errors using grids
6. Evaluate the circumstances for proper grid selection
7. Debate the advantages and disadvantages of the use of grids in relation to patient radiation exposure

OUTLINE

Scatter Radiation and Image Contrast
Grids
  Cleanup of scatter radiation
  Grid construction
  Grid performance
Grid types
Grid problems
Grid selection
Grids and patient dose
Alternative to grid use

Contrast is one of the most important characteristics of image quality. Contrast is the light, dark, and shades of gray on the radiograph. These variations actually make up the radiographic image. Scatter radiation emitted from tissue through the Compton effect fogs image contrast and makes the manifest image less visible. The two types of devices that reduce scatter from reaching the film are beam-restricting devices (Chapter 17) and radiographic grids.

. . . .

SCATTER RADIATION AND IMAGE CONTRAST

From x-ray interaction with tissue, the Compton effect(151) produces scatter radiation, which not only results in the lack of useful information recorded in the latent image but also increases film fog, which reduces **image contrast.** Contrast is one of the most important characteristics of film or image quality. Contrast is the number of shades of gray and the difference between light and dark areas on the image. Contrast and other characteristics that affect radiographic quality are discussed in detail in Chapter 19.

The intensity of scatter (see Chapter 17) is a function of kVp level, beam or field size, and thickness of irradiated tissue. Even though scatter radiation reaching the film is reduced when kVp is low, there is a disadvantage with low-kVp levels. Low-kVp levels increase patient radiation dose because of increased absorption of low-energy x-rays. Beam-restricting devices (see Chapter 17) are efficient in reducing scatter radiation, but alone their effect is not adequate. Even under the most favorable conditions more than half the remnant x-rays exiting the film side of the patient are from scatter radiation. Figure 18-1 illustrates that scatter x-rays are emitted from the patient in all directions.

If a student radiographer imaged a long bone using only primary-beam x-rays, the image would be sharp (Figure 18-2, *A*). The change in optical density from dark to light corresponding to bone and soft tissue would be very abrupt, and therefore the radiographic contrast would be high. On the other hand, if the radiograph were taken with only scatter radiation and no primary-beam x-rays reached the film, the image would be dull gray (Figure 18-2, *B*). The radiographic contrast would be very low. In the normal situation, x-rays arriving at the image receptor consist of both primary and scattered x-rays. If the radiograph were properly exposed, the image would appear as in Figure 18-2, *C*, and the image would have moderate contrast. The loss of contrast results from the presence of scattered x-rays. The more scattered x-rays there are, the lower the contrast will be.

There are two approaches to reducing the amount of scattered x-rays in the remnant beam—use of **beam-**

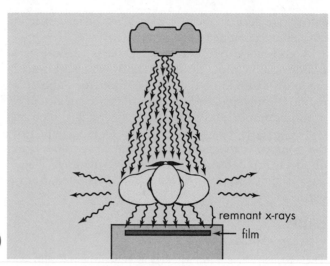

FIGURE 18-1 When primary x-rays interact with a patient, secondary scattered x-rays are emitted from the patient in all directions.

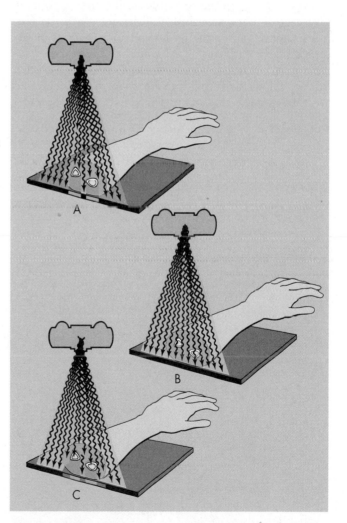

FIGURE 18-2 Radiographs of a cross section of long bone. **A,** High contrast would result from using only primary photons. **B,** No contrast would result from using only scattered photons. **C,** Moderate contrast would result from using both primary and scattered photons.

restricting devices and use of a **grid.** Beam-restricting devices are discussed in Chapter 17.

A grid is a carefully fabricated series of sections of radiopaque material (**grid material**), which are usually made of lead, alternating with sections of radiolucent material (**interspace material**), which are usually made of aluminum or plastic. The grid is designed to transmit only those x-rays whose direction is straight from the source to the image receptor. X-rays that travel obliquely are absorbed in the grid material. Figure 18-3 is a schematic of how a grid **cleans up** scatter radiation.

GRIDS
Cleanup of Scatter Radiation

The cleanup of scatter radiation reaching the film was first demonstrated in 1913 by Gustave Bucky. Over the years, Bucky's grid has been improved by more precise manufacturing, but the basic principle has not changed. X-rays exiting the patient that strike the radiopaque grid material are absorbed and do not reach the film. For instance, a typical grid may have grid strips approximately 50 μm thick separated by interspace material approximately 350 μm thick. Consequently, up to 12.5% of all x-ray photons striking the grid interact with radiopaque grid material and are absorbed.

Question: A grid is constructed with 50 μm grid strips and a 350 μm interspace. What percentage of incident x-rays will be absorbed by the grid?

Answer: The **line pairs** are 350 μm plus 50 μm or 400 μm in size. The part of the grid that absorbs x-ray photons is the lead strip area, which is 50 μm in size.

$$\frac{50 \ \mu m}{350 \ \mu m + 50 \ \mu m} = 0.125 \text{ or } 12.5\%$$ of the grid absorbs x-ray photons and conversely 12.5% of incident x-rays will be absorbed by the grid

Primary-beam x-rays striking on the interspace material are transmitted through to the film. Scattered x-rays striking interspace material may or may not be absorbed, depending on their angle of incidence and the physical characteristics of the grid. If the deviation of a scattered x-ray is great enough to cause it to intersect the grid material, it will be absorbed. If the deviation is slight, the scattered x-ray will be transmitted like a primary x-ray. Laboratory measurements show that high-quality grids can absorb 80% to 90% of the scatter radiation. Such a grid is said to exhibit good **cleanup** properties.

Grid Construction

Grid ratio. Grid ratio can be understood by reference to Figure 18-4. The following are three important dimensions in a grid:
1. The thickness of the grid material (T).
2. The thickness of the interspace material (D).
3. The height of the grid (h).

The **grid ratio** is the height divided by the interspace thickness as follows:

$$\text{Grid ratio} = h/D$$

High-ratio grids are more effective in cleaning up scatter radiation than are low-ratio grids. This is because the angle of deviation allowed by high-ratio grids is less than that permitted by low-ratio grids (Figure 18-5).

Unfortunately, grids with high ratios are more expensive to manufacture than low-ratio grids. High-ratio grids are made by reducing the width of the interspace or increasing the height of the grid material or by a combination of both. With all grids, higher exposure

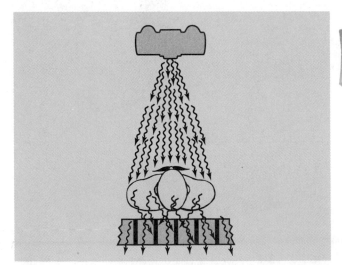

FIGURE 18-3 The only x-rays transmitted through a grid are those traveling in the direction of the interspace. X-rays scattered obliquely throughout the interspace are absorbed.

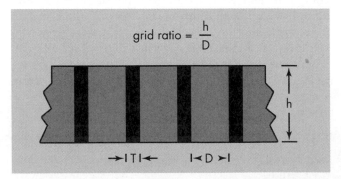

grid ratio = $\dfrac{h}{D}$

FIGURE 18-4 Grid ratio is defined as the height of the grid strip divided by the thickness of the interspace material.

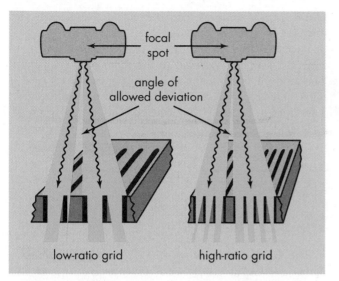

focal
spot

angle of
allowed deviation

low-ratio grid   high-ratio grid

FIGURE 18-5 High-ratio grids are more effective than low-ratio grids in cleaning up scatter radiation because the angle of deviation they allow is smaller.

factors are required with higher grid ratios to transmit a sufficient number of x-rays through to the image receptor. The result of higher grid ratios is higher patient dose.

Generally, grid ratios range from 5:1 to 16:1. The higher ratio grids are used in high-kVp radiography. An 8:1 or 10:1 grid is frequently used in general-purpose equipment. A 5:1 grid will clean up approximately 85% of the scatter radiation, whereas a 16:1 grid may clean up as much as 97%.

Question: A certain grid is made of lead 30 μm thick sandwiched between fiber interspace material 300 μm thick. The height of the grid is 2.4 millimeters. What is the grid ratio?

Answer: Grid ratio = h/D

$$= 2400 \ \mu m/300 \ \mu m$$

$$= 8:1 \text{ is the grid ratio}$$

Grid frequency. The number of grid strips or grid lines per inch or per centimeter is called the *grid frequency*. Grids with high frequencies show less distinct grid lines on a radiograph than grids with low frequencies. If the thickness of the grid strips is held constant, the higher the frequency of a grid, the thinner its strips of interspace material must be and the higher the grid ratio. In addition, the higher the grid frequency, the higher the radiographic technique required, resulting in higher patient dose. The greater technical factors and patient dose result because as grid frequency increases, there is relatively more grid material to absorb radiation. The disadvantage of increased patient dose with high-frequency grids is compensated for by using high-speed intensifying screens, which reduces patient dose significantly.

Most grids have frequencies in the range of 60 to 110 lines per inch (25 to 45 lines per centimeter). Grid frequency can be calculated if the thicknesses of the grid material and the thickness of the interspace material are known. Grid frequency is computed by dividing the thickness of one line pair, which is the thickness of the grid material (T) plus the thickness of the interspace material (D), and is expressed in μm (microns) into 1 centimeter:

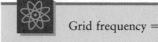

$$\text{Grid frequency} = \frac{10{,}000 \ \mu m/centimeter}{(T + D) \ \mu m/line \ pair}$$

Question: What is the grid frequency of the previously described grid, which has a grid strip thickness of 30 μm (microns) and an interspace thickness of 300 μm?

Answer: If 1 line pair = 300 μm + 30 μm = 330 μm, how many line pairs are in 10,000 μm (10,000 μm = 1 centimeter)?

$$\frac{10{,}00 \ Mm/cm}{330 \ Mm/line \ pair} = 30.3 \text{ lines/cm}$$

30.3 lines/centimeter × 2.54 centimeter/inch = 77 lines/inch

Grids are designed for mammography as well. Grid ratios of 2:1 to 4:1 are used. These low-ratio grids have grid frequencies of approximately 200 lines/inch (80 lines/centimeter).

Interspace material. The purpose of the interspace material is to maintain a precise separation between the delicate strips of the grid. The interspace material of most grids is either **aluminum** or **plastic fiber,** and there are conflicting reports as to which is better. Aluminum has a higher atomic number than plastic and therefore may provide some selective filtration of scattered x-rays not absorbed in the grid material. Aluminum also has the advantage of producing less visible grid lines on the radiograph. On the other hand, use of aluminum as interspace material increases the absorption of primary x-rays in the interspace, especially at low kVp. Higher mAs factors are required, which results in higher patient dose. At low kVp levels, patient dose may be increased by 20% or more. For this reason fiber-interspace grids are usually preferred to aluminum-interspace grids. Still, **aluminum** has two additional advantages over fiber. First, it is **nonhygroscopic;** that is, it does not absorb moisture as plastic fiber will. Fiber-interspace grids can become warped if they absorb moisture. Second, aluminum-interspace grids are easier to manufacture because aluminum is easier to form and roll into sheets of precise thickness than is fiber.

Lead strips. Theoretically the grid strip should be infinitely thin and have high x-ray scatter absorption properties. There are several possible materials out of which to form these strips. **Lead** is the most widely used because it is easy to shape and is relatively inexpensive. The high atomic number and high mass density of lead contributes to making it the material of choice in the manufacture of grids. Tungsten, platinum, gold, and uranium have all been tried, but none has the overall desirable characteristics of lead. Regardless of its composition, the grid is encased completely by a thin cover of aluminum. The aluminum casing provides rigidity for the grid and helps to seal out moisture.

Grid Performance

Contrast improvement factor. The largest single factor responsible for poor radiographs is scatter radiation. The radiographic grid removes the scattered x-rays in the beam, which is the source of poor image contrast.

The characteristics of grid construction previously described, especially the grid ratio, are usually specified when identifying a grid. Grid ratio, however, does not relate the ability of the grid to improve radiographic contrast. This property of the grid is specified by the **contrast improvement factor (k).**

> ### Contrast Improvement Factor (k)
> The contrast improvement factor of a grid is the ratio of the contrast of a radiograph made with the grid to the contrast of a radiograph made without the grid.

A contrast improvement factor of 1 indicates no improvement whatsoever. Most grids have contrast improvement factors of between 1.5 and 2.5. In other words the radiographic contrast is approximately doubled when grids are used. Mathematically the contrast improvement factor (k) is expressed as follows:

> ### Contrast Improvement Factor (k)
> $$k = \frac{\text{Radiographic contrast with grid}}{\text{Radiographic contrast without grid}}$$

Question: An aluminum step wedge is placed on a tissue phantom 20 centimeters thick, and a radiograph is made. Without a grid the measure of contrast is 1.1. With a 12:1 grid, radiographic contrast is 2.8. What is the contrast improvement factor of this grid?

Answer: $k = \dfrac{2.8}{1.1}$

   $= 2.55$ is the contrast improvement factor

The contrast improvement factor is usually measured at 100 kVp, but it should be realized that k is a complex function of the x-ray emission spectrum, the patient thickness, and the area irradiated. Generally the contrast improvement factor is higher for high-ratio grids.

Other factors, such as lead content, also influence this measure of grid performance.

Bucky factor. Although the use of a grid improves contrast, a penalty is paid in the form of patient dose. The amount of remnant radiation penetrating a grid is much less than the remnant radiation hitting the grid. Therefore to produce the same optical density when using a grid, the technique must be increased. The amount of increase is calculated using the **Bucky factor (B).**

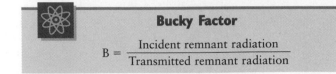

> ### Bucky Factor
> $$B = \frac{\text{Incident remnant radiation}}{\text{Transmitted remnant radiation}}$$

The Bucky factor, sometimes called *grid factor,* is named for Gustave Bucky, the inventor of the grid. It is an attempt to measure the penetration of both primary and scatter radiation through the grid. Table 18-1 gives representative values of the Bucky factor for several commonly used grids.

The following two generalizations can be made from the data presented in Table 18-1:

1. The higher the grid ratio, the higher the Bucky factor. The penetration of primary radiation through a grid is independent of grid ratio. Penetration of scatter through a grid becomes less likely with increasing grid ratio, and therefore the Bucky factor increases.

2. The Bucky factor increases with increasing kVp. At high kVp, more scatter radiation exits the patient. This scatter radiation has a more difficult time penetrating the grid, and thus the Bucky factor increases.

Whereas the contrast improvement factor measures an improvement in image quality when using grids, the Bucky factor measures how much of an increase in technique will be required compared with nongrid exposure. The Bucky factor also indicates how much of an increase in patient dose accompanies the use of a particular grid. With increasing the Bucky factor, radiographic technique and patient dose increase proportionately.

Selectivity. The ideal grid would be constructed so that all primary x-rays would be transmitted and all

TABLE 18-1

Approximate Bucky Factor for Grids

Grid Ratios	Bucky Factor at		
	70 kVp	**90 kVp**	**120 kVp**
No grid	1	1	1
5:1	2	2.5	3
8:1	3	3.5	4
12:1	3.5	4	5
16:1	4	5	6

TABLE 18-2

A Summary of Grid Characteristics

Grid ratio	$\dfrac{\text{Height of grid (h)}}{\text{Thickness of interspace material (D)}}$
Grid frequency	$\dfrac{1\ cm}{\text{Thickness of grid material minus thickness of interspace material}}$ or $\dfrac{1\ cm}{(T \times D)\ \mu m/\text{line pair}}$
Contrast improvement factor (k)	$k = \dfrac{\text{Contrast with grid}}{\text{Contrast without grid}}$
Bucky factor (B)	$B = \dfrac{\text{Remnant radiation before grid}}{\text{Remnant radiation after grid}}$
Selectivity (Σ)	$\Sigma = \dfrac{\text{Primary radiation after grid}}{\text{Scatter radiation after grid}}$

scattered x-rays would be absorbed. The ratio of transmitted primary radiation to transmitted scatter radiation is called the *selectivity* of the grid and is usually identified by a Greek sigma (Σ).

Selectivity (Σ)

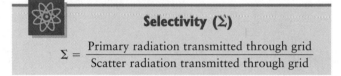

$$\Sigma = \frac{\text{Primary radiation transmitted through grid}}{\text{Scatter radiation transmitted through grid}}$$

Selectivity is primarily a function of the construction characteristics of the grid rather than the characteristics of the x-ray beam. This is not the case for the contrast improvement factor. Selectivity is related to grid ratio, but the total lead content in the grid has the primary influence on selectivity. Figure 18-6 shows how two grids

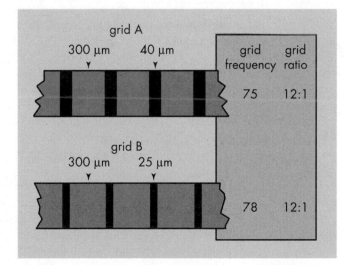

FIGURE 18-6 Because grids A and B have the same height and interspace thickness, they have identical ratios. Grid A has 60% more lead but slightly lower frequency. Grid A has higher selectivity and therefore a higher contrast improvement factor.

can have the same grid ratio yet greatly different lead content. This is usually accomplished with a small loss in grid frequency. The heavier a grid is, the more lead it contains, the higher its selectivity, and the more efficient it is in cleaning up scatter radiation. Of course, the lead must be properly arranged. A flat sheet of lead with high mass would make a very poor grid.

The biomedical engineer or medical physicist will take into account grid ratio, grid frequency, contrast improvement factor, and selectivity in setting up apparatus for a particular radiographic site.

The relationships among these grid characteristics are complicated; however, a few general rules regarding them follow:

1. High-ratio grids have high contrast improvement factors. As the grid absorbs scatter radiation, contrast is improved on the radiograph.
2. High-frequency grids have thin strips of interspace material.
3. Heavy grids have high selectivity and high-contrast improvement factors. The heavier the grid, the more lead it contains, the higher its selectivity, and the more efficient it is in cleaning up scatter radiation. Table 18-2 summarizes grid characteristics.

Grid Types

Linear parallel grid. The simplest type of grid is the linear grid diagrammed in cross section in Figure 18-7. In the linear grid, all lead grid strips are parallel. This type of grid is the easiest to manufacture, but it has some properties that are clinically undesirable.

The undesirable absorption of primary x-rays by the grid is called *grid cutoff.* Grid cutoff may be partial or complete and can result in reduced optical density or total absence of film exposure. The term is derived from the fact that the **primary x-rays are cut off** from getting to the film. Grid cutoff can occur with

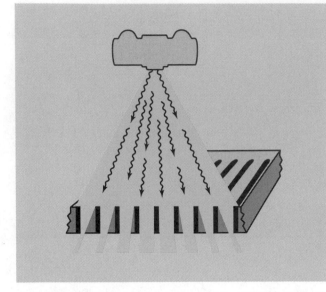

FIGURE 18-7 Linear grid is constructed with parallel grid strips. At a short SID, some grid cutoff may occur.

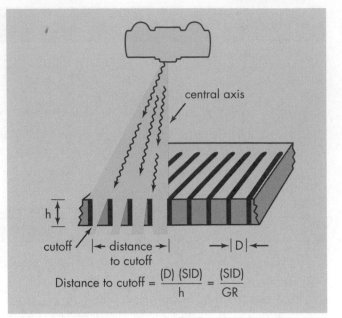

$$\text{Distance to cutoff} = \frac{(D)\,(SID)}{h} = \frac{(SID)}{GR}$$

FIGURE 18-8 With a linear grid, optical density decreases toward the edge of the film. Grid cutoff will occur according to the equation below.

any type of grid if the grid is improperly positioned, but it is most common with linear grids. Figure 18-8 illustrates that the attenuation of primary x-rays becomes greater as one approaches the edges of the grid. The lead strips in 14 × 17 inch grids are 17 inches long. Across the 14-inch dimension, a variation in optical density may be observed because of the primary x-ray attenuation. The optical density reaches a maximum along the center line of the film and decreases toward the sides.

Linear grid cutoff is most pronounced when the grid is used *at a short source-to-image receptor distance (SID)* or *with a large image receptor* (14 × 17). The distance from the **central axis** at which complete cutoff (Figure 18-8) will occur is given by the following equation. The central axis is the line drawn parallel to the lead strips in the center of the grid.

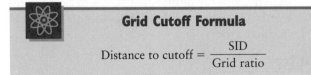

Grid Cutoff Formula

$$\text{Distance to cutoff} = \frac{SID}{\text{Grid ratio}}$$

The radiographs in Figure 18-9 were taken with a 8:1 focused grid at 100- and 75-centimeter SID. They demonstrate increasing degrees of grid cutoff with decreasing SID, and increasing grid cutoff with off-centering or lateral decentering.

Question: A 16:1 parallel grid is positioned for chest radiography at 180-centimeter SID. What is the distance from the central axis to complete grid cutoff?

Answer: Distance to cutoff $= \dfrac{180}{16} = 11.3$ centimeters

Distance to edge of grid $= (14 \div 2) \times 2.54$

$= 17.8$ centimeters

The image will not satisfactorily cover a 14 × 17 inch film. Grid cutoff will occur 6.5 centimeters from the edges of the image receptor.

Crossed grid. Linear grids clean up scatter radiation in only one direction, which is along the axis of the grid. Crossed grids are made to overcome this deficiency. These grids have lead grid strips running parallel to both the long and short axes of the grid (Figure 18-10). They are usually made by sandwiching two linear grids together with their grid strips perpendicular to one another. They are not too difficult to manufacture and therefore are not expensive; however, they have restricted application. Bucky's original grid was crossed. Crossed grids are much more efficient than linear grids in cleaning up scatter radiation. In fact a crossed grid has a higher contrast improvement factor than a linear grid of twice the grid ratio. A 6:1 crossed grid will clean up more scatter radiation than a 12:1 linear grid. This advantage of the crossed grid increases as the kVp of operation is increased. A crossed grid identified as having a grid ratio of 6:1 is constructed with two 6:1 linear grids.

There are two serious disadvantages to using crossed grids. First, positioning the grid is critical; the central ray of the x-ray beam must coincide with the center of the grid. Second, tilt-table techniques are possible only

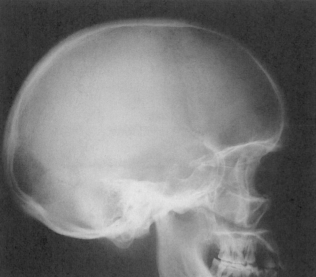

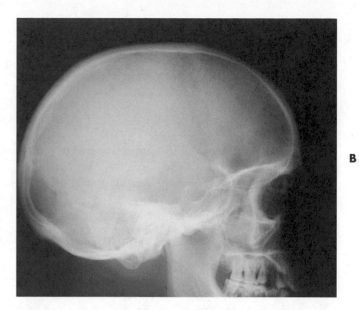

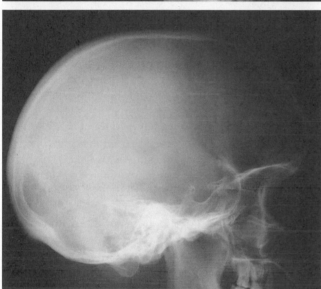

FIGURE 18-9 These radiographs were taken with a 8:1 grid focused to 100 centimeters. The techniques were **A,** 100-centimeters SID, on center; **B,** 100-centimeters SID, 8 centimeters off laterally; **C,** 75-centimeters SID, 8 centimeters off laterally. *(Courtesy Alex Backus.)*

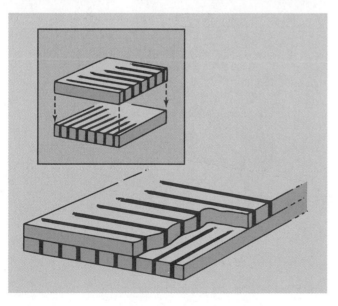

FIGURE 18-10 Crossed grids are made by sandwiching two linear grids together so that their grid strips are perpendicular.

if the tube and table are properly aligned. If the table is horizontal and the tube is angled, grid cutoff occurs.

Focused grid. The main disadvantage of linear and crossed grids is grid cutoff. The focused grid is designed to minimize this deficiency. The lead grid strips of a focused grid run only along one axis and are tilted so that they lie on imaginary lines of the divergent x-ray beam (Figure 18-11).

Focused grids, however, are more difficult to manufacture than linear grids. They are characterized by all the properties of linear grids except they have less grid cutoff. The radiographer must take care when positioning focused grids because of their source-to-image distance limitations. Every focused grid will be marked with its intended focal distance and the side of the grid that should face the x-ray tube.

Remember: if radiographs are made at distances other than those specified by the manufacturer of the grid, cutoff will occur.

A focused grid intended for use at 100-centimeter SID will usually have sufficient latitude to produce acceptable radiographs when used at an SID between 90 and 110 centimeters. High-ratio grids have less positioning latitude than low-ratio grids.

Moving grids. A shortcoming of the grids previously discussed is that they produce grid lines on the radiograph. Grid lines are the images made when primary x-rays are absorbed in the grid strips. Even though the grid strips are very small, their images are still observable. One can demonstrate the presence of grid lines simply by radiographing a grid.

A major improvement in grid development occurred in 1920. Hollis E. Potter hit on a very simple idea—move the grid while the x-ray exposure is being made.

The grid lines disappear at little cost of increased technique. A device that does this is now called a ***moving grid,*** although the terms *Potter-Bucky diaphragm,* ***Bucky diaphragm,*** and ***Bucky grid*** are still widely used (Figure 18-12). Moving grids are usually focused grids. They are placed in a mechanism that is moved at the time of x-ray exposure. The following are three basic types of moving grid mechanisms: (1) **single stroke,** (2) **reciprocating,** and (3) **oscillating.**

- **Single-stroke grid.** A single-stroke mechanism causes the grid to move continuously across the film while the x-ray exposure is being made. Usually it is spring loaded and requires a manual cocking of the mechanism before each exposure. Exposure times no shorter than perhaps 200 milliseconds can be accommodated. The spring mechanism of the moving grid will be designed for the shortest possible exposure time. Longer exposure times are accommodated so that it moves more slowly. Single-stroke moving grids are difficult to use because they require cocking before exposure and are not used in modern radiographic equipment.

- **Reciprocating grid.** A reciprocating grid is a moving grid that is motor driven. During the x-ray exposure it moves back and forth several times. The total distance of drive is approximately 2 centimeters. The main advantage this type of moving-grid mechanism has over the single-stroke grid is that it does not require resetting after each exposure. This is the most commonly used grid in modern radiographic equipment.

- **Oscillating grid.** An oscillating grid has some of the characteristics of both the single-stroke and the reciprocating grids. An oscillating grid is positioned in a frame with 2- to 3-centimeter tolerance

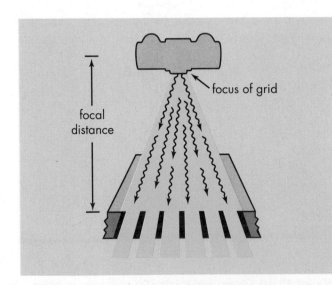

FIGURE 18-11 A focused grid is made so that the grid strips are parallel to the primary x-ray path across the entire film.

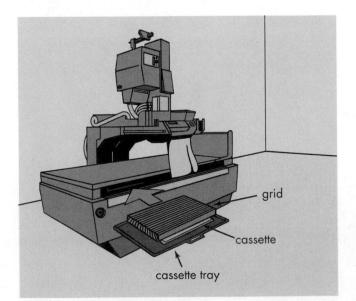

FIGURE 18-12 Moving grid mechanism.

on all sides between the frame and grid. Delicate springlike devices located in the four corners hold the grid centered in the frame. A powerful electromagnet pulls the grid to one side and releases it at the beginning of the exposure. Thereafter the grid oscillates in a circular fashion around the grid frame, coming to rest after 20 to 30 seconds.

The main difference between reciprocating and oscillating grids is their pattern of motion. The motion of a reciprocating grid is to and fro, whereas that of an oscillating grid is circular.

Disadvantages of moving grid. The grids available in the early days of radiography when the moving-grid mechanism was developed contained large, thick lead grid strips and therefore produced very objectionable grid lines. Because today's grids are of much higher quality, with thinner grid strips and grid frequencies of over 100 lines per inch (40 lines per centimeter), most radiologists find stationary grids perfectly acceptable. Moving grids require a bulky mechanism that is subject to failure. The distance between the patient and the film is increased with moving grids because of this mechanism; that extra distance may create an unwanted increase in magnification and image blur. Moving grids often introduce motion into the film-holding device, which can result in additional image blur.

If not properly designed, moving grids can produce a **stroboscopic effect** when used with **half-** or **full-wave-rectified** x-ray generators because of synchronization between x-ray pulsation and grid movement. This effect results in the presence of pronounced grid lines. Also, the exposure time is longer with moving grids than with stationary grids.

However, the advantages of moving grids far outweigh the disadvantages. The types of motion blur are discussed for descriptive purposes only. The motion blur generated by moving grids that function properly is undetectable. Only malfunctioning moving-grid systems create problems, and those problems occur infrequently. The moving grid is universally used. Table 18-3 is a summary of the characteristics of the most popular commercially available grids.

Grid Problems

Most grids in x-ray rooms are the moving type. The grids are permanently mounted in the moving mechanism just below the tabletop or just behind the upright Bucky. To be effective, of course, the grid must move side to side, perpendicular to the lead strips. If the grid is installed incorrectly and moves in the same direction as the lead strips, grid lines will appear on the radiograph.

Stationary grids are either taped or slipped on the front surface of a cassette. Formerly they were built into specially designed grid cassettes. Stationary grids are used for mobile radiography and non-Bucky radiography of thick anatomic parts.

The most frequent error in the use of grids is improper positioning. For the grid to function correctly, it must be precisely positioned relative to the x-ray tube target and to the central axis of the x-ray beam. There are five situations that must be avoided. Most are characteristic of focused grids. Only one is a problem with linear and crossed grids.

1. **Off-level error.** A properly functioning grid must lie in a plane perpendicular to the central axis of the x-ray beam (Figure 18-13). The **central axis** of the x-ray beam is composed of the x-rays traveling along the center of the useful x-ray beam.

   Despite its name, an **off-level grid** error can be produced by having an improperly positioned radiographic tube head and not an improperly positioned grid. If the x-rays reach the grid at an angle, all incident x-rays will be angled and grid cutoff will occur across the entire radiograph, which

	TABLE 18-3			
Construction Characteristics of Some of the More Popular Grids				
Type	**Interspace**	**Grid Frequency (lines/inch)**	**Grid Ratio**	
Focused	Aluminum	145	8:1 to 14:1	
Focused	Aluminum	103	6:1 to 12:1	
Parallel	Aluminum	103	6:1	
Focused	Aluminum	85	5:1 to 12:1	
Parallel	Aluminum	85	5:1 and 6:1	
Parallel	Aluminum	196	2:1 and 3.5:1	
Crossed-focused	Aluminum	85	5:1 and 6:1	
Crossed-parallel	Aluminum	85	5:1 and 6:1	
Focused	Fiber	80	5:1, 8:1, and 12:1	
Crossed-focused	Fiber	80	5:1 and 8:1	
Focused	Fiber	60	6:1	
Parallel	Fiber	60	6:1	

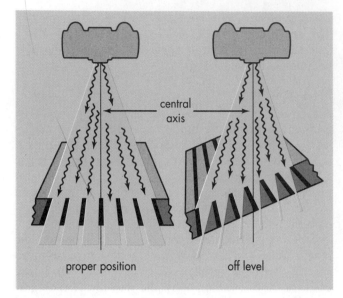

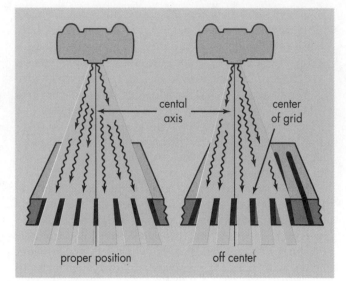

FIGURE 18-13 If a grid is off level so that the central axis is not perpendicular to the grid, partial cutoff will occur over the entire film.

FIGURE 18-14 When a focused grid is positioned off center, partial grid cutoff will occur over the entire film.

results in lower optical density. This condition can be prevented.

Remember: pay careful attention to the use of grids and the positioning of the x-ray tube head. The x-ray beam must be perpendicular to the grid.

2. **Off-center error.** A grid can be perpendicular to the central x-ray beam and still produce grid cutoff if it is shifted laterally. This is a problem with focused grids, as shown in Figure 18-14, where an off-center grid is shown with a properly positioned grid.

Remember: the center of a focused grid must be positioned directly under the x-ray tube target so that the central axis x-ray beam passes through the central axis of the grid.

Any lateral shift will result in grid cutoff across the entire radiograph, resulting in lower optical density. This error in positioning is called *lateral decentering*. As with off-level grids, this condition is more a matter of positioning the tube head than the grid. In practice, it means that the radiographer must carefully line up the center of the **light-localized field** with the center of the **cassette holder.** Marks on both, and sometimes on the table, are provided so that this can be done quickly and easily.

3. **Off-focus error.** A major problem with using a focus grid arises when radiographs are taken at SIDs unspecified for that grid. Figure 18-15 illustrates what happens when a focused grid is not used at the proper focal distance.

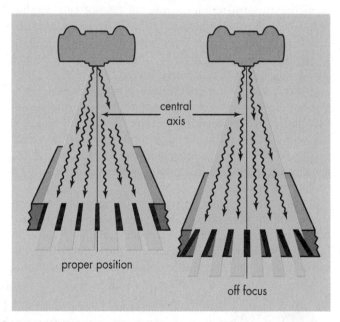

FIGURE 18-15 If a focused grid is not positioned at the specific focal distance, grid cutoff will occur and the radiographic density will decrease from the central axis.

Remember: grid cutoff occurs at any distance that is not within the specifications for that grid; however, the closer the grid is to the tube the more severe the grid cutoff.

In Figure 18-15 the grid cutoff is not uniform across the film but rather is more severe at the periphery.

This condition is not normally a problem if all chest radiographs are taken at 180-centimeter SID and table radiographs at 100-centimeter SID.

Occasionally, table radiographs are taken at an SID other than 100 centimeter, with a grid having a 100-centimeter focal distance. Positioning the grid at the proper focal distance is more important with high-ratio grids. More positioning latitude is possible with low-ratio grids.

4. **Upside-down grid error.** The upside-down grid error need occur only once and it will be noticed immediately. A radiographic image taken with an upside-down focused grid shows severe grid cutoff on either side of the central axis (Figure 18-16). Every focused grid has a clear label on one side and sometimes on both. The label indicates the **tube-side** or **film-side** and the prescribed focal distance. With just moderate attention, upside-down grid error will not occur.

Grid Selection

Modern grids are so well manufactured that many radiologists do not find the grid lines of stationary grids objectionable. Moving-grid mechanisms are also well-designed, and image blur does not occur with their use. Therefore it is appropriate to use moving grids for most radiographic procedures. When moving grids are used, focused grids are most common.

Focused grids are generally far superior to linear grids, but they require attention when used. When focused grids are used, the x-ray equipment must be in good adjustment and properly calibrated. The source-to-image receptor distance indicator, the source-to-tabletop distance indicator, and the light-localizing collimator must all be properly adjusted.

Selection of a grid with the proper ratio depends on an understanding of the following three interrelated factors: (1) kVp, (2) degree of cleanup, and (3) patient dose. When using high kVp, use high-ratio grids. Of course, the choice of grid will also be influenced by the size and shape of the part of the anatomy being radiographed. As grid ratio increases, the amount of cleanup also increases. Figure 18-17 shows the approximate percentage of scatter radiation and primary radiation transmitted as a function of grid ratio. Note that the difference between a grid ratio of 12:1 and a grid ratio of 16:1 is small. Difference in patient dose is large and, therefore 16:1 grids are not often used.

> Remember: as a general rule, grid ratios up to 8:1 are satisfactory at tube potentials below 90 kVp. Grid ratios above 8:1 are used when kVp exceeds 90.

Many general-purpose x-ray rooms have installed an 8:1 grid. Managers and biomedical engineers find the 8:1 grid a good compromise between the desired levels of scatter radiation cleanup and patient dose. In departments where high-kVp technique for chest radiography is used, 16:1 grids can be used in chest units.

Grids and Patient Dose

One disadvantage that accompanies the use of x-ray grids is increased patient dose. For a given examination, using a grid may require several times more radiation exposure to the patient than not using one. Use of a moving grid instead of a stationary grid with similar physical characteristics requires approximately 15%

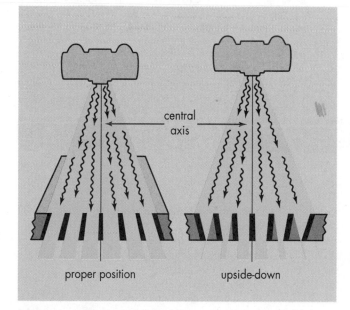

FIGURE 18-16 A focused grid positioned upside down should be detected on the first radiograph. Complete grid cutoff will occur except in the region of the central axis.

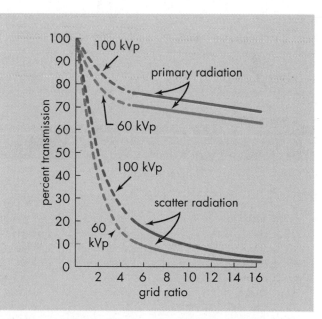

FIGURE 18-17 As grid ratio increases, scatter radiation decreases faster than transmission of primary radiation. Therefore as grid ratio increases, attenuation (clean up) of scatter radiation also increases.

more radiation to the patient. Table 18-4 is a summary of approximate patient doses for various grid techniques with a 200-speed image receptor.

Low-ratio grids are used during mammography. All mammographic equipment is equipped with a 2:1 to a 4:1 ratio moving grid. Even at the low kVp used for mammography, considerable scatter radiation occurs. Use of such grids greatly improves image contrast, with no loss of spatial resolution. Patient dose still is a concern, but modern intensifying screens and the efficiency of rare-earth imaging systems compensate for the increase in patient dose. Grids should be chosen so that the increase in contrast will enhance diagnostic interpretation. The following three factors must be remembered when selecting a grid:

1. Patient dose increases with increasing grid ratio.
2. High-ratio grids are usually used for high-kVp examinations.
3. Patient dose at high kVp when x-rays are transmitted through tissue is less than that at low kVp when x-rays are absorbed in tissue.

In general, compared with the use of low-kVp and low-ratio grids, the use of high-kVp and high-ratio grids will result in lower patient dose and radiographs of equal quality.

One additional disadvantage of using grids is the increased radiographic technique required. When a grid is used, the technique factors must be increased over what they were for nongrid examinations; either the time of exposure or the mA or the kVp must be increased. Table 18-5 presents approximate changes in technique factors required by standards grids. Usually mAs is increased rather than kVp. Often standard kVp factors are used within a department and mAs is changed to compensate for differences in patient size.

Table 18-6 summarizes the clinical factors that should be considered in the selection of various types of grids.

Alternative to Grid Use

An alternative technique to radiographic grid use is the **air-gap technique.** The use of the air-gap technique is another method of reducing scatter radiation and enhancing image contrast. In the air-gap technique the image receptor is moved 10 to 15 centimeters from the patient (Figure 18-18). A portion of the scattered x-rays

TABLE 18-4

Approximate Entrance Skin Dose (mrad) for Examination of the Adult Pelvis with a 200-speed Receptor

	Entrance Dose (mrad)		
Type of grid	70 kVp	90 kVp	110 kVp
Nongrid	85	70	50
5:1	270	215	145
8:1	325	285	205
12:1	425	395	290
16:1	520	475	365
5:1 crossed	535	405	295
8:1 crossed	585	530	405

TABLE 18-5

Approximate Change in Radiographic Technique for Standard Grids

Grid Ratio	mAs Increase	kVp Increase
nongrid	1×	0
5:1	2×	8 to 10
8:1	4×	13 to 15
12:1	5×	20 to 25
16:1	6×	30 to 40

TABLE 18-6

Clinical Considerations in Grid Selection

Type of Grid	Degree of Scatter Removal	Off Center	Off Focus	Positioning Latitude kVp Level	Application
5:1 linear	+	Very wide	Very wide	Up to 80	Inexpensive and easy to use
6:1 linear	+	Very wide	Very wide	Up to 80	Inexpensive and suited for bedside radiography
8:1 linear	++	Wide	Wide	Up to 100	General stationary grid use
10:1 linear	+++	Wide	Wide	Up to 100	Proper alignment required
5:1 crossed	+++	Narrow	Very wide	Up to 100	5-degree tilt limitation
12:1 linear	++++	Narrow	Narrow	Over 110	Proper alignment critical
6:1 crossed	++++	Narrow	Very wide	Up to 110	Proper alignment critical
16:1 linear	+++++	Narrow	Narrow	Over 100	Proper alignment critical
8:1 crossed	+++++	Narrow	Wide	Up to 120	Proper alignment critical

Adapted from *Characteristics and applications of x-ray grids,* Cincinatti, OH, Liegel-Florsheim.

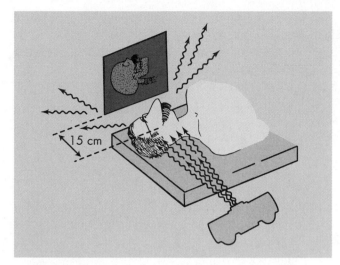

FIGURE 18-18 To apply the air-gap technique, one positions the film 10 to 15 centimeters from the patient. A large fraction of the scattered x-rays will not interact with the film, the exact amount depends on exposure factors.

generated in the patient are scattered away from the film and are not detected. Since fewer scattered x-rays interact with the image receptor, the contrast is enhanced. Generally, when using an air-gap technique, the technique factors are about the same as those for an 8:1 grid. Therefore the patient dose is higher than that of the nongrid technique and is approximately equivalent to that of an intermediate grid technique.

One disadvantage of the air-gap technique is image magnification because of the part distance from the image receptor. The air-gap technique has found application, particularly in areas of chest radiography and **cerebral angiography.** The magnification that accompanies these techniques is usually acceptable. In chest radiography, however, some radiographers will increase the SID from 180 to 300 centimeters. This results in very little magnification and a sharper image. Of course, the technique factors must be increased, but the patient dose does not increase (Figure 18-19).

The air-gap technique is not effective with high-kVp radiography because in high-kVp radiography the direction of the scattered x-rays is toward the film. At tube potentials below approximately 90 kVp, the scattered x-rays are directed more to the side and therefore have a higher probability of being scattered away from the film. Nevertheless, in some departments, 120 to 140 kVp air-gap chest radiography is used with good results.

The air-gap technique is sometimes called *air filtration,* but Figure 18-18 shows that air filtration is an improper name for this procedure. In the air-gap technique the air does not act as a filter of low-energy scattered x-rays; rather the distance between the patient and the film permits the scattered x-rays to escape before they reach the film.

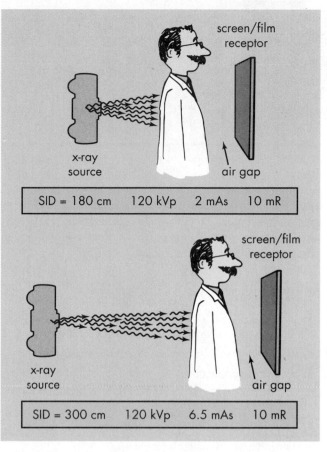

FIGURE 18-19 Two chest radiographs with SID increased from 180 cm to 300 cm.

SUMMARY

Contrast is one of the most important characteristics making up the radiographic image. Scatter radiation is the primary factor that reduces image contrast on a radiograph. Beam-restricting devices and grids are the two types of devices that reduce the amount of scatter reaching the film. Refer to Table 18-2 for the summary of the grid characteristics.

The two main components of grid construction are the interspace material (aluminum or plastic fiber) and grid material (lead strips). Problems arise with the use of grids, including off-level, off-centering, and upside-down grid errors. Grids are selected for use in particular situations. Under 90 kVp, grid ratios of 8:1 and lower are used. Above 90 kVp, grid ratios greater than 8:1 are used.

In all cases the use of a grid compared with nongrid use increases patient dose. However, use of grids combined with use of high-speed rare-earth intensifying screens reduces patient radiation dose to the lowest possible level. Table 18-7 summarizes the changes in grid ratio and changes in mAs required. This table must be memorized.

TABLE 18-7

Changes in Grid Ratio and mAs

Grid Ratio	mAs Increase
No grid	1 × (old mAs times 1)
5:1	2×
8:1	4×
12:1	5×
16:1	6×

An alternative to using a grid is the air-gap technique, in which the image receptor is moved 10 to 15 centimeters from the patient. Scatter is reduced with this technique because scatter exiting the patient escapes in the air space between the patient and the film.

REVIEW QUESTIONS

1. _____ of the remnant x-rays exiting the film side of the patient are from scatter radiation.
2. Why do low kVp levels increase patient dose?
3. a. Define contrast.
   b. What is the effect of scatter radiation on contrast?
4. Describe what Gustave Bucky invented.
5. Write the symbol for microns.
6. What is the grid ratio for a certain grid made with 20 microns of lead between 200 microns of aluminum interspace material and a height of 2.5 millimeters?
7. a. How is grid frequency calculated?
   b. What is the grid frequency of the grid in question 6?
8. Grid frequencies in mammographic grids are _____.
9. Why is lead used as the grid strip material of choice?
10. State the contrast improvement factor.
11. A step wedge is placed on a tissue phantom and two radiographs are made, one without a grid and one with a 10:1 grid. The contrast on the step-wedge image measures 1.25 without a grid and measures 2.8 with the grid. What is the contrast improvement factor of this 10:1 grid?
12. What is the difference in Bucky factor at 70 kVp between no grid and a 5:1 grid? Refer to Table 18-1.
13. Define selectivity.
14. Explain why high-ratio grids have high-contrast improvement factors.
15. Draw cross-sectional diagrams of a linear grid and a focused grid.
16. A 16:1 parallel grid is positioned for 14 × 17 chest radiography at 180-centimeters SID. What is the width of the unexposed area around the radiograph?
17. Gustave Bucky's original grid was a _____ grid.
18. Explain one example of how grid cutoff can occur.
19. What is the advantage of a moving grid?
20. Grid ratios up to _____ are satisfactory for tube potentials below _____. Grid ratios above _____ are used when kVp exceeds _____.

19

Radiographic Quality

OBJECTIVES

At the completion of this chapter the student will be able to:

1. Define radiographic quality, resolution, noise, and speed
2. Interpret the characteristic curve and define portions of the characteristic curve including toe, shoulder, and straight-line portion
3. Distinguish the geometric factors affecting radiographic quality
4. Analyze the subject factors affecting radiographic quality
5. Examine the tools and techniques available to the radiographer to create high-quality films

OUTLINE

Definitions
  Radiographic quality
  Resolution
  Noise
  Speed
Film Factors
  Quality control
  Sensitometry and densitometry of radiographic film
  Contrast and the characteristic curve
  Speed and the characteristic curve
  Latitude

Geometric Factors
  Magnification
  Distortion
  Focal-spot blur
  Heel effect
Subject Factors
  Subject contrast
  Motion unsharpness
Tools to Improve Radiographic Quality
  Patient positioning
  Image receptors
  Selection of technique factors

adiographic quality is defined as the exactness of representation of the patient's anatomic structures on the radiograph. High-quality radiographs are required so that radiologists can make accurate diagnoses. Radiographers have the knowledge and expertise to produce high-quality radiographs for the radiologist. This chapter describes the three major interrelated categories of radiographic quality—(1) film factors, (2) geometric factors, and (3) subject factors.

DEFINITIONS

In preparation for this important chapter on radiographic quality, first examine the following definitions carefully.

Radiographic Quality

Radiographic quality is the exactness of representation of the anatomic structure on the radiograph within the useful density range. A radiograph that exactly reproduces the anatomic part is called a *high-quality radiograph,* and high quality is needed by radiologists to be able to make accurate **diagnoses.** Poor-quality radiographs contain information that is difficult for the human eye to interpret, which can lead to repeated x-rays or missed diagnoses.

Resolution

One of the three important characteristics of radiographic quality is resolution. Resolution is the ability to visually detect separate objects on a radiograph. Spatial resolution refers to the bone versus soft tissue interface. Radiographs have excellent spatial resolution. *Detail* or *visibility of detail* are terms commonly used when referring to spatial resolution. Detail is defined as the degree of sharpness of structural lines on a radiograph. Visibility of detail allows the viewer to see detail because image contrast and optical density are adequate. *Spatial resolution,* the preferred term, is measured in line pairs per millimeter (lp/mm). One other term for resolution is *contrast resolution,* which refers to contrast differences between similar tissues such as the liver and spleen.

Noise

Radiographic noise is the undesirable fluctuation in the optical density of the image. Relate image noise to the "snow" on a television screen or the background noise in an audio system. Noise is a term borrowed from electrical engineering, and often it is inherent in a system. On the radiographic image, some noise is inherent; however, other noise is controllable and contributes to the deterioration of the radiographic image. Radiographic noise has the following three components:

(1) film graininess, (2) structure mottle, and (3) quantum mottle. Film graininess refers to the distribution and size of the silver-halide crystals in the emulsion of the film. Film graininess is inherent noise on a radiograph. Structure mottle is similar to film graininess but instead refers to the phosphor of the radiographic screen rather than silver-halide crystals. Structure mottle is equally inherent and because intensifying screens are so carefully manufactured, it contributes little to radiographic noise. Quantum mottle is the principal cause of radiographic noise. Quantum mottle refers to the randomness with which a low number of x-ray photons interact with the intensifying screens. The use of very fast intensifying screens may result in increased quantum mottle. If an image is formed with a few x-rays, the radiographic noise will be higher than if the image is formed by many x-rays. Quantum mottle is evident using low mAs, high kVp, and fast-image receptors.

Speed

The ability of an x-ray film to respond to an x-ray exposure is the measure of its **sensitivity** or its **speed.** In general, resolution and noise are affected by image-receptor speed. The following rules apply to film-screen combinations.

1. Fast-image receptors (400, 600, and above) have high noise and low resolution.
2. Slow-image receptors (50, 100, 200, and 300) have low noise and high resolution.

The quality of a radiograph relates directly to the radiographer's understanding of the basic principles of x-ray physics and his or her evaluation of the factors affecting radiograph quality. Figure 19-1 is a chart showing the factors affecting radiographic quality. Each is considered in detail. The following discussion begins with the process of quality control and how necessary it is to the production of optimal radiographs. How film factors affect radiographic quality follows the discussion of quality control.

FILM FACTORS
Quality Control

Every diagnostic imaging department in hospitals, most doctor's offices with x-ray equipment, and most clinics with x-ray suites is required by medical accrediting commissions to ensure that the x-ray equipment and radiographic film processing follow **quality control** guidelines. A program of quality control (QC) is designed to make sure the radiologist is provided with an optimal x-ray image and that the radiographer follows radiation safety procedures. Preventative maintenance and testing of x-ray equipment are done within a QC program by biomedical engineers and specially trained radiographers. Equipment QC is discussed in later chapters. Processing QC is checked daily, usually by the QC radiographer.

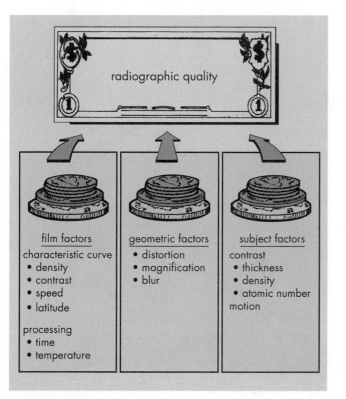

FIGURE 19-1 Organizational chart of principal factors affecting radiographic quality.

Sensitometry and Densitometry of Radiographic Film

Processing QC has two specific parts—sensitometry and densitometry. Sensitometry is performed when a **step-wedge** image is flashed onto an x-ray film to simulate an exposure or, if that device is not available, the aluminum step-wedge may be imaged. The step-wedge image shows the shades of gray, which demonstrate radiographic contrast or variations in optical density. The **densitometer** measures the light transmitted through the step-wedge increments. The film-screen manufacturer's representative helps departments set up their QC programs. Usually, these representatives set up the parameters for optical density, and the QC radiographer tests daily that the step-wedge increments or optical density falls within the set parameters.

Sensitometry and densitometry are important because the daily testing and recording identifies any changes that may indicate processing problems. A problem with even one processor in an imaging department could affect the output of the whole department.

Sensitometry and Densitometry of Radiographic Film

Sensitometry and densitometry are used for processing QC in imaging departments. Sensitometry and densitometry are also used by film manufacturers to determine the characteristics of x-ray film. The testing is similar, but the optical density (OD) numbers for film

characteristics are plotted on **semi-logarithmic** graph paper rather than on a daily record as with processor QC. When the optical density of film is plotted onto semilogarithmic graph paper, the result is a **characteristic curve.**

Characteristic curve. The two principal measurements involved in sensitometry and densitometry are the exposure to the film and the percentage of light transmitted through the processed film. Such measurements are used to describe the relationship between **optical density** and **radiation exposure.** This relationship plotted on a graph is called a *characteristic curve* or sometimes the *H & D curve* after Hurter and Driffield, who first described this relationship. A typical characteristic curve is shown in Figure 19-2.

At high and low exposure levels, large variations in exposure result in only a small change in optical density. These portions of the characteristic curve are called the *toe* and *shoulder.* At intermediate exposure levels, small changes in exposure result in large changes in optical density. This intermediate region, called the *straight-line portion,* is the region in which the optical density numbers from a properly exposed radiograph appear.

QC radiographers and manufacturers' technical specialists determine the optical density and **base plus fog** on radiographs by simple tests and calculations. When the characteristic curve is plotted from densitometry numbers, **contrast, gradient,** and **speed** can be easily determined. Contrast, gradient, and speed characteristics of the film are interpreted from the slope and position of the curve on the graph.

To perform sensitometry and densitometry, an aluminum step wedge or **penetrometer** and a **densitometer,**

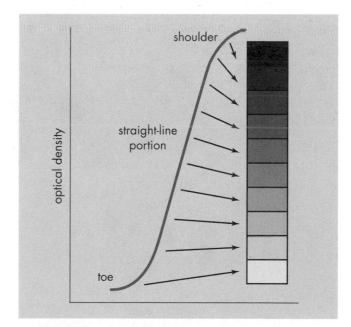

FIGURE 19-2 Characteristic curve of radiographic film is the graphic relationship between optical density and exposure.

a device that measures optical density, are used. The steps involved are outlined in Figure 19-3.

First the aluminum step wedge is exposed at a standard technique (e.g., 70 kVp with 2.5-millimeters aluminum total filtration). When processed, the film will have areas of increasing optical density that correspond to thinner penetrometer steps. The processed film is analyzed in the densitometer, a device that has a light source focused through a pinhole. The x-ray film is positioned between the pinhole and a light sensor, and the amount of light transmitted through each step of the radiographic step-wedge image is measured. Data are recorded and, when plotted on semilogarithmic graph paper, results in a characteristic curve.

Radiographic film is sensitive over a wide range of exposures. Screen film, for example, will respond to radiation intensities from under 1 to over 1000 mR. Consequently the exposure values for a characteristic curve including such a large range of values are presented in logarithmic fashion. It is not the absolute exposure that is of interest but rather the change in optical density over each exposure interval. Therefore the **log of relative exposure** is used as the scale along the x-axis.

Figure 19-4 shows the exposure in mR, log of relative exposure, and mAs for a representative screen-film combination. The log relative exposure scale is usually presented in increments of 0.3 because the log of 2 is 0.3. An increase in log relative exposure of 0.3 results from doubling the exposure. This can be done by doubling the mAs.

Optical density. It is not enough to say that optical density is the degree of blackening of a radiograph or that a clear area of the radiograph represents low opti-

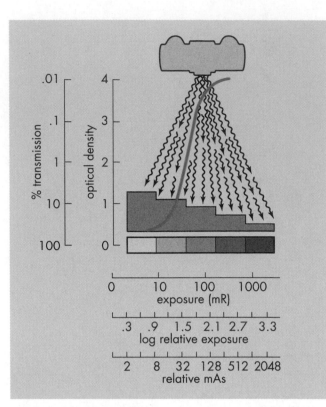

FIGURE 19-4 Relationship among exposure, log relative exposure, and relative mAs for typical screen-film combination. Relationship between percent transmission and optical density is shown along the y-axis.

cal density and a black area represents high optical density. Optical density is the numerical value calculated between the level of light incident on a processed step-wedge image (I_o) and the level of light transmitted through that film (I_t).

Optical Density

The optical density (OD) is defined as follows:

$$OD = log_{10} \times \left(\frac{I_o}{I_t}\right)$$

Question: The lung field of a chest radiograph transmits only 0.15% of incident light as determined with a densitometer. What is the optical density?

Answer: 0.15% = 0.0015

$$OD = log_{10} \frac{1}{0.0015}$$

$$OD = 2.8$$

Optical density is a logarithmic function. Logarithms allow a wide range of values to be expressed by small numbers. Radiographic film contains optical densities

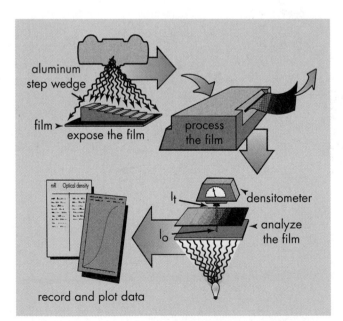

FIGURE 19-3 Steps involved in construction of a characteristic curve.

ranging from near 0 (clear) to 4 (black). An optical density of 4 actually means that only 1 in 10,000 light photons (10^4) is capable of penetrating the x-ray film. Table 19-1 shows the range of light transmission as it corresponds to various levels of optical density.

High-quality glass has an optical density of 0, which means that all incident light is transmitted. Unexposed x-ray film allows no more than about 80% of light to be transmitted through it. Most unexposed and processed radiographic film has an optical density in the range of 0.1 to 0.15, which corresponds to 79% and 71% transmission of light.

These optical densities in unexposed film are due to **base density** and **fog density** (Figure 19-5). The base density is the optical density inherent in the base of the film. The base density is due to the composition of the base and the tint added to the base. The tint is added to prevent eye fatigue because radiologists have to look directly into the illuminator or **viewbox** as they read radiographs.

Base Density
Base density has a value of approximately 0.05 OD.

Fog density has been previously described as the development of silver grains that contain no useful information. Fog density results from inadvertent exposure of film during storage, undesirable chemical contamination, and improper processing.

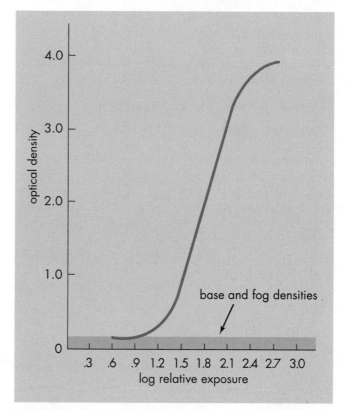

FIGURE 19-5 Base and fog densities do not contribute to diagnostic information on the radiograph and should be as low as possible.

Fog Density
Fog density on a processed radiograph should not exceed 0.05 OD.

Higher fog density levels reduce the contrast of the radiograph.

Question: The light incident on the radiograph of a long bone has a relative value of 1500. If the light transmitted through the radiopaque bony structures on the film has an intensity of 480, and the light transmitted through the radiolucent soft tissue on the film has an intensity of 2, what are the approximate respective optical densities? Refer to Table 19-1 if necessary.

Answer:
$$OD = \log_{10}\left(\frac{I_o}{I_T}\right)$$

a. For bone: $OD = \log_{10} \times \dfrac{1500}{480}$

$$= 0.5 \text{ OD for bone}$$

b. For soft tissue: $OD = \dfrac{\log_{10} 1500}{2}$

$$= 2.9 \text{ OD for soft tissue}$$

The useful range of optical densities is approximately 0.25 to 2.5. Most radiographs, however, show image

TABLE 19-1

Relationship of Optical Density of Radiographic Film to Light Transmission Through the Film

Percent of Light Transmitted ($I_t/I_o \times 100$)	Fraction of Light Transmitted (I_t/I_o)	Optical Density ($\log I_t/I_o$)
100	1	0
50	$\frac{1}{2}$	0.3
32	$\frac{8}{25}$	0.5
25	$\frac{1}{4}$	0.6
12.5	$\frac{1}{8}$	0.9
10	$\frac{1}{10}$	1
5	$\frac{1}{20}$	1.3
3.2	$\frac{4}{125}$	1.5
2.5	$\frac{1}{30}$	1.6
1.25	$\frac{1}{80}$	1.9
1	$\frac{1}{100}$	2
0.5	$\frac{1}{200}$	2.3
0.32	$\frac{2}{625}$	2.5
0.125	$\frac{1}{800}$	2.9
0.1	$\frac{1}{1000}$	3
0.05	$\frac{1}{2000}$	3.3
0.032	$\frac{1}{3125}$	3.5
0.01	$\frac{1}{10,000}$	4

patterns in the range of 0.5 to 1.25 optical density. Attention to this part of the characteristic curve is essential. However, very low optical density may be too light to contain an image pattern, whereas very high optical density is usually viewed with a **hot light**.

Contrast and the Characteristic Curve

When a high-quality exposed and processed radiograph is placed on an illuminator, it is easily seen that the image is formed by the differences in optical density. These optical density differences are called *radiographic contrast*. A radiograph that has sharp differences in optical density is a **high-contrast radiograph**. If the optical density differences are less distinct, the radiograph is of **low contrast**. Figure 19-6 illustrates the difference between high contrast and low contrast with a photographic scene of a vicious dog.

Radiographic contrast is the product of the following two separate factors:

1. **Film contrast,** which is inherent in the film and influenced by processing.
2. **Subject contrast** is determined by the size, shape, and x-ray–attenuating characteristics of the anatomic part.

Radiographic contrast can be greatly affected by changes in either film contrast or subject contrast. In the clinical setting, it is usually best to standardize the film contrast and alter the subject contrast according to the needs of the examination. Subject contrast is dealt with in greater detail later. Film selection is generally limited by the intensifying screen used. Screen-film images always have higher contrast than direct-exposure images. All these factors require some judgment on the part of the radiographer.

The best control the radiographer can exercise is exposing the film properly so that the optical densities lie within the diagnostically useful range, which is **0.5 to 2.5 OD**. Outside this range, contrast is lost because the image is in either the toe or the shoulder of the characteristic curve (Figure 19-7). It is important to expose the film so that the optical densities lie within the diagnostically useful range. Standardized film processing is necessary for consistent film contrast and good radiographic quality. Deviation from manufacturer's recommendations for film-screen combinations, improper exposure techniques, and lack of processing quality control will result in inconsistent film quality.

The characteristic curve of a film shows the degree of contrast for that particular film.

 Contrast on the Characteristic Curve
Film contrast is equal to the slope of the straight-line portion of the characteristic curve.

If this slope had a value of 1, then the straight-line portion of the characteristic curve would be angled 45 degrees. An increase of 1 unit along the log relative exposure axis would result in an increase of 1 unit along the optical density axis. The contrast would be 1. Film that has a contrast of 1 is low-contrast film. Film with a contrast higher than 1 reflects the differences in x-ray exposure to the film. Film with a contrast of 3, for instance, would show large optical density differences over a small range of x-ray exposure.

From the appearance of the characteristic curve, radiographers (with help from the manufacturer's representative), should be able to distinguish high-contrast film from low-contrast film. Figure 19-8 shows the char-

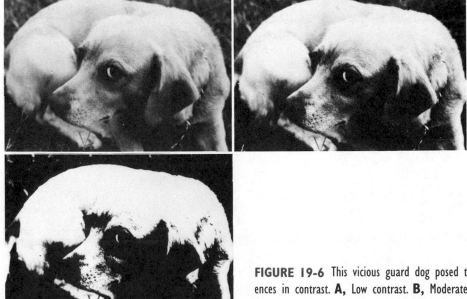

FIGURE 19-6 This vicious guard dog posed to demonstrate differences in contrast. **A,** Low contrast. **B,** Moderate contrast. **C,** High contrast.

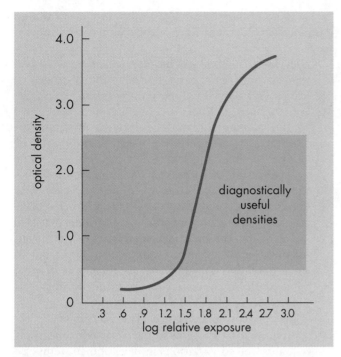

FIGURE 19-7 If the exposure of the film results in densities that lie in the toe or shoulder regions, where the slope of the curve is less, contrast is reduced.

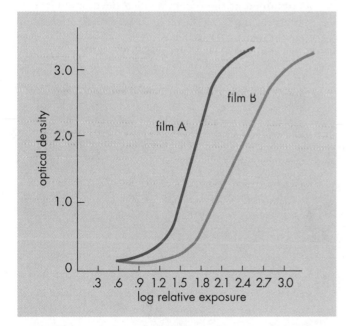

FIGURE 19-8 Slope of the straight-line portion of the characteristic curve is greater for film **A** than for film **B**. Film **A** has higher contrast.

acteristic curves for two different types of x-ray film. Film *A* has higher contrast than film *B*, as shown by the fact that the slope of the straight-line portion of the characteristic curve is steeper for *A* than for *B*.

Several methods are used to numerically specify film contrast. The one most often used is **average gradient**.

The average gradient is the slope of a straight line drawn between the two points on the characteristic curve at optical densities 0.25 and 2.0 above base and fog densities. The equation for average gradient is as follows:

$$\text{Average gradient} = \frac{OD_2 - OD_1}{LRE_2 - LRE_1}$$

OD_2 is the optical density of 2 plus base and fog densities. OD_1 is the optical density of 0.25 plus base and fog densities. LRE_2 and LRE_1 are the log relative exposures associated with OD_2 and OD_1. This method is diagrammed in Figure 19-9 for a film having a combined base and fog density of 0.1.

Most radiographic films have an average gradient in the range of 2.5 to 3.5. The average gradient of x-ray film is usually much larger than 1, especially with the use of film-screen radiography, which inherently improves subject contrast. Film-screen radiography is used almost exclusively in modern imaging departments.

Film contrast may also be identified by **gradient**. The gradient is the slope of the tangent at any point on the characteristic curve (Figure 19-10). **Toe gradient** is probably more important than average gradient, since many clinical optical densities appear in the toe region of the characteristic curve.

Question: A radiographic film has a base density of 0.06 and a fog density of 0.11. At what optical densities should one evaluate the characteristic curve to determine the film contrast?

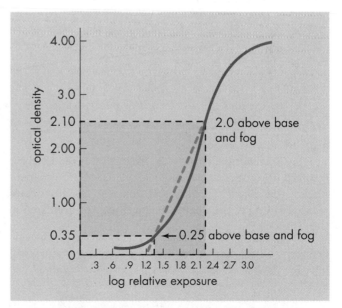

FIGURE 19-9 Average gradient is the slope of the line drawn between the points on the characteristic curve that correspond to density levels 0.25 and 2 above the combined base and fog densities.

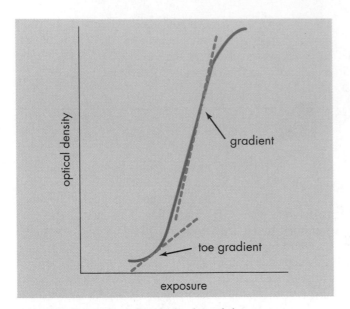

FIGURE 19-10 The gradient is the slope of the tangent at any point on the characteristic curve.

Answer: The curve should be evaluated at optical densities 0.25 and 2 above base plus fog densities. Therefore at optical densities of:

$$0.06 + 0.11 + .25 = 0.42 \text{ OD}$$

$$0.06 + 0.11 + 2.0 = 2.17 \text{ OD}$$

Question: If optical densities of 0.42 and 2.17 on the characteristic curve in the preceding example correspond to log relative exposures of 0.95 and 1.75, what is the average gradient?

Answer: Average gradient $= \dfrac{OD_2 - OD_1}{LRE_2 - LRE_1}$

$$= \frac{2.17 - 0.42}{1.75 - 0.95}$$

$$= \frac{1.75}{0.8}$$

$$= 2.19 \text{ is the average gradient}$$

Note that the numerator in the expression for average gradient always equals 1.75.

Film processing. Proper film processing is required for optimal film contrast because the degree of development affects fog density and optical density. The important factors affecting the degree of development are listed in the box below.

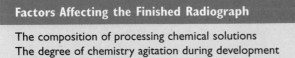

Factors Affecting the Finished Radiograph

The composition of processing chemical solutions
The degree of chemistry agitation during development
The development time
The development temperature

Two factors that the QC radiographer examines daily are **development time** and **development temperature.**

- **Development time.** As development time is varied, the characteristic curve for any film changes in shape and position along the log relative exposure axis (Figure 19-11).

  If the characteristic curves were analyzed for contrast, speed, and fog level, each would be shown to vary as in Figure 19-12.

  Speed and fog increase with longer development time. Contrast increases and then decreases with development time. The development time recommended by the manufacturer is the time that will result in maximum contrast, relatively high levels of speed, and low levels of fog. When development time extends much beyond the recommended period, the film contrast decreases and the fog level increases.

- **Development temperature.** The relationships just described for variations in development time apply equally well to variations in development temperature. If the average gradient, speed, and fog level for the characteristic curves representative of various temperatures were plotted, the results would appear also as in Figure 19-12. Maximum contrast is obtained at the recommended development temperature. The fog level increases with increasing temperature.

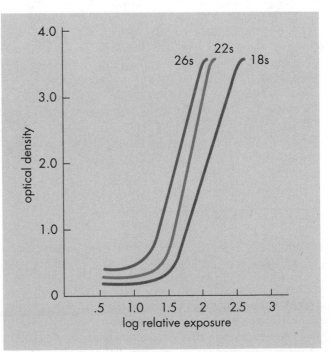

FIGURE 19-11 As development time increases, changes occur in the shape and relative position of the characteristic curve.

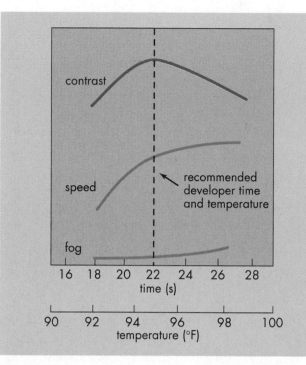

FIGURE 19-12 Analysis of characteristic curves at various development times and temperatures yields these relationships for contrast, speed, and fog for 90-second automatically processed film.

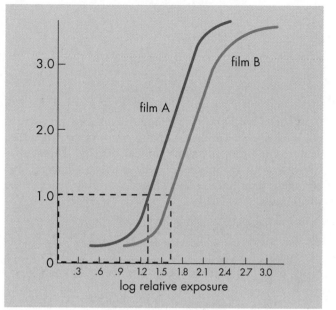

FIGURE 19-13 Speed of a film is the reciprocal of the exposure, in roentgens, needed to produce a density of 1. Film A is faster than film B (Speed A = $\frac{1}{1.3}$ = 0.78; speed B = $\frac{1}{1.6}$ = 0.63).

Within a small range, a change in either time or temperature can be compensated for by a change in the other. However, a small change in either time or temperature alone can result in a large change in the sensitometric characteristics of the x-ray film.

Monitoring of time and temperature for film development is very important for rapid processing. If the processing time of an automatic processor is optimized at 90 seconds, a variation of 5 seconds in development time can result in significant changes in radiographic quality.

Speed and the Characteristic Curve

The ability of an x-ray film to respond to x-ray exposure is a measure of its **sensitivity** or **speed.** An exposure of less than 1 mR can be detected with film-screen combinations. Several mR are necessary to produce a measurable response with direct-exposure film.

The characteristic curve of an x-ray film is also useful in identifying **film speed.** Figure 19-13 shows the characteristic curves of two different x-ray films. Since film A requires less exposure than film B to produce any optical density, film A is faster than film B. The characteristic curves of fast films are positioned to the left of those of slow films along the log relative exposure scale. X-ray films are identified as either fast or slow, according to their sensitivity to x-ray exposure. The identification of a given film as so many times faster than another film is important information for the radiographer. If

film A were twice as fast as film B, film A would require only half the mAs required by film B to produce a given optical density. In addition, the image on film A might be of lesser quality because of increased radiographic noise.

In sensitometry the optical density specified for determining film speed is 1, and the speed is measured in reciprocal roentgens. The following is the definition of film speed:

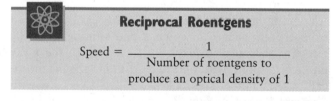

Reciprocal Roentgens

$$\text{Speed} = \frac{1}{\text{Number of roentgens to produce an optical density of 1}}$$

Question: The characteristic curve of a given film-screen shows that 25 mR are needed to produce an optical density of 1 on that image-receptor. What is the image-receptor speed?

Answer: $\text{Speed} = \frac{1}{25 \text{ mr}} = \frac{1}{0.025 \text{ R}} = 40R$

Question: How much exposure is required to produce an optical density of 1 on a 600-speed image receptor?

Answer: $\text{Speed} = \frac{1}{\text{Exposure}}$

$$\text{Exposure} = \frac{1}{\text{Speed}}$$

$$= \frac{1}{600}$$

$$= 0.00167R$$

$$= 1.7 \text{ mR} = 600 \text{ speed}$$

When a radiographer changes from one film-screen combination to another, a change in mAs may be necessary to maintain the same optical density. If image receptor-speed is doubled, mAs must be halved. No change is required in kVp. This relationship is expressed as follows:

$$\frac{\text{New image-receptor speed}}{\text{Old image-receptor speed}} = \frac{\text{Old mAs}}{\text{New mAs}}$$

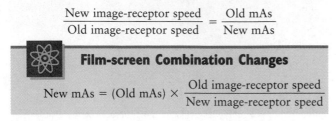

Film-screen Combination Changes

$$\text{New mAs} = (\text{Old mAs}) \times \frac{\text{Old image-receptor speed}}{\text{New image-receptor speed}}$$

Question: A PA chest requires 120 kVp at 8 mAs with a 100-speed image receptor. What radiographic technique should be used with a 250-speed image receptor?

Answer: $\text{New mAs} = (8 \text{ mAs}) \times \dfrac{100}{250}$

$$= 3.2 \text{ mAs}$$

Therefore the new technique is 120 kVp at 3.2 mAs.

Changing from one film-screen combination to another is so commonly done in imaging departments that it is recommended that the above formula be memorized.

Latitude

An additional image-receptor feature easily obtained from the characteristic curve is the **latitude**. Latitude refers to the range of exposures over which the x-ray film will respond with optical densities in the diagnostically useful range. Figure 19-14 shows two films with different latitudes. Film *B* responds to a much wider range of exposures than film *A* and is said to have a wider latitude than film *A*.

Films with a wide latitude are said to have **long gray scale,** and those with narrow latitude have **short gray scale.** From Figure 19-14 it should be clear that *latitude and contrast are inversely proportional*—high-contrast film has narrow latitude, and low-contrast film has wide latitude.

GEOMETRIC FACTORS

Making a radiograph is similar in many ways to taking a photograph. Proper exposure time and intensity are required for both. Images are recorded in both because

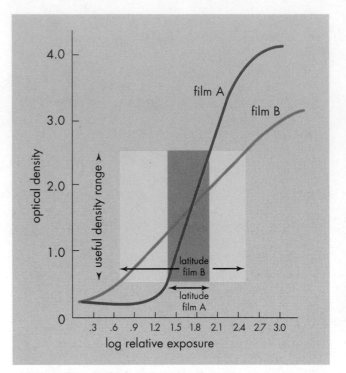

FIGURE 19-14 Latitude of a film is the exposure range over which it responds with diagnostically useful optical densities.

the x-rays and the visible-light photons travel in straight lines. In that regard an x-ray image may be considered analogous to a **shadowgraph.** Figure 19-15 shows the familiar shadowgraph that can be made to appear on a wall if light is shown on a properly positioned hand. The sharpness of the shadow image on the wall is a function of a number of geometric factors. For example, the closer to the wall the hand is placed, the sharper the shadow. Similarly, the farther from the hand the light source is, the sharper the shadow.

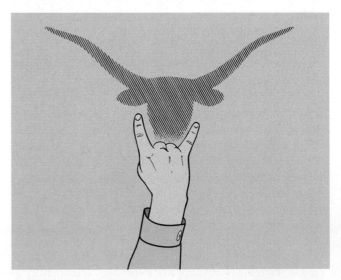

FIGURE 19-15 A shadowgraph is analogous to a radiograph. *(Dedicated to Xie Nan Zhu, Guangzhou, Peoples' Republic of China.)*

These geometric conditions also apply to the production of high-quality radiographs. There are three principal geometric factors that affect radiographic quality—two similar to shadowgraph geometry and one specific to the x-ray tube. The three principal geometric factors are as follows:

1. Magnification
2. Distortion
3. Focal-spot blur

Magnification

All images on the radiograph are larger than the object they represent, which is called *magnification.* For most clinical examinations one should maintain the smallest magnification possible. During some situations, however, magnification is desirable and is carefully planned as part of the radiographic examination. This is called *magnification radiography.* It is presented in Chapter 22.

Quantitatively, magnification is measured and expressed by the magnification factor (MF), which is defined as follows:

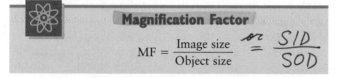

Magnification Factor

$$MF = \frac{Image\ size}{Object\ size} \text{ or } = \frac{SID}{SOD}$$

The MF depends on distance from the **source** to the image or **SID.** For most radiographs taken at an SID of 100 centimeters, the MF will be approximately 1.1. For radiographs taken at 180 centimeters (40 inches) SID, the MF will be approximately 1.05.

Question: If a heart measures 12.5 centimeters from side to side at its widest point, and its image on a chest radiograph measures 14.7 cm, what is the MF?

Answer: $MF = \dfrac{14.7\ centimeters}{12.5\ centimeters} = 1.176$ is the MF

In the usual radiographic examination, it is not possible to determine the object size. The image size may be measured directly from the radiograph. In such situations the MF can be determined from the ratio of the SID to the source-to-object distance (SOD):

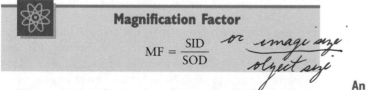

Magnification Factor

$$MF = \frac{SID}{SOD} \text{ or } \frac{image\ size}{object\ size}$$

Figure 19-16 shows that this method of calculating the MF results from the basic geometric relationship between **similar triangles.** If two right triangles have a common **hypotenuse,** the ratio of the height of one to its **base** will be the same as the ratio of the height of the

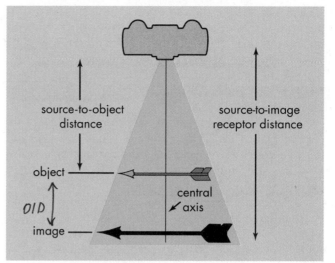

FIGURE 19-16 Magnification can be measured by the ratio of image size to object size or SID to SOD.

other to its base. This is the situation that generally is encountered in radiography. The SID is known and can be measured directly. The SOD can be estimated relatively accurately by a radiographer who has a good foundation in human anatomy. The image size can be measured accurately; therefore the object size can be calculated as follows.

$$MF = \frac{Image\ size}{Object\ size} = \frac{SID}{SOD}$$

$$Object\ size = (Image\ size)\frac{SOD}{SID}$$

Question: A renal calculus or kidney stone measures 1.2 centimeters on the radiograph. The SID is 100 centimeters and the SOD is estimated at 92 centimeters. What is the size of the calculus?

Answer: Object size = $1.2 \times \dfrac{92}{100}$

= 1.1 centimeters is the measurement of the kidney stone

Question: A lateral film of the lumbar spine taken at 100 cm SID and 75 cm SOD results in the image of a vertebral body with maximum and minimum dimensions of 6.4 centimeters and 4.2 centimeters. What is the object size?

Answer: $MF = \dfrac{100}{75} = 1.33$

Therefore the object size is

$\dfrac{6.4}{1.33} \times \dfrac{4.2}{1.33} = 4.81$ centimeters $\times$ 3.16 centimeters

The MF will be the same for objects positioned off the central axis of the grid or film as for those lying on the central axis (Figure 19-17). Magnification occurs with an increase in object-to-image distance (OID). An increase in OID reduces the SOD. Because the SOD is inversely proportional to the SID, reducing the SOD increases the MF.

The MF is appropriate for use with the off-axis subject. In Figure 19-17 the projection lines indicate that the two triangles of interest, although not right triangles, are still similar triangles; therefore the ratio of height to base is the same in both.

In summary, there are two factors that affect magnification: large SID and small OID.

> **Remember: to Minimize Magnification Use The Following:**
> 1. **Large SID.** Use as large a source-to-image receptor distance as possible.
> 2. **Small OID.** Place the object as close to the image receptor as possible.

The SID is a standard distance in most imaging departments: 180 centimeters for chest imaging (72 inches) and 100 centimeters (40 inches) for routine Bucky examinations. Figure 19-18 shows the value of the MF for these three SIDs and for OIDs varying from 0 to 75 centimeters. There are three familiar clinical examinations that routinely minimize magnification. Most chest radiographs are taken at 180 centimeters SID from the posterioanterior projection. This projection results in a smaller heart-to-image receptor distance than with an an-

terioposterior projection. Magnification of the heart is reduced because of the large SID and the small OID.

Many dentists now take **bite-wing** and **periapical** exposures at 40-centimeters SID rather than at 20-centimeters SID, which is the technique that prevailed for years. Using the 40-centimeters SID, known as ***long-cone technique*** dental radiography, has many advantages over the short-cone technique. One such advantage is less magnification. Figure 19-19 shows periapical radiographs of the bicuspid taken at 20- and 40-centimeter SID. The difference in magnification is great even though the OID is small in each case.

Mammography units are designed for 50- to 70-centimeters SID. This is a relatively short SID, but it is necessary, considering the low kVp and low radiation intensity of mammography units. Such units have a device for compression of the breast to reduce OID magnification and spread breast tissue.

Distortion

The previous discussion concerning magnification assumed the anatomy was perpendicular to the central x-ray beam at a fixed OID. If any one of these conditions is changed, as they all are in most clinical examinations, the magnification will not be the same over the entire object. Unequal magnification of different portions of the same object is called *distortion*. Distortion of anatomy can produce inaccurate diagnosis. Two conditions contribute to image distortion: object thickness and object position.

> **Distortion is Caused by the Following:**
> 1. The thickness of the object
> 2. The position of the object

Object thickness. Thick objects are distorted and thin objects are not. With a thick object the OID changes across the object. Consider, for instance, two rectangular structures of different thicknesses (Figure 19-20). Because of the change in OID across the thicker structure, the image of that structure will be more distorted than the image of the thinner structure.

Consider the images produced by a disk and a sphere of the same diameter (Figure 19-21). When positioned on the central axis, the images of both objects will appear as circles. The image of the sphere will appear less distinct because of its varying thickness. When these objects are positioned laterally to the central axis, the disk still appears circular. The sphere appears not only less distinct but also elliptical because of its thickness. This distortion resulting from object thickness is shown more dramatically in Figure 19-22 by the image of an irregular object. Irregular objects such as those shown in Figure 19-22, show significant distortion. Many areas on the human body may be perfect examples of irregular object distortion.

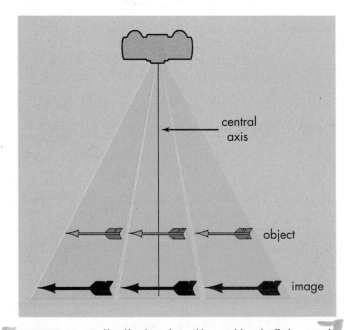

FIGURE 19-17 Magnification of an object positioned off the central x-ray axis is the same as that for an object on the central axis if the objects are in the same plane.

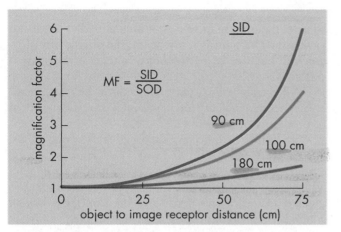

FIGURE 19-18 Graph showing value of magnification factor at 90-, 100-, and 180-centimeters SID for various object-to-image receptor distances

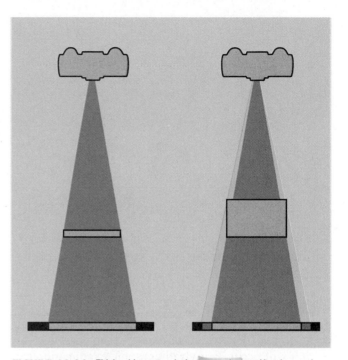

FIGURE 19-20 Thick objects result in unequal magnification and therefore more distortion than thin objects.

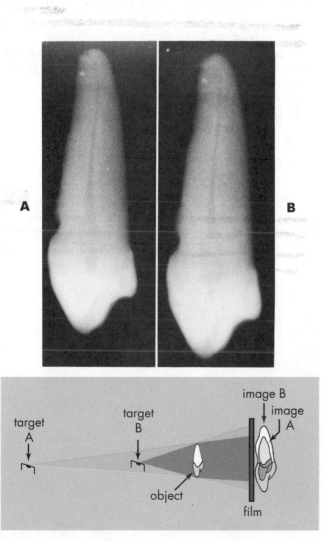

FIGURE 19-19 Periapical radiographs of a bicuspid. **A,** 40-centimeters SID. **B,** 20-centimeters SID. The long-cone technique results in noticeably less magnification.

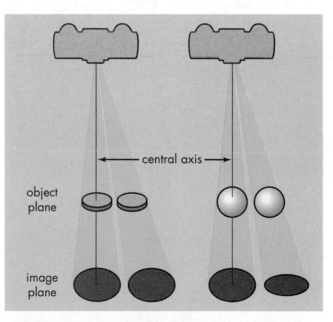

FIGURE 19-21 Object thickness influences distortion. Radiographs of a disk or sphere will appear as circles if the object is on the central axis. If they are lateral to the central axis, the disk will appear as a circle and the sphere as an ellipse.

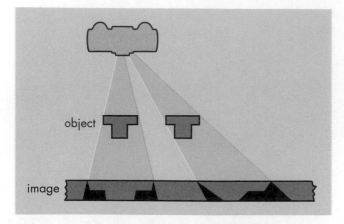

FIGURE 19-22 Irregular objects such as these, or the human body, can cause considerable distortion when radiographed off the central axis.

Object position. If the object plane and the image plane are parallel, the image will be undistorted, but if the object plane and image plane are not parallel, distortion will occur. Every radiographic examination can possibly be distorted if the patient is not properly positioned.

Figure 19-23 is an example of gross distortion and shows that the image of an inclined object can be smaller than the object itself. In such a condition the image is **foreshortened.** The amount of foreshortening—

the amount of reduction in image size—increases as the angle of inclination increases. If an inclined object is not located on the central x-ray beam, the degree of distortion will be affected by the object's angle of inclination and its lateral position from the central axis. Figure 19-24 illustrates this situation and shows that the image of an inclined object can be severely foreshortened or considerably magnified.

With multiple objects positioned at various OIDs, **spatial distortion** can occur. Spatial distortion is the misrepresentation in the image of the actual spatial relationships among objects. Figure 19-25 demonstrates this condition for two arrows of the same size, one of which lies on top of the other. Because of the position of the arrows, only one image should be seen, which represents the superimposition of the arrows.

However, unequal magnification of the two objects causes arrow *A* to appear larger than arrow *B* and to be positioned more laterally. This distortion is minimal for objects lying along the central x-ray beam. As object position is shifted laterally from the central axis, spatial distortion is more significant.

Magnification and distortion illustrate the projection nature of x-ray images; a single image is not enough to define the three-dimensional configuration of a complex object. Most x-ray examinations include two or more projections of the same part.

Focal-Spot Blur

So far the discussion of the geometric factors affecting radiographic quality has assumed that x-rays are emitted from a point target. In actual practice there is not a point source of radiation but rather a square or rectangular source varying in size from approximately 0.1 to 1.5 millimeters on a side, depending on the type of x-ray tube in use.

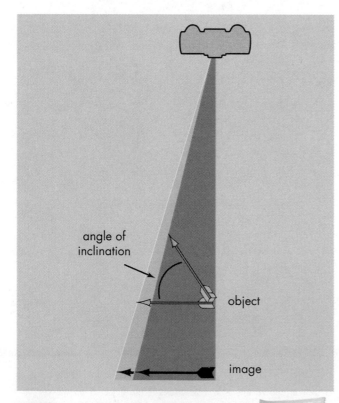

FIGURE 19-23 Inclination of an object results in a foreshortened image.

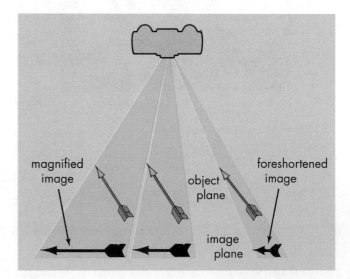

FIGURE 19-24 An inclined object positioned lateral to the central x-ray beam may be severely distorted by magnification or foreshortening.

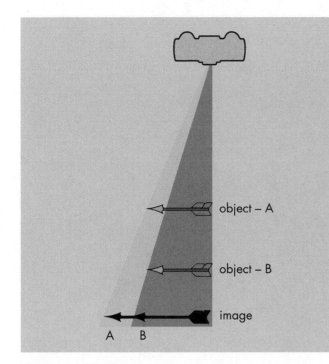

FIGURE 19-25 When objects of the same size are positioned at different distances from the film, spatial distortion occurs. *OID*

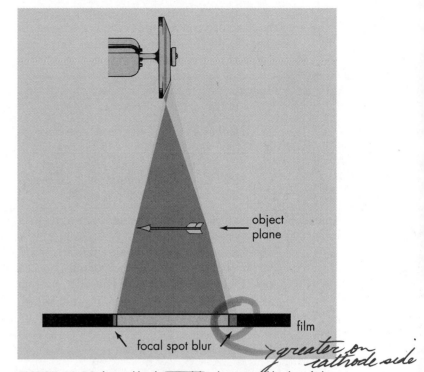

FIGURE 19-26 Image blur is caused by the measurable size of the focal spot. *= size of the area the e⁻ hit on the anode*

greater on cathode side

focal spot projected on to patient and image receptor

Figure 19-26 illustrates the result of using x-ray tubes with different **effective focal spots**. The point of the object arrow in Figure 19-26 will not appear as a point in the image plane because the x-rays used to image that point originate throughout the target. This phenomenon is called *focal-spot blur.* As shown in the illustration, it is greater on the cathode side of the image. Focal-spot blur is undesirable and is the most important factor in determining spatial resolution.

Three conditions result in focal-spot blur: large effective focal spot, short SID, and long OID.

Focal-spot Blur is Caused by the Following:

1. Large effective focal spot
2. Short SID
3. Long OID

The geometric relationships governing magnification also influence focal-spot blur. As the geometry of the source, object, and image are altered to produce greater magnification, they also produce increased focal-spot blur.

The region of focal-spot blur can be calculated using the formula relating to similar triangles. If an arrowhead were positioned near the x-ray tube target, the size of the focal-spot blur would be larger than that of the effective focal spot (Figure 19-27, *A*). Generally the object is much closer to the film and therefore the focal-spot blur is much smaller than the effective focal spot (Figure 19-27, *B*).

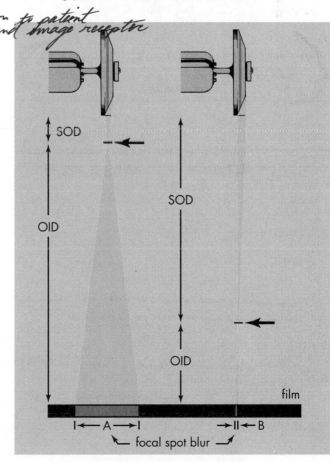

FIGURE 19-27 Focal-spot blur is small when OID is small.

From these drawings, there are two similar triangles. Therefore the ratio of SOD to OID is the same as the ratio of the sizes of the effective focal spot and the focal-spot blur.

$$\frac{SOD}{OID} = \frac{\text{Effective focal spot}}{\text{Focal-spot blur}}$$

Therefore focal-spot blur can be computed as follows:

$$\text{Focal-spot blur} = (\text{effective focal spot}) \frac{OID}{SOD}$$

Question: An x-ray tube target having a 1.6 mm effective focal spot is used to image an object in a chest cavity estimated to be 8 cm from the anterior chest wall. If the radiograph is taken posterior-anterior at 180 cm SID, with a tabletop film separation of 5 cm, what will be the size of the focal-spot blur?

Answer: Focal-spot blur $= (1.6 \text{ mm}) \times \dfrac{8 + 5}{180 - (8 + 5)}$

$= (1.6 \text{ millimeters}) \times \dfrac{13}{167}$

$= (1.6 \text{ millimeters}) (0.078)$

$= 0.125$ millimeters is the focal-spot blur size

Remember: to minimize focal-spot blur, use small focal spot when applicable and position the patient so that the anatomy under examination is close to the image receptor.

The SID is usually fixed but should be as large as possible. High-contrast objects that are smaller than the focal-spot blur cannot normally be imaged.

The terms *penumbra* and *geometric unsharpness* were used in the past to describe focal-spot blur. These terms were borrowed from the scientific disciplines of astronomy and mathematics and have been replaced in radiography by the term *focal-spot blur.*

Heel Effect

The heel effect, introduced in Chapter 10, is described as a *varying intensity across the x-ray field caused by attenuation of x-rays in the heel of the anode.* Another characteristic of the heel effect is unrelated to x-ray intensity but affects focal-spot blur.

The size of the effective focal spot is not constant across the radiograph. A tube said to have a 1-millimeter focal spot has a smaller effective focal spot on the anode side and a larger effective focal spot on the cathode side (Figure 19-28). This variation in focal-spot size results in a variation in focal-spot blur. *The focal-spot blur is small on the anode side and large on the cathode side.* Consequently, images toward the cathode

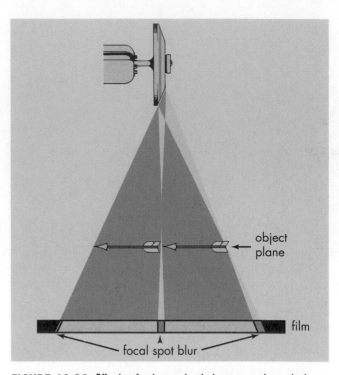

FIGURE 19-28 Effective focal-spot size is largest on the cathode side, and therefore focal-spot blur is greatest on the cathode side.

side of a radiograph have higher blur and poorer spatial resolution than those to the anode side. This situation is clinically significant when x-ray tubes with small target angles are used at short SIDs. Table 19-2 lists radiographic examinations that should be performed with the heel effect in mind.

SUBJECT FACTORS

The third group of factors affecting radiographic quality concerns the patient. These factors are associated not so much with the positioning of the patient as with the patient's size, shape, and tissue composition.

Subject Contrast

The contrast of a radiograph viewed on an illuminator is called *radiographic contrast.* As indicated previously,

TABLE 19-2		
Examinations that Can Take Advantage of the Heel Effect		
Examination	**Position Toward the Cathode (−)**	**Position Toward the Anode (+)**
PA chest	Abdomen	Neck
Abdomen	Abdomen	Pelvis
Femur	Hip	Knee
Humerus	Shoulder	Elbow
AP thoracic spine	Abdomen	Neck
AP lumbar spine	Abdomen	Pelvis

radiographic contrast is a function of the film contrast and the subject contrast. In fact the radiographic contrast is simply the product of the film contrast and the subject contrast.

Radiographic Contrast

Radiographic contrast =
Film contrast × subject contrast

Question: Film that has a film contrast of 3.1 is used to radiograph a long bone having a subject contrast of 4.5. What is the radiographic contrast?

Answer: Radiographic contrast = (3.1) (4.5)

= 13.95

In practice, however, subject contrast is difficult to determine quantitatively. Subject contrast can be determined based on the factors listed in the box below.

Several of these factors are discussed in Chapter 13 in their relation to the attenuation of an x-ray beam. The effect of each on subject contrast is a direct result of differences in attenuation in body tissues.

Factors Affecting Subject Contrast

Patient thickness
Tissue mass density
Atomic number
Object shape
Kilovoltage

Patient thickness. Given a standard composition, a thick body section will attenuate more x-rays than a thin body section (Figure 19-29). The same number of x-rays is incident on each section. If the same number of x-rays exit each section, the subject contrast would be 1. Since more x-rays are transmitted through thin body sections than through thick ones, subject contrast will be greater than 1. The degree of subject contrast is directly proportional to the number of x-rays leaving sections of the body.

Tissue mass density. Sections of the body may have equal thicknesses yet different **mass densities.** Tissue mass density is an important factor affecting subject contrast. Consider, for example, the radiograph of slices of an orange, kiwi, a piece of celery, and a chunk of carrot (Figure 19-30). The materials have similar thick-

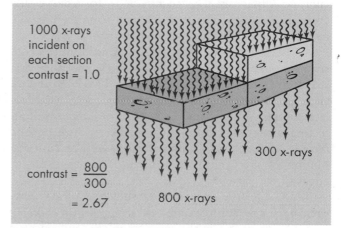

FIGURE 19-29 Variation in thickness of body part contributes to subject contrast.

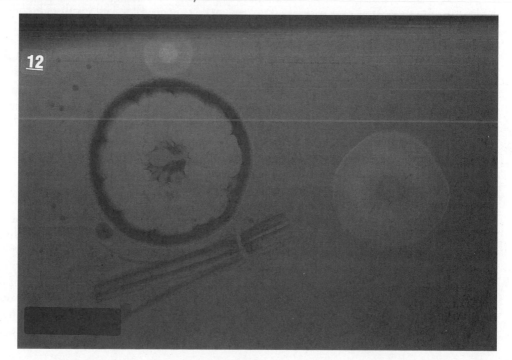

FIGURE 19-30 Radiograph of an orange, a Kiwi, a piece of celery, and a chunk of carrot shows the effect of subtle differences on mass density. *(Courtesy Marcy Barnes.)*

nesses and chemical composition. But because of the differences in densities, they will be imaged differently. The effect of mass density on subject contrast is demonstrated in Figure 19-31.

Atomic number. Another important factor affecting subject contrast is the atomic number of the tissue being radiographed. In Chapter 13, it is shown that Compton interactions are independent of the atomic number of tissue being radiographed, but photoelectric interactions vary in proportion to the cube of the atomic number. In the diagnostic range of x-ray energies the photoelectric effect varies because of kVp output. With higher x-ray energy, fewer interactions occur, so more x-rays are transmitted without interaction.

Shape of anatomy. The shape of the anatomic structure influences the radiographic quality not only through its geometry but also through its contribution to subject contrast. Obviously, if a structure had a form that would coincide with the shape of the x-ray beam there would be maximum subject contrast (Figure 19-32, *A*).

All other anatomic shapes have reduced subject contrast because of the change in thickness that they present across the x-ray beam. Figure 19-32, *B* and *C*, show examples of two shapes that result in reduced subject contrast. This characteristic of the subject itself affecting subject contrast is sometimes termed ***absorption blur.*** It reduces both spatial resolution and contrast resolution of any anatomic structure, especially at the edges of the part.

Kilovoltage. The magnitude of subject contrast, however, is greatly controlled by the kVp of operation. In fact, kVp is probably the most important influence on subject contrast, and the radiographer can learn to take advantage of optimizing subject contrast by changes in kVp.

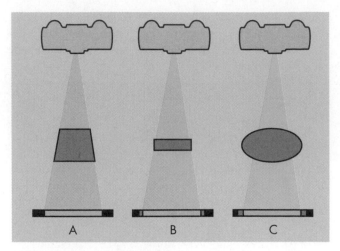

FIGURE 19-32 Shape of the structure under investigation contributes to absorption blur.

Figure 19-33 shows a series of radiographs of an aluminum step wedge taken at kVps ranging from 40 to 100. Low kVp results in high subject contrast, called *short-scale contrast,* since the radiographic image will appear either black or white with few shades of gray. On the other hand, high kVp results in low subject contrast, or **long-scale contrast,** since the radiographic image will display many shades of gray.

It would be easy to jump to the conclusion that low-kVp techniques are always more desirable than high-kVp techniques. There are two major disadvantages to low-kVp radiography.

As kVp is lowered for any radiographic examination, the x-ray beam becomes less penetrating and thus requires a higher mAs to produce acceptable optical density. The result is higher patient dose.

Remember: a radiographic technique that produces low subject contrast (higher kVp) allows for wide latitude in exposure factors.

Subject contrast can be greatly enhanced by the use of contrast media. The high atomic number of iodine (Z = 53) and barium (Z = 56) result in extremely high subject contrast. Contrast media are effective because they accentuate subject contrast through increased photoelectric absorption.

Motion Unsharpness

Movement of either the patient or the x-ray tube during exposure results in a blurring of the radiographic image. This loss of radiographic quality, called ***motion unsharpness,*** may result in repeated radiographs.

Normally, motion of the x-ray tube is not a problem. In **tomography** the x-ray tube is deliberately moved during exposure to blur the images of structures on either side of the plane of interest. Tomography is described in Chapter 22.

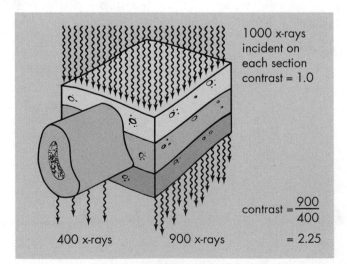

1000 x-rays incident on each section
contrast = 1.0

400 x-rays   900 x-rays

$$contrast = \frac{900}{400}$$
$$= 2.25$$

FIGURE 19-31 Variation in tissue mass density contributes to subject contrast.

TOOLS TO IMPROVE RADIOGRAPHIC QUALITY

The radiographer has the tools available to produce high-quality radiographs. Proper patient preparation, the selection of proper imaging devices, and proper radiographic technique are complex, related concepts. For any given radiographic examination, proper interpretation and application of each of these concepts must be made. A small change in one may require a compensating change in another.

Patient Positioning

Proper patient positioning requires that the anatomic structure under investigation be placed as close to the image receptor as practical and that the axis of this structure lie in a plane parallel to the plane of the image receptor. The central axis of the x-ray beam should be directed to the center of the anatomy. Finally the patient must be effectively instructed to hold still to minimize motion blur.

To be able to position patients properly, the radiographer must have a good knowledge of human anatomy. If multiple structures are being radiographed and are to be imaged with uniform magnification, the structures must be the same distance from the film. The various techniques that are described in textbooks on radiographic positioning are designed to produce radiographs with minimal image distortion and maximum image resolution.

Image Receptors

Usually a standard type of film-screen combination is used in imaging departments for a given examination. Generally, **extremity** and **soft tissue** radiographs are taken with the fine-detail film-screen combinations. For most other radiographs faster film-screen systems are used. The new, structured-grain x-ray films produce excellent images with limited patient dose when used with high-resolution intensifying screens.

The following general principles regarding these imaging devices should be considered when selecting the proper combination for any particular examination:

1. Use of rare-earth intensifying screens decreases patient dose by a factor of at least 20 times compared with direct-exposure film.
2. As the speed of the image receptor increases, spatial resolution is decreased and radiographic noise increases, which results in reduced radiographic quality.
3. Direct exposure x-ray film always results in lower contrast than screen-film combinations but is rarely used in modern departments, except for studies of arthritic pathology.
4. Low-contrast imaging procedures allow for a wider margin of error in producing an acceptable radiograph.

FIGURE 19-33 Radiographs of an aluminum step wedge, demonstrating change in contrast with varying kVp. *(Courtesy Eastman Kodak.)*

Patient motion is usually the cause of motion blur. Motion blur can be reduced by careful patient instructions by the radiographer: "Take a deep breath and hold it. Don't move." The most important factor in reducing voluntary motion is patient cooperation.

Motion unsharpness is primarily affected by four factors. By observing the guidelines listed in the box below, the radiographer can reduce motion unsharpness. Note that the last two items in this list have the same relation to motion unsharpness as to focal-spot blur. With the use of low ripple power and high-speed image receptors, motion has been eliminated as a common clinical problem.

Procedures for Reducing Motion Unsharpness

Use the shortest possible exposure time
Restrict patient motion by instructing the patient or by using restraining devices
Use a large SID
Use a small OID

Selection of Technique Factors

Before each examination the radiographer exercises judgment in selecting the radiographic technique factors of kVp, mA, and exposure time. The considerations that determine the value of each of these factors are complex and related. Few generalizations are possible. However, one generalization that can be made for all radiographic exposures is that the time of exposure should be as short as possible. Image quality is improved with short exposure times. One of the reasons three-phase and high-frequency generators are better than single-phase generators is that shorter exposure times are possible.

Remember: keep exposure times as short as possible.

Since time is to remain at a minimum, the selection of kVp, mA, and the resulting mAs may be considered.

The kVp primarily influences the quality of the x-ray beam, but it also has an effect on quantity. As the kVp is increased, the penetrability of the x-ray beam and the total number of x-rays emitted at any x-ray energy are also increased. The mAs affects only the radiation quantity. As mAs is increased, the quantity of radiation is increased proportionately.

The radiographer should strive for the most favorable radiographic contrast and optical density by exposing the patient with the proper quantity and quality of radiation.

The primary control of radiographic contrast is kVp. As kVp is increased, both the quantity and quality of radiation increases; more x-rays are transmitted through the patient so that a higher portion of the primary beam reaches the film. Thus kVp also affects optical density. Of those x-rays that interact with the patient, the relative number of Compton interactions increases with increasing kVp, resulting in less differential absorption and reduced subject contrast.

Furthermore, with increased kVp there is an increase in the percentage of scatter radiation and consequently higher fog density on the radiograph. The result of increased kVp is loss of contrast. When radiographic contrast is low, however, latitude is high, and there is greater margin for error in the selection of technical factors.

The principal advantages to the use of high kVp are the great reduction in patient dose and the wide latitude of exposures allowed in the production of a diagnostic radiograph. Figure 19-34 shows a series of chest radiographs that demonstrates the increased latitude that results from high-kVp technique. The technique factors are indicated on each radiograph. To some extent the use of grids can compensate for the loss of contrast accompanying high-kVp technique.

As mAs is increased, the radiation quantity increases, and therefore the number of x-rays arriving at the image receptor increases, which results in higher optical density and lower radiographic noise. The primary control of optical density is mAs. In a secondary

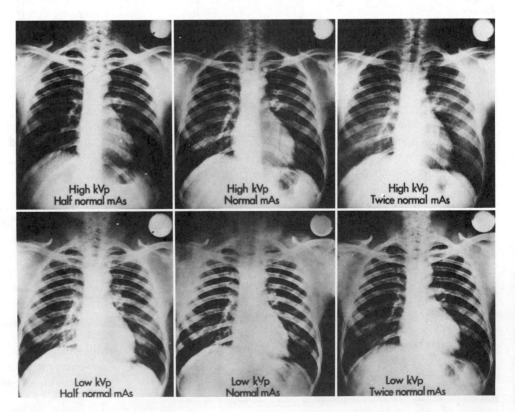

FIGURE 19-34 Chest radiographs demonstrating two advantages of high-kVp technique—greater latitude and margin for error. *(Courtesy Eastman Kodak.)*

way the mAs also influences contrast. Recall that maximum contrast is obtained only when the film is exposed over a range that results in optical densities along the straight-line portion of the characteristic curve. Low mAs will result in low optical density and reduced radiographic contrast. High mAs will result in high optical density and a loss of radiographic contrast.

A number of other factors influence optical density and radiographic contrast and therefore radiographic quality. A change in SID results in a change in optical density because x-ray intensity varies with distance. Adding filtration to the x-ray tube head reduces the intensity but increases the quality. Table 19-3 summarizes the principal factors that influence the making of a radiograph.

The most important resource for a radiographer when learning technical factors for radiographic examinations is the QC personnel within his or her place of employment. If they are not available, the representatives of the film-screen manufacturer can formulate accurate technique charts for each radiographic room. With the results of a few test films entered into a computer, the manufacturer's representative can prepare a print-out of a technique chart. The resulting chart may have to be fine-tuned with data from actual examinations but is generally accurate.

SUMMARY

Radiographic quality is the exactness of representation of the anatomic structure on the radiograph. Characteristics that make up radiographic quality are as follows:

1. High resolution or the ability to detect separate structures on the radiograph
2. Low noise or elimination of optical densities that do not reflect anatomic structures
3. Proper speed of the film-screen combination, which limits patient dose but produces a high-resolution, low-noise radiograph

These characteristics and three other factors combine, which results in a high-quality radiograph. The three factors are film factors, geometric factors, and subject factors. Film factors involve quality control in film processing and characteristics of film. The graph on semilogarithmic paper resulting from sensitometry and densitometry data of film optical density is the characteristic curve. The characteristic curve shows film contrast (slope of the straight-line portion), speed (determined on the log of relative exposure scale—fast speed film is to the left and slow speed film is to the right), and latitude (range of exposures in the diagnostically useful range of the characteristic curve). Geometric factors of radiographic quality involve preventing magnification and distortion, as well as using object thickness, position, focal-spot blur, and the heel effect advantageously. Subject factors that involve radiographic quality depend on the patient. A radiographer must prevent motion blur by encouraging patient cooperation. Also,

TABLE 19-3

Principal Factors Affecting the Making of a Radiograph*

	Patient Dose	Magnification	Focal-spot Blur	Motion Blur	Absorption Blur	Radiographic Density	Radiographic Contrast
Film speed	−	0	0	−	0	+	0
Screen speed	−	0	0	−	0	+	0
Grid ratio	+	0	0	0	0	−	+
Processing time and temperature	0	0	0	0	0	+	−
Patient thickness	+	+	+	+	+	−	−
Field size	+	0	0	0	0	+	−
Use of contrast media	0	0	0	0	0	−	+
Focal-spot size	0	0	+	0	0	0	0
SID	−	−	−	−	−	−	0
OID	0	+	+	+	0	0	0
Screen-film contact	0	0	−	0	0	0	+
mAs	+	0	0	0	0	+	−
Time	+	0	0	+	0	+	−
kVp	+	0	0	0	0	+	−
Voltage waveform	+	0	0	0	0	+	−
Total filtration	−	0	0	0	0	−	−

*As the factors in the left-hand column are increased while all other factors remain fixed, the cross-referenced conditions are affected as shown: +, increase; −, decrease; 0, no change.

by measuring patient thickness, recognizing tissue density, examining anatomy shape, and evaluating optimal kVp levels, a radiographer can create a high-quality radiograph. Finally, it is important for a radiographer and student radiographer to use as resources the following people knowledgeable in all aspects of quality control and quality radiographic imaging: (1) manufacturer's representatives and (2) quality-control radiographers.

REVIEW QUESTIONS

1. The exactness of representation of the anatomic structure on the radiograph is _____.

2. _____ is the ability to visually detect separate objects on a radiograph.

3. Contrast resolution is the contrast differences between _____ _____.

4. Radiographic noise is the undesirable _____ in the _____ _____ on a radiographic image.

5. Define quantum mottle.

6. MATCH
   Low noise, high resolution   Fast-image receptors
   High noise, low resolution   Slow-image receptors

7. Quality control in imaging departments refers to _____ and _____.

8. List the equipment used in sensitometry and densitometry.

9. What is the importance of processor quality control in an imaging department?

10. Have the manufacturer's representative help construct a characteristic curve from the data obtained from sensitometry and densitometry of a film-screen combination used in your department.

11. Using Table 19-1, solve the following problem. The intensity of light emitted by a viewbox is 1000. The intensity of the light transmitted through the film is 1. What is the optical density on the film? Will it be light, gray, or black?

12. In relation to contrast, when the characteristic curve shows a steep slope then there is _____ contrast on a film, when the characteristic curve shows a lesser slope there is _____ contrast on the film.

13. Base and fog densities on a given radiograph are 0.35. At densities 0.25 and 2 above base and fog densities, the characteristic curve shows log relative exposure values of 1.3 and 2. What is the average gradient?

14. List the factors affecting the finished radiograph in relation to film processing.

15. X-ray films *A* and *B* require 15 mR (3.9 C/kg) and 45 mR (12 C/kg) to produce an optical density of 1. What is the speed of each?

16. What are the three principal geometric factors that affect radiographic quality?

17. Calculate the inches for SIDs of 180 cm and 100 cm.

18. To minimize magnification of an anatomic part, use _____ and _____.

19. Distortion is caused by _____ and _____.

20. List and explain the five factors that affect subject contrast.

21. See Table 19-3 to complete the following exercise: justify each factor in the left-hand column in relation to the column headings (patient dose to radiographic contrast) in relation to the effect on radiographic quality.

Additional Reading

Eastman Kodak Company: *Introduction to Medical Radiographic Imaging,* Rochester, NY, 1993, Eastman Kodak.

Hedrich WR: Effect of quantum mottle on radiographic image quality, *Radiol Technol* 67(5):401, May-June, 1996.

Kattan KR: More on quality assurance (and ICUs), *Appl Radiol* 23(8):7, August, 1995.

Mosby's radiographic instructional series: radiographic imaging [slide set], St Louis, 1996, Mosby.

Nelson MT: Continuous quality improvement (CQI) in radiology: an overview, *Appl Radiol* 23(7):11, July 1994.

Pirtle OL: Study shows inconsistency in film processing quality, *Radiol Technol* 64(3):154, January-February, 1993.

Sprawls Perry Jr: *Minimizing radiographic blur,* Rochester, NY, Eastman Kodak.

20 Radiographic Exposure

OBJECTIVES

At the completion of this chapter the student will be able to:

1. List the four prime exposure factors
2. Discuss the relationship between mAs and kVp in relation to beam **quality** and **quantity**
3. Describe equipment characteristics that are secondary factors in changing the quantity and quality of the x-ray beam

OUTLINE

Exposure Factors
  Kilovolt/peak
  Milliampere
  Exposure time
  Milliampere seconds
  Distance

Equipment Characteristics
  Focal-spot size
  Filtration
  High-voltage generation

Exposure factors are a few of the tools that radiographers use to create high-quality radiographs of diagnostic value. Radiographic quality and its many components are discussed in Chapter 19. This chapter introduces the student radiographer to the factors that are under the radiographer's control—the prime factors. The prime exposure factors are kVp, mA, exposure time, and distance from source to image receptor (SID).

EXPOSURE FACTORS

Radiographic **exposure factors** are selected by the radiographer for the production of properly exposed film. **Kilovolt peak** (kVp) and **milliampere second** (mAs) are the exposure factors used to control x-ray quality and quantity. Focal-spot size, distance, and filtration are secondary factors that require consideration during all radiographic examinations.

Kilovolt Peak

The effects of kVp on the x-ray beam are described in previous chapters. For the purpose of understanding kVp as an exposure technique factor, remember that kVp is the primary control of beam quality and therefore **beam penetrability**. A higher quality x-ray beam is one with higher energy that is more likely to penetrate the anatomy of interest. With increasing kVp, more x-rays are produced, and they have a greater penetrabiity. Unfortunately, because they are of higher energy, they produce more scatter radiation as well. The kVp selected greatly determines the number of x-rays in the remnant beam and therefore the resulting optical density. Finally, and perhaps most important, kVp controls the scale of contrast on the finished radiograph.

Milliampere

Principally the mA station selected for patient exposure determines the number of x-rays produced and therefore the **radiation quantity**. Recall that the unit of electric current is the ampere (A). One A is equal to one coulomb (C) of electrostatic charge flowing each second in a conductor.

$$1 \text{ A} = 1 \text{ C/s} = 6.3 \times 10^{18} \text{ electrons per second}$$

Therefore when one selects the 100-mA station on the operating console, 6.3×10^{17} electrons flow through the x-ray tube each second.

Question: What is the electron flow from cathode to anode when the 500-mA station is selected?

Answer: 500 mA = 0.5 A

$= (0.5 \text{ A}) (6.3 \times 10^{18} \text{ electrons/sec/A})$

$= 3.15 \times 10^{18} \text{ electrons per second}$

The more electrons flowing through the x-ray tube, the more x-rays produced. This relationship is directly proportional. When one changes from the 200-mA station to the 300-mA station, the number of electrons flowing through the x-ray tube is increased by 50% and therefore so is patient exposure. A change from 200 mA to 400 mA would be a 100% increase or a doubling of the x-ray tube current and x-ray exposure.

Remember: changes in mA change x-ray quantity proportionately.

Question: At 200 mA the x-ray quantity is an **entrance skin exposure** (ESE) or patient dose of 752 mR. What will be the ESE at 500 mA?

Answer: $\text{ESE} = 752 \text{ mR} \times \dfrac{500 \text{ mA}}{200 \text{ mA}}$

$= 1880 \text{ mR}$ is the entrance skin exposure at 500 mA

A change in mA does not change the kinetic energy of electrons flowing from cathode to anode. It simply changes the number of electrons. Consequently the energy of the x-rays produced is not changed, only the number. Therefore x-ray quality remains fixed with the change in mA stations.

Often, x-ray units are identified by the maximum x-ray tube current possible. Radiographic units designed for private physicians' offices normally have a maximum capacity of 600 mA. The available mA stations may be 600 milliampere, 400 milliampere, 300 milliampere, 200 milliampere, 100 milliampere, and 50 mA. High-powered **special-procedures equipment** may have a capacity of 1200 mA. The available mA stations are those previously listed plus 1200 milliampere, 1000 milliampere and 800 milliampere.

Exposure Time

Radiographic exposure times are usually kept as short as possible. The purpose is not only to minimize patient radiation exposure but to minimize the unsharpness that can occur because of patient motion.

Remember: short exposures reduce patient motion unsharpness.

Radiation exposure of the patient is necessary to produce a diagnostic radiograph. Therefore, when exposure time is reduced, mA must be increased proportionately to provide the required x-ray intensity. On older x-ray units, exposure time is expressed in fractional seconds, whereas most modern equipment identifies exposure time in milliseconds (ms). Table 20-1 shows how the different units of time are related.

An easy way to identify an x-ray machine as either **single-phase, three-phase** or **high-frequency** is to note the shortest exposure time possible. Single-phase units

TABLE 20-1

Relationships Among Different Units of Exposure Time

Fractional	Seconds (s)	Milliseconds (ms)
1.0	1.0	1000
$\frac{4}{5}$	0.8	800
$\frac{3}{4}$	0.75	750
$\frac{2}{3}$	0.67	667
$\frac{3}{5}$	0.6	600
$\frac{1}{2}$	0.5	500
$\frac{2}{5}$	0.4	400
$\frac{1}{3}$	0.33	333
$\frac{1}{4}$	0.25	250
$\frac{1}{5}$	0.2	200
$\frac{1}{10}$	0.1	100
$\frac{1}{20}$	0.05	50
$\frac{1}{60}$	0.017	17
$\frac{1}{120}$	0.008	8

cannot produce an exposure time less than half a cycle or its equivalent $\frac{1}{120}$ of a second (8 milliseconds). Three-phase and high-frequency generators can normally provide an exposure as short as 1 millisecond.

The radiographer selects exposure time. It is always selected with consideration of the mA station. The mAs is the product of the exposure time and tube current.= mA

mAs

$$mA \times time = mAs$$

Milliampere Seconds *optical density*

Milliampere and time (seconds) are usually combined and used as one factor—mAs—in radiographic technique selection. Indeed, many x-ray consoles may not allow the separate selection of mA and exposure time; such units permit only mAs selection.

The mAs determines the number of x-rays in the primary beam, and therefore mAs principally controls radiation quantity in the same way that mA and exposure time do. It does not influence radiation quality. The mAs is the key factor in the control of optical density on the radiograph.

Question: A radiographic technique calls for 600 mA at 200 milliseconds. What is the mAs?

Answer: 600 mA × 200 milliseconds = 600 mAs × 0.2 seconds

= 120 mAs

mA and time are directly proportional. An increase in mA requires a corresponding decrease in time. Time and

mA can be used to compensate for each other. This is described by the following:

mA and Time

$$\frac{\text{Time (first exposure)}}{\text{Time (second exposure)}} = \frac{\text{mA (second exposure)}}{\text{mA (first exposure)}}$$

Question: A radiograph of the abdomen requires 300 mA and 500 milliseconds. The patient is unable to hold his or her breath, which results in motion unsharpness. A second exposure is made with an exposure time of 200 milliseconds. Calculate the new mA that is required.

Answer: $\frac{x}{300 \text{ mA}} = \frac{500 \text{ milliseconds}}{200 \text{ milliseconds}}$

(200 milliseconds)x = (500 milliseconds) (300 mA)

(0.2 seconds)x = (0.5 second) (300 milliseconds)

(0.2 seconds)x = 150 mAs

$$x = \frac{150 \text{mAs}}{0.2 \text{ second}}$$

$$x = 750 \text{ mA}$$

Or

$$\text{new mA} = \frac{\text{Original mAs}}{\text{New time}}$$

$$\text{new mA} = \frac{0.5 \text{ second} \times 300 \text{ mA}}{0.2 \text{ second}}$$

new mA = 750 mA

If the high-voltage generator is properly calibrated, the same mAs and, therefore, the same optical density can be produced with various combinations of mA and time (Table 20-2). Note how many different combinations of factors equal the same mAs.

Milliampere seconds is the product of x-ray tube current and exposure time. Since x-ray tube current is electron flow per unit time, mAs is therefore simply a mea-

TABLE 20-2

Product of Milliampere (mA) and Time (ms) for 10 mAs

mA	Times	Milliseconds	Seconds	Equals	mAs
100	×	100	$\frac{1}{10}$	=	10
200	×	50	$\frac{1}{20}$	=	10
300	×	33	$\frac{1}{30}$	=	10
400	×	25	$\frac{1}{40}$	=	10
600	×	17	$\frac{1}{60}$	=	10

sure of the total number of electrons conducted through the x-ray tube for a particular exposure.

$$\text{mAs} \times \text{seconds (s)} = \text{C/s} \times \text{s} = \text{C}$$

On modern x-ray equipment one can occasionally select only mAs rather than mA and exposure time. On some radiographic equipment the exposure factors are automatically adjusted to the highest mA at the shortest exposure time allowed by the high-voltage generator. Such a design is called a *falling-load generator.*

Question: A radiographer selects a technique of 200 mAs. The operating console is automatically adjusted to the maximum mA station, 1000 mA. What will be the exposure time?

Answer: $\dfrac{200 \text{ mAs}}{1000 \text{ mA}} = 0.2$ second = 200 milliseconds

Varying the mAs changes only the number of electrons conducted during an exposure, not the energy of those electrons. Therefore only the x-ray quantity is affected by changes in mAs. The relationship is directly proportional; a doubling of the mAs will double the x-ray quantity.

Question: A cervical spine examination calls for 68 kVp at 30 mAs and results in an entrance skin exposure (ESE) of 114 mR. The next patient is examined at 68 kVp at 25 mAs. What will be the ESE?

Answer: $\dfrac{25}{30} = .83$

$.83 \times 114 = 95$ mR

Distance

Distance affects skin entrance exposure (mR) of the image receptor according to the **inverse square law,** which is discussed in Chapter 5 in relation to electromagnetic radiation. The source-to-image receptor distance (SID) selected largely determines the intensity (mR) of the x-ray beam at the image receptor. Distance has no effect on radiation quality or kVp. The following relationship is derived from the inverse square law and is called the *direct square law* or *distance maintenance law.* It relates a change in mAs to a change in SID to produce the same optical density:

Direct Square Law

$$\frac{\text{mAs (second exposure)}}{\text{mAs (first exposure)}} = \frac{(\text{SID})^2 \text{ (second exposure)}}{(\text{SID})^2 \text{ (first exposure)}}$$

Question: An examination requires 100 mAs at 180-centimeters SID. If the distance is changed to 90-centimeters SID, what should be the new mAs?

Answer: $\dfrac{x}{100} = \dfrac{90^2}{180^2}$

$$x = 100 \left(\frac{90}{180}\right)^2$$

$$= 100 \left(\frac{1}{2}\right)^2$$

$$= 100 \, \frac{1}{4}$$

= 25 mAs is the new factor at 90 centimeters

When preparing to make a radiographic exposure, the radiographer selects specific settings for each of the factors described: kilovoltage, mAs, and SID. The control panel selections are based on an evaluation of the patient, the thickness of the anatomic part, and the type of imaging devices used.

Standard SIDs have been in use for many years now. For tabletop radiography, 100 centimeters is common. This was first recommended by Glenn Files in 1945 as 40 inches target-to-film-distance. Before that, first 20 inches (50 centimeters), then 25 inches (63 centimeters), and finally 36 inches (90 centimeters) was recommended. With advances in generator design and image receptors, even larger SIDs are anticipated. Tabletop radiography at 120 centimeters and chest radiography at 250 centimeters are now more common. The use of longer SID is based on achieving less magnification, less focal-spot blur, and improved spatial resolution.

EQUIPMENT CHARACTERISTICS
Focal-Spot Size

Most x-ray tubes are equipped with two possible focal-spot sizes. On the operating console, they are usually identified as large and small. Conventional tubes have two focal spots of 0.6 millimeter/1.2 millimeters or 0.5 millimeter/1 millimeter available. X-ray tubes used in special procedures or magnification radiography have 0.3 millimeter/1 millimeter focal spots. Most mammography tubes have 0.1-millimeter/0.4-millimeter focal spots. The smaller focal spots are called *microfocus tubes* and are designed specifically for imaging very small microcalcifications at relatively short SIDs.

For large anatomic parts and grid imaging, the large focal spot is used. This ensures that a sufficient mAs can be produced to image dense body parts. The large focal spot also provides for a shorter possible exposure time, which minimizes motion unsharpness and prevents filament burnout.

One difference between the large and small focal spots is the capacity to produce x-rays. Far more x-rays can be produced with the large focal spot. With the small focal spot, electron interaction occurs over a much smaller area of the anode. The resulting heat load of the small focal spot limits the capacity of the equipment to produce x-rays.

A small focal spot is reserved for fine-detail radiography in which the quantity of x-rays is relatively unimportant. They will normally be used during extremity radiography and in examination of other thin body parts. Changing the focal spot for a given kVp or mAs does not change x-ray quantity or quality.

Also, with the increased use of fast-imaging systems (400 to 800 speeds), small focal spot can be used more often with safety.

Filtration

All x-ray beams are affected by the **inherent filtration** properties of the glass envelope of the x-ray tube. For general-purpose tubes the value of inherent filtration is approximately 0.5 millimeters aluminum equivalent. The **variable-aperture light-localizing collimator** usually provides an additional 1 millimeter aluminum equivalent. Most of this is provided by the reflective surface of the mirror of the collimator. To meet the **required total filtration of 2.5 millimeter aluminum,** the manufacturer inserts an additional 1-millimeter aluminum thickness between the tube housing and the collimator.

Some x-ray units have selectable added filtration as shown in Figure 20-1. Usually the equipment is placed into service with the lowest allowable added filtration. Radiographic technique charts are formulated at the lowest filtration position. If any higher filter position is used, a radiographic technique chart must be developed at that position.

High-Voltage Generation

The high-voltage generation is determined by the type of x-ray apparatus available. It is important to understand how the various high-voltage generators affect radiographic technique and patient exposure.

Three basic types of high-voltage generators are available: (1) single-phase, (2) three-phase, and (3) high-frequency. The radiation quantity and quality produced in the x-ray tube are influenced by the type of high-voltage generator. Review Figure 9-25 for the shape of the voltage waveform associated with each type of high-voltage generator. Table 20-3 lists the percent ripple of various types of high-voltage generators, the variation in their output, and the change in the radiographic technique for two common examinations associated with each generator.

Half-wave rectification. A half–wave rectified generator has 100% voltage ripple. The radiation quality is the same as that for full-wave rectification, but the radiation quantity is only half. During exposure with a half–wave rectified generator, x-rays are produced and emitted only half of the time. During each negative half-

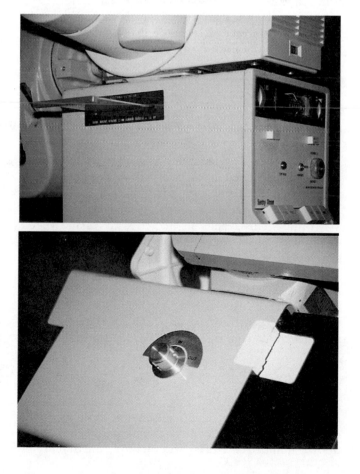
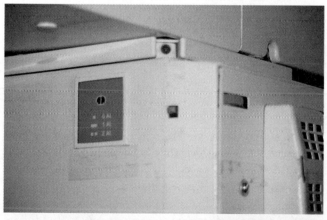
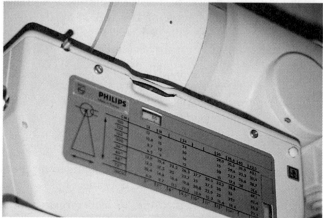

FIGURE 20-1 Four examples of selectable added filtration.

TABLE 20-3

Characteristics of the Various Types of High-Voltage Generators

Generator Type	% Ripple	Equivalent Technique (kVp/mAs) Chest	Abdomen
Half-wave	100	120/40	75/80
Full-wave	100	120/20	75/40
Three φ, six-pulse	14	115/6	72/43
Three φ, 12-pulse	4	115/4	72/30
High-frequency	<1	112/3	70/24

TABLE 20-4

Factors Influencing X-ray Quantity and Quality

Increase	Quantity	Quality
kVp	Increase	Increase
mAs	Increase	No change
mA	Increase	No change
Exposure time	Increase	No change
Distance	Decrease	No change
High-voltage generator	Increase	Increase
Filtration	Decrease	Increase

cycle of power, no x-rays are emitted. Some mobile x-ray systems and most dental x-ray units are half-wave rectified, but few general-purpose x-ray units have this type of high-voltage generator.

Full-wave rectification. The voltage waveform for full-wave rectification is identical to half-wave rectification except there is no dead time. During exposure, x-rays are always being emitted, although the emission is pulsed. The radiation quality does not change when going from half-wave to full-wave rectification, but the radiation quantity doubles. Consequently the required exposure time for full-wave rectification is only half that for half-wave rectification.

Three-phase power. Three-phase power comes in two principal forms, six-pulse or 12-pulse. The difference is determined by the manner in which the high-voltage step-up transformer is engineered. The difference between the two forms is minor but does cause a detectable change in x-ray quantity and quality. Three-phase power is more efficient than single-phase power. More x-rays are produced per mAs, and the average energy of those x-rays is higher. Consequently, three-phase power results in higher x-ray quantity and quality. The radiation emitted is constant rather than pulsed.

High-frequency generation. High-frequency generators were developed in the early 1980s and are increasingly used, especially with low-power x-ray systems. The voltage waveform is nearly constant with less than 1% ripple. This results in higher x-ray quantity and quality compared with the other types of high-voltage generators.

At the present time, high-frequency generators are being increasingly used with mammography systems and mobile x-ray machines. It is likely that most high-voltage generators of the future will be the high-frequency type regardless of the required power levels.

SUMMARY

Exposure factors (mAs, kVp, and distance) are used by radiographers to produce high-quality radiographs of diagnostic value. The exposure factors influence quantity (or number of x-rays) and quality (penetrability of the x-ray beam). Table 20-4 summarizes the effects of primary and secondary factors on the quantity and quality of the beam.

REVIEW QUESTIONS

1. kVp is used to control beam _____ and therefore beam _____.

2. mAs is used to control x-ray _____.

3. One ampere is equal to _____ of electromagnetic charge per second flowing in a conductor.

4. If the mA station on the control panel was changed from 100 to 200, the number of electrons flowing from the cathode to the anode would increase by _____ or would _____ the x-ray tube current and x-ray exposure.

5. Explain the following statement: mA does not change the kinetic energy of electrons flowing across the x-ray tube.

6. Why is it important to keep exposure times as short as possible?

7. Write three mA and second exposure factors that equal 100 mAs. Explain the advantages of each exposure factor choice.

8. An increase in mA requires a corresponding decrease in exposure time. Calculate the new technique of equal optical density using the following data. A hand technique of 100 mA at 50 milliseconds needs to be changed to 25 milliseconds, a shorter exposure time, to accommodate a pediatric patient. What will the new mA be?

9. What is the shortest exposure time available on single-phase, three-phase, and high-frequency radiographic equipment?

10. Using the direct square law calculate the following: an examination requires 150 mAs at 100-centimeters SID. If the distance is changed to 180-centimeters, what would the new mAs be?

11. Who first recommended the 40-inch target-to-film distance?

12. What are the two types of focal spots available in x-ray tubes? Explain how each is typically used.

13. Required total filtration for the x-ray tube is _____.

14. List the three types of high-voltage generators manufactured.

15. Using Table 20-3, make a list of the generator type and the percentage ripple.

16. Explain how a change in kVp influences x-ray beam quantity and quality.

17. Explain how a change in mAs influences x-ray beam quantity and quality.

18. Explain how high-voltage generation influences x-ray beam quantity and quality.

19. Explain how a change in filtration influences x-ray beam quantity and quality.

20. Assess the radiographic units at your clinical site(s). What filtration is used? What type of high-voltage generation are the units?

Additional Chapter Assignment:

Prepare a mAs and time chart for use in the routine diagnostic room at your clinical site.

Additional Reading

Eastman Kodak Company: *Introduction to medical radiographic imaging,* Rochester, NY, 1993, Eastman Kodak.

Mosby's radiographic instructional series: radiographic imaging [slide set], St Louis, 1996, Mosby.

CHAPTER 21 Radiographic Technique

OBJECTIVES

At the completion of this chapter the student will be able to:

1. List the four patient factors and explain their affects on radiographic technique
2. Discuss the four image quality factors of optical density, contrast, image detail, and distortion and how they are used to describe the characteristics of a radiograph
3. Identify the three types of technique charts
4. Explain the three types of automatic-exposure controls.

OUTLINE

Patient Factors
   Thickness of part
   Body composition
   Pathology
Image Quality Factors
   Optical density
   Contrast
   Image detail
   Distortion

Exposure-technique Factors
   Technique guides
   Automatic-exposure techniques

R

adiographic technique is the combination of factors used to expose an anatomic part to produce a radiograph. The radiographer needs to assess the patient factors, which include the anatomic thickness, body composition, and pathology. Image quality factors are characteristics of the radiograph that are considered the language of radiography. The image quality factors of optical density, contrast, detail, and distortion are the criteria that the radiographer uses to evaluate the quality of the finished radiograph. The prime factors, or exposure-technique factors, of kVp, mAs, and SID are the fundamental factors that the radiographer uses during the radiographic examination to correctly expose the radiograph.

PATIENT FACTORS

Perhaps the most difficult task for the radiographer is to evaluate the patient. The patient's size, shape, and physical condition greatly influence the required radiographic technique. The general size and shape of a patient is called the *body habitus*. There are four categories that describe body habitus (Figure 21-1). The **sthenic** patient is the average patient. Radiographic technique charts are based on the sthenic patient. The **hyposthenic** patient is thin and requires less radiographic technique. The **hypersthenic** patient is big in frame and requires more radiographic technique. The **asthenic** patient is very small and requires much less radiographic technique. Recognition of body habitus is essential to radiographic technique selection. Once body habitus is established then the thickness and composition of the anatomy is determined.

Thickness of Part

The thicker the patient, the more radiation required to penetrate through the patient to the image receptor. For this reason, the radiographer must use **calipers** to measure the thickness of the anatomy being irradiated. Patient thickness cannot be guessed visually.

Table 21-1 shows an example of how the mAs changes when patient thickness changes and the kVp is fixed.

Body Composition

The thorax and the abdomen of a patient may have the same thickness, but the radiographic technique used on the thorax and the abdomen will be considerably different. The radiographer must estimate the **mass density** of the anatomy and the range of mass densities of the anatomy being radiographed. Generally speaking, when only soft tissue is being imaged, low kVp and high mAs will be used. With extremities that have both soft tissue and bone, however, low kVp will be used because the body part is thin.

When imaging the chest, it is important to take advantage of the **high subject contrast.** Lung tissue has very low mass density, the bony structures have high mass density, and the mediastinal structures have intermediate mass density. Consequently, high kVp and low mAs can be used. This results in an image with satisfactory contrast for all anatomic parts and low patient radiation exposure.

These variations in tissue mass density are often described by their degree of **radiolucency** or **radiopacity** (Figure 21-2).

> Remember: radiolucent tissue attenuates few x-rays and appears black on the radiograph. Radiopaque tissue absorbs x-rays and appears white on the radiograph.

Table 21-2 shows the relative degree of radiolucency for various body habitus and tissues.

Pathology

The type of pathology and the degree of pathology influence radiographic technique. This is where the patient examination request form is necessary. The radi-

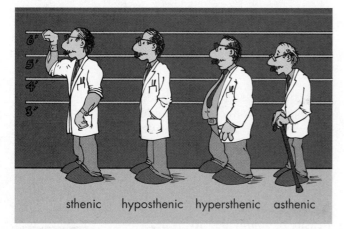

FIGURE 21-1 The four general states of body habitus.

TABLE 21-1
mAs Changes for Centimeters of Patient Thickness for an Anteroposterior Abdominal Examination

	Patient thickness	
kVp	in cm	mAs
80	16	12
80	18	15
80	20	22
80	22	30
80	24	45
80	26	60
80	28	90
80	30	120

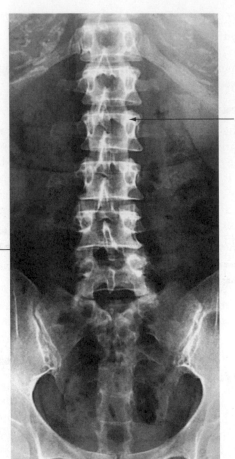

radiopaque

radiolucent

FIGURE 21-2 Radiolucent tissue such as fat and muscle appear black. Radiopaque structures such as bone appear white. *(Courtesy Mesa College Class of 1977.)*

TABLE 21-2

Relative Degrees of Radiolucency

	Body Habitus	Tissue Type
Radiolucent (Black)	Asthenic	Lung
	Hyposthenic	Fat
	Sthenic	Muscle
Radiopaque (White)	Hypersthenic	Bone

TABLE 21-3

Classifying Pathology

Radiolucent	Radiopaque
Active tuberculosis	Aortic aneurysm
Atrophy	Ascites
Bowel obstruction	Atelectasis
Cancer	Cirrhosis
Degenerative arthritis	Hypertrophy
Emphysema	Metastases
Osteoporosis	Pleural effusion
Pneumothorax	Pneumonia
	Sclerosis

ographer should not hesitate to seek more information from the referring physician, the radiologist, or the patient regarding the suspected pathology because pathology affects technique selection.

Some pathology is **destructive,** and causes the tissue to be more radiolucent. Other pathology can increase mass density or composition and cause the tissue to be more radiopaque. Practice and experience will guide your clinical judgment. A list of pathology classifications is shown on Table 21-3.

IMAGE QUALITY FACTORS

The phrase *image quality factors* refers to the characteristics of the radiographic image. Image quality factors include optical density, contrast, image detail, and distortion. These factors provide a means for the radiographer to produce, review, and evaluate radiographs. Image quality factors are considered the language of radiography and often it is difficult to separate one factor from another.

Optical Density

Optical density (OD), sometimes called **radiographic density** or simply **density,** is described as the blackening of the finished radiograph. Optical density can be present in varying degrees, from complete black, where no light is transmitted through the radiograph on the **viewbox,** to almost clear. Black is numerically equivalent to an optical density of 3 or greater, whereas clear is less than 0.2.

The blackening on the radiograph is a result of development of the silver-bromide crystals in the film emulsion. Film blackening relates directly to the amount of exposure received from x-rays, the conversion into visible light within the intensifying screens, and the film processing time, temperature, and chemical concentration.

Optical density is defined in Chapter 19 as follows:

$$OD = \log_{10} \times \frac{I_o}{I_t}$$

I_o is the incident light and I_t is the transmitted light.

Optical density is the logarithm to the base 10 of the ratio of light incident on a film (I_o) to the light transmitted through the film (I_t). Figure 21-3 shows a step-wedge radiograph. The amount of light transmitted through the radiograph is determined by the optical density of the film. This is discussed in more detail in Chapter 19.

In medical radiography most problems with images relate to the optical density of a radiograph being too dark or too light. A radiograph that is too dark has a high optical density resulting from **overexposure.** This situation is caused by too much radiation being converted to light in the intensifying screen and reaching the film.

A radiograph that is too light has been exposed to too little radiation, resulting in **underexposure** and a low optical density. Either of these conditions can result in unacceptable image quality, which may require that the examination be repeated. Figure 21-4 shows clinical

examples of the two extremes of overexposure and underexposure.

Optical density can be controlled in radiography by two major factors—**mAs** and **SID.** A significant number of problems would arise if one continually changed the distance from the x-ray source to the image receptor. Therefore SID is usually fixed at 100 or 180 centimeters for mobile examinations, 100 centimeters for table studies, and 180 centimeters for upright chest examinations. Figure 21-5 illustrates the change in optical density at these SIDs when other exposure technique factors remain constant.

When distance is fixed, however, as is usually the case, mAs becomes the primary variable technique factor that is used to control optical density. Figure 21-6 shows how optical density increases with increasing mAs.

Optical density increases directly with mAs, which means that if the optical density is to be increased on a radiograph, the mAs needs to be increased accordingly. When the optical density of the radiograph is the only characteristic that is to be changed, the appropriate factor to adjust is the mAs.

Optical density can be affected by other factors, but mAs becomes the factor of choice for its control. The mAs must be increased by approximately 30% to produce a perceptible increase in optical density. Less than that will not produce a visible change. As a general rule, when only mAs is changed, it should be halved or doubled (Figure 21-7). If at least a ½x or 2x change in mAs is not required, the repeat examination is probably not required.

An increase in optical density on the finished radiograph is accomplished with a proportionate increase in mAs, and the same is true for kilovoltage in a qualified manner. As kVp is increased, the quality of the beam is increased and more x-rays are able to penetrate the anatomic part of interest. This results in more remnant radiation exposing the image receptor.

Other qualitative factors change when kVp is used to adjust for optical density. This makes it much more difficult to optimize optical density with kVp. It takes the eye of an experienced radiographer to determine if optical density is the only factor to be changed or if contrast should also be changed to optimize the radiographic image.

Technique changes involving kVp become complicated. A change in kVp affects penetration, scatter, patient dose, and especially contrast. It is generally accepted that if the optical density on the radiograph is to be increased using kVp, an increase in kVp of 15% would be equivalent to doubling the mAs. This is known as the *fifteen-percent rule.* Figure 21-8 illustrates the optical density change when applying this rule. If only optical density is to be changed, the fifteen-percent rule should not be used because a 15% change in kVp will change image contrast.

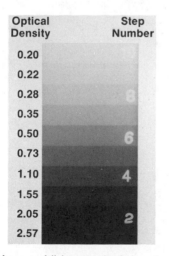

Optical Density	Step Number
0.20	
0.22	
0.28	8
0.35	
0.50	6
0.73	
1.10	4
1.55	
2.05	2
2.57	

FIGURE 21-3 Amount of light transmitted through a radiograph is determined by the density of a film. This step-wedge radiograph shows a representative range of densities.

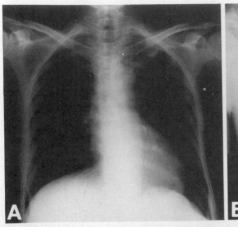

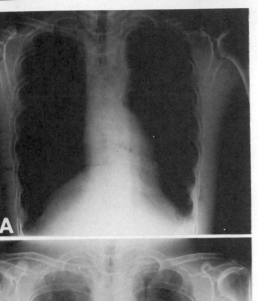

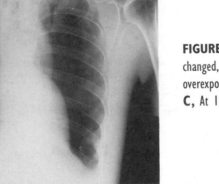

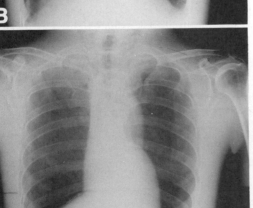

FIGURE 21-4 **A,** Overexposed radiograph of the chest is too black to be diagnostic. **B,** Likewise, underexposed chest radiograph is unacceptable because there is no detail to the lung fields.

FIGURE 21-5 **A,** If the exposure technique factors are not changed, a radiograph at less than 100-centimeters SID will be overexposed. **B,** A chest radiograph taken at 100-centimeters SID. **C,** At 180-centimeters SID the radiograph is underexposed.

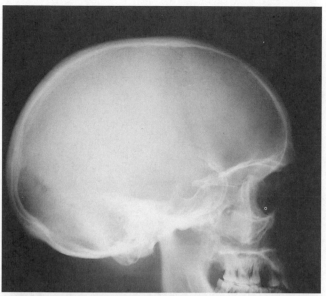

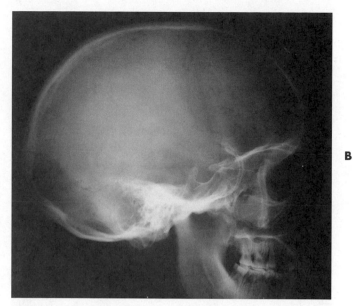

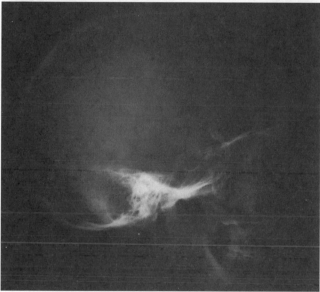

FIGURE 21-6 Optical density is determined principally by mAs, as shown by these lateral skull radiographs. **A,** 70 kVp/20 mAs. **B,** 70 kVp/40 mAs. **C,** 70 kVp/80 mAs. *(Courtesy Alex Backus.)*

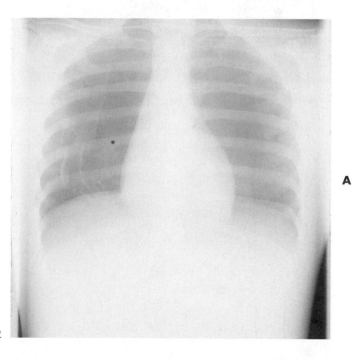

FIGURE 21-7 These chest radiographs illustrate the degree of change in optical density with changing mAs. **A,** 2.5 mAs.   *cont'd.*

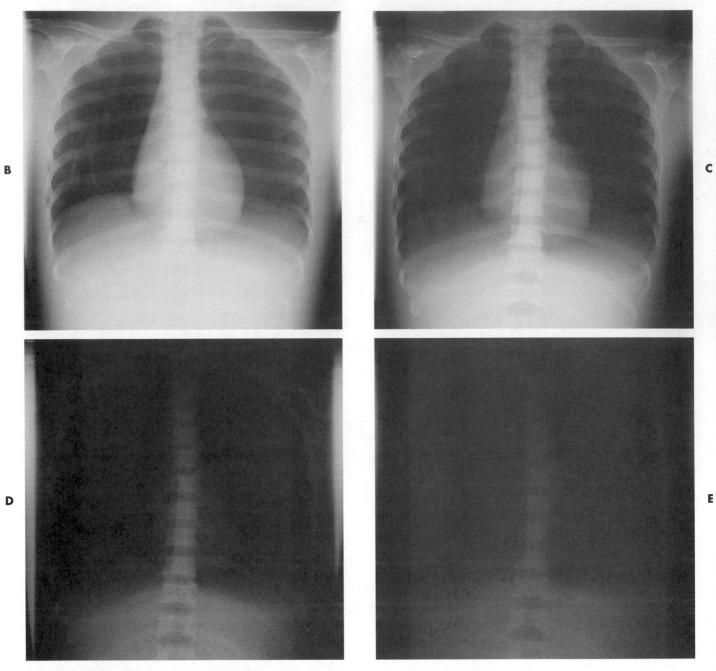

FIGURE 21-7, cont'd B, 5 mAs. **C,** 10 mAs. **D,** 20 mAs. **E,** 30 mAs. *(Courtesy John Lampignano.)*

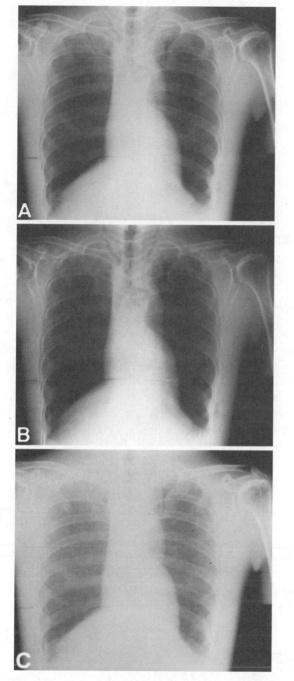

FIGURE 21-8 A, A chest radiograph taken at 70 kVp. **B,** If the kilovoltage is increased 15% to 80 kVp, overexposure occurs. **C,** Similarly, at 15% less, 60 kVp, the radiograph is underexposed.

The simplest way to increase or decrease optical density on a radiograph is to increase or decrease the mAs. This reduces other possible factors that could affect the finished image. The various factors that affect optical density are listed in Table 21-4.

Contrast

The function of contrast in the image is to make anatomic detail more visible. Contrast, therefore, is one

TABLE 21-4

Technique Factors Affecting Optical Density

Factor Increased	Effect on Optical Density
mAs	Increases
kVp	Increases
SID	Decreases
Thickness of part	Decreases
Mass density	Decreases
Development time in processor	Increases
Image receptor speed	Increases
Collimation	Decreases
Grid ratio	Decreases

of the most important factors in radiographic quality evaluation. The radiographer should be able to examine the finished radiograph and determine that sufficient contrast is present to produce the best possible image detail.

Contrast is defined as the difference in optical density between adjacent anatomic structures or the variation in optical density present on a radiograph. The difference in optical density between adjacent structures is the most important factor.

Figure 21-9 shows an image of a spinal column and pelvis and illustrates the difference in optical density between adjacent structures. High contrast is visible at the bone–soft tissue interface along the spinal column. The soft tissues of the psoas muscle and kidneys exhibit much less contrast, although details of those structures are readily visible. The low-contrast resolution of the soft tissues can be enhanced with reduced kVp but only at the expense of higher patient dose.

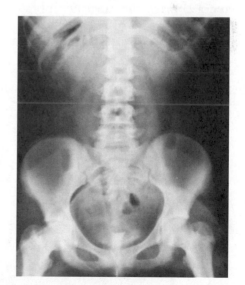

FIGURE 21-9 Radiograph of the abdomen showing the vertebral column with its inherent high contrast. The kidneys, pelvis, and psoas muscle are low-contrast tissues that are better visualized with low kVp.

Contrast on a radiograph is necessary for the outline or border of a structure to be visible. Contrast is the result of differences in attenuation of the x-ray beam as it passes through various tissues of the body. The penetrating ability of the beam is important, since relative penetrability among tissues determines the image contrast.

The penetrability of the primary x-ray beam is controlled by kilovoltage. Thus kVp becomes the major factor for control of radiographic contrast. To obtain adequate contrast, the anatomic part must be adequately penetrated. Penetration becomes the key to understanding radiographic contrast. Compare the radiographs shown in Figure 21-10. Figure 21-10, *A*, shows high contrast or short scale, whereas Figure 21-10, *B*, shows low contrast or long scale.

The terminology for describing radiographic contrast must be studied carefully. Consider the terms *short scale* and *long scale* of contrast. **Scale of contrast** means the range of optical densities from the whitest to the blackest part of the radiograph. For example, think of using scissors to cut a small patch to represent each optical density on the radiograph and then arranging the patches in order from the lightest to darkest. The result would be a scale of optical densities.

High-contrast radiographs produce shorter scales. They exhibit black to white in just a few steps. Low-contrast radiographs produce longer scales and have the appearance of many shades of gray. Figure 21-11 presents two radiographs of a step wedge, which demonstrates scale of contrast. The one taken at 50 kVp shows that only five steps are visible. At 90 kVp, all 13 steps are visible because of the long scale of contrast.

Often the radiographer is required to increase or decrease contrast because of an unacceptable image. To increase contrast, make the range of optical densities more black and white with a greater difference in adjacent structures. In other words, a radiograph with a

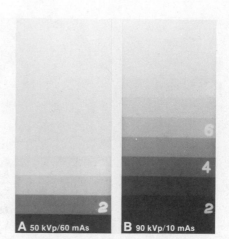

FIGURE 21-11 Images of a step wedge exposed at low kVp, **(A)** and high kVp, **(B)** illustrate the meaning of short scale and long scale of contrast, respectively.

shorter contrast scale will be produced. Accomplishing this requires a reduction in kVp.

To reduce contrast, one must produce a radiograph with longer scale contrast and therefore with more grays. This is done by increasing kVp. Normally a 4-kVp change is required to visually affect the scale of contrast in the 50- to 90-kVp range. At lower kVp a 2-kVp change may be sufficient, whereas at higher kVp a 10-kVp change may be required (Figure 21-12).

The phrases *high contrast, high degree of contrast,* and *a lot of contrast* all define short scale of contrast and are obtained by the use of low-kVp exposure techniques. **Low contrast** and **low degree of contrast** are the same as long scale of contrast and result from high-kVp exposure techniques. These relationships in radiographic contrast are summarized in Table 21-5.

In addition to kilovoltage, many other factors influence radiographic contrast. The mAs is a secondary influence on contrast. If the mAs is too high or two low, the predominant optical densities will fall on the shoul-

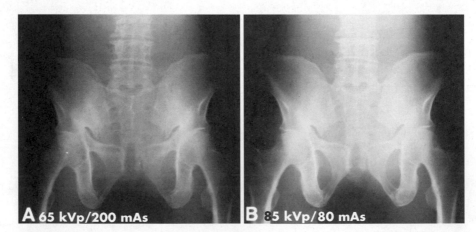

FIGURE 21-10 Radiographs of a pelvis phantom demonstrate long scale of contrast **(A)** and short scale of contrast, **(B).**

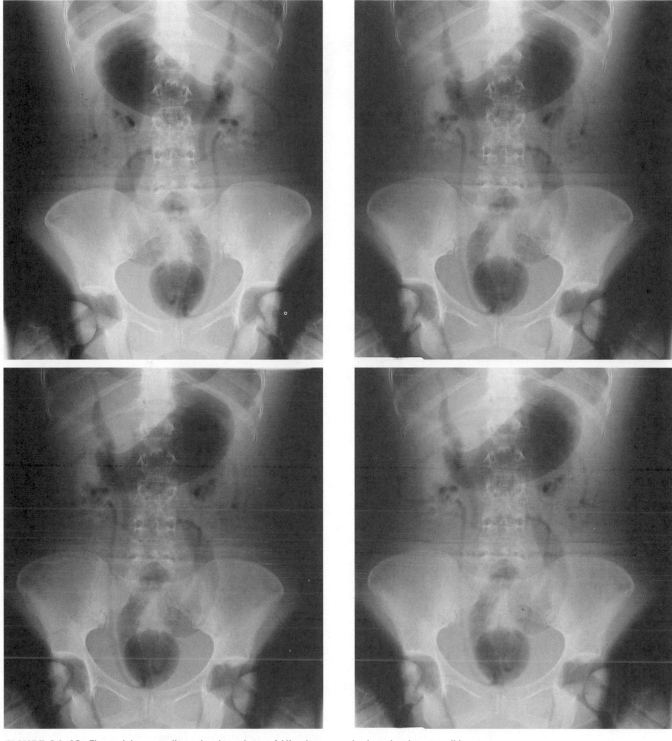

FIGURE 21-12 These abdomen radiographs show that a 4-kVp change results in a barely perceptible difference in contrast. *(Courtesy Lil Rossadillo.)*

cont'd.

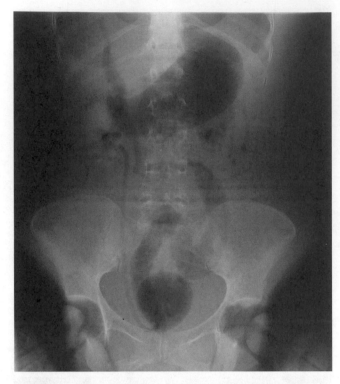

FIGURE 21-12, cont'd These abdomen radiographs show that a 4-kVp change results in a barely perceptible difference in contrast. *(Courtesy Lil Rossadillo.)*

TABLE 21-5

The Relationship Between kVp and Scale of Contrast

High Kilovoltage Produces	Low Kilovoltage Produces
Long scale	Short scale
Low contrast	High contrast
Less contrast	More contrast

der or toe of the characteristic curve, respectively. Radiographic contrast is low on the shoulder and toe regions because the slope of the characteristic curve is low in these regions. All structures look the same despite differences in subject contrast.

The use of intensifying screens results in shorter contrast scales when compared with nonscreen exposures. Collimation removes some scatter radiation from the radiograph, producing a radiograph of shorter scale contrast. Grids also help reduce the amount of scatter that reaches the film, thus producing radiographs of shorter scale contrast. Grids with high ratios will increase the contrast. The exposure-technique factors that affect contrast are summarized in Table 21-6.

A typical clinical problem faced by a radiographer is the adjustment of image contrast. An image is made but

TABLE 21-6

Exposure-technique Factors that Affect Radiographic Contrast

An Increase in This Factor	Will Result in the Following Change in Contrast
kVp	Decreases
mAs	Decreases
Development time	Decreases
Image receptor used	Variable
Beam restriction	Increases
Grid ratio	Increases

the contrast scale is either too long (too many grays) or too short (too much black and white). Usually it is the latter and a longer scale of contrast is required.

To solve such a problem apply the fifteen-percent rule. Increase the kVp by 15% while reducing the mAs by one half.

Question: A patient's knee measures 14 centimeters and an exposure is made at 62 kVp/12 mAs. The resulting contrast scale is too short. What should the repeat technique be?

Answer: Increase kVp by 15%

$$62 \text{ kVp} \times 0.15 = 9.3 \text{ kVp}$$

Therefore new kVp = 62 + 9 = 71 kVp

Reduce mAs by ½

$$12 \text{ mAs} \times 0.5 = 6 \text{ mAs}$$

Repeat technique = 71 kVp/6 mAs

A less abrupt technique compensation for a change in contrast scale may be required. An increase of 5% in kVp may be accompanied by a 30% reduction in mAs to produce the same optical density at a slightly reduced contrast scale. This is known as the *five-percent rule.* The proper technique compensation by the radiographer is a judgment call. The anatomic part, body habitus, suspected pathology, and x-ray image receptor characteristics must all be considered by the skillful radiographer. With practice and experience this will become routine.

Question: A modest reduction in image contrast is required for a knee exposed at 62 kVp/12 mAs. What technique should be tried?

Answer: Apply the five-percent rule.

$$62 \text{ kVp} \times 0.05 = 3.1 \text{ kVp}$$

$$62 + 3 = 65 \text{ kVp}$$

$$12 \text{ mAs} \times 0.30 = 3.6 \text{ mAs}$$

$$12 - 4 = 8 \text{ mAs}$$

Repeat technique = 65 kVp/8 mAs

Image Detail

The phrase *image detail* describes the sharpness of small structures on the radiograph. With adequate detail, even the smallest parts of anatomy are visible and the radiologist can more readily detect tissue abnormalities. Image detail must be evaluated by the following two means: (1) sharpness of image detail and (2) visibility of image detail.

Sharpness of image detail refers to the structural lines or borders of tissues in the image and the amount of clarity or blur of the image. The factors that generally control the sharpness of detail are the geometric factors discussed in Chapter 19—focal-spot size, SID, and OID.

Sharpness of image detail is also influenced by the type of intensifying screens used and the presence of motion.

To produce the sharpest image detail, one should use the smallest appropriate focal spot and the longest standard SID and place the anatomic part as close to the image receptor as possible. Figure 21-13 shows two radiographs of a foot. Figure 21-13, *A,* was taken with a 1-millimeter focal spot, and Figure 21-13, *B,* was taken with a 2-millimeter focal spot. The difference in sharpness of image detail is clear.

Visibility of image *detail* describes the ability to see the detail on the radiograph. Loss of visibility refers to any factor that causes the deterioration or obscuring of the image detail. For example, fog reduces the ability to see structural lines on the image. An attempt to produce the best defined image can be accomplished by using all the correct factors, but if the film is fogged by light or radiation, the detail present will not be fully visible (Figure 21-14). One might conclude that good detail would have been present but that the visibility of image detail was poor.

The assumption is that any factor that affects optical density and contrast affects the visibility of image detail.

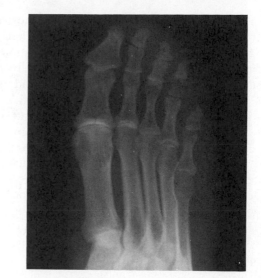

FIGURE 21-14 Same radiograph as shown in 21-13, *A,* except the visibility of image detail is reduced because of safelight fog.

Key factors that provide the best visibility of image detail are collimation, use of grids, and all other methods that prevent scatter radiation from reaching the image receptor.

Distortion

The fourth image quality factor is distortion. Distortion is the misrepresentation of object size and shape on the finished radiograph. Because of the position of the x-ray tube, the anatomic part of interest, and the image receptor, the final image may misrepresent the object.

Poor alignment of the image receptor or the x-ray tube can result in **elongation** of the image. Elongation means the object or part of interest appears larger than normal. Poor alignment of the anatomic part may also

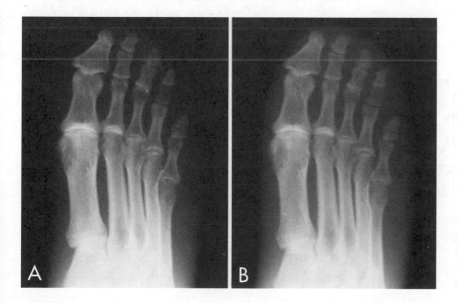

FIGURE 21-13 Radiograph **A** was taken with a 1-millimeter focal spot and exhibits far greater detail than **B,** which was taken with a 2-millimeter focal-spot x-ray tube.

result in **foreshortening** of the image. Foreshortening means that the anatomic part appears smaller than normal. Figure 21-15 provides examples of elongation and foreshortening. Many body parts are naturally foreshortened as a result of shape (e.g., ribs and facial bones).

Distortion can be minimized by proper alignment of the tube, the anatomic part of interest, and the image receptor. This alignment is fundamentally important for **patient positioning**. A discussion of these principles is presented in Chapter 19.

Table 21-7 summarizes the principal radiographic image quality factors. The primary controlling technique factor for each image quality factor is given, as well as secondary technique factors that influence each image quality factor.

EXPOSURE-TECHNIQUE FACTORS

Kilovoltage, milliamperage, exposure time, and source-to-image receptor distance (SID) are the principal exposure-technique factors. It is important for the radiographer to know how to manipulate these exposure-technique factors to produce the desired optical density, radiographic contrast, image detail, and lack of distortion on the finished radiograph.

Technique Guides

It is not necessary, however, to become creative with each new patient. For each radiographic unit a guide or chart should be available that describes standard methods for the radiographer to use to produce high-quality images consistently. Such an aid is called a *radiographic technique chart*. Radiographic technique charts are written tables that provide a means for determining the specific technical factors to be used for a given radiographic examination.

For a radiographic technique chart to meet with success, the radiographer must understand its purpose, how it was constructed, and how it is to be used. Most important, the radiographer must know how to make adjustments for body habitus and pathologic processes.

TABLE 21-7

Principal Radiographic Image Quality Factors

Factor	Controlled By	Influenced By
Optical density	mAs	kVp
		Distance
		Thickness of part
		Mass density
		Development time/ temperature
		Image receptor speed
		Collimation
		Grid ratio
Contrast	kVp	mAs
		Development time/ temperature
		Image receptor speed
		Collimation
		Grid ratio
Detail	Focal-spot size	SID
		OID
		Motion
		All factors related to density and contrast
Distortion	Patient positioning	Alignment of tube, anatomic part, and image receptor

When used properly, the radiographic technique chart allows for consistently good diagnostic images. The scale of contrast and optical density are more predictable than if no standard chart is used.

Radiographic technique charts can be prepared to accommodate all types of facilities. Historically the four principal types of charts are based on **variable kilovoltage, fixed kilovoltage, high kilovoltage,** and **automatic exposure.** The following three of these charts are in common use today: (1) fixed-kVp chart, (2) high-kVp chart, and (3) automatic-exposure chart. Each of these charts provides the radiographer with a guide in the selection of exposure factors for all patients and all examinations.

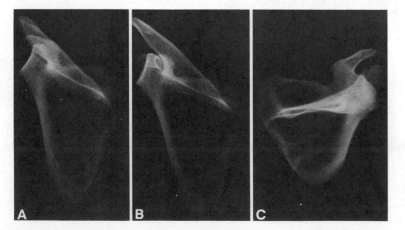

FIGURE 21-15 A, Normal projection of the scapula. **B,** Elongation of the scapula. **C,** Foreshortening of the scapula.

Most facilities select a particular type for use and then prepare similar charts for each radiographic examination room. The type of chart selected usually depends on the technical director of radiology, the type of equipment available, the screen-film combination, and the accessories available.

Radiographic technique charts and their use become an important issue in patient protection. Radiographers are required to use their skills in producing the best possible image with a single exposure. Repeat examinations serve only to increase the radiation dose to the patient. The preparation of these charts becomes an important and challenging task, and, once in use, the charts must constantly be evaluated and changed when necessary.

The preparation of a chart does not require that it be created completely from scratch. Many authors have guides that can be used in preparation of specific charts. It is important that radiographic technique charts from books and pamphlets not be used as printed. Each radiographic unit is unique in its radiation characteristics. Therefore a specific chart should be prepared and tested for each examination room.

Before the preparation of the radiographic technique chart begins, the x-ray equipment must be calibrated by a service engineer, and the processing system must be thoroughly evaluated. The total filtration also should be determined. Although 2.5 millimeters aluminum is the prescribed standard, one may find 3 millimeters aluminum total filtration or more available on the collimator housing. This significantly alters contrast and will make a considerable difference in any technique chart. The type of grid to be used should be known and the collimator or beam restrictor checked for accurate light field and x-ray beam coincidence. It is very important that all variables are reduced to a minimum. When a radiographic technique chart is found to be inadequate, all the above factors should be checked.

Variable-kVp technique chart. The variable-kVp radiographic technique chart, of historical interest only, used a fixed mAs and a kVp that varied according to the thickness of the anatomic part. Kilovoltage varied with the thickness of the anatomic part by 2 kVp per centimeter. The basic characteristic of the variable-kVp chart was the short scale of contrast resulting from the lower kVp values that were used. Generally, exposures made with this method provided radiographs of shorter contrast scale for small anatomic parts and variable scale of contrast for medium and large anatomic parts. With the anatomic part such as an abdomen, because of large variations in tissue thickness from patient to patient, there were varying scales of contrast. For example, the abdomen radiograph may have demonstrated short scale of contrast for asthenic patients using lower kVp and long scale of contrast for hypersthenic patients using high kVp. Radiologists tend to prefer similar scales of contrast for similar anatomic examinations or similar procedures.

There are approximate procedures for establishing a base kVp when beginning to formulate a variable-kVp technique chart. The beginning kVp depends on the voltage ripple as follows.

Beginning kVp = 2 × thickness of anatomy (cm) + 30 (single phase)

To begin preparation of a variable-kVp radiographic technique chart, select the body part for examination. For example, if the knee is chosen, use a knee phantom for all test exposures. First, measure the thickness of the knee phantom accurately, using a caliper designed for that purpose. Multiply the part thickness by 2 and add 30; this indicates a kVp with which to begin if the high-voltage generator is single phase. If the high-voltage generator is three phase or high frequency, 25 or 23, respectively, are the additive factors.

Question: A phantom knee measures 12 centimeters thick. What single-phase kVp should be used to begin construction of a variable-kVp technique chart?

Answer: 12 × 2 = 24

24 + 30 = 54 kVp

The kilovoltage setting for examination of the knee will be 54 kVp. The next task is to select the optimal mAs at this kVp. This will depend on the image receptor characteristics and effectiveness of scatter radiation control. For example, when using a 200-speed image receptor with an 8:1 grid, make test exposures at 54 kVp with 9 mAs, 12 mAs, and 20 mAs (Figure 21-16). Select the radiograph that produces the best optical density, or make additional exposures at other mAs values if necessary.

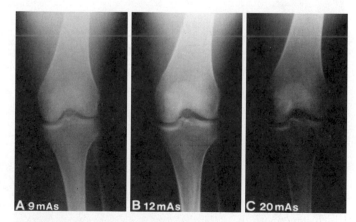

FIGURE 21-16 Radiographs of a knee phantom taken at 54 kVp. The radiograph obtained at 12 mAs **(B)** was selected to begin the variable-kVp chart.

The result of this exercise is the first line of the variable-kVp technique chart. The kVp and mAs to be used when radiographing a knee measuring 12 centimeters have been established at 54 kVp and 12 mAs, as shown in Table 21-8.

At this point the chart can be expanded to include knees with other thicknesses. To prepare a variable-kVp radiographic technique chart for other anatomic parts, the same procedure is used. When completed and ready to use on patients, one must be ready for some minor adjustments and continuing refinement of each chart.

Fixed-kVp technique chart. The fixed-kVp radiographic technique chart is the one used most often in modern diagnostic imaging departments. Developed by Arthur Fuchs, it is a method for selecting exposures that produce radiographs with a longer scale of contrast. In addition, fixed-kVp charts produce scales of contrast that are consistent within anatomic regions. The kVp is selected as the optimum required for penetration of the anatomic part. This usually results in somewhat higher kVp values for most examinations than with the variable-kVp technique.

Once selected the kVp is fixed at that level for each type of examination and not varied according to different thicknesses of the anatomic part. The mAs, however, is changed according to the thickness of the anatomic part to provide the proper optical density. For example, all examinations of the knee might require 60 kVp with mAs adjusted to accommodate for differences in thickness.

One benefit of this technique is that on average, the patient receives a lower radiation dose. There is greater latitude and more consistency with exposures of the same anatomic part. Measurement of the part is not as critical because part size is grouped as small, medium, or large. For most examinations of the trunk of the body, the optimal kVp is approximately 80. For most distal extremities, the optimum would be approximately 60 kVp.

To prepare a fixed-kVp radiographic exposure chart, the first step is to separate anatomic part thickness into three groups—small, medium, and large. It is also necessary to identify the range of thickness that is to be included in each group. Using the abdomen as an example, small might be 14 to 20 centimeters; medium, 21 to 25 centimeters; and large, 26 to 32 centimeters. For test exposures, use a medium-size phantom and begin with 80 kVp using varied mAs increments (Figure 21-17). Again, the optical density selected depends on the type of image receptor and available scatter-radiation control devices.

Once the proper optical density has been established, the chart can then be expanded to include small and large anatomic parts. For small anatomy, one should reduce the mAs by 30%. For large anatomy, one should increase the mAs by 30%. For a part that is swollen as a result of trauma, a 50% increase may be required. Table 21-9 presents the results of a representative procedure.

Fixed-kVp charts can also be calculated with specific mAs values for every 2 centimeters thickness. This approach is more accurate than the subjective *small, medium,* and *large* labels.

High-kVp Chart. The kVp selected for high-kVp charts is generally greater than 100. Examples of high-kVp radiography are radiographs for barium sulfate procedures using 120 to 135 kVp for each exposure. High-kilovoltage exposure techniques ensure adequate penetration of the barium.

This type of exposure technique could also be used for routine chest radiography to provide improved visualization of the various tissue mass densities present in the lung fields and mediastinum. Lower or more conventional kVp settings provide increased subject contrast between bone and soft tissue. When 120 kVp is selected for chest radiography, however, all skeletal tissue will be penetrated and the radiograph will exhibit all the different mass densities present.

To prepare a high-kVp chart, the procedure is basically the same as for preparing the fixed-kVp technique chart. All exposures for a particular anatomic part would use the same kVp. Obviously the mAs would be much less than that used for the fixed-kVp chart.

Test exposures are made using a phantom to determine the appropriate mAs for adequate optical density. Figure 21-18 shows a chest radiograph made at 120 kVp. Notice the improved visualization of the tissue markings of the bronchial tree and the mediastinal structures compared with the low-kVp radiographs of Figure 21-8. An additional advantage to using the high-kVp exposure technique is the reduced patient radiation dose.

AUTOMATIC-EXPOSURE TECHNIQUES

The appearance of the operating console of an x-ray machine is changing in response to our ability to

TABLE 21-8

Variable-kVp Chart for Examination of the Knee

Knee-AP/Lat	Part Thickness (cm)	Kilovoltage
mAs: 12	$8 \times 2 + 30$	46
SID: 100 centimeters	9	48
Grid: 12:1	10	50
Collimation: to part	11	52
Image receptor speed: 200	$12 \times 2 + 30$	54
	13	56
	14	58
	15	60
	16	62

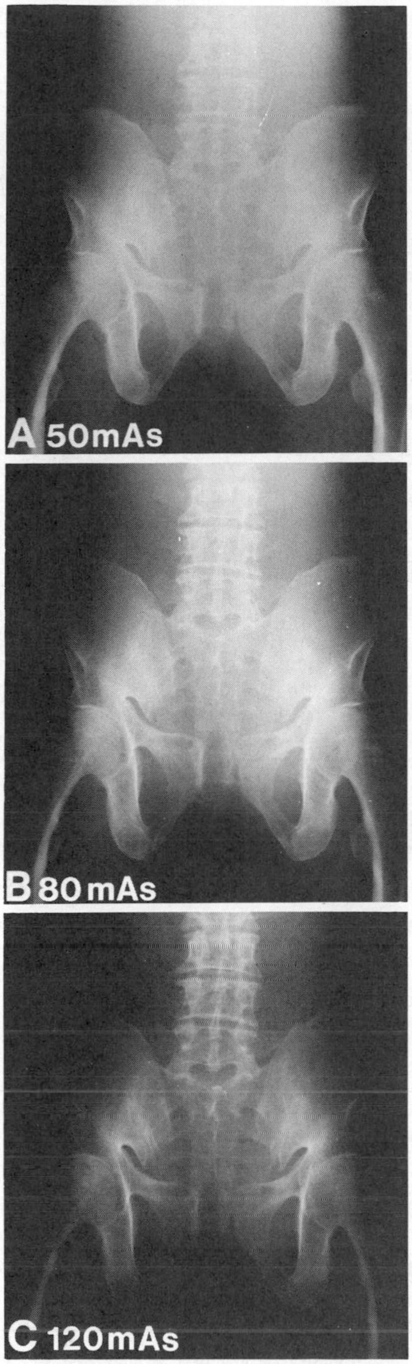

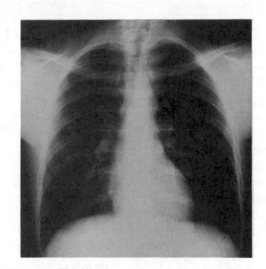

FIGURE 21-17 Radiographs of an abdomen phantom used to construct a fixed-kVp chart. All exposures were taken at 80 kVp. **B,** From this series, 80 mAs was selected to begin the chart.

TABLE 21-9

Fixed-kVp Chart for Examination of the Abdomen

Abdomen AP	Part Thickness (cm)	Required mAs
kVp: 80	Small: 14 to 20	50
SID: 100 centimeters	Medium: 21 to 25	80
Grid: 12:1	Large: 26 to 31	110
Collimation: to part		
Image receptor speed: 200		

FIGURE 21-18 High-kVp chest radiograph illustrating the improved visualization of mediastinal structures.

incorporate computer-assisted technology. Several automated-exposure techniques are now available, but the radiographer still has the responsibility of identifying certain characteristics of the patient and the anatomy to be imaged.

Computer-assisted automatic-exposure systems use an electronic exposure timer, such as described in Chapter 9. The radiation intensity is measured by either a photo cell or an ionization chamber and terminates the exposure when the proper optical density on the image receptor has been reached. The principles associated with automatic-exposure systems have already been described, but the importance of using radiographic exposure charts with these systems has not been covered.

Automatic-control x-ray systems are not completely automatic. It is incorrect to assume that because the radiographer does not have to select kVp, mA, and time for each examination, a less-qualified or less-skilled operator can use the system.

Generally the radiographer must use a guide for the selection of kVp and optical density setting. Sometimes only optical density as a function of patient size must be selected. The kVp selection is similar to that of the fixed-kVp method. Optical density selections are numerically scaled to allow for different thicknesses of the anatomic part.

Patient positioning must be accurate, and positioning must include anatomy to cover the photo cell. The specific body part must be placed over the photo-timing device to ensure proper exposure. However, if part of the photo cell does not cover anatomy and raw beam exposes the photo-timing device, the exposure will terminate prematurely. As a result, some body parts laying close to the edge of the body do not photo time accurately, for example, the clavicle. In addition to the accuracy in positioning, it is recommended that the anatomic part be measured before each examination for determination of the appropriate optical density selection.

The factors shown in Table 21-10 must be considered when preparing the radiographic exposure chart for an automatic x-ray system. The kVp is selected according to the specific anatomic part being examined. The optical density control is set according to the part thickness. The specific accessories to be used, such as film, screens, and grids, will determine to a great extent the previous selections. It is critical to ensure that collimation confines the x-ray beam only to the anatomic part under investigation or to the image receptor, whichever is smaller. Excessive scatter radiation will affect the response of the automatic-exposure control and reduce image contrast.

Photo timing. The earliest automatic-exposure system was the photo timer. The photo timer incorporates a device to sense the amount of radiation falling on the image receptor. Through an electronic feedback circuit the radiation exposure is terminated when a sufficient number of x-rays have reached the image receptor.

To image with the use of a phototimer, the radiographer selects the appropriate kVp, and the photo timer does the rest. Exposure will be terminated when the image receptor has received the appropriate radiation exposure.

Photo timers usually have two or three exposure sensors available for control (Figure 21-19). For instance, three radiation sensing cells may be available, and the radiographer is responsible for selecting which of the sensors to use for the examination. During a chest examination, if the mediastinum is the region of interest, only the central sensing cell will be used. If the lung

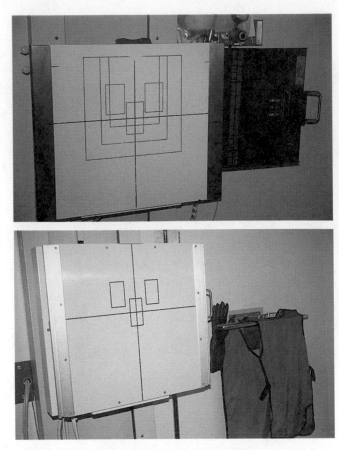

FIGURE 21-19 These vertical chest stands show the position of three independent photo timers. The additional dimensions indicate the standard image receptor sizes.

fields are of principal importance, the two lateral cells will be activated.

Most photo timers have a 2-second safety override. Should the photo timer itself fail to terminate the exposure, the secondary safety circuit will terminate the exposure at 2 seconds.

In addition to the selection of the exposure cells the radiographer will usually have a three- to seven-position dial labeled *optical density* or simply *density*. Each step on the dial is calibrated to increase or decrease the average optical density of the image receptor by 0.1. This control can be used to accommodate any unusual patient characteristics or to overcome the slowly changing calibration or sensitivity of the photo timer.

Programmed exposure. Microprocessors are being incorporated ever more frequently into operating consoles. A microprocessor allows the operator to digitally select any kVp or mAs, and the microprocessor will automatically activate the appropriate mA station and exposure time.

With falling-load generators, the microprocessor begins the exposure at a maximum value and then causes the tube current to be reduced during exposure. The

TABLE 21-10
Factors to Consider When Constructing a Radiographic Exposure Chart for Automatic Systems

Factor for Selection	Rationale for Selection
Kilovoltage	To select for each anatomic part
Density control	To adjust according to the thickness of part
Collimation	To reduce patient dose and ensure proper response of automatic exposure control
Accessory selection	To optimize the radiation dose-image quality ratio

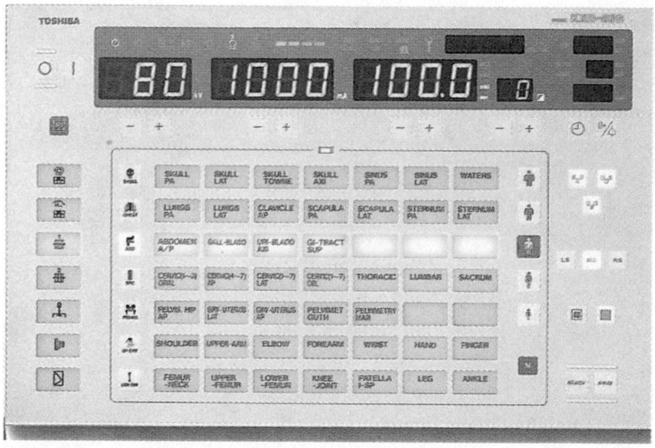

FIGURE 21-20 APR operating console with AP abdomen automatic exposure control selected. *(Courtesy Toshiba Medical Systems.)*

overall objective is to minimize exposure time to reduce motion blur.

Anatomically programmed radiography. The ultimate in patient exposure control is termed *anatomically programmed radiography (APR)*. APR also uses microprocessor technology. Rather than have the radiographer select a desired kVp and mAs, graphics on the console or on a video-touch screen guide the radiographer (Figure 21-20). To produce an image, the radiographer simply touches a picture, a written description of the anatomy to be imaged, and an indication of body habitus. The microprocessor selects the appropriate kVp and mAs automatically. The whole process is photo timed, which results in near-flawless radiographs. Thus fewer retakes are necessary.

The principle of APR is similar to automatic exposure with the radiographic technique chart stored in the microprocessor of the control unit. The service engineer loads the controlling programs during installation and calibrates the exposure control circuit for the general conditions of the facility. The radiographer need only select the part and its relative size before each exposure. The programmed instructions, however, must be continuously adjusted by the radiographer until the entire panel of examinations is optimized for best image quality.

SUMMARY

Radiographic technique is the combination of factors used to expose an anatomic part to produce a radiograph. Radiographic technique is characterized by the following three groups of factors: (1) patient factors, (2) image quality factors, and (3) exposure-technique factors.

Patient factors are the anatomic thickness, body composition, and the pathology within the human body. These factors affect radiographic technique. Body thickness is measured by calipers. The larger the thickness the more radiographic technique used, the smaller the thickness the lower the radiographic technique used. Radiographers recognize body habitus of sthenic, asthenic, hyposthenic, and hypersthenic as a way to determine body composition and thus proper radiographic technique. Pathology within the body may be either radiolucent, which may necessitate a decrease in technique, or radiopaque, which necessitates an increase in technique.

Image quality factors are the characteristics of the finished radiographs that define the quality of the image. The image quality factors are: (1) optical density, (2) contrast, (3) image detail, and (4) distortion. Optical density (OD) is the blackening of the radiograph and is defined as the log of the incident light over the transmitted light through the radiograph. Optical density increases directly with increases in mAs. A 30% change in mAs is required to produce a perceptible increase in optical density. Contrast is defined as the difference in optical density between adjacent anatomic structures. Because relative penetrability of the beam determines image contrast and penetrability is controlled by kVp, kVp becomes the major factor for the control of radiographic contrast. High kVp produces long-scale, low-contrast images, whereas low kVp produces short-scale, high-contrast images. Image detail is the sharpness of the image on the radiograph. To produce the sharpest image detail, use the smallest focal spot, the longest standard SID, and the least OID. Visibility of detail refers to the ability to see the detail on the radiograph. *Distortion* refers to the misrepresentation of object size on the radiograph. Table 21-7 summarizes the image quality factors and their primary and secondary influences.

The principal exposure-technique factors are kVp, mAs, and SID. The two most common technique charts for use by radiographers to produce consistently high-quality radiographs are the fixed-kVp chart and the high-kVp chart. The high-kVp chart is used for barium studies and chest radiographs with kVp from 120 to 135. The fixed-kVp chart uses approximately 60 kVp for extremity radiography and approximately 80 kVp for examinations of the trunk of the body. Even with automatic-exposure controls, radiographic exposure charts are required. It is recommended that the anatomic part be measured before examination even with automatic-exposure controls to determine the appropriate optical density selection. Anatomically programmed radiography uses microprocessor technology to program in the technique chart into the control unit. The radiographer selects an anatomic display of the part under examination, and the microprocessor selects the appropriate kVp and mAs automatically.

REVIEW QUESTIONS

1. What are the three groups of variables or factors that determine the quality of the finished radiograph?

2. How does body habitus affect the selection of technical factors?

3. Describe the two classifications of pathology and how technical factors may be affected by each classification.

4. Name the tool used to measure the thickness of an anatomic part when a radiographer is determining technical factor selection.

5. Radiopaque tissue such as _____ appears _____ on the radiograph.

6. How does the radiographer determine the type of pathology a patient may have before a radiographic examination?

7. List and define the four image quality factors that characterize the finished radiograph.

8. Write the formula for optical density (OD).

9. Identify the numerical equivalent range of optical densities from black to clear.

10. What is the relationship between optical density and mAs?

11. The mAs must be changed by _____ to produce a perceptible increase on optical density on the radiograph.

12. As SID is increased, OD _____.

13. Define contrast. Give an example of tissues with high contrast and an example of tissues with low contrast.

14. kVp determines beam _____.

15. High kVp produces _____ scale or _____ contrast, and low kVp produces _____ scale or _____ contrast.

16. List the three ways to produce the sharpest image detail.

17. Define elongation and foreshortening.

18. The primary controller of OD is _____, of contrast is _____, of detail is _____, and of distortion is _____.

19. List and discuss the four radiographic exposure charts.

20. The high-kVp chart is used for which two types of radiographic examinations? The fixed-kVp chart generally requires which two kVp ranges?

Additional Readings

Eastman T: Technique charts improve x-ray quality, *Radiol Technol* 65(3):183, January-February 1994.

Euganeo Kathleen D, Evantach Alan B: *Radiographic exposure and technique*, St Louis, 1992, Mosby.

Mosby's radiographic instructional series: radiographic imaging [slide set], St Louis, 1996, Mosby.

Warner R: Using technique factors to predict patient ESE, *Radiol Technol* 65(1):21, September-October 1993.

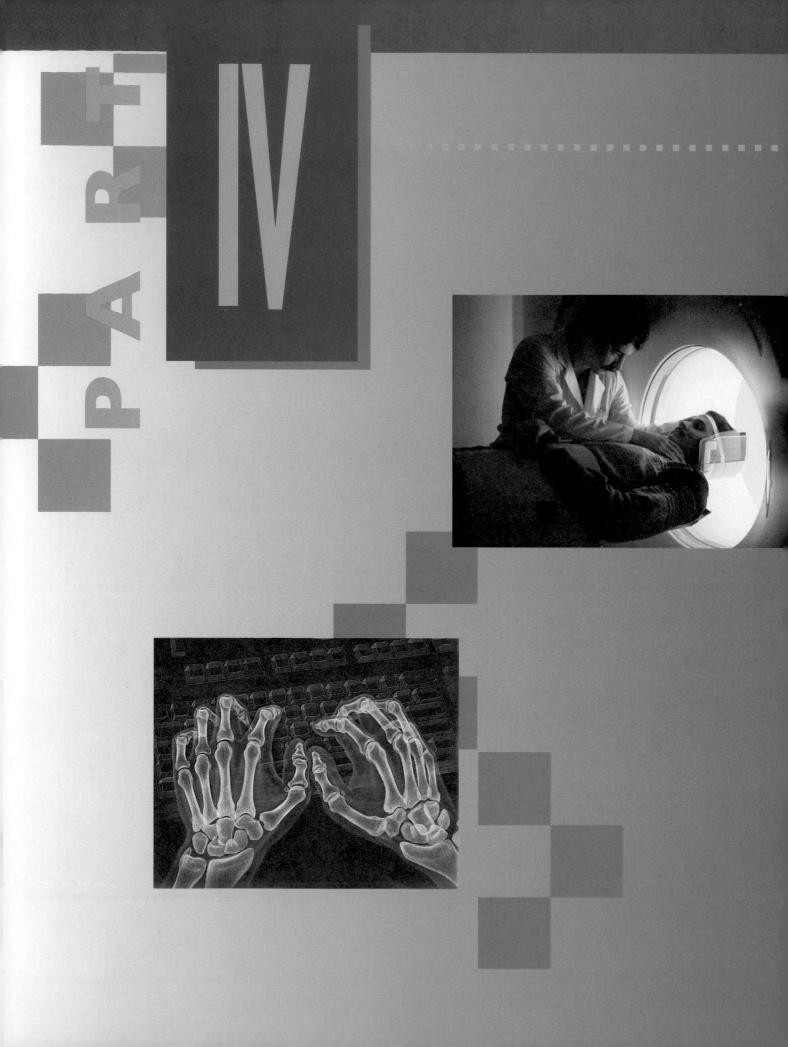

PART IV

SPECIAL X-RAY IMAGING

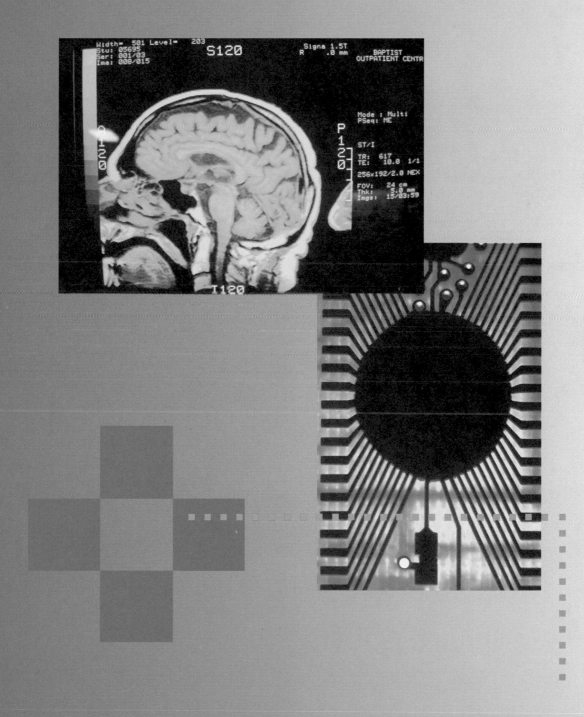

22 Alternative Film Procedures

OUTLINE

Tomography
    Linear tomography
    Multidirectional tomography
    Zonography
    Panoramic topography
    Practical considerations

Stereoradiography
    Making stereoradiographs
    Viewing stereoradiographs
Magnification Radiography

Many areas of x-ray diagnosis require special equipment and techniques to obtain diagnostic information. The equipment and procedures discussed in this chapter include tomography, stereoradiography, and magnification radiography. These x-ray examinations are not routine and therefore require the radiographer to be specially trained for these alternative film procedures.

TOMOGRAPHY

In a conventional radiograph of the chest or abdomen the images of all the structures on the film are seen with equal exactness. Although the images seem clear, the structures in fact are superimposed on one another. This superimposition can mask the structure of interest. When a diagnosis cannot be determined because of superimposition, the radiologist may order **tomography.**

Tomographic x-ray equipment appears similar to conventional radiographic equipment in most features. Note, however, a vertical rod fixes the x-ray tube head to the table Bucky device (Figure 22-1). The rod attachment is the feature unique to tomography, which links the tube to the radiographic image receptor to enable both to move at the same time.

The tomographic examination is designed to bring into focus only that anatomy lying in a plane of interest while blurring structures on either side of the plane. Actually the anatomy is not focused in the normal sense, but rather its radiographic contrast is enhanced by the blurring of the structures above and below.

Since the introduction of computed tomography (CT) and magnetic resonance imaging (MRI) with their excellent contrast resolution, tomography is less frequently used. Tomography is now applied principally to high-contrast procedures such as imaging calcified stones in the soft tissue of the kidney. Table 22-1 lists common linear tomographic examinations and related data.

One early attempt to reduce patient dose during tomography was a technique known as **simultaneous multifilm tomography.** During simultaneous multifilm tomography, a book cassette was loaded with four to six films in stacked fashion (Figure 22-2). The screen-film combination of each page of the book was adjusted so that optical density remained constant throughout. The separation of one film from another could be varied but was usually 0.5 to 1 centimeter. In effect, simultaneous multifilm tomography accomplished with one exposure the same objective that conventional tomography does with four to six exposures.

There are five basic types of tomographic movements: linear, circular, elliptical, hypocycloidal, and trispiral.

Linear Tomography

The simplest tomographic examination is linear tomography. During linear tomography (Figure 22-3), the x-ray tube is mechanically attached to the image receptor and moves in one direction while the image receptor moves in the opposite direction. With linear tomography, the x-ray tube and the image receptor remain in the same plane during motion (Figure 22-3, *A*). Equipment designed especially for linear tomography is constructed so that the x-ray tube and the image receptor move in arcs during the exposure (Figure 22-3, *B*). This arc method results in higher-quality tomographs; however, the equipment is expensive and has limited use.

Other aspects of the linear tomographic examination are shown in Figure 22-4. The **fulcrum** is the imaginary pivot point about which the x-ray tube and the image receptor move. The fulcrum lies in the **object plane,** and only those anatomic structures lying in this plane will be clearly imaged. The farther from the object plane an anatomic structure is, the more blurred its image will be.

The angle of movement is known as the *tomographic angle.* The tomographic angle determines the **section thickness,** which is the thickness of tissue that will not be blurred. The determination of the section thickness is made by selecting the proper tomographic angle. The plane of the section is determined by adjusting the height of the x-ray tube from the table or by repositioning the patient between exposures with an adjustable table.

Figure 22-5 illustrates how anatomic structures in the object plane are imaged while structures above and below this plane are not. The examination begins with the x-ray tube and the image receptor positioned on opposite sides of the fulcrum. The exposure begins as the

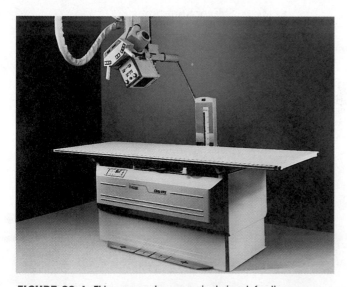

FIGURE 22-1 This tomography system is designed for linear movement. *(Courtesy Picker International.)*

TABLE 22-1

Linear Tomography

Examination	Projection	Tube Movement	kVp	mAs*	Slice Thickness
Cervical spine	Anteroposterior	Linear	approximately 75		3 to 5 millimeters
	Lateral	Thin cut	approximately 75		2 millimeters
Thoracic spine	Anteroposterior	Linear	approximately 75		5 millimeters
Lumbar spine	Anteroposterior	Linear	approximately 75		5 millimeters
Chest	Anteroposterior	Linear	approximately 90		2 to 5 centimeters
Intravenous pyelogram	Anteroposterior	Linear	approximately 75		1 centimeter
Wrist	Anteroposterior	Linear	approximately 60		2 millimeters

*Usually automatic exposure control

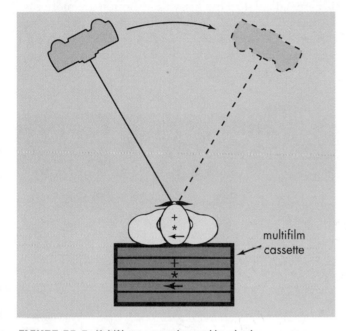

FIGURE 22-2 Multifilm tomography provides simultaneous tomographic views of different object planes within the body.

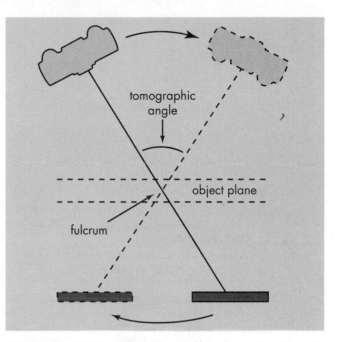

FIGURE 22-4 Relationship of fulcrum, object plane, and tomographic angle.

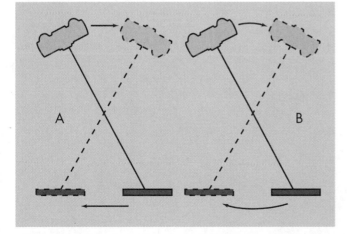

FIGURE 22-3 **A,** Cassette tray and tube head of a general-purpose x-ray table altered for tomography to move in a plane. **B,** Tray and tube of a table designed specifically for tomography to move in an arc.

x-ray tube and image receptor move simultaneously in opposite directions. The image of an anatomic structure lying in the object plane, such as the arrow, will have a fixed position on the radiograph throughout the tube travel. The images of structures lying above or below the object plane, such as the ball and box, will have varying positions on the image receptor, according to the tomographic movement. Consequently the ball and box in Figure 22-5 will be blurred. The larger the tomographic angle, the more blurred the images of structures above and below the object plane appear. The farther from the object plane an anatomic structure is, the more blurred it will be.

The blurring of anatomic structures lying outside the object plane is simply an example of **motion blur** or **unsharpness** caused by the moving x-ray tube. In theory, only objects lying precisely in the object plane—the

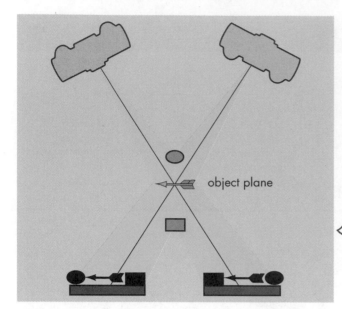

FIGURE 22-5 Only objects lying in the object plane are properly imaged. Objects on either side of this plane are blurred because they are imaged across the film.

plane of the fulcrum—will be clearly imaged. Objects lying outside this plane exhibit increasing motion blur with increasing distance from the object plane. Objects within a section of tissue between two parallel planes are in focus. This thickness of tissue that will be imaged is called the ***tomographic layer.***

The section thickness is controlled by the tomographic angle. The larger the tomographic angle, the

thinner the section (Figure 22-6). Table 22-2 shows the relationship between tomographic angle and section thickness. Figure 22-7 graphically shows this relationship. When the tomographic angle is very small (e.g., 0 degrees), the section thickness is the entire anatomic structure. This would be a conventional radiograph. When the tomographic angle is 10 degrees, the section thickness is approximately 6 millimeters. Structures lying farther than approximately 3 millimeters from the object plane will appear blurred.

Linear anatomic structures will be imaged better if they are positioned with their length parallel to the x-ray tube motion. This is illustrated with a tomographic phantom (Figure 22-8). Linear structures that lie perpendicular to the x-ray tube motion are more easily blurred. Figure 22-9 shows this effect in foot tomograms taken parallel to the long axis of the patient and perpendicular to the long axis of the patient.

TABLE 22-2

Approximate Values for Section Thickness During Linear Tomography as a Function of Tomographic Angle

Tomographic Angle (degrees)	Section Thickness (mm)
0	Infinity
2	31
4	16
6	11
10	6
20	3
35	2
50	1

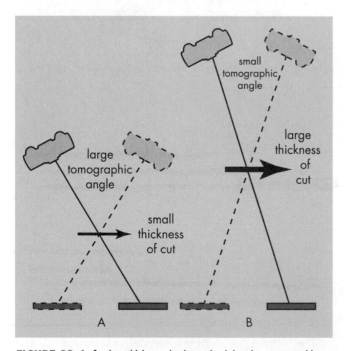

FIGURE 22-6 Section thickness is determined by the tomographic angle. **A,** A large tomographic angle results in a small thickness of cut. **B,** A small tomographic angle results in a large thickness of cut.

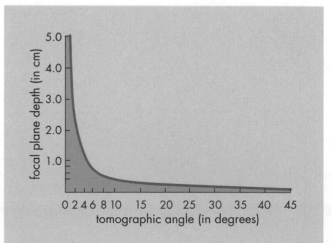

FIGURE 22-7 Section thickness becomes thinner as the tomographic angle is increased.

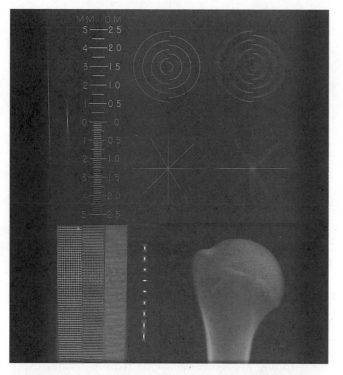

FIGURE 22-8 This phantom image shows increased blur of objects perpendicular to the motion of the x-ray tube. *(Courtesy Sharon Glazer.)*

Multidirectional Tomography

Linear tomograms sometimes appear streaked. This occurs when linear structures such as long bones lie outside the object plane and are oriented in the direction of x-ray tube and image-receptor movement. Another disadvantage of linear tomography is that the in-focus section is not very distinct and the degree of blurring varies over the radiograph. This effect occurs during large-angle tomography because the distance from x-ray tube to the patient and the angulation of the x-ray beam change during exposure. A lack of uniform optical density across the radiograph results. If sharper tomograms are needed, a multidirectional motion is necessary.

Actually a tomogram can be produced if the x-ray tube and image receptor move synchronously in any pattern or direction. Because of engineering considerations, the following four multidirectional movements are used: (1) circular, (2) elliptical, (3) hypocycloidal, and (4) trispiral (Figure 22-10). For a given tomographic angle, the hypocycloidal and trispiral movements will result in the sharpest tomographic image. The circular tomographic movement is the poorest of the four, but it is considerably better than linear tomography for the production of sharp, thin-sectioned tomograms. These multidirectional tomography units, however, are out-of-date and have been replaced by computed tomography and magnetic resonance imaging.

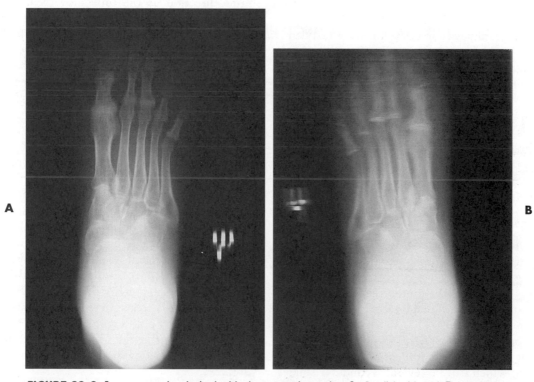

FIGURE 22-9 Foot tomographs obtained with the x-ray tube motion. **A,** Parallel with and **B,** perpendicular to the long axis of the patient. *(Courtesy Cheryl Pressley.)*

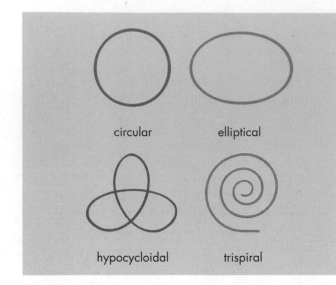

FIGURE 22-10 Multidirectional tomography movements for tube head and film tray.

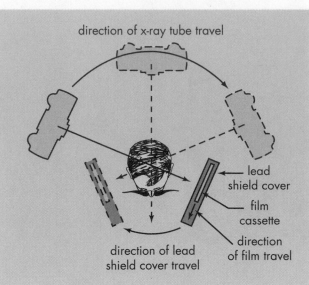

FIGURE 22-11 The x-ray source-image receptor motion for panoramic tomography.

Zonography

If the tomographic angle is less than about 10 degrees, the section thickness will be quite large (Table 22-2). This type of tomography is called **zonography** because a relatively large zone of tissue is imaged. Zonography is used when the subject contrast is so low that thin-section tomography would result in a poor image. Zonography is used for chest examinations with tomographic angles of 1 to 5 degrees.

Panoramic Tomography

Panoramic tomography was first developed for fast dental surveys. Recently, panoramic examinations have been done of curved bony structures of the head like the mandible. For this procedure the x-ray tube and image receptor move around the head as shown in Figure 22-11. The x-ray beam is collimated to a slit and the image receptor is likewise slit collimated. During the examination, the image receptor rotates to expose the entire length of the film and revolves around the patient with the slit collimator exposing the film. Figure 22-12 is an example of the panoramic image.

Practical Considerations

The principal advantage to tomography is **improved radiographic contrast.** By blurring overlying and underlying tissues, the subject contrast of tissue of the tomographic layer is enhanced. The more irregular the movement of the x-ray tube and image receptor, the greater the contrast enhancement.

The principal disadvantage of tomography is increased patient dose. The x-ray tube is on during the entire tube travel, which can be several seconds. A single **nephrotomographic** exposure, for example, can result in a patient dose of 1000 mrad (10 mGy). Furthermore,

most tomographic examinations require several exposures to make certain that the area of interest is imaged. A 16-film tomographic examination can result in a patient dose of several rad.

Grids are used during a tomographic examination for the same reason that they are used during conventional radiography. During tomography, linear grids must be used, and the grid lines must be oriented in the same direction as the tube movement. For linear tomography, this usually means that the grid will be positioned with its grid lines parallel with the length of the table. For multidirectional tomography, the grid must change with the movement of the tube head (Figure 22-13) while the image receptor remains fixed. During multidirectional tomography, the grid rotates over the image receptor.

STEREORADIOGRAPHY

During the early part of the twentieth century, the **stereoscope** was a popular device (Figure 22-14). When two photographs are inserted, the stereoscope provides great depth perception. Today the use of a stereoscope is mostly limited to children's toys.

Similarly, **stereoradiography** was popular in imaging departments. Today its use is limited. Stereoradiography involves making two radiographs of the same object and viewing them stereoscopically. The viewing is done with a specially constructed stereoscope that allows each eye to view a different radiograph. Stereoradiography provides a three-dimensional image instead of the flat image obtained with conventional radiography (Figure 22-15).

Stereoradiography can be particularly helpful in locating **foreign bodies** and identifying calcified lesions in

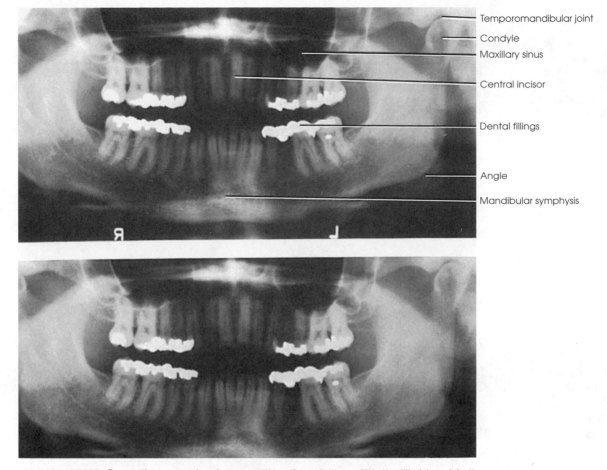

Temporomandibular joint

Condyle

Maxillary sinus

Central incisor

Dental fillings

Angle

Mandibular symphysis

FIGURE 22-12 Panoramic tomography of the mandible. *(From Ballinger PW: Merrill's Atlas of Radiographic positions and radiologic procedures, vol 2, ed 8, St Louis, 1995, Mosby.)*

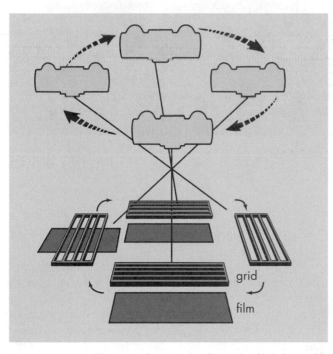

grid

film

FIGURE 22-13 Movement of x-ray tube, film, and grid during multidirectional tomography.

dense or thick body sections where interpretation of conventional radiographs might be difficult. Stereoradiography also provides information on the location of internal body structures.

The principal disadvantage of stereoradiography is that it requires twice the patient exposure. Additionally, it takes practice to produce good stereoradiographs, and considerable patient cooperation is required. Three-dimensional computed tomography and magnetic resonance images have largely replaced stereoradiography.

Making Stereoradiographs

Stereoradiographs involve the exposure of two films with the x-ray tube shifted in position between the two. The radiographer must carefully shift the tube to produce a good stereoradiograph.

The tube shift depends on a number of factors, principally the SID, the viewing distance, and the **interpupillary** distance. These factors are interrelated. A good rule of thumb assumes an interpupillary distance of 65 millimeters and a viewing distance of approximately 65 centimeters. These values are in the ratio of 1:10. One to ten is approximately what the ratio of the

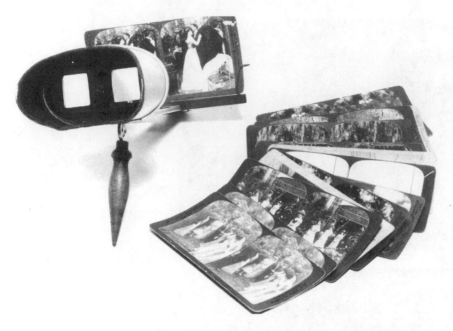

FIGURE 22-14 Early twentieth-century stereoscopes. (Courtesy Sharon Briney-Glaze.)

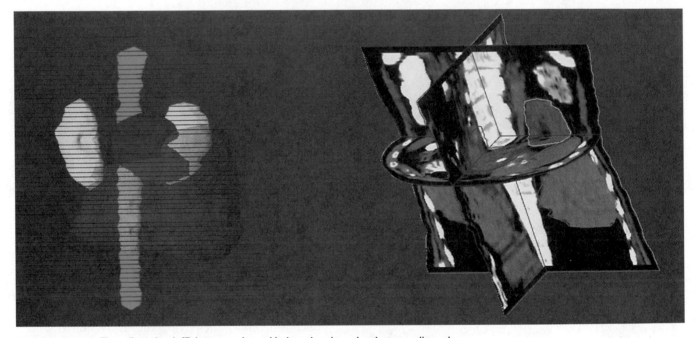

FIGURE 22-15 Three-dimensional CT images such as this have largely replaced stereoradiography. *(Courtesy Randall Ten Haken.)*

tube shift to SID should be (Figure 22-16). To calculate the degree of tube shift, use the following formula:

$$\text{Tube shift} = 0.1 \times \text{SID}$$

Question: Chest stereoradiographs are made at 180-centimeters SID. What should the amount of tube shift on either side of the midline be?

Answer: Tube shift = 0.1 × 180 centimeters

= 18 centimeters

Therefore the shift should be 9 centimeters to each side of the midline.

When using grids while making stereoradiographs, one must take care that the tube shift is in the same direction as the grid lines. With low-ratio grids and large SIDs, a tube shift across the grid lines is usually acceptable. The tube shift should also be across any dominant linear structures like long bones. If the direction of the tube shift is the same as the direction of the linear structure, the stereoscopic effect will be lessened.

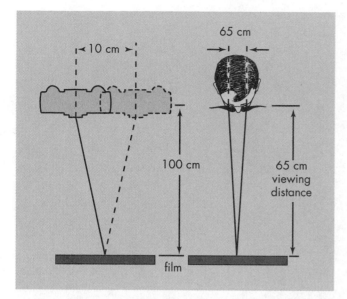

FIGURE 22-16 Degree of tube shift required to make a stereoradiograph depends on the SID, the interpupillary distance, and the viewing distance.

The stereoscopic effect will be lost if there is any patient movement between exposures. This should be carefully explained for patient cooperation.

Stereoradiography takes practice and patience. The procedural steps are listed in the box below.

Viewing Stereoradiographs

Stereoradiographs are normally viewed in stereoscopes specially designed for such radiographs. These stereoscopes are optical devices incorporating lenses, prisms, and mirrors.

The important requirement for viewing stereoradiographs is the proper placement of the film (Figure 22-17). The radiographs should be viewed in the same position in which the radiographs were taken. When

---

Follow These Steps in Sequence for Stereoradiography

1. Properly position the patient and line up the image receptor and x-ray tube as though a single radiograph were to be taken.
2. Determine the SID and the appropriate tube shift distance using the equation on p. 288.
3. Shift the tube half the required distance from the midline and expose the film. The film should be marked to identify the direction of the tube shift.
4. Change films and mark the new film.
5. Shift the tube an equal distance to the opposite side of the midline and expose the second radiograph.
6. Process both radiographs under identical conditions.
7. View them stereoscopically.

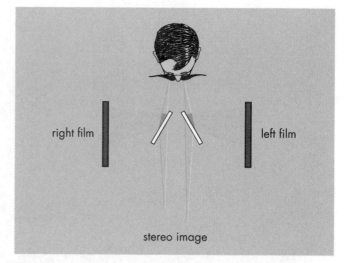

FIGURE 22-17 Basic principle used in viewing a stereograph.

viewing, the eyes are the x-ray tube. The radiographs should be positioned side by side along the direction of the tube shift and not perpendicular to it. The right eye should view the film made when the tube was shifted to the right of center, and the left eye should view the film made when the tube was shifted to the left of center.

Many radiologists are proficient at cross-eyed stereoscopy. This technique requires no special viewing equipment. The stereoradiographs are positioned in reverse order to their normal relationship and viewed by crossing the eyes.

The purpose of stereoradiography is to produce a three-dimensional image. Three-dimensional images are now routine in computed tomography and magnetic resonance imaging. Both CT and MRI provide a volume of data and can be viewed from any direction. Such a technique results in **virtual reality,** which offers exceptional promise for the future.

X-ray holography and stereograms may become routine for future three-dimensional imaging. Christopher Taylor created the first stereograms in 1979, and now they abound in novelty shops (Figure 22-18). To see this three dimensional image, hold this book up, cross your eyes (and your fingers) and focus on an object across the room. While so focused, slowly bring your eyes down to this image and a reddish ram should appear. Approximately 2% of the population—including this author—is stereoblind and will never see the ram.

MAGNIFICATION RADIOGRAPHY

Magnification radiography is a technique used principally by **vascular** radiologists and **neuroradiologists.** Magnification radiography allows radiologists to see small vessels. Conventional radiography minimizes the object-to-image receptor distance (OID). Magnification radiography increases OID.

FIGURE 22-18 See text on p. 289 in order to find the ram in this stereogram.

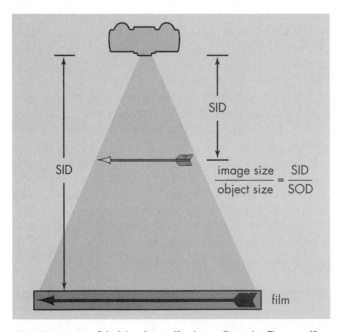

FIGURE 22-19 Principle of magnification radiography. The magnification factor is equal to the ratio of image size to object size.

In magnification radiography the principles of magnification from Chapter 19 are used. To obtain a magnified radiograph, the OID is measured (Figure 22-19).

The degree of magnification is given by the **magnification factor (MF),** described in Chapter 19 as follows:

$$MF = \frac{SID}{SOD} = \frac{Image\ size}{Object\ size}$$

SID is the source-to-image receptor distance and SOD is the source-to-object distance.

Question: A magnified radiograph of the **sella turcica** is taken at 100 centimeters SID with the object positioned 25 centimeters from the image receptor. If the image of the sella turcica measures 16 millimeters, what is its actual size?

Answer:

$$MF = \frac{Image\ size}{Object\ size}$$

$$\text{Object size} = \frac{\text{Image size}}{\text{MF}}$$

$$\text{MF} = \frac{100}{(100 - 25)}$$

$$= 1.33$$

$$\text{Object size} = \frac{16 \text{ mm}}{1.33}$$

$$= 12 \text{ mm}$$

For magnification radiography the use of a small focal spot is recommended. The focal-spot blur resulting from an unnecessarily large focal spot can destroy the diagnostic value of the radiograph. Grids are not needed for magnified radiography because the large OID results in a significant air gap so that the scatter radiation misses the image receptor.

The principal disadvantage of magnification radiography, like so many specialized techniques, is increased patient dose. To obtain a magnification factor of 2, one must position the patient halfway between the x-ray tube and the image receptor. Radiation intensity is related to the square of the distance. A magnification factor of 2 relates to a 4 times increase in patient dose.

SUMMARY

Although CT and MRI have replaced much of the plain-film tomographic examinations, nephrotomography is still frequently done even in modern departments. The emphasis is generally on linear techniques with thin 1-centimeter sections or cuts through the kidney. There are multidirectional tomographic units in use with movements illustrated in Figure 22-10. Zonography is defined as thick-slice tomography with a tomographic angle of less than 10 degrees. Panoramic tomography was originally developed for dental radiography but has found application for radiographing the mandible and other facial structures.

Tomographic image blur theory, which is diagrammed in Figure 22-5, describes the object plane as the plane that is clearly imaged. The image plane also contains the fulcrum point (see Figure 22-4), which is the imaginary pivot point from which the tube and image receptor move. The tomographic angle is the angle of movement and determines the section thickness or the thickness of the object plane. The principal advantage of tomography is improved radiographic contrast. By blurring the structures above and below the object plane, the subject contrast of the tomographic layer is enhanced.

Stereoradiography is a procedure that produces a three-dimensional image of an anatomic structure. The step-by-step procedure is listed in the box on p. 289.

Magnification radiography is a technique used mainly for special procedures to highlight fine vascular detail. Magnification radiography increases OID to magnify small structures. The actual size of the structure can be calculated using the magnification factor formula.

All the alternative plain film procedures discussed in this chapter have the disadvantage of increasing patient dose. As a result, it is important to be careful when positioning patients and when selecting technical factors in order to limit repeated radiographs.

REVIEW QUESTIONS

1. Why is tomography necessary as an alternative to conventional radiographs?
2. Describe tomographic image blur theory.
3. What two imaging procedures have replaced most tomographic examinations?
4. From Table 22-1, indicate the slice thickness required for intravenous pyelograms? What is the anatomy of interest?
5. List the five types of tomographic movements. Using Figure 22-10 copy and label the multidirectional tube movements.
6. Describe the equipment alterations required for tomography.
7. Define fulcrum, object plane, and tomographic angle.
8. Describe the relationship between tomographic angle and section thickness.
9. Explain how tomography improves subject contrast.
10. Are linear structures that lie perpendicular to the tube motion more or less easily blurred?
11. What was the advantage of using a book cassette for tomography?
12. Give two examples of anatomic structures that are best imaged using panoramic tomography.
13. What is the relationship between grid lines and tomographic direction?
14. Define stereoradiography. List two ways stereoradiography is used.
15. Explain the calculation for tube shift in stereoradiography.
16. What are the steps in performing stereoradiography?
17. Describe the stereoradiographic viewing method.
18. When is magnification radiography used?
19. The 4th lumbar vertebra is radiographed at an SID of 150 cm and an SOD of 50 cm. The width of L4

on the radiograph measures 72 mm. What is the true width of L4?

20. What is the major disadvantage of tomography, stereoradiography, and magnification radiography?

Additional Reading

Caldwell EW: The stereoscope in roentgenology, *Am J Roentgenol.* 5:554, 1918.

23 Mammography

OBJECTIVES

At the completion of this chapter the student will be able to:

1. Discuss the differences between soft tissue radiography and conventional radiography
2. List the anatomic parts of the breast
3. Describe the recommended intervals for breast and mammographic examinations
4. Discuss the advantages of mammographic compression
5. Describe the composition of the tube target in a mammographic unit
6. Indicate tube filtration used in mammography
7. List the grid ratio and line pairs per millimeter used in a mammographic grid
8. Describe the image receptors used in mammography

OUTLINE

Mammography
  Soft tissue radiography
  History and development of mammography
  Breast cancer
  Anatomy of the breast
  Technical factors
Mammographic Compression

Mammographic Equipment
  Target composition
  Focal spot
  Filtration
  Grids
  Phototimers
  Image receptors
Alternative Techniques
  Magnification mammography
  Charged couple device

Breast cancer is the leading cause of death from cancer in women. Each year about 175,000 new cases of breast cancer are reported in the United States, with one-quarter of these cases resulting in death. These statistics indicate that one out of every nine women will develop breast cancer during her life. Physicians and scientists believe that early detection of breast cancer leads to more effective treatment and fewer deaths. X-ray mammography has proved to be an accurate and simple breast cancer detection method. However, mammography is not a simple process to perform. Mammography requires exceptional knowledge, skill, and patient care by the radiographer and the support staff. As well, the federal government has recently mandated regulations in the Mammography Quality Standards Act (MQSA), which sets standards for image quality and examination procedures.

MAMMOGRAPHY
Soft Tissue Radiography

Radiographic examination of soft tissues, called *soft tissue radiography,* requires techniques that differ from conventional radiography. This is due to the substantial differences in the anatomic structures being imaged. In conventional radiography the subject contrast is great because of the large differences in mass density and atomic number among bone, muscle, fat, and lung tissue.

In soft tissue radiography, only muscle and fat structures are imaged. These tissues have similar atomic numbers (see Table 13-3) and similar mass densities (see Table 13-5). Consequently, in soft tissue radiography the techniques are designed to enhance differential absorption in very similar tissues.

History and Development of Mammography

A prime example of soft tissue radiography is **mammography,** the radiographic examination of the breast. As a distinct type of radiographic examination, mammography was first attempted in the 1920s. The lack of adequate equipment, however, prevented its development at that time. In the late 1950s, Robert Egan demonstrated a successful mammographic technique, which used low kVp, high mAs, and **direct-exposure film.**

In the 1960s, **xeroradiography** was developed by Wolf and Ruzicka with a substantially lower dose than what was needed using direct-exposure film. Xeroradiographs showed exceptional detail and were easily read. Finally, with lower dose and simplified detection of lesions, mammography was applied to widespread population screening.

Since that time, mammography has undergone much change and development. The continued spread of the high standards of mammography is primarily because of the efforts of the American College of Radiology

(ACR) volunteer accreditation program. Now there is a federally mandated Mammography Quality Standards Act (MQSA).

Breast Cancer

The principal motivation for continuing the development and improvement of mammography equipment and techniques is the incidence of breast cancer. Breast cancer is the leading cause of cancer death in women and the leading cause of death from all causes for women in the 40-to-50 age group. Each year about 175,000 new cases of breast cancer are reported in the United States and the incidence is rising. One quarter of these result in death. Equally frightening is the knowledge that one out of every nine women will develop breast cancer during her life.

Physicians and scientists believe that early detection of breast cancer leads to more effective treatment and fewer deaths. X-ray mammography has proved to be an accurate breast cancer detection method. However, mammography requires exceptional knowledge, skill, and patient care by the radiographer and support staff. With continuing development of mammographic x-ray units and imaging systems, the image quality is being improved and the patient dose reduced.

There are two types of mammographic examinations. **Diagnostic mammography** is performed on patients with symptoms or elevated risk factors. Two or three views of each breast may be required. **Screening mammography** is performed on asymptomatic women using one view, the medial lateral oblique (MLO). Screening mammography in patients 50 years and older has been shown to reduce cancer mortality. The American Cancer Society recommends women perform **breast self-examination** (BSE) monthly. In breast self-examination a woman is taught by her health-care professional to check her breasts regularly for lumps, thickening of the skin, or any changes in size or shape. It is also recommended that a woman have a physician examine her breasts annually. In Table 23-1 the recommended intervals for breast examination using self-examination, physician examination, or mammographic examination are listed. The **baseline** mammo-

TABLE 23-1
Recommended Intervals for Breast Examinations

Examination	<40 Years Old	40 to 49 Years Old	≥50 Years Old
Breast self-examination	Monthly	Monthly	Monthly
Physician physical examination	Annually	Annually	Annually
X-ray mammography			
High risk	Baseline	Annually	Annually
Low risk	Baseline	Biannually	Annually

graphic examination is done as the first examination of the breasts. This mammogram is saved in file and never discarded. Radiologists may use this baseline mammogram for comparison with all future mammograms.

High-risk individuals are those women who have a family history of breast cancer. Low-risk individuals are women who do not have a pronounced family history of breast cancer.

Anatomy of the Breast

Normal breasts consist of three principal types of tissue—fibrous, glandular, and adipose (fat) as shown in Figure 23-1. In a premenopausal woman the fibrous and glandular tissues are structured into various ducts, glands, and connective tissues. These are surrounded by a thin layer of fat. The radiographic appearance of glandular and connective tissue is very dense. Postmenopausal breasts are characterized by a degeneration of this fibroglandular tissue and an increase in the adipose tissue. Adipose tissue is less dense radiographically and requires less exposure.

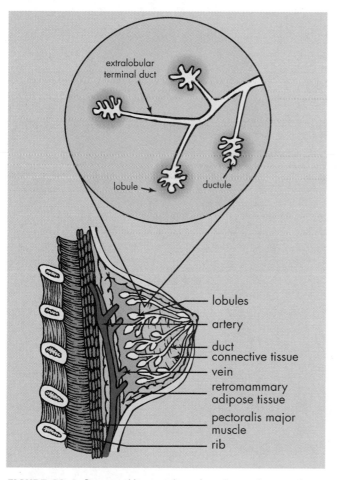

FIGURE 23-1 Breast architecture determines the requirements for x-ray apparatus and image receptors.

Technical Factors

If a malignancy is present, it will be seen as a distortion of the normal ductal and connective tissue patterns and may have associated deposits of **microcalcifications.** These calcific deposits appear as small grains of varying sizes. The sizes of interest for breast cancer detection are microcalcifications less than 500 μm.

Because the mass density and atomic number of soft tissue components of the breast are so similar, conventional radiographic technique is useless. In the 70 to 100 kVp range, Compton scattering predominates with soft tissue. Thus differential absorption within soft tissues is minimal. Low kVp is used to maximize the photoelectric effect and therefore enhance differential absorption.

Recall that x-ray absorption in tissue occurs principally by photoelectric effect and Compton effect. The degree of absorption is determined by the mass density and the atomic number of tissue. Absorption caused by differences in mass density is simply proportional. Absorption caused by differences in the atomic number, however, is directly proportional for Compton interactions and proportional to the cube of the atomic number for photoelectric interaction. Furthermore, at low x-ray energy, photoelectric absorption be-comes increasingly more frequent than Compton scattering.

Therefore x-ray mammography requires a low-kVp technique. As kVp is reduced, however, the penetrability of the x-ray beam is also reduced, which in turn requires an increase in the mAs. If the kVp is too low, an inordinately high mAs is required. High mAs could be unacceptable because of the increased patient dose. Technique factors of approximately 24 to 28 kVp are used as an effective compromise between the increased dose at the low kVp range and reduced image quality at the high-kVp range.

MAMMOGRAPHIC COMPRESSION

Although it may be difficult for patients to understand, compression of the breast is vital for an adequate mammographic examination (Figure 23-2). Primarily, compression holds the breast in position and prevents motion blur. Compression also separates overlying tissue, preventing superimposition of structures. By using compression, all tissue is brought closer to the image receptor. All mammographic units have a built-in compression device, which is designed to be parallel to the film holder and image receptor. The compressed breast has more uniform thickness. The thick tissues near the chest wall and the thinner tissue near the nipple are equally exposed with proper compression. The optical density of the image is more uniform. Because the tissue is thinner when using compression, there is less scatter radiation so contrast resolution is improved. There is also less radiation dose to the patient with thinner anatomy being radiographed.

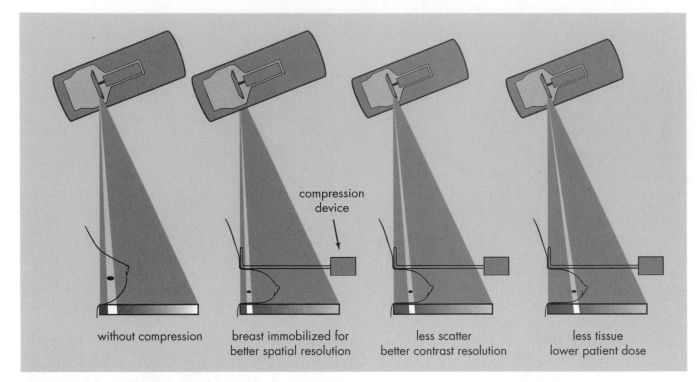

| without compression | breast immobilized for better spatial resolution | less scatter better contrast resolution | less tissue lower patient dose |

FIGURE 23-2 Use of compression in mammography has many advantages.

TABLE 23-2

Advantages of Compression during Mammography

Effect	Result
Immobilizes breast	Reduces motion blur
Less thickness tissue	Separates overlying tissue (superimposition)
Uniform thickness	Equal optical density on mammogram
Reduces scatter radiation	Improves contrast resolution
Position closer to image receptor	Improves spatial resolution
Thinner tissue	Reduces radiation dose

Table 23-2 lists the advantages of compression during mammography.

MAMMOGRAPHIC EQUIPMENT

Acceptable mammograms cannot be performed with conventional x-ray units. Therefore specially designed mammography units are used. Nearly all x-ray manufacturers now produce mammographic units. Figure 23-3 shows three models. Mammographic units are designed for flexibility in patient positioning. The units also have a compression device, a low-ratio grid, automatic-exposure control, and a microfocus x-ray tube for magnification mammography.

Target Composition

Mammographic x-ray tubes are manufactured with a **tungsten,** a **molybdenum,** or a **rhodium** target. Figure

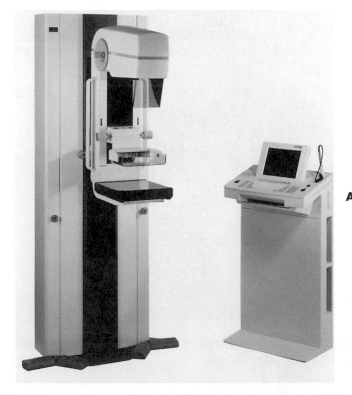

A

FIGURE 23-3 Representative dedicated mammography units. **A,** The Lorad. *(Courtesy Lorad Medical Systems.)*

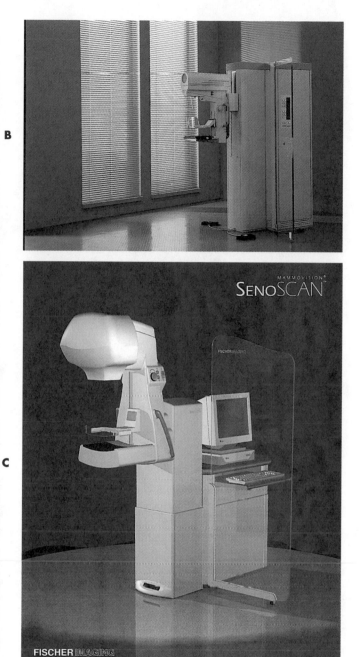

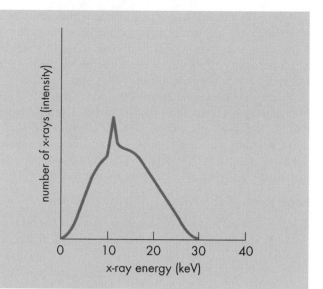

FIGURE 23-4 X-ray emission spectrum for a tungsten-target x-ray tube operated at 30 kVp.

FIGURE 23-3, cont'd B, The Philips Mammo Diagnost. **C,** Fischer Imaging. *(B, Courtesy Philips Medical Systems; C, Courtesy Fischer Medical Systems.)*

23-4 shows the x-ray emission spectrum from a tungsten-target tube filtered with 3 millimeters aluminum and operating at 30 kVp. Note that the bremsstrahlung spectrum predominates and that the only characteristic x-rays present are those from L-shell transitions. These L-characteristic x-rays are of no value in mammographic imaging because their energy (approximately 12 keV) is too low to penetrate the breast. These photons are all absorbed and contribute to patient dose.

The useful x-rays for enhancing differential absorption in breast tissue and for maximizing radiographic contrast are in the 20 to 30 keV range. The tungsten target supplies sufficient x-rays in this energy range.

Figure 23-5 shows the emission spectrum from a molybdenum-target tube filtered with 30 μm of molybdenum. There is an absence of bremsstrahlung x-rays. The spike shown in Figure 23-5 is characteristic of K-shell interactions, with an energy of approximately 20 keV. Molybdenum has an atomic number of 42 compared with 74 for that of tungsten. This difference in atomic number is responsible for the differences in emission spectra.

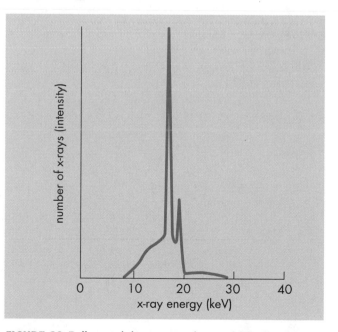

FIGURE 23-5 X-ray emission spectrum for a molybdenum-target x-ray tube operated at 30 kVp.

The x-ray emission spectrum from a rhodium target (Figure 23-6) appears similar to that from a molybdenum target. However rhodium has a slightly higher atomic number (Z = 45). With a slightly higher K-edge (23 keV), more bremsstrahlung x-rays are produced.

Bremsstrahlung x-rays are produced more easily in high-Z target atoms than low-Z target atoms. Molybdenum and rhodium K-characteristic x-rays have energy corresponding to their K-shell electron binding energy. This just happens to be within the range of energies that are most effective for mammographic imaging.

Focal Spot

Focal-spot size is an exceedingly important characteristic of mammography tubes because of the higher de-

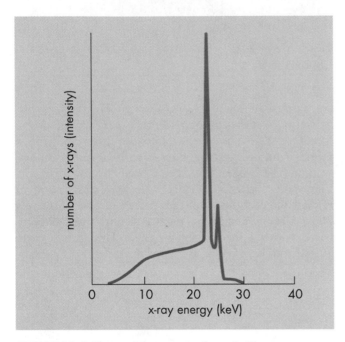

FIGURE 23-6 X-ray emission spectrum for a rhodium-target x-ray tube operated at 30 kVp.

mands for spatial resolution. Imaging microcalcifications requires small focal spots. Mammography x-ray tubes usually have stated focal-spot sizes (large/small) of 0.6/0.3, 0.5/0.2, and 0.4/0.1 millimeters.

In general the smaller the better, however, the shape of the focal spot is also important (Figure 23-7). A circular focal spot is preferred, but rectangular shapes are common.

Heel effect. The heel effect is important to mammography. The conical shape of breasts requires that the radiation intensity near the chest wall be higher than the intensity to the nipple side so that a uniform exposure of the image receptor occurs. This is accomplished by positioning the cathode toward the chest wall (Figure 23-8). In practice, this is not necessary because **compression** ensures a uniform thickness of tissue is imaged. When the cathode is positioned to the chest wall, the spatial resolution of tissue near the chest wall is reduced because of the increased focal-spot blur created by the larger effective focal-spot size. Some manufacturers of mammography equipment use a relatively long source-to-image receptor distance (SID), 60 to 70 centimeters, with the anode to the chest wall (Figure 23-9). Some manufacturers tilt the x-ray tube and claim that to be the best arrangement because the focal spot is made effectively smaller (Figure 23-10).

Filtration

At the low x-ray tube kVp for mammography, it is important that the x-ray tube window does not attenuate the x-ray beam. Therefore mammography x-ray tubes have either a **beryllium** (Z = 4) window or a very thin **borosilicate** glass window. Inherent filtration is usually 0.1-aluminum equivalent. The proper type and thickness of filtration must be installed as added filtration. Under no circumstances should total beam filtration be less than 0.5-millimeter aluminum equivalent.

FIGURE 23-7 Pinhole-camera images of a circular focal spot (**A**) and a rectangular-shaped focal spot (**B**). *(Courtesy Donald Jacobsen.)*

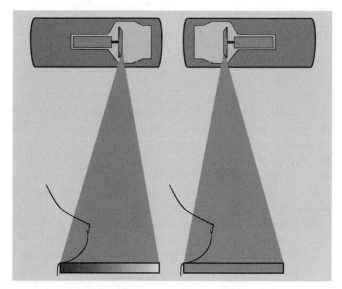

FIGURE 23-8 Heel effect can be used advantageously in mammography by positioning the cathode toward the chest wall to produce a more uniform optical density.

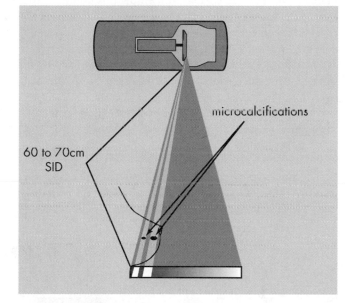

FIGURE 23-9 If the anode is positioned toward the chest wall, spatial resolution of objects, such as microcalcifications, will be improved because of less focal-spot blur.

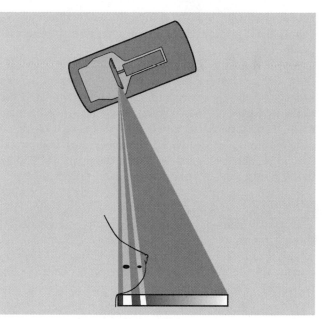

FIGURE 23-10 By tilting the x-ray tube in its housing, the effective focal spot is made even smaller, further improving spatial resolution.

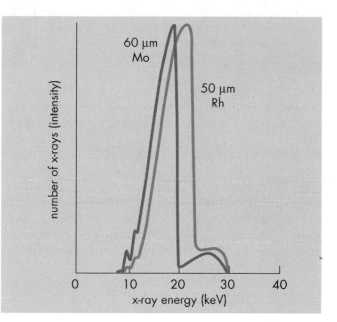

FIGURE 23-11 Emission spectrum from a tungsten-target x-ray tube filtered by molybdenum and rhodium.

For a tungsten target x-ray tube, a molybdenum or rhodium filter should be used. The purpose of filter is to reduce the higher energy bremsstrahlung x-rays (Figure 23-11).

If a molybdenum-target x-ray tube is used, molybdenum filtration of 30 μm or rhodium filtration of 50 μm is recommended. These combinations provide the molybdenum characteristic x-rays for imaging along with the shaped bremsstrahlung x-ray emission spectrum.

If a rhodium-target x-ray tube is used, it should be filtered with 50 μm Rh. This combination provides a slightly higher quality x-ray beam of greater penetrability. The use of rhodium as a target or filter is designed for thicker, more dense breasts.

Mammography x-ray tubes are manufactured with various target/filter combinations. The most common ones are molybdenum-molybdenum, molybdenum-rhodium, rhodium-rhodium, and tungsten-rhodium. By selecting the appropriate filter, one can shape the x-ray emission spectrum to be compatible with the image receptor used and the breast characteristics of each patient.

Some research has suggested that 50 μm rhodium (Z = 45) is a better filter for imaging thicker and denser breasts when the x-ray tube target is tungsten. Look again at Figure 23-11, which shows the emission spectrum from a tungsten target tube designed for screen-film mammography filtered by either molybdenum or rhodium. The radiographer selects the proper filter after determining the patient's breast characteristics.

Grids

The use of grids during mammography is routine. Although mammographic image contrast is high because of the low kVp used, it is not high enough. Many departments use moving grids with a ratio of 4:1 to 5:1 focused to the SID to increase image contrast. A grid frequency of at least 30 lines per centimeter is necessary.

Use of such grids does not compromise spatial resolution, but it does increase patient dose. Use of a 4:1 ratio grid approximately doubles the patient dose when compared with nongrid screen-film mammography. The dose is acceptably low, however, and the improvement in contrast is significant.

Phototimers

Phototimers for mammography are designed to not only measure x-ray intensity at the image receptor but also x-ray quality. These phototimers are referred to as *automatic-exposure control devices (AEC),* and they are positioned underneath the Bucky device and the image receptor (Figure 23-12). The following three types are used: (1) transmission ionization chamber, (2) photomultiplier tube, and (3) solid-state diode. Each type has at least two detectors. The detectors are filtered differently, which allows the AEC to determine the beam quality passing through the breast. This allows an assessment of breast composition.

Accurate performance of the AEC is necessary to ensure **reproducible** images at low radiation dose. The

phototimer should have at least three possible positions to accommodate various breast sizes.

Image Receptors

Three types of image receptors have been used for mammography—direct-exposure film, xerox, and screen-film. Screen-film is used at the present time. In 1990 the Xerox Corporation discontinued the manufacture and marketing of its mammography products. The use of xeromammography is only of historical interest. Direct-exposure mammography has the disadvantage of excessively high patient dose. Consequently, this technique is also a thing of the past.

Screen-film combinations. Radiographic intensifying screens and films have been especially designed for x-ray mammography and are combined into a single-emulsion film matched with a single screen. Double-emulsion low-crossover films matched with two screens are available. They use half the dose of single-emulsion systems, but the image quality is compromised because of the blur from **crossover.** Regardless of the type of film and screen used, they must be spectrally matched. Most manufacturers have special film emulsions coupled with rare-earth screens.

The screen-film combination is placed in a specially designed cassette that has a low-Z front cover for low attenuation. The latching or spring mechanism is designed to produce especially close screen-film contact.

Remember: (1) The emulsion surface of the film must always be next to the screen. (2) The cassette must be positioned so that the film is closest to the x-ray tube.

The position of the screen and film in the cassette is important (see Figure 23-13). X-rays interact primarily with the entrance surface of the screen. If the screen is

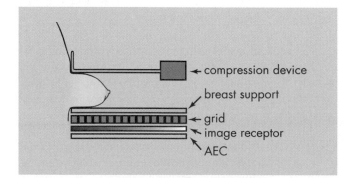

FIGURE 23-12 The relative position of an AEC device.

compression device
breast support
grid
image receptor
AEC

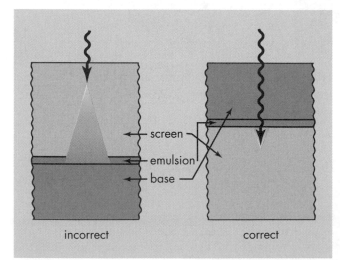

screen
emulsion
base

incorrect

correct

FIGURE 23-13 Spatial resolution improves when the x-ray film is placed between the x-ray tube and the intensifying screen.

between the x-ray tube and the film, excess screen blur results. If, on the other hand, the film is between the x-ray tube and the screen, with the emulsion side to the screen, spatial resolution is better.

ALTERNATIVE TECHNIQUES

Magnification Mammography

Magnification techniques are frequently used in mammography, producing images 1½ times normal size. "Mag" views may be taken as additional views in a mammographic examination if a previously seen lesion has to be further evaluated. Special equipment is required for magnification mammography, such as microfocus tubes, adequate compression, and patient positioning devices. Effective focal-spot size should not exceed 0.3 millimeters. Magnification mammography should not be used routinely because of the following:

1. Normal mammograms are adequate for most patients.
2. The breast may not be completely imaged.
3. Patient dose may be doubled.

Charged Couple Device

A recent development that promises improved digital radiographic imaging has special application for digital mammography. The image receptor is a **charged couple device (CCD)**, which is a remarkable solid-state device. The CCD is an image receptor similar to that used in

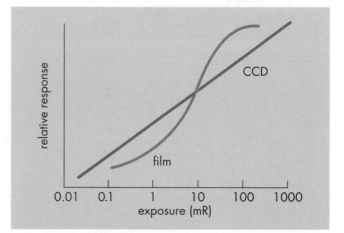

FIGURE 23-15 CCD has a linear response, not the curvilinear response of screen-film.

personal camcorders. It is the result of research in the military and in astronomy. As with screen-film mammography, the remnant x-ray beam interacts with an intensifying screen. Here the similarity ceases. The light from the intensifying screen is captured either by a fiberoptic bundle or a lens system and is directed to the CCD (Figure 23-14). The CCD is a solid-state device that converts visible light photons to electrons. The electron signal is read in pixel-fashion to form an image. Because the CCD is an electronic device, it has electronic noise. The noise is reduced by cooling the detector to 225 K (−25° C) thermoelectrically. The CCD has image characteristics similar to that of film except that its response to x-rays is linear (Figure 23-15). The principal advantage to CCD imaging is its digital format, which allows for converting the image after retrieval.

SUMMARY

Breast cancer is the leading cause of death in women between 40 and 50 years old. This is the principal reason mammographic equipment and techniques have improved over the years. This is also the principal reason that the Mammography Quality Standards Act, which is a federal mandate regulating mammography procedures in hospitals and clinics, was recently instituted.

Anatomically the breast consists of three different tissue types—fibrous tissue, glandular tissue, and adipose tissue. The percentage of tissue types varies in women of different ages. Premenopausal women have breasts composed mainly of fibrous and glandular tissue surrounded by a thin layer of fat. These breasts are dense and difficult to image. For postmenopausal women the glandular tissue turns to fat. Because of its predominant fatty content, the older breast is easier to image.

Table 23-1 outlines the recommended intervals of breast self-examination, physician examination of the

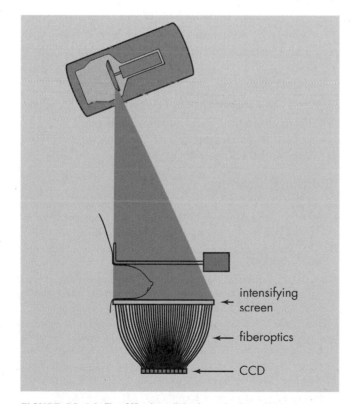

FIGURE 23-14 The CCD views light from the intensifying screen and converts that to a digital image.

TABLE 23-3	
Features of a Mammographic Unit	
High-voltage Generator	High Frequency
Target/filter	W/60 μm Mo
	W/50 μm Rh
	Mo/30 μm Mo
	Mo/50 μm Rh
	Rh/50 μm Rh
kVp	20 to 35 kVp in 1-kVp increments
Compression	Low Z, auto adjust and release
Grids	Ratio of 3:1 to 5:1, 30 lines per centimeter
Exposure control	Automatic to account for tissue thickness and composition
Focal spot: large/small	0.4 millimeter/0.1 millimeter
Magnification	Up to 2×
SID	50 to 80 centimeters

breasts, and mammographic examination for women of various age groups. Diagnostic mammography is often performed every 6 months on women who have an elevated risk of breast cancer or who have a known lesion.

Compression is an important factor in producing high-quality mammograms. Compression is performed for the reasons listed in Table 23-2.

Radiographic equipment is specially designed for mammographic examinations. Mammographic tube targets are made of tungsten, molybdenum, or rhodium. The kVp range of mammography is between 20 and 35 kVp. This is the most useful range for maximizing radiographic contrast of soft tissue. The x-ray beam should be filtered with 30 to 60 microns of molybdenum or rhodium to accentuate the characteristic x-ray emission. Small focal spots are used (0.4 to 0.1 millimeters) because of the demand for increased spatial resolution when imaging microcalcifications. Moving grids (4:1 or 5:1) and the use of film-screen systems (single-emulsion film) further increase radiographic contrast and image detail. Phototimers are designed with three positions to accommodate imaging of various sizes of breast tissue.

Table 23-3 summarizes all the technical aspects of mammographic equipment.

■ ■
REVIEW QUESTIONS

1. How is soft tissue radiography different from conventional radiography?
2. What success did Robert Egan have in the development of mammographic technique in the 1950s?
3. What do ACR and MQSA denote?
4. What is the difference between diagnostic and screening mammography?
5. List the recommended intervals for high-risk x-ray mammography.
6. Describe three types of breast tissue.
7. Define microcalcification.
8. Explain why mammography requires a low-kVp technique.
9. List the six advantages of mammographic compression.
10. Name the three materials used for mammographic tube targets.
11. What sizes of focal spots are used for mammography? Why?
12. What is the best target-filter combination for imaging dense breast tissue?
13. What grid ratio and grid frequency are used for mammographic imaging?
14. In magnification mammography, images are magnified _____ times the normal size.
15. For mammographic cassettes, the latching mechanism is designed for close film-screen contact. This minimizes _____.
16. The emulsion surface of the film must always be toward the _____.
17. The cassette must be positioned so that the film is _____ to the x-ray tube.
18. Why is it important that x-rays interact primarily with the entrance surface of the screen?
19. The long SID for mammography suggested by some manufacturers ranges from _____ to _____ centimeters.
20. In mammography, phototimers have _____ positions to accommodate various breast tissue sizes and thicknesses.

Additional Reading

Beam CA, Layde PM, Sullivan DC: Variability in the interpretation of screening mammograms by US radiologists. Findings from a national sample, *Arch Intern Med* 156(2):209, January 1996.

Bird RE: Increasing the sensitivity of screening mammography, *Appl radiol* 22(2):72, February 1993.

Eklund GW, Cardenosa G, Parsons W, et al: *Mammography: positioning and technical considerations for optimal image quality,* St Louis, 1992, Mosby.

Hendrick RE: What primary care physicians should know about radiation exposure, image quality, and accreditation of mammography providers, *Women's Health Issues* 1(2):79, Winter 1991.

Kruse BD, Leibman AJ, McCain L: Breast imaging and the augmented breast, *Plast Surg Nurs* 12(3):109, Fall 1992.

Mammography update, *Appl Radiol* 21(7):53, July 1992.

Monticcolo DL, Sprawls P, Kruse BD, Peterson JE: Optimization of radiation dose and image quality in mammography: a clinical evaluation of rhodium versus molybdenum, *South Med J* 89(4):391, April 1996.

Peart O: Helping patients overcome their fear of mammography, *Radiol Technol* 66(1):34, September-October, 1994.

Peart O: Stereotactic localization pinpointing breast lesions, *Radiol Technol* 63(4):234, March-April, 1992.

Rothenberg LN, Haus AG: Physicists in mammography—a historical perspective, *Med Phys* 22:1923, November 1995.

Rubin E: Breast cancer in the 90's, *Appl Radiol* 22(3):23, March 1993.

Smith PE: Breast cancer prevention and detection update, *Semin Oncal Nurs* 9(3):150, August 1993.

Vyborny CJ: Quality control in mammography: the radiologist's role, *Appl Radiol* 23(5):11, May 1994.

Wagner AJ, Frey GD: Quantitative mammography contrast threshold test tool, *Med Phys* 22(2):127, February 1995.

24 Mammography Quality Control

OBJECTIVES

At the completion of this chapter the student will be able to:

1. Define quality control
2. List the members of the quality-control team in radiology
3. Indicate the quality-control tasks relating to the radiologist and the medical physicist
4. Itemize the mammographer's quality control duties on a weekly, monthly, and annual basis
5. List the processor quality-control steps

OUTLINE

Quality-Control Team
  Radiologist
  Medical physicist
  Mammographer

Quality-Control Duties for the Mammographer
  Daily tasks
  Weekly tasks
  Monthly tasks
  Quarterly tasks
  Semiannual tasks

ammography has been a screening and diagnostic tool for breast disease for many years, but there are challenges in producing high-quality mammographic images. A team of radiology workers, including the radiologists, medical physicists, and mammographers, works together using a quality-control program to produce excellence in mammographic imaging. Each member of the team has specific tasks that relate to quality control. This chapter identifies the team responsibilities in maintaining mammographic quality control.

■ ■ ■ ■ ■ ■ ■ ■ ■ ■ ■ ■ ■ ■ ■ ■ ■ ■

QUALITY-CONTROL TEAM

Quality control (QC) is an equipment and processing evaluation program in diagnostic imaging departments, radiologic clinics, and anywhere else that uses x-ray mammographic equipment. QC involves testing, record keeping, and evaluating imaging equipment and image processing. QC begins with the manufacturer's examination of equipment. Evaluation of the equipment continues in the workplace with the radiologist, medical physicist, and QC mammographer all working together. In mammography, QC is a high priority.

The American College of Radiology (ACR) has endorsed and the Mammography Quality Standards Act (MQSA) subsequently has outlined a QC program of specific duties required by the radiologist, the medical physicist, and the mammographer (Figure 24-1). Each of these individuals plays an important role in ensuring the patient is receiving the best mammographic care with the least radiation risk.

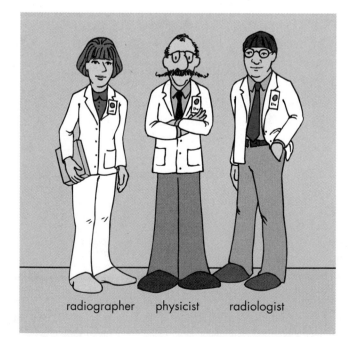

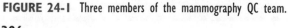

FIGURE 24-1 Three members of the mammography QC team.

Radiologist

The primary responsibility for mammography QC lies with the radiologist. The radiologist's responsibilities often fall under the more broad area of **quality assurance (QA).** QA may be thought of as an overall plan intended to link the different aspects of QC and to generate an assurance that all evaluations are being carried out on the highest level.

The radiologist also supervises patient education and patient tracking. Patient tracking ensures that any mammogram with a positive diagnosis is followed up. The radiologist or a staff member calls the physician's office to ensure the appropriate procedure is followed after the mammogram. Quality patient care is the ultimate goal of any mammography facility. The radiologist has the final responsibility to meet this goal. **Continuous quality improvement (CQI)** is an extension of the QA/QC program. Continuous quality improvement is the administrative plan for QA/QC evaluation processes.

Medical Physicist

The medical physicist, as a member of the mammography QC team, has many tasks. Primarily the physicist is responsible for QC evaluation of the mammographic equipment. The physicist's annual evaluation is summarized in the box below.

The medical physicist understands how the technical aspects of the imaging chain affect the resulting images. Occasionally the medical physicist may pass information directly to the service engineer or serve as an intermediary between the imaging facility and the service engineer. The aim of this portion of the QC program is to ensure that equipment functions properly and that the highest quality images are produced with the lowest dose to the patient.

Medical physicists also advise mammographers in their portions of comprehensive QC programs. The physicist also evaluates the QC program annually. All

---

Annual QC Evaluation Performed by the Medical Physicist

Mammographic unit assembly inspection
Collimation assessment
Evaluation of focal-spot size
kVp accuracy
kVp reproducibility
Beam quality assessment (half-value layer)
Automatic-exposure control performance assessment
Automatic-exposure control reproducibility
Uniformity of screen speed
Breast entrance exposure
Average glandular dose
Image quality evaluation
Artifact evaluation

procedures are reviewed to ensure compliance with current recommendations and standards, and charts and records are thoroughly reviewed.

Mammographer

The mammographer plays an extremely important role in a mammography QC program. The mammographer is the most hands-on member of the QC team and is responsible for the day-to-day execution of QC and for watching all control charts and logs for any trends that might indicate a problem. The 11 specific tasks required of the mammographer responsible for QC may be broken into categories that reflect how often they are done. Table 24-1 outlines these tasks and gives an estimate of the time it takes to perform them.

QUALITY-CONTROL DUTIES FOR THE MAMMOGRAPHER

The 11 tasks of the QC staff are well defined and have recommended performance standards. A full understanding of these tasks, as well as the reasons for the recommended performance levels, is necessary for the mammographer to maintain a thorough and proper QC program.

Daily Tasks

Darkroom cleanliness. The first task each day is to wipe the darkroom clean. A clean darkroom minimizes artifacts on the films (Figure 24-2). First the floor should be mopped with a damp mop. Next, all unnecessary items should be removed from counter tops and work surfaces. A clean, damp towel should be used to wipe off the processor feed tray and all counter tops and work surfaces. Even the passbox should be cleaned

TABLE 24-1

Elements of a Mammographic QC Program

Task	Minimum Frequency	Approximate Time to Carry Out Procedure (minutes)
Darkroom cleanliness	Daily	<5
Processor quality control	Daily	10
Screen cleanliness	Weekly	5
Viewboxes and viewing conditions	Weekly	<5
Phantom images	Monthly	10
Visual checklist	Monthly	<5
Repeat analysis	Quarterly	15 to 30
Analysis of fixer retention in film	Quarterly	<5
Darkroom fog	Semi-annually	15
Screen-film contact	Semi-annually	5
Compression	Semi-annually	<5

daily. Hands should be kept clean to minimize fingerprints and handling artifacts. Overhead air vents and safelights should be wiped or vacuumed weekly before the other cleaning procedures are performed.

Eating or drinking in the darkroom is prohibited. Food or drink should not be taken into the darkroom at any time. There should be nothing stored on the counter top that is used for loading and unloading cassettes. There should be no shelves above the counter tops in the darkroom. These are sites for dust to collect, and this dust will eventually fall onto cassettes and the work surfaces.

Processor quality control. The first step in a processor QC program is to establish operating control levels for the processing system. Before any films are processed, one should verify that the processor chemical system is working according to preset specifications. The processor tanks and racks should be cleaned and the processor supplied with the proper replenisher, fixer, developer, and developer starter fluids, as specified by the manufacturer. The developer temperature, as well as the developer and fixer replenishment rates, should also be set to the levels specified by the manufacturer.

Once the processor has been allowed to warm up and the developer is at the correct temperature and stable, the test may continue. A new box of film should be set aside to carry out the daily processor QC. This is called *control film*. A sheet of control film is exposed with a sensitometer such as that shown in Figure 24-3.

The sensitometric strip is always processed in exactly the same manner. The least exposed end is fed into the processor first. The same side of the feed tray is used with the emulsion-side down. The delay between exposure and processing should be similar each day.

Next a densitometer is used to measure and record the optical densities of each of the steps on the sensitometric strip. This process should be repeated each day for 5 consecutive days. The average optical density is then determined for each step from the five different strips.

Once the averages have been determined, the step that has an average optical density closest to 1.2 but not less than 1 is found and marked as the **mid-density (MD)** step for future comparison. This is sometimes referred to as the *speed index*.

The step with an average density closest to 2.2 and the step with an average density closest to but not less than 0.45 is found and marked for future comparison. The difference between these two steps is recorded as the **density difference (DD)**, which is sometimes referred to as the *contrast index*.

Finally the average density from an unexposed area of the strips is recorded as the **base plus fog (B+F)**. The three values that have now been determined are recorded on the center lines of the appropriate control chart. An example is given in Figure 24-4.

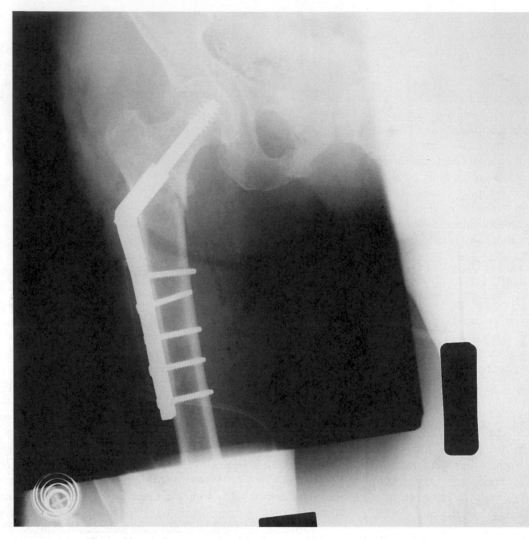

FIGURE 24-2 These white specks were produced by dust trapped between the film and the screen. *(Courtesy Linda Shields.)*

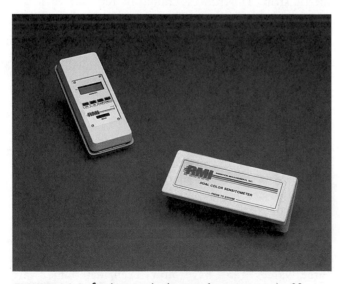

FIGURE 24-3 Sensitometer-densitometer for mammography QC. *(Courtesy Grammex RMI.)*

Once the control values have been established, the daily processor QC begins. At the beginning of each day, before any films are processed, a sensitometric strip is exposed and processed following the guidelines given in the previous discussion. The MD, DD, and B+F are each determined from the appropriate predetermined steps and plotted on the control charts.

The MD is determined to evaluate the constancy of image-receptor speed and the DD to evaluate the constancy of image contrast. These values are allowed to vary within ±0.15 of the control values. If either value is out of this control limit, the point should be circled, the cause of the problem corrected, and the test repeated. If the value cannot be brought within the control limits, no clinical images should be processed. If either value falls outside a +0.1 range of the control value, the test should be repeated. If the value continues to remain outside this range, the processor may be used for clinical processing but should be monitored closely

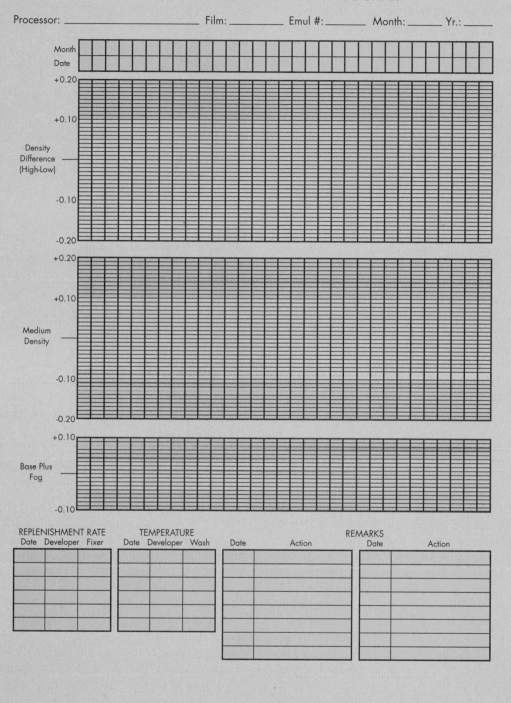

FIGURE 24-4 An example of the type of processor QC record that should be maintained for any processor.

while attempting to identify the problem. The B+F is determined to evaluate the level of fog present in the processing chain. This value is allowed to vary within +0.03 of the control value. Any time the value exceeds this limit, steps should be taken as described for the MD and DD values.

When a new box of film must be opened and dedicated for processor QC, a crossover must be performed with the old film. Five strips from each of the old and new boxes of film should be exposed and processed at the same time. The optical densities should be read on each film for the three predetermined steps and the B+F. The five values for each of the old and the new set of films should be averaged for each of the predetermined steps. The difference between the old and new values of MD, DD, and B+F should be determined, and the control values adjusted to the new values. If the B+F of the new film exceeds the B+F of the old film by more than 0.02, the cause should be investigated and remedied.

There are a few important points to note here. The use of strips exposed more than an hour or two before processing is unacceptable, since these strips may be less sensitive to changes in the processor. The proper combination of film, processor, chemistry, developer temperature, **immersion time**, and replenishment rate should be used as recommended by the film manufacturer. QC should also be performed on the densitometer, sensitometer, and thermometer in order that their proper calibrations are maintained. A log of these evaluations should be maintained.

Weekly Tasks

Screen cleanliness. Screens are cleaned to ensure that mammographic cassettes and intensifying screens are free of dust and dirt particles, which can resemble microcalcifications and result in misdiagnoses. Intensifying screens should be cleaned using the material and methods suggested by the screen manufacturer. If a liquid cleaner is used, screens should be allowed to air dry while standing vertically before the cassettes are closed or used (Figure 24-5). If compressed air is used, the air supply should be checked to ensure that no moisture, oil, or other contaminants are present. If dust or dirt artifacts are noticed, the screens should be cleaned immediately.

It is also necessary to have each screen-cassette combination clearly labeled. The identification should be on the exterior of the cassette, as well as on the edge of the screen, so it will be legible on the processed film. This will enable the mammographer to identify specific screens that have been found to contain artifacts.

Viewboxes. Cleaning viewboxes is a weekly task done to ensure that the viewboxes and viewing conditions are maintained at an optimal level. Viewbox surfaces should be cleaned with window cleaner and soft paper towels to ensure that all marks are removed. The view-

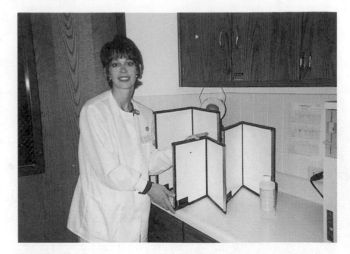

FIGURE 24-5 The proper way to dry screens after cleaning is to position them vertically. *(Courtesy Linda Joppe.)*

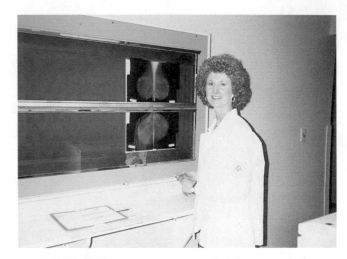

FIGURE 24-6 Mammograms must be masked for proper viewing. *(Courtesy Lois Depouw.)*

boxes should be visually inspected for uniformity of luminance and to ensure that all masking devices are functioning properly. Room illumination levels should be visually checked as well, so that no sources of bright light are present in the room or are reflected from the viewbox surface.

Any marks that are not easily removed should be removed with an appropriate cleaner. If the viewbox luminance appears to be nonuniform, all of the interior lamps should be replaced. Mammography viewboxes have considerably higher luminance levels than conventional viewboxes. As a result, all mammograms and mammography test images should be completely masked for viewing, so that no extraneous light from the viewbox enters the eye. **Masking** can be provided simply by cutting black paper to the proper size (Figure 24-6). Ambient light in the area of the viewbox should also be low and diffuse.

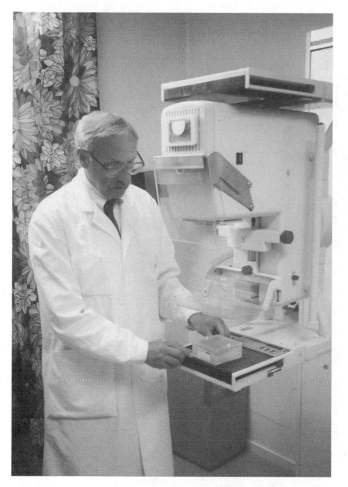

FIGURE 24-7 Analysis of an image of the ACR mammography phantom by a medical physicist scores the detection limits of the system for fibers, specks, and masses. *(Courtesy Art Haus.)*

Monthly Tasks

Phantom images. Phantom images are taken to ensure that film density, contrast, uniformity, and image quality resulting from the x-ray imaging system and film processor are at optimal levels. Using a standard film and a cassette designated as the control or phantom cassette, an image should be taken of an ACR/MQSA **accredited phantom.**

The phantom should be placed on the image receptor assembly so that the edge of the phantom is aligned with the chest wall edge of the receptor (Figure 24-7). The compression device is in contact with the phantom, and the phototimer sensor is positioned similarly for all future phantom images. The technique selected for imaging the phantom is the technique used for a 50% fatty, 50% dense, 4.5-centimeter compressed breast. When the exposure is made, the time or mAs is recorded. The film is then processed just like a clinical mammogram.

With a densitometer, the optical densities are determined for the density disk and for the background im-

mediately adjacent to the density disk. The time or mAs recorded earlier, the background density, and the optical density difference is plotted on a phantom control chart (Figure 24-8). The exposure time or mAs should stay within a range of ±0.15. The background density of the film should be greater than 1.2 with an allowed range of ±0.2. A good target value is approximately 1.4. The density difference should be approximately 0.4 with an allowed range of ±0.05. However, this is defined for 28 kVp, so slightly different densities should be expected at other kVps.

The next step is to score the phantom image. Scoring the phantom involves determining the number of fibers, speck groups, and masses visible in the phantom image. A radiograph and conceptual drawing of the ACR accreditation phantom are shown in Figure 24-9. These results should also be plotted on the phantom control chart.

The objects on the phantom image are counted from the largest object to the smallest, with each object group receiving a score of 1, 0.5, or zero. A **fiber** may be counted as 1 if its entire length is visible at the correct location and with the correct orientation. A fiber may be given a score of 0.5 if more than half of its length is visible at the correct location and with the correct orientation. The score is zero if less than half of the fiber is visible.

Using a magnifying glass, a **speck group** may be counted as a full point if four or more of the six specks are visible. A score of 0.5 may be given to a speck group if at least two of the six specks are visible. If fewer than two specks in group are visible, the score is zero.

A **mass** may be counted as a full point if a density difference is seen at the correct location with a circular border. A score of 0.5 may be given to a mass if a density difference is seen at the correct location but the shape is not circular. If there is only a hint of a density difference, the score is zero.

Next a magnifying glass is used to check the image for nonuniform areas or artifacts (Figure 24-10). If any artifacts are found that resemble the phantom objects, they should be subtracted from the score given for that object. Never subtract below the next full integer point. For example, if a score of 3.5 or 4 was given, the score cannot be subtracted below 3. The score of phantom objects counted on subsequent phantom images for each type object should not decrease by more than 0.5. The minimum number of objects required to pass ACR accreditation is four fibers, three speck groups, and three masses.

Phantom images should be taken initially after calibration to determine the control values of the phantom objects for future comparison. Phantom images should also be taken after any maintenance is performed on the imaging equipment. Any time the phantom image results in any of the factors exceeding the control values,

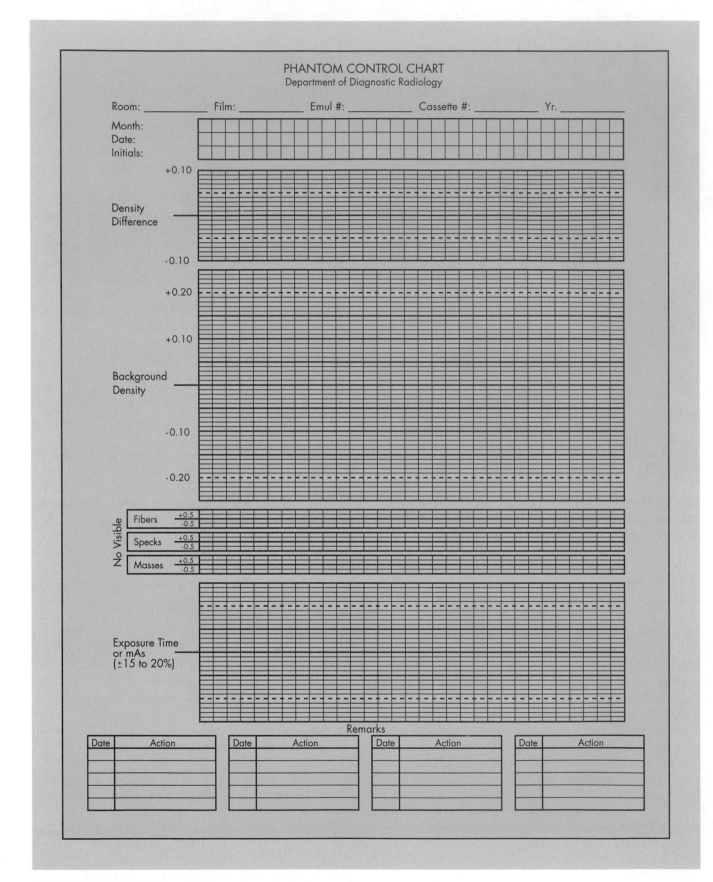

FIGURE 24-8 A phantom control chart.

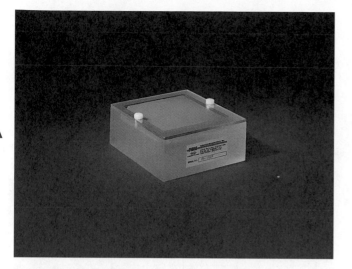

A

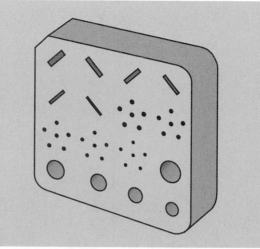

B

FIGURE 24-9 The ACR accreditation phantom **(A)** and its schematic image **(B)** are shown. **(A,** *Courtesy Grammex RMI.)*

FIGURE 24-10 These are really gross artifacts caused by processor rollers that have not been cleaned. A phantom image containing such artifacts would result in an unacceptable score. *(Courtesy Cristl Thompson.)*

the cause should be investigated and corrected as soon as possible. The phantom images should always be viewed by the same person, on the same mammography viewbox, under the same viewing conditions, using the same type of magnifier used for mammograms, and at the same time of day.

Visual checklist. The visual check is a monthly task done to ensure the imaging system lights, displays, and mechanical locks and detents are functioning properly

and to confirm the optimal level of the equipment's mechanical rigidity and stability. An example of a visual checklist is given in Figure 24-11. Mammography staff reviews all the items on the list and indicates the condition of each. This will help to ensure patient safety, high-quality images, and operator convenience. If any item on the list fails visual inspection, immediate steps should be taken to remedy the problem. Date and initial the checklist.

Quarterly Tasks

Repeat analysis. The repeat analysis is a procedure to determine the number and cause of repeated mammograms. Repeat analysis will also identify ways to improve efficiency, reduce costs, and reduce unnecessary patient exposure. Approximately 250 patients are needed for this evaluation to be valid.

The QC mammographer begins by discarding all rejected films. All rejected films are then collected for the next quarter or until 250 patients have been examined. The rejected films are sorted into different categories such as poor positioning, patient motion, too light, and the other categories shown on the reject analysis form shown in Figure 24-12.

Next the total number of films repeated and the total number of films exposed are counted. The repeat rate is computed as follows:

$$\text{Repeat rate} = \frac{\text{Number of repeated films}}{\text{Total number of films}} \times 100$$

The repeat rate for each category is determined by dividing the number of repeated films in a given category by the total number of repeats. The overall repeat rate should be ≤2%, and the rates for each category should be from 2 to 5%. A high overall rate or a single cate-

MAMMOGRAPHY QUALITY CONTROL VISUAL CHECKLIST

Room #: _____ Tube: _____

Month: J F M A M J J A S O N D

		J	F	M	A	M	J	J	A	S	O	N	D
C-ARM	SID indicator or marks												
	Angulation indicator												
	Locks (all)												
	Field light												
	High tension cable/other cables												
	Smoothness of motion												
CASSETTE HOLDER	Cassette lock												
	Compression device												
	Compression scale												
	Amount of compression												
	Grid												
CONTROL BOOTH	Exposure control												
	Observation window												
	Panel switches/lights/meters												
	Technique charts												
	Gonad shield/aprons/gloves												
	Cones												
	Cleaning solution												
OTHERS	Pass = √ Month:												
	Fail = X Date:												
	Not applicable = NA R.T.												

FIGURE 24-11 This checklist contains items that should be inspected monthly by the mammographer.

gory higher than the others indicates a problem that should be investigated. It is important to note that all repeated films should be included in the analysis, not just those rejected by the radiologist.

Question: A mammography service examined 327 patients during the third calendar quarter of 1996. 719 films were exposed during this period, eight of which were repeats. What is the repeat rate?

Answer: Repeat rate $= \dfrac{8}{719} \times 100$

$= 1.1\ \%$

Archival quality check. An archival quality check is a quarterly task done to determine the amount of residual fixer in the processed film. The result is used as an indicator of the film's storage quality. One sheet of unexposed film is processed. Next, one drop of residual hypo test solution is placed on the emulsion side of the film and allowed to stand for 2 minutes. The excess solution is blotted off and the stain compared with a hypo estimator, which comes with the test solution, using a white sheet of paper as a background. The matching number from the hypo estimator is recorded. The comparison must be made immediately after blotting, which prevents the spot to darken.

The hypo estimator provides an estimate of the amount of residual hypo in grams per square meter (Figure 24-13). If the comparison results in an estimate of more than 0.05 grams per square meter, the test must be repeated. If elevated residual hypo is then indicated, the source of the problem should be investigated and corrected.

MAMMOGRAPHY REPEAT ANALYSIS

From _____ To _____

Cause	Number of Films	Percentage of Repeats
1. Postitioning		
2. Patient Motion		
3. Light Film		
4. Dark Film		
5. Black Film		
6. Static		
7. Fog		
8. Incorrect Patient I.D., or Double Exposure		
9. Mechanical		
10. Miscellaneous		
11. Good Film (no apparent problem)		
12. Clear Film		
13. Wire Localization		
14. Q.C.		

	Totals	
Rejects (All; 1-14)	%	
Repeats (1-11)	%	

Total Film Used	

FIGURE 24-12 Reject analysis form.

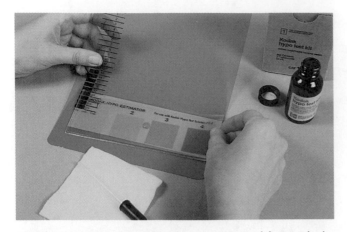

FIGURE 24-13 Analysis to determine the amount of fixer retained on the film. *(Courtesy Eastman Kodak.)*

Semiannual Tasks

Darkroom fog. Darkroom fog analysis ensures that darkroom safelights and other sources of light inside and outside of the darkroom do not fog mammographic films. Fog results in a loss of contrast and therefore a loss of diagnostic information. The darkroom fog test is done in a new darkroom and anytime safelight bulbs or filters are changed, and as a QC test, under the MSQA, every 6 months.

Safelight filters should be checked. If they are faded or cracked, the filter should be replaced. The wattage and distance of the bulbs from work surfaces should also be checked against the recommendations of the film manufacturer. To check for light leaks, all lights should be turned off for 5 minutes to allow the eyes to adjust to the darkness. Light leaks are searched for around the door, passbox, processor, and in the ceiling. Light leaks are often visible from only one perspective, so the radiographer may have to move around the darkroom. Any leaks should be corrected before proceeding.

If fluorescent lights are present, they should be turned on for at least 2 minutes and then turned off. A piece of film should then be loaded into the cassette in total darkness, and a image should be taken as previously described. The film should be taken to the darkroom and placed, emulsion side up, on the countertop, with an opaque object covering one half of the image (left or right). The safelights should then be turned on for 2 minutes with the half-covered film on the countertop.

After 2 minutes have passed, the film should be processed and optical densities should be measured very near both sides of the line separating the covered and uncovered portions of the film. The difference in the two optical densities represents the amount of fog created by the safelights or by fluorescent-light afterglow. This value is recorded.

Safelight fog should not exceed 0.05. Excessive fog levels should be investigated. The background optical density (unfogged) of the phantom is in the range specified previously (1.2 to 1.5).

Screen-film contact. The screen-film contact test evaluates the contact between the screen and the film in each cassette. Poor screen-film contact results in image blur, which causes a loss of diagnostic information in the mammogram.

New cassettes should always be tested before being placed into service. All cassettes and screens should be completely cleaned and allowed to air dry for at least 30 minutes before being loaded with film for this test. After loading, the cassettes should be allowed to sit upright for 15 minutes to allow any trapped air to escape. The cassette to be tested should be placed on top of the cassette holder assembly with the test tool being placed directly on top of the cassette. An appropriate test tool is made of copper wire mesh of at least 40 wires per inch grid density (Figure 24-14). The compression paddle should be raised as high as possible. A manual tech-

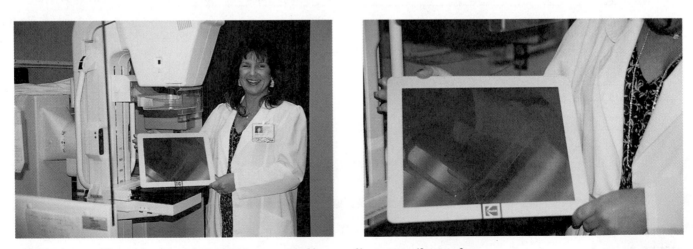

FIGURE 24-14 Wire-mesh test tool for evaluating mammographic screen-film contact. *(Courtesy Susan Sprinkle.)*

nique between 25 and 28 kVp should be selected that will result in an optical density between 0.7 and 0.8 near the chest wall. The exposure should be at least 500 milliseconds.

A piece of acrylic should be placed between the x-ray tube and cassette if the above parameters cannot be met under normal circumstances. If this is done, the acrylic should be placed as close as possible to the x-ray tube to reduce scatter radiation reaching the cassette.

The film should be processed regularly and viewed from a distance of at least 3 feet. Dark areas on the film indicate poor screen-film contact (Figure 24-15). If any cassettes are found to have such poor screen-film contact, they should be cleaned and tested again. If the poor contact persists, the problem should be investigated and the cassette removed from service until corrections can be made.

Compression check. The compression test is done to ensure that the mammographic system can provide adequate compression in the manual and power-assisted modes for an adequate amount of time. It must also be shown that the equipment does not allow too much compression to be applied.

Firm compression is absolutely necessary for high-quality mammography as is discussed in Chapter 23. Compression reduces the thickness of tissue that the x-rays must penetrate and thus reduces scatter radiation. Spatial resolution is improved because compression reduces focal-spot blur and patient motion. Finally, compression serves to make the thickness of the breast more uniform, which results in a more uniform optical density.

To check the compression device, a sponge is placed on the cassette holder assembly. A flat bathroom scale is centered under the compression device. Another sponge is placed over the scale without covering the readout area (Figure 24-16). The compression device should be engaged automatically until it stops, the degree of compression should be recorded, and the device then released.

The procedure should be repeated using the manual drive, again recording the compression. Never exceed 40 pounds of compression in the automatic mode. Both modes should be able to compress between 25 and 40 pounds and hold this compression for at least 15 seconds. If either mode fails to reach these levels, the equipment should be properly adjusted.

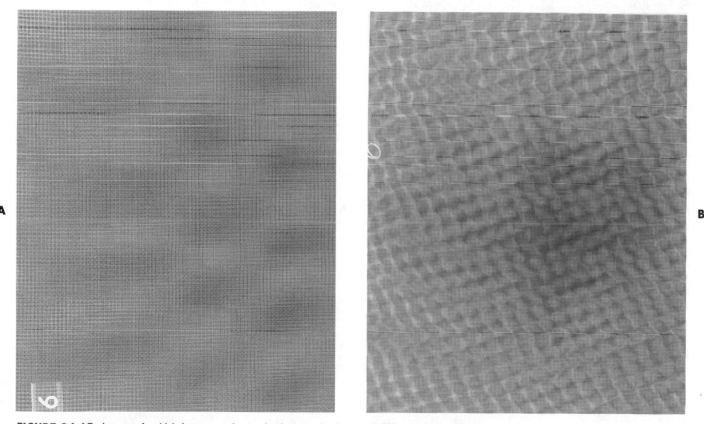

A   **B**

FIGURE 24-15 Images of a high-frequency wire mesh phantom showing good **(A)** and poor **(B)** film-screen contact. *(Courtesy Sharon Glaze.)*

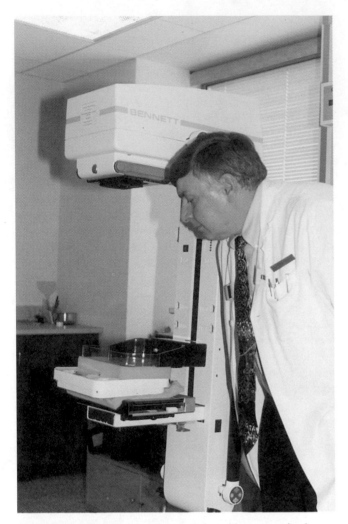

FIGURE 24-16 Testing breast compression with a conventional bathroom scale. *(Courtesy Edward Nickoloff.)*

SUMMARY

Quality control in mammography is part of an overall equipment and processing evaluation analysis and includes testing, record keeping, and evaluation of results. The three QC team members are the radiologist, who has specific duties of administration and tracking diagnostic results; the medical physicist, who examines and tests equipment; and the mammographer, who performs many testing and evaluation functions involving equipment, processing, and mammographic images.

The daily, weekly, and annual duties and responsibilities of the QC mammographer are listed by time intervals. Daily routines include maintaining darkroom cleanliness and performing the steps of processor QC. Processor QC includes sensitometry and densitometry, as well as graphing results on a daily basis. The following steps are involved:

1. Check processor temperature
2. Prepare sensitometric strip
3. Process sensitometric strip
4. Measure processed strip (densitometry)
   a. Optical density of step of mid-density range (closest to 1.2 but not less than 1) called the *speed index*
   b. Optical density of two steps, one closest to 2.2 and one closest but not less than 0.45. The difference between these two steps is known as the density difference or *contrast index*
   c. Optical density from the unexposed area called the *base plus fog*
   d. Log and graph this data on the processing QC charts
   e. Examine for normal values

Weekly routines include intensifying screen and viewbox cleaning. Monthly tasks involve exposing phantom images and performing equipment checks. Review Figure 24-8, for analysis of phantom objects—fibers, speck groups, and masses. Four times a year a repeat analysis is done based on 250 mammographic examinations. A repeat rate of less than or equal to 2% is normal. Greater repeat rates should be investigated. Also, an archival check of film quality is performed quarterly.

Semi-annually the darkroom fog check is done and screen-film contact tests are performed on all mammographic cassettes. Finally the compression test is done using a bathroom scale under the compression paddle. Compression should never exceed 40 pounds of pressure. The automatic and manual modes should compress between 25 to 40 pounds of compression for 15 seconds. Annually, the health physicist surveys the mammography equipment.

REVIEW QUESTIONS

1. Define quality control.
2. List two aspects of the radiologists' duties involving mammographic QC.
3. Name the 13 annual evaluation tests performed by the medical physicist.
4. What task of the mammographic QC radiographer takes up the greatest amount of time?
5. Which member of the QC team would track the patients' positive diagnoses?
6. Which member would notice a temperature error in the developer solution?
7. Define base plus fog.
8. Density difference on the processor QC chart is used to evaluate the constancy of image _____.
9. Mid-density on the control chart is used to evaluate the constancy of _____ _____ _____.

10. Describe how to clean intensifying screens. How often is this task performed?

11. Explain how mammographic viewboxes are different from conventional viewboxes.

12. What is masking?

13. What are the three objects on the mammographic phantom?

14. List the process for scoring the phantom objects.

15. Name the reject film categories listed on Figure 24-12.

16. The archival quality of mammographic film has to do with _____ retention on the film.

17. How do you check for light leaks in the darkroom?

18. What is the acceptable fog value for 2 minutes of safelight exposure of film?

19. Describe the device used to check screen-film contact.

20. What is the maximum pounds of compression allowable on mammographic equipment?

Additonal Reading

Beam CA, Layde PM, Sullivan DC: Variability in the interpretation of screening mammograms by US radiologists. Findings from a national sample, *Arch Intern Med* 156(2):127, February 1995.

Eklund GW, Cardenosa G, Parsons W, et al: *Mammography: positioning and technical considerations for optimal image quality,* St Louis, 1992, Mosby.

Farria DM, Dassett LW, Kimme-Smith C, DeBruhl N: Mammography quality assurance from A to Z, *Radiographics* 14(2):371, March 1994.

Haus AG: *Screen-film processing systems and quality control in mammography,* Rochester, NY, January 1992, Eastman Kodak.

Haus Arthur G: *Medical physicist's role under MQSA,* Rochester, NY, 1994, Eastman Kodak.

Kimme-Smith C: Selection and acceptance testing of breast imaging equipment, *Appl Radiol* 22(9):25, September 1993.

Langer TG, de Paredes ES, Agarwal S, Smith D: QA in mammography: QA physics part 1, *Appl Radiol* 21(2):17, February 1992.

Langer TG, de Paredes ES, Agarwal S, Smith D: QA in mammography: QA physics part 2, *Appl Radiol* 21(3):69, March 1992.

Monticcolo DL, Sprawls P, Kruse BD, Peterson JE: Optimization of radiation dose and image quality in mammography: a clinical evaluation of rhodium versus molybdenum, *South Med J* 89(4):391, April 1996.

25 Fluoroscopy

OBJECTIVES

At the completion of this chapter the student will be able to:

1. Discuss the history of fluoroscopy
2. Explain visual physiology in relation to fluoroscopic illumination
3. Describe the parts of the fluoroscopic image intensifier
4. Calculate flux gain and brightness gain
5. List the approximate kVp levels for seven common fluoroscopic examinations
6. Discuss the role of the television monitor and television image in forming the fluoroscopic image

OUTLINE

History of Fluoroscopy
Fluoroscopy and Visual Physiology
    Illumination
    Human vision
Image Intensification
    Image-intensifier tube
    Multifield intensification

Fluoroscopic-image Monitoring
    Television monitoring
Spot Filming

The primary function of the fluoroscope is to aid the radiologist in viewing dynamic studies of the human body. Dynamic studies are examinations that show the motion of circulation or that show the motion of hollow internal structures. During fluoroscopy, the radiologist generally uses contrast media to highlight the anatomy. The radiologist then views a continuous image of the internal structure while the x-ray tube is on. If the radiologist observes something during the fluoroscopic examination and would like to preserve that image for further study, a radiograph called a *spot film* can be taken with little interruption of the dynamic examination.

HISTORY OF FLUOROSCOPY

Thomas A. Edison invented the fluoroscope in 1896. The original fluoroscope was a zinc-cadmium sulfide screen placed above the patient's body in the x-ray beam (Figure 25-1). The radiologist stared directly into the screen, viewing a very faint yellow-green fluoroscent image. Later, optics were designed to remove the radiologist from the direct beam; however, only one individual could view the image at a time. In addition, radiologists had to adapt their eyes to the dark before fluoroscopy, which meant wearing red goggles for up to 30 minutes before an examination. In these early days of fluoroscopy, examinations were done in a completely darkened room. In 1941, William Chamberlain's studies on the poor illumination from fluoroscopic screens resulted in the development of the image intensifier in the 1950s.

The modern fluoroscopic system is shown in Figure 25-2. The x-ray tube is usually under the patient couch. Over the patient couch is the image intensifier and other image-detection devices. Some fluoroscopes are operated remotely from outside the x-ray room. There are many different arrangements for fluoroscopy.

In all cases, fluoroscopy requires the operator to view a dimly illuminated image. As a result, fluoroscopy requires knowledge of image illumination and visual physiology.

FLUOROSCOPY AND VISUAL PHYSIOLOGY

Fluoroscopy is a dynamic process in which images are viewed in dimly lit examination rooms. The radiologist must adapt not only to moving images but also to viewing dim images in low light.

Illumination

The principal advantage of image-intensified fluoroscopy over earlier fluoroscopy is the increased image brightness. Just as it is much more difficult to read a book in dim illumination than in bright illumination, it is much harder to interpret a dim fluoroscopic image than to interpret a bright one.

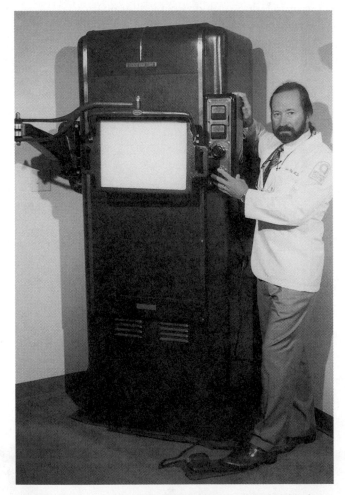

FIGURE 25-1 Brian Peck, MD, Medical Director of the Arthritis Center, with the Picker T-10 unit. The machine was graciously donated by Mrs. Rose Coshak in honor of her husband, the late Dr. Morris Coshak.

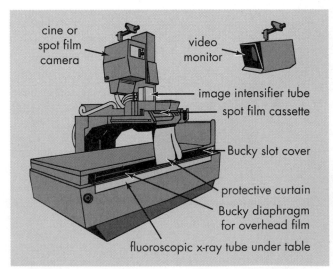

FIGURE 25-2 Fluoroscope and associated parts.

Illumination levels are measured in units of lamberts (L) and millilamberts (mL) (1 L = 1000 mL). Figure 25-3 lists some approximate illumination levels from a movie theater to a bright snowy day. Radiographs are viewed under illumination levels of 10 to 1000 mL. Modern image-intensified fluoroscopy is performed at the same illumination levels as radiographs.

Human Vision

The structures in the eye responsible for vision are called *rods* and *cones*. Figure 25-4 is a cross section of the human eye that identifies its principal parts and its appearance on MRI. Light incident on the eye must first pass through the **cornea**, a transparent protective covering, and then through the **lens,** where the light is focused onto the **retina.**

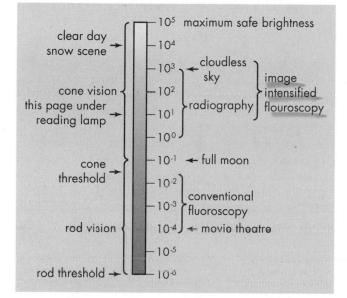

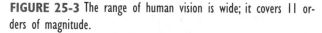

FIGURE 25-3 The range of human vision is wide; it covers 11 orders of magnitude.

Between the cornea and the lens is the **iris**, which behaves like the diaphragm of a photographic camera to control the amount of light admitted to the eye. In the presence of bright light the iris contracts and allows only a small amount of light to enter. During dark conditions, such as a darkened movie theater, the iris **dilates** and allows more light to enter.

When light arrives at the retina, it is detected by the rods and the cones. Rods and cones are small structures. There are more than 100,000 of them per square millimeter of retina. The cones are concentrated on the center of the retina in an area called the *fovea centralis.* Rods, on the other hand, appear on the periphery of the retina.

The rods are sensitive to low light. The threshold for rod vision is approximately 10^{-6} mL. Cones, on the other hand, are less sensitive to light; their threshold is only approximately 10^{-2} mL, but they are capable of responding to intense light levels, whereas rods cannot.

Consequently, cones are used primarily for daylight vision, which is called *photopic vision,* and rods are used for night vision, which is called *scotopic vision.* This aspect of visual physiology explains why dim objects are more readily viewed if they are not looked at directly. Astronomers and radiologists are familiar with the fact that a dim object can be seen better if viewed peripherally where rod vision dominates.

The ability of the rods to perceive small objects is much worse than that of the cones. This ability to perceive fine detail is called *visual acuity.* Cones are also much more able to detect differences in brightness levels than rods. This property of vision is termed *contrast perception.* Furthermore, cones are sensitive to a wide range of wavelengths of light. Cones perceive color, but rods are essentially color blind.

The visual features distinguishing rods from cones emphasize that cone vision is preferred over rod vision. During fluoroscopy, maximum image detail is desired

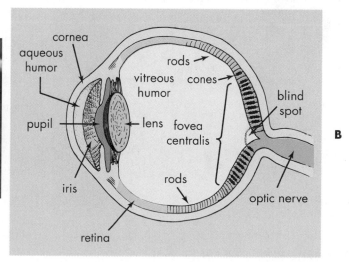

FIGURE 25-4 The human eye's appearance on MR image **(A)** and the parts responsible for vision **(B).** **(A,** *Courtesy Helen Schumpert.)*

and image brightness must be high. This is the principal reason that the image intensifier was developed to replace the conventional fluorescent screen. The fluorescent screen had to be viewed in a dark room after 15 minutes of dark adaptation (Figure 25-5). The image intensifier raises the illumination into the cone-vision region where visual acuity is greatest.

IMAGE INTENSIFICATION
Image-Intensifier Tube

The image-intensifier tube is a complex electronic device that receives the remnant x-ray beam, converts it into light, and increases the light intensity. Figure 25-6 illustrates the x-ray image-intensifier tube. The tube is usually contained in an evacuated glass envelope for structural support. When installed, the tube is mounted inside a metal container to protect it from rough handling.

X-rays that exit the patient hit the image-intensifier tube, are transmitted through the glass envelope, and interact with the **input phosphor.** The input phosphor is cesium iodide (CsI). When an x-ray interacts with the input phosphor, its energy is converted into visible light, which is similar to the effect of radiographic intensifying screens. The CsI crystals are grown as tiny needles

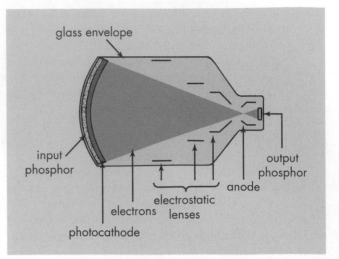

FIGURE 25-6 The image-intensifier tube converts the pattern of the x-ray beam into a bright visible-light image.

and are tightly packed as a 100 to 200 μm layer. This results in microlight pipes with little dispersion and excellent spatial resolution.

The next active element of the image-intensifier tube is the **photocathode**, which is bonded directly to the input phosphor with a thin, transparent, adhesive layer. The photocathode is composed of cesium and antimony compounds that emit electrons when stimulated by light. This process is known as *photoemission.* Thus the photocathode is a photoemissive surface. The terminology is similar to **thermionic emission,** which refers to electron emission after heat stimulation. Photoemission is electron emission after light stimulation. The number of electrons emitted by the photocathode is directly proportional to the intensity of light falling on it. Consequently, this number of electrons is proportional to the intensity of the incident x-rays.

The image-intensifier tube is approximately 50 centimeters long. A potential difference of about 25,000 volts is maintained across the tube between photocathode and anode so that the electrons of photoemission will be accelerated to the anode.

On the other side of the anode is the output phosphor where the electrons interact and produce light. The anode is a circular plate with a hole in the middle to allow the electrons through to the output phosphor.

If there is to be an accurate image pattern, the electron path from photocathode to output phosphor must be precise. The engineering aspects of maintaining proper electron travel are called *electron optics* because the electrons emitted over the face of the image-intensifier tube must be focused just like visible light. The devices responsible for this control, called *electrostatic focusing lenses,* are located along the length of the image-intensifier tube. The electrons arrive at the output

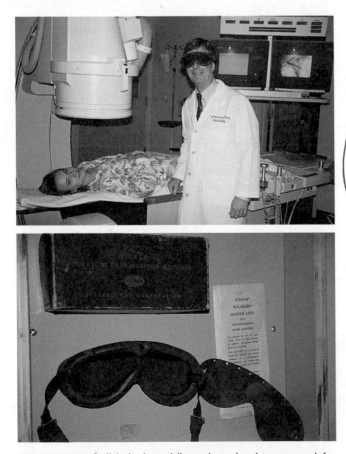

FIGURE 25-5 Radiologist is modeling red goggles that were used for fluoroscopic dark adaptation. *(Courtesy Ben Archer.)*

phosphor with high kinetic energy and contain the image of the input phosphor in minified form.

When these high-energy electrons interact with the output phosphor, a considerable amount of light is produced. The **output phosphor** usually is made of zinc-cadmium sulfide. Each photoelectron that arrives at the output phosphor results in approximately 50 to 75 times as many light photons as were necessary to create it. The entire sequence of events from initial x-ray interaction to output image is summarized in Figure 25-7. This ratio of the number of light photons at the output phosphor to the number of x-rays at the input phosphor is the **flux gain.**

$$\text{Flux gain} = \frac{\text{Number of output light photons}}{\text{Number of input x-ray photons}}$$

The increased illumination of the image is due to the multiplication of the light photons at the output phosphor compared with the x-rays at the input phosphor and the image minification from input phosphor to output phosphor. The ability of the image-intensifier tube to increase the illumination level of the image is called its **brightness gain.** The brightness gain is simply the product of the **minification gain** and the flux gain.

$$\text{Brightness gain} = \text{Minification gain} \times \text{Flux gain}$$

The minification gain is the ratio of the square of the diameter of the input phosphor to the square of the diameter of the output phosphor. Output phosphor size is fairly standard at 2.5 or 5 centimeters. Input phosphor size varies from 10 to 35 centimeters and is used to identify image-intensifier tubes.

Question: What is the brightness gain for a 17-centimeter image-intensifier tube having a flux gain of 120 and a 2.5-centimeter output phosphor?

Answer:

$$\text{Brightness gain} = \frac{17^2}{2.5^2} \times 120$$

$$= 46 \times 120$$

$$= 5520$$

The brightness gain of most image intensifiers is 5000 to 20,000. As an image intensifier ages, patient dose increases to maintain brightness. Ultimately the image intensifier must be replaced.

When image intensifiers were introduced, brightness gain was the increased illumination compared with the standard conventional fluoroscent screen at that time, which was a Patterson B-2. Now it is defined as the ratio of the illumination intensity at the output phosphor, measured in **Candela** per meter squared (cd/m²) to the radiation intensity to the input phosphor, measured in milliroentgen per second (mR/sec). This quantity is called the *conversion factor* and is approximately 10^{-2} times the brightness gain. The proper way to express intensification is with the conversion factor.

$$\text{Conversion factor} = \frac{\text{Output phosphor illumination (cd/m}^2)}{\text{Input exposure rate (mR/s)}}$$

Image intensifiers have conversion factors ranging from 50 to 300. This corresponds to brightness gains at 5000 to 30,000.

Figure 25-8 demonstrates some of the modes of operation for an image-intensifier tube. Fluoroscopic images are viewed on a television monitor. The spot-film camera uses 105-millimeter film and is becoming increasingly popular. The cineradiography camera is used almost exclusively in cardiac catheterization.

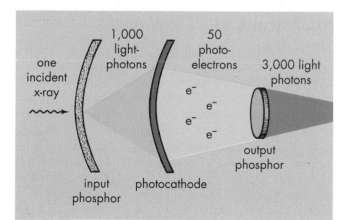

FIGURE 25-7 In an image-intensifier tube, each incident x-ray that interacts with the input phosphor results in a large number of light photons at the output phosphor. The image intensifier shown here has a gain of 3000.

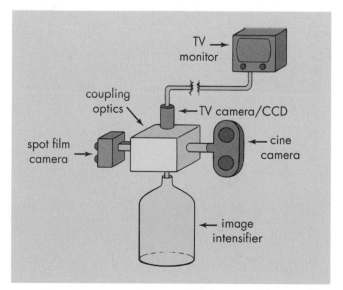

FIGURE 25-8 Some possible modes of operation with an image-intensifier tube.

Multifield Image Intensification

Most image intensifiers are of the multifield type. These multifield image intensifiers provide for considerably more flexibility for all fluoroscopic examinations and are standard components in digital fluoroscopy. Dual-field tubes come in a varied range of sizes, but perhaps the most popular is the 25- to 17-centimeters (25/17) design. Trifield tubes of 25/17/12 or 23/15/10 are also often used.

These numeric dimensions refer to the diameter of the input phosphor of the image-intensifier tube. The operation of a typical multifield tube is illustrated by the 25/17 type shown in Figure 25-9. In the 25-centimeter mode the photoelectrons from the entire input phosphor are accelerated to the output phosphor. When switched to the 17-centimeter mode, the voltage on the electrostatic focusing lenses is increased, and this causes the electron focal point to move further from the output phosphor. Consequently, only electrons from the center 17-centimeter diameter of the input phosphor are incident on the output phosphor.

The principal result of this change in focal point is to reduce the field of view and thereby magnify the image. Use of the smaller dimension of a multifield image-intensifier tube always results in a magnified image with a magnification factor in direct proportion to the ratio of the diameters. A 25/17 tube operated in the 17-centimeter mode will produce a magnified image 1.5 times larger than the image produced in the 25-centimeter mode.

Question: How magnified is the image of a 25/17/12 image intensifier in the 12-centimeter mode compared with the 25-centimeter mode?

Answer:

$$MF = \frac{25}{12} = 2.1$$

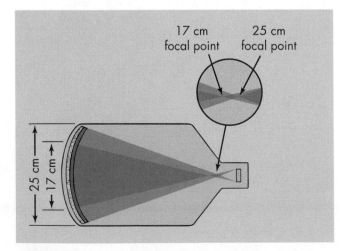

FIGURE 25-9 A 25/17 image-intensifier tube produces a magnified image in the 17-centimeter mode.

This magnified image comes at a price. When operating in the magnified mode, the minification gain is reduced and there are fewer photoelectrons incident on the output phosphor. A dimmer image results.

To maintain the same level of brightness, the x-ray tube mA is automatically increased, but this increases the patient dose. The increase in dose is approximately equal to the ratio of the area of the input phosphor used or 2.2 times ($25^2 \div 17^2$) the dose obtained in the wide field of view mode.

Question: A 23/15/10 image-intensifier tube is used in the 10-centimeter mode. How much higher is the patient dose in this mode compared with the 23-centimeter mode?

Answer: $23^2/10^2 = 5.3$ times as high

This increase in patient dose results in better image quality. The patient dose is higher because more x-ray photons per unit area are used to form the image. This results in lower noise and higher **contrast resolution.**

That portion of any image resulting from the periphery of the input phosphor is inherently unfocused and suffers from **vignetting,** which is a reduction in brightness at the periphery.

Because only the central region of the input phosphor is used in the magnification mode, spatial resolution is also better. In the 25-centimeter mode a cesium-iodide (CsI) image-intensifier tube can image approximately 0.125-millimeter objects (4 lp/mm); in the 10-centimeter mode, the resolution is approximately 0.08 millimeters (6 lp/mm).

The concept of spatial resolution as measured in lp/mm was first introduced in Chapter 16 and is discussed more completely in Chapter 29. At this stage, it is sufficient to know that good spatial resolution is associated with higher lp/mm.

FLUOROSCOPIC-IMAGE MONITORING

The brightness of the fluoroscopic image primarily depends on the anatomic structure being examined, the kVp, and the mA. Fluoroscopic kVp and mA can be controlled by the operator. The influence of kVp and mA on fluoroscopic image quality is similar to their influences on radiographic image quality. In general, high kVp and low mA are preferred for fluoroscopy.

The precise fluoroscopic technique will be determined by the training and experience of the radiologist and radiographer. Table 25-1 shows fluoroscopic kVp for several common examinations. The fluoroscopic mA is not given because that will vary according to patient body characteristics and the response of the fluoroscopic system. Fluoroscopic equipment also allows the radiologist to select an image brightness level that is maintained automatically by the automatic-brightness

TABLE 25-1

Fluoroscopic and Spot-Film kVp for Fluoroscopic Contrast Examinations

Examination	kVp
Gall bladder	65 to 75
Nephrostogram	70 to 80
Myelogram	70 to 80
Barium enema (air contrast)	80 to 90
Upper GI	100 to 110
Small bowel	110 to 120
Barium enema	110 to 120

control (ABS), the automatic-exposure control (AEC), or the automatic-gain control (AGC).

FLUOROSCOPIC IMAGE MONITORING
Television Monitoring

When a **television monitoring system** is used in fluoroscopy, the output phosphor of the image-intensifier tube is coupled directly to a television camera tube. The **vidicon** (Figure 25-10) is the television camera tube most often used in television fluoroscopy. It has a sensitive input surface the same size as the output phosphor of the image-intensifier tube. The television camera tube converts the light image into an electrical signal. The signal is then sent to the television monitor where it is reconstructed as an image on the television screen.

A significant advantage to the use of television monitoring is the electronic control of brightness level and contrast. With television monitoring, several observers can view the fluoroscopic image at the same time. It is even common to place monitors outside the examination room for others to observe.

Television monitoring also allows for storage of the image in its electronic form for playback and image manipulation. Television monitoring is an essential part of the digital fluoroscopic equipment described in Chapter 28.

Television camera. The television camera consists of a cylindrical housing approximately 15 millimeters in diameter and 25 centimeters in length. The housing contains the television camera tube, which is the heart of the camera. It also contains electromagnetic coils for steering the electron beam inside the tube. There are a number of such television camera tubes available for television fluoroscopy, but the vidicon and its modified version the **plumbicon** are used most often.

Figure 25-11 shows a typical vidicon. The **glass envelope** serves the same function that it does for the x-ray tube—to maintain a vacuum and provide mechanical support for the internal elements. The internal elements are the cathode, its **electron gun**, assorted **electrostatic grids**, and a **target assembly** that serves as an anode.

The electron gun is a heated filament that supplies a constant electron current by thermionic emission. These electrons are formed into an electron beam by the control grid, which helps to accelerate the electrons to the anode. The electron beam is further accelerated and focused by additional electrostatic grids. The size of the electron beam and its position are controlled by external electromagnetic coils known as *deflection coils, focusing coils,* and *alignment coils.*

At the anode end of the tube the electron beam passes through a wire meshlike structure and interacts with the target assembly. The target assembly consists of three layers sandwiched together. The outside layer is the face plate, or **window**, the thin part of the glass envelope. Coated on the inside of the window is a thin layer of metal or graphite called the *signal plate.* The signal plate is thin enough to transmit light yet thick enough

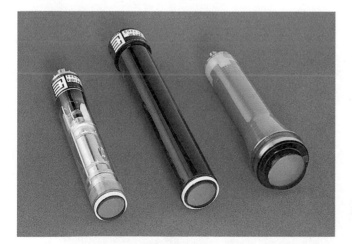

FIGURE 25-10 These three variations of a vidicon television camera are approximately 1 inch in diameter by 6 inches in length. The right tube uses electrostatic electron beam deflection rather than electromagnetic. *(Courtesy Picker International Inc.)*

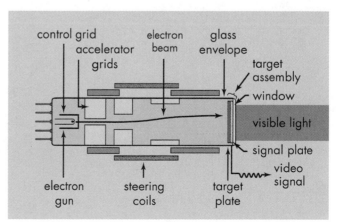

FIGURE 25-11 A vidicon television camera tube and its principal parts.

to be an efficient electrical conductor. Its name derives from the fact that it conducts the video signal out of the tube into the external video circuit.

Applied to the inside of the signal plate is a photoconductive layer of antimony trisulfide. This layer is called the *target,* or *photoconductive layer,* and it is this layer with which the electron beam interacts. Antimony trisulfide is photoconductive because, when illuminated, it conducts electrons; when dark, it behaves as an insulator.

The mechanism of the target assembly is complex but can be described simply as follows. When light from the output phosphor of the image-intensifier tube strikes the window, it will be transmitted through the signal plate to the target. If the electron beam is incident on the same part of the target at the same time, some of its electrons will be conducted through the target to the signal plate and conducted from there out of the tube as the video signal. If that area of the target is dark, there will be no video signal. The magnitude of the video signal is proportional to the intensity of light (Figure 25-12).

Coupling the television camera. Image intensifiers and television camera tubes are manufactured so that the output phosphor of the image-intensifier tube is the same diameter as the window of the television camera tube, usually 2.5 or 5 centimeters. Two methods are commonly used to attach, or couple, the television camera tube to the image-intensifier tube (Figure 25-13).

The simplest method is to use a bundle of fiber optics. The fiber-optics bundle is only a few millimeters thick and contains thousands of glass fibers per square millimeter of cross section. One advantage of this type of coupling is its small size, which makes it easy to manipulate the image-intensifier tower. This coupling is also rugged and can withstand rough handling.

The principal disadvantage is that it cannot accommodate auxiliary imaging devices such as cine or spot-film cameras. With this type of coupling, cassette-loaded spot films are necessary.

To accept a cine or spot-film camera a lens coupling is required. This type of coupling results in a much larger assembly that must be handled with care. It is absolutely essential that the lenses and mirror remain precisely adjusted. Malposition results in a blurred image. The **objective lens** accepts the light from the output phosphor and converts it into a parallel beam. When recording an image on film, this beam is interrupted by a **beam-splitting mirror** so that only a portion is transmitted to the television camera, whereas the remainder is reflected to a film camera. The amount of reflected image is determined by the film and camera system. This system allows the fluoroscopist to view the image while it is being filmed.

Usually the beam-splitting mirror is retracted from the beam when a film camera is not in use. Both the television camera and the film camera are coupled to lenses that focus the parallel light beam onto the film and target of the respective cameras. The alignment of these **camera lenses** is the most critical part of the optical chain. Although the lenses are shown as simple convex lenses, it should be understood that each is a compound lens system consisting of several separate lens elements.

Television monitor. The video signal is amplified and transmitted by cable to the television monitor where it is transformed back into a visible image. The television monitor forms one end of a closed-circuit television system. The other end is the television camera. There are two immediately obvious differences between closed-circuit television fluoroscopy and a home television set. There is no audio or channel selection in fluoroscopy.

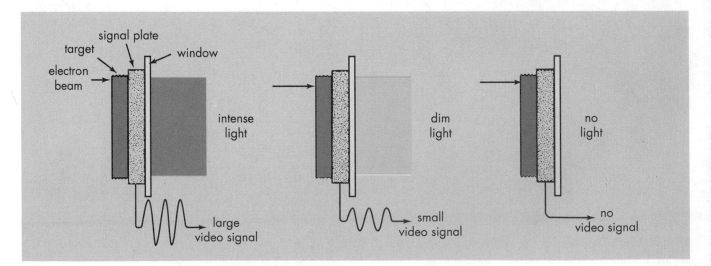

FIGURE 25-12 The target of a television camera tube conducts electrons, which creates a video signal only when illuminated.

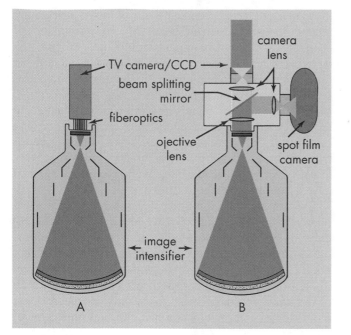

FIGURE 25-13 Television camera tubes are coupled to an image-intensifier tube in two ways. **A,** Fiber optics. **B,** Lens system.

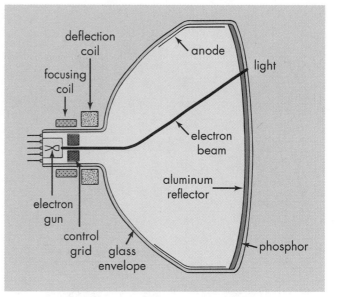

FIGURE 25-14 A television picture tube (CRT) and its principal parts.

There are usually only two controls that the radiographer will manipulate—contrast and brightness.

The heart of the television monitor is the **television picture tube** or cathode-ray tube (CRT) (Figure 25-14). It has many similarities to the camera tube—a glass envelope, an electron gun, and external coils for focusing and steering the electron beam. It is different from a camera tube in that it is very much larger and its anode assembly consists of a fluorescent screen with graphite lining.

The video signal received by the picture tube is modulated. **Modulation** means that the magnitude of the video signal is directly proportional to the light intensity received by the television camera tube. Unlike the television camera tube, the electron beam of the television picture tube varies in intensity according to the modulation of the video signal.

The intensity of the electron beam is modulated by a **control grid** attached to the electron gun. This electron beam is focused onto the output fluorescent screen by the external coils. Here the electrons interact with an output phosphor and produce a burst of light. The phosphor is composed of linear crystals aligned perpendicularly to the glass envelope to reduce **lateral dispersion.** It is usually backed by a thin layer of aluminum that transmits the electron beam but reflects the light.

Television image. The image on the television monitor is formed in a complex way but can be described rather simply. It involves transforming the visible-light image of the output phosphor of the image-intensifier tube into an electrical video signal that is created by a constant electron beam in the television camera tube. The

video signal then modulates, or varies, the electron beam of the television picture tube and transforms that electron beam into a visible image at the fluorescent screen of the picture tube.

Both electron beams, the constant one of the television camera tube and the modulated one of the television picture tube, are finely focused pencil beams that are precisely and synchronously directed by the external electromagnetic coils of each tube. The beams are synchronous because they are both always at the same position at the same time and move in precisely the same fashion.

The movement of these electron beams produces a **raster pattern** on the screen of a television picture tube (Figure 25-15). Although the following discussion relates to a picture tube, remember that the same electron-beam pattern is occurring in the camera tube.

The electron beam begins in the upper-left corner of the screen and moves to the upper-right corner, creating a line of varying intensity of light as it moves. This is called an *active trace.* The electron beam then is **blanked,** or turned off, and it returns to the left side of the screen as shown. This is the **horizontal retrace.** A series of active traces is followed by horizontal retraces until the electron beam is at the bottom of the screen. The electron beam, when it completes its trace, is a **television field.**

At the bottom of the screen, the electron beam is blanked again and undergoes a **vertical retrace** to the top of the screen. The beam describes a second television field, the same as the first except that each active trace lies between two adjacent active traces of the first

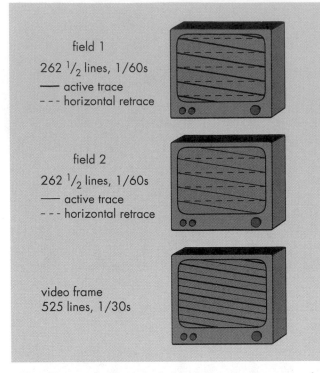

field 1
262 ¹/₂ lines, 1/60s
—— active trace
- - - horizontal retrace

field 2
262 ¹/₂ lines, 1/60s
—— active trace
- - - horizontal retrace

video frame
525 lines, 1/30s

FIGURE 25-15 A video frame is formed from a raster pattern of two interlaced video fields.

field. This movement of the electron beam is termed *interlace,* and two interlaced television fields form one **television frame.**

In the United States, our power is supplied at 60 Hz and therefore there are 60 television fields per second and 30 television frames per second. The flickering of home movies shown at 16 frames per second does not appear on the television image. Flickering is not detectable by the human eye at rates above about 20 frames per second. At a frame rate of 30 per second, each frame is 33 milliseconds long.

In the television camera tube, as the electron beam reads the optical signal, the signal is erased. In the television picture tube, as the electron beam creates the television optical signal, it immediately fades, hence the term *fluorescent screen.* Therefore each new television frame represents 33 milliseconds of new information.

Standard broadcast and closed-circuit television are called *525-line systems* because they have 525 lines of active trace per frame. Actually there are only about 480 lines per frame because of the time required for retracing. Other special purpose systems have 875 or 1000 lines per frame and therefore have better **spatial resolution.** These high-resolution systems are particularly important for digital fluoroscopy.

Vertical resolution is determined by the number of lines. **Horizontal resolution** is determined by a property called *bandwidth* or *bandpass.* Bandpass is expressed

in frequency (Hz) and describes the number of times per second that the electron beam can be modulated or changed. A 1-MHz bandpass would indicate that the electron beam intensity could be changed a million times each second. The higher the bandpass, the better the horizontal resolution.

The objective of television designers is to create a television frame having equal horizontal and vertical resolution. Commercial television systems have a bandpass of about 3.5 MHz. Those used in fluoroscopy are about 4.5 MHz. 1000-line, high-resolution systems have a bandpass of about 20 MHz.

Even though these numbers may seem to indicate a relatively high resolution, the television monitor remains the weakest link in image intensified fluoroscopy. A 525-line system can do no better than about 2 lp/mm, but the image intensifier is good to about 5 lp/mm. Therefore, to take advantage of the superior resolution of the image intensifier, the image must be recorded on film through an optically coupled photographic camera.

SPOT FILMING

The conventional **cassette-loaded spot film** is used with image-intensified fluoroscopes. The spot film is positioned between the patient and the image intensifier (Figure 25-16). During fluoroscopy the cassette is parked in a lead-lined shroud so that it is not unintentionally exposed. When a cassette spot-film exposure is desired, the radiologist must actuate a control that properly positions the cassette in the x-ray beam and changes the operation of the x-ray tube from low fluoroscopic mA to high radiographic mA. Sometimes a second or two is required for the rotating anode to be energized to a higher speed.

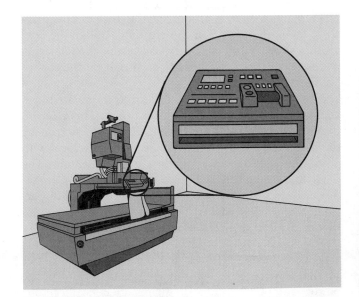

FIGURE 25-16 The cassette-loaded spot film is positioned between the patient and the image intensifier.

The spot film is masked by a series of lead diaphragms to allow several image formats. When the entire film is exposed that is called *one on one*. When only half of the film is exposed at a time, two images result, which is called *two on one*. Four-on-one and six-on-one modes are also available, with the images becoming smaller.

Exposures with spot films require more patient dose, and the delay necessary before exposure can be made is undesirable. However, spot films do provide a familiar format for the radiologist to have high image quality.

The **photo-spot camera** is similar to a movie camera except that it exposes only one frame when activated. It receives its image from the output phosphor of the image-intensifier tube and therefore requires less patient exposure than the spot film. It does not require significant interruption of the fluoroscopic examination nor is there the additional heat load on the x-ray tube associated with spot films.

The photo-spot camera uses film sizes of 70 and 105 millimeters. As a general rule, the larger film format results in better image quality but at increased patient dose. Even with 105 millimeter spot films, however, the patient dose is only approximately half of that with spot films.

The trend in spot filming is use of the photo-spot camera. The photo-spot camera provides adequate image quality without interruption of the fluoroscopic examination and at a rate of up to 12 images per second.

SUMMARY

The original fluoroscope invented by Edison was a zinc-cadmium sulfide screen placed in the x-ray beam directly above the patient. The radiologist stared directly into the screen and viewed a faint yellow-green fluoroscopic image. It was not until the 1940s that the poor illumination from the fluorescent screen was investigated by Chamberlain. As a result, the image intensifier was finally developed in the 1950s.

In the past fluoroscopy required radiologists to adapt their eyes to the dark before the examination. Dark adaptation in the human eye uses rod vision or scotopic vision, which has low visual acuity. The image from the modern fluoroscopic unit is bright enough to be perceived by the cone vision or photopic vision. Cone vision has visual acuity and contrast perception. When viewing the modern fluoroscopic image, the radiologist is able to see fine anatomic detail and differences in brightness levels of anatomic parts.

The x-ray tube in a fluoroscopic unit is under the patient table, and the image intensifier and other devices are above the patient. The image intensifier is a complex device that receives the remnant x-ray beam, converts it to light, and increases the light intensity for better viewing. The input phosphor converts the x-ray beam into light. When stimulated by light the photocathode then emits electrons and the electrons are directed toward the output phosphor and anode. Located along the intensifier tube are electrostatic focusing lenses that focus the electrons emitted from the photocathode. The photoelectrons arriving at the output phosphor are 50 to 75 times as bright because of the action of the focusing lenses.

The following is a list of the formulas relating to fluoroscopy:

$$\text{Flux gain} = \frac{\text{Number of output light photons}}{\text{Number of input x-ray photons}}$$

$$\text{Minification gain} = \frac{(\text{Diameter of input phosphor})^2}{(\text{Diameter of output phosphor})^2}$$

$$\text{Brightness gain} = \text{Minification gain} \times \text{Flux gain}$$

Brightness gain or intensification is also expressed as the conversion factor:

$$\text{Conversion factor} = \frac{\text{Output phosphor illumination (candella/meter}^2)}{\text{Input exposure rate (mR/s)}}$$

The vidicon is the television camera used in fluoroscopy. The television camera is attached to the image intensifer with a lens coupling to accomodate a cine or a spot-film camera. The lens of the lens coupling receives light from the output phosphor and converts it to a parallel beam. When recording an image on film, a beam-splitting mirror separates the beam so that only a portion is transmitted to the television camera and the remainder is reflected to a film camera. The video signal, the signal to the television, forms the fluoroscopic image on the monitor. Spot films can be taken by a multiformatted system using cassettes. One on one, two on one, or four on one can be formatted for spot-film images. The photo-spot camera is similar to a movie camera, but it exposes only one frame when activated. Film sizes of 70 millimeters or 105 millimeters are used in the photo-spot camera.

Generally, high kVp and low mAs are preferred for fluoroscopic technique factors. Table 25-1 lists the kVp levels for common fluoroscopic examinations. MAs is determined by the anatomic part, patient characteristics, and type of fluoroscopic automatic-brightness control used.

REVIEW QUESTIONS

1. Who invented the fluoroscope in 1896? What was the phosphor used on the fluoroscopic screen?
2. Draw a diagram showing the relationship between the x-ray tube, the patient table, and the image intensifier.

3. What is the difference between rod and cone vision? When is visual acuity greater? Define photopic and scotopic vision.

4. What is the kVp setting for the following fluoroscopic examinations: barium enema, gall bladder, upper GI, and air-contrast barium enema?

5. Draw the cross section of the human eye and label the following parts: cornea, lens, and retina.

6. Explain the difference between photoemission and thermionic emission.

7. Diagram the image-intensifier tube and discuss the function of each part.

8. A 23-centimeter image-intensifier tube has an output phosphor size of 2.5 centimeters and a flux gain of 75. What is its brightness gain?

9. Define vignetting.

10. The electron gun in a vidicon is a heated filament that supplies a constant electron current by _____ _____.

11. Why is the television monitor considered the weakest link in image-intensified fluoroscopy?

12. The cassette spot film is positioned between the _____ and the _____.

13. When using the photo-spot camera, the larger the film format, the better the image quality but at increased _____ .

14. What is the primary function of the fluoroscope?

15. If the radiologist observes something during the fluoroscopic examination and would like to preserve that image a _____ _____ can be taken.

Additional Reading

Chamberlain WE: Fluoroscopes and fluoroscopy, *Radiology* 38:383, 1942.

26

Introduction to Angiography and Interventional Radiology

OBJECTIVES

At the completion of this chapter the student will be able to:

1. State the meaning of the initials RT (CV) (ARRT)
2. Discuss the Seldinger technique for vascular access
3. Describe the most common route of vascular access
4. List the four sections of an angiographic guidewire
5. Name the four catheters most commonly used in angiointerventional radiography
6. Discuss the type of contrast media most often in use today during angiointerventional procedures
7. List the step-by-step preparation and monitoring of a patient having an angiointerventional procedure
8. Name the three risks of arteriography
9. Describe the five types of equipment in the angiointerventional suite

OUTLINE

Types of Angiointerventional
  Procedures
Basic Principles
  Arterial access
  Guidewires
  Catheters
  Contrast media
  Patient preparation and monitoring
  Risks of arteriography

Angiointerventional Suite
  Personnel
  Equipment

In previous years, myleography and venograms were considered special procedures. In recent years, there has been rapid development in the area of vascular imaging and theraputic intervention through vessels. As a result, special procedures have been replaced to bring about suites of rooms and complex equipment that have been specially designed for the expanded field of angiointerventional radiology.

The radiographers trained in these areas can now be registered by the American Registry of Radiologic Technologists as certified vascular technologists, which is writtten as RT (CV) (ARRT) after their name.

. . . .

TYPES OF ANGIOINTERVENTIONAL PROCEDURES

Angiointerventional procedures began in the 1930s with **arteriography** (using catheters to enter and highlight an artery with contrast media) and **cardiac catheterization** (using catheters to enter and highlight the coronary arteries with contrast media). The early 1960s saw the introduction of **transfemoral selective coronary angiography** (entering select coronary arteries through a femoral approach) and **percutaneous transluminal angioplasty** (PTA) (enlargement of vessel diameter by using a ballon catheter).

Angiography refers to the many ways to image vessels injected with contrast media. **Angioplasty, thrombolysis, embolization, vascular stents,** and **biopsy** are **interventional** therapeutic procedures conducted in and through vessels. Table 26-1 lists the types of imaging and interventional procedures likely to be conducted in an angiointerventional suite.

BASIC PRINCIPLES
Arterial Access

In 1953, Sven Ivar Seldinger described a method of arterial access that uses a catheter and makes surgery of the vessel unnecessary. The Seldinger needle is an 18-gauge hollow needle with a stylet. Once the Seldinger needle is inserted and pulsating arterial blood returns, the stylet is removed and a guidewire is then inserted into the artery. With the guidewire in the vessel, the Seldinger needle is removed and a catheter is threaded onto the guidewire. Under fluoroscopic view, the catheter is then advanced into the artery.

The common femoral artery is most often used for arterial access in angiography. The common femoral artery can be palpated by locating the pulse below the inguinal ligament, which passes between the pubis and the anterior superior iliac spine.

Guidewires

Guidewires allow the safe introduction of the catheter into the vessel. Once the catheter is in place, the guidewire allows the radiologist to position the catheter within the vascular network.

Guidewires are made of stainless-steel wire, which contains a stiff inner wire tapered at the end to a soft tip. Additionally, there is another fine core wire that joins both ends of the guidewire and prevents loss of sections of the wire should it break. The trailing end of the guidewire is stiff and allows maneuverability along the length of the guidewire. Conventional guidewires are 145 centimeters long. Catheters overlaying the guidewire are usually 100 centimeters long. Wires are additionally categorized by length to the beginning of the tapered tip, configuration of the tip, stiffness of the guidewire, and coating.

The J-tip for guidewires is a variation of the tip configuration and is used for **atherosclerotic** vessels that are filled with obstructions. The J-tip deflects off edges of **plaques** and helps prevent **dissection** of the artery. The coatings on guidewires are materials designed to reduce friction and include Teflon, **heparin** coatings, and **hydrophilic polymers.**

Catheters

Just like guidewires, catheters are designed in many different shapes and sizes. Usually, catheter diameter is categorized in French (Fr) sizes, with 3 Fr equaling 1 millimeter in diameter. Figure 26-1 illustrates four catheter shapes. The shaped tip of the catheter is required for selective catheterization of openings into specific arteries. The H1, or headhunter tip, is used for the femoral approach to the **brachiocephalic** vessels. The Simmons catheter is highly curved for approach to sharply angled vessels such as the **celiac axis.** The C2, or Cobra catheter, has an angled tip joined to a gentle curve and is used for introduction into **renal** and **mesenteric** arteries. Pigtail catheters have side holes for ejecting contrast media into a compact bolus. The jet effect is minimized with the curved pigtail, which prevents injury to the vessel.

TABLE 26-1

Representative Procedures Conducted in an Angiointerventional Suite

Imaging Procedures	Interventional Procedures
Angiography	Stent placement
Aortography	Embolization (vascular occulsion to stop bleeding)
Arteriography	Intravascular stent
Cardiac catheterization	Thrombolysis (declotting)
Myelography	Balloon angioplasty
Venography	Atherectomy (removal of vascular plaque)

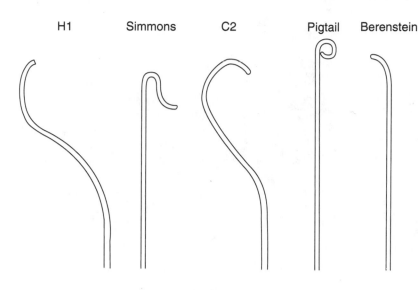

H1   Simmons   C2   Pigtail   Berenstein

FIGURE 26-1 Catheter shapes. *(From Wojtowycz M: Handbook of interventional radiology and angiography, ed 2, St Louis, 1995, Mosby.)*

Once the catheter is introduced into the vessel, the guidewire is removed. The catheter must then immediately be flushed to prevent clotting of blood within the catheter. Heparinized saline is generally used to flush catheters.

Contrast Media

Vessels under investigation in angiography are injected with radiopaque contrast media. In the past, ionic compounds have been used for contrast injections; however, more recently nonionic contrast media has been introduced. The new agents, because of their low concentration of ions (**low-osmolality**), cause fewer physiologic problems and fewer adverse reactions for a patient undergoing angiographic injection.

Patient Preparation and Monitoring

Before angiography the patient is visited by the radiologist to establish rapport and to obtain informed consent. A physical examination is also preliminary to angiography to assess the patient's medical history and allergies and to conclude whether a femoral approach is possible. Orders are written for intravenous hydration and a diet of clear liquids. The patient may be premedicated in the angiography suite.

During the procedure, monitoring by electrocardiography, automatic blood pressure measurement, and pulse oximetry is mandatory. The code cart for life-threatening emergencies must be accessible. After the procedure, when the catheter is removed, manual compression on the femoral site is required. The patient is instructed to remain immobile for 4 hours after the angiographic procedure while vital signs are frequently monitored and the puncture site inspected.

Risks of Arteriography

The most common problem relating to angiography is continued bleeding at the puncture site. Of course, there is also a risk for a hypersensitivity reaction to the contrast media, and there are risk factors related to kidney failure. For these risks to be minimized, it is important to obtain a complete patient medical, surgical, and allergy history before any angiographic procedure.

ANGIOINTERVENTIONAL SUITE
Personnel

Unlike a conventional x-ray room, the angiointerventional facility requires a suite of rooms (Figure 26-2). The procedure room itself should be not less than 20 feet along any wall and not less than 500 square feet. Such a size is required to accommodate the amount of equipment required and the large number of people involved in most procedures. The procedure room will normally have at least three means of access. Patient access should be through a door wide enough to accommodate a bed. Access to the central room does not normally require a door. An open passageway is adequate.

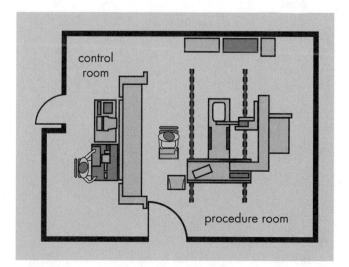

FIGURE 26-2 Typical layout for an angiointerventional suite.

Doors interfere with personnel movement. A door leading to an adjacent surgical suite is necessary for the well-planned angiointerventional suite.

The procedure room should be finished with consideration for maintaining a clean and sterile environment. The floor, walls, and all counter and cabinet surfaces must be smooth and easy to clean. The control room should be large, perhaps 100 square feet. This room should connect directly with processing and viewing areas.

A radiographer can specialize in many different fields (Figure 26-3). The radiographer who specializes in angiointerventional radiography is highly skilled. The American Registry of Radiologic Technologists offers an examination in angiointerventional radiography. Once the examination is passed, the radiographer may add (CV) after the RT (R). There may be two or three radiographers in the angiographic suite setting up runs, as well as the interventional radiologist who performs the procedure and a radiology nurse who carefully monitors the patient. During procedures when the patient has to be highly medicated, an anesthesiologist may also be present in the angiointerventional suite.

Equipment

X-ray tube. The x-ray apparatus for an angiointerventional suite is generally more massive, flexible, and expensive than that required for conventional radiographic and fluoroscopic imaging. Advanced radiographic and fluoroscopic equipment is required (Figure 26-4). Generally, two ceiling track-mounted radiographic x-ray tubes are required with an image-intensified fluoroscope mounted on a C or an L arm.

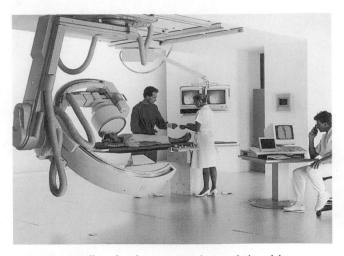

FIGURE 26-4 X-ray imaging apparatus in a typical angiointerventional suite. *(Courtesy Philips Medical Systems.)*

The angiointerventional x-ray tube has a small target angle, a large-diameter massive anode disk, and cathodes designed for magnification and serial radiography. Table 26-2 describes the specifications for such a typical x-ray tube.

A small focal spot of not greater than 0.3 millimeter is necessary for the spatial resolution requirements of magnification radiography of small vessels in the brain. Neuroangiography of contrast-filled vessels as small as 1 millimeter is possible with proper geometry and patient positioning. With an SID equalling 100 centimeters and an OID equaling 40 centimeters the radiographer can take advantage of the air gap to improve image contrast. Using a 0.3-millimeter focal spot results in a focal-spot blur of 1.2 millimeters.

Question: A left cerebral angiogram is performed with a 0.3-millimeter focal spot at 100-centimeters SID. The artery to be imaged is 20 centimeters from the image receptor. What is the magnification factor, focal-spot blur, and approximate spatial resolution?

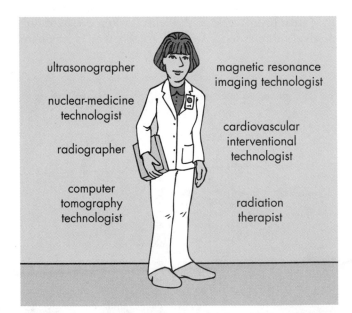

FIGURE 26-3 A radiographer can be any of the following imaging specialists.

TABLE 26-2

Specifications for a Typical Angiointerventional Radiographic X-ray Tube.

Feature	Size	Why
Focal spot	1.0 millimeter/ 0.3 millimeter	Large for heat load; small for magnification
Anode disk size	5 inches diameter 2 inches thick	To accommodate heat load
Power rating	80 kW	For rapid sequence, serial radiography
Anode heat capacity	1 MHU	To accommodate head load

Answer: $MF = \dfrac{SID}{SOD} = \dfrac{100 \text{ cm}}{80 \text{ cm}} = 1.25$

Focal-spot blur $= (EFS)\dfrac{OID}{SID} =$

$$(0.3)\,\dfrac{20}{100} = .06 \text{ mm}$$

Approximate spatial resolution =

$2 \times$ focal-spot blur = .12 millimeters

Spatial resolution for the above procedure can be approximated multiplying the focal-spot blur by two. Figure 26-5 shows geometry that results in 0.5-millimeter focal-spot blur images of a 10-millimeter vessel. A 0.5-millimeter vessel will be too blurred to be seen. Any vessel larger than 1 millimeter will be imaged.

All of the other essential characteristics of an angiointerventional x-ray tube are based on required tube loading. The size and construction of the anode disk determines the anode heat capacity, which in turn influences the power rating. An x-ray tube with a minimum 80-kW rating with 1-MHU heat capacity is required.

High voltage generator. High-frequency generators are often used in all x-ray examinations including angiointerventional procedures, but angiointerventional procedures, require higher power than may be available even with high-frequency generators. High-voltage generators with three-phase, 12-pulse power capable of at least 100 kW with low ripple are needed for the high power requirements.

Patient couch. Whereas most general fluoroscopy imagers have a tilt-table, angiointerventional imagers do not. During general fluoroscopy head-down and head-up tilting of the patient is often necessary for manipulation of contrast. Only myelography as an angiointerventional procedure requires a tilt-table and therefore that procedure is often done in general fluoroscopy.

Other angiointerventional procedures do not require a tilt-table and therefore use a stationary patient couch with a floating or moveable table top (Figure 26-6). Controls for couch positioning are located on the side of the table and duplicated on a floor switch. The floor switch is necessary to accommodate patient positioning while maintaining a sterile field.

The patient couch may also have a computer-controlled **stepping** capability. This feature is necessary to allow imaging from the abdomen to the feet after a single injection of contrast medium. An additional requirement of this stepping feature is the ability to preselect the time and position of the patient couch to coincide with the image receptor.

Image receptor. Three different types of image receptors are used in angiointerventional procedures. The cinefluorographic camera is used during cardiac catheterization. The serialographic changer has been the principal image receptor for many years, but digital fluoroscopy is rapidly making these devices obsolete (see Chapter 28). Photofluorographic cameras (Figure 26-7) were described in Chapter 25.

Cine camera. In cinefluorography the television camera tube is replaced with a movie camera that records the image on film for later playback. Cinefluorography is used most often in certain angiographic procedures,

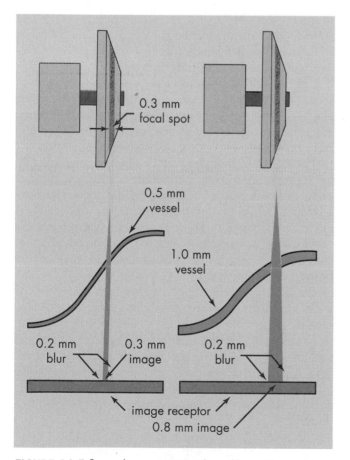

FIGURE 26-5 For a given geometry, such as this resulting in 0.5-millimeter focal-spot blur, the vessels must be twice the size of the focal-spot blur.

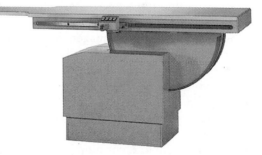

FIGURE 26-6 Typical angiointerventional patient couch with a floating, rotating and tilting top. (*Courtesy Continental X-ray Corporation.*)

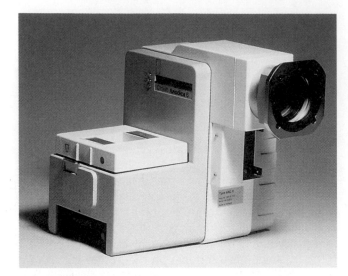

FIGURE 26-7 This 105 mm photofluorographic spot film camera captures images from the output phosphor of an image intensifier in either single or rapid serial fashion. *(Courtesy of Odelft.)*

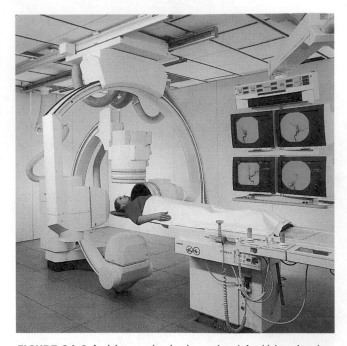

FIGURE 26-8 Angiointerventional suite equipped for biplane imaging. *(Courtesy Siemans Medical Systems.)*

especially those associated with cardiac catheterization. The patient dose is much higher than that required for recording images electronically, but the image quality is also higher.

Both 16- and 35-millimeter film movie cameras are used for cinefluorography. The 35-millimeter film format requires more patient exposure than the 16-millimeter film format, but the image quality is also better.

Cine cameras are driven by **synchronous motors** controlled by the line voltage, which is 60 Hz. Therefore they have frame rates of 7.5, 15, 30, and 60 frames per second. Naturally, the higher the frame rate, the higher the radiation dose. High frame rates are necessary for cardiac studies, but 7.5 frames per second may be adequate for other examinations.

Cinefluorographic systems are **synchronized** (i.e., the x-ray tube is energized only during the time when the cine film is in position for exposure). The x-ray tube is not energized during the time between frames when the film is advancing because this would result in considerably excessive and unnecessary patient exposure.

Serial changer. The serial changer has been the principal unique angiographic imager since the 1950s. Production of these devices has dwindled because of the emergence of digital fluoroscopy. Serial changers, referred to as *rapid film changers* or simply *film changers*, are often used in pairs with two orthogonal x-ray sources in a configuration called *biplane imaging* (Figure 26-8). There are two types of serialographic changers—roll film and cut film.

The roll-film changer predates automatic processing and was designed to replace bulky cassette changers. Up

to 12 images per second are possible, but processing, viewing, and storage of the roll of images are difficult. Because of this deficiency, this type of film changer was quickly replaced by cut-film changers.

Cut-film changers incorporate a supply magazine of sheets of film, an exposure chamber, and a receiving magazine for exposed film. The supply and receiving magazines are lead lined to protect the unprocessed film from radiation.

The exposure chamber contains two radiographic intensifying screens to accommodate 35 × 35 centimeter double-emulsion film. Before exposure the screens are separated while a film from the supply magazine is moved into position. During exposure the screens are pressed against the film to ensure good screen-film contact. After exposure the screens separate and the exposed film is moved to the receiving magazine. Precise mechanical and electrical synchronization with the x-ray generator, exposure timer, and x-ray tube are essential.

Normally up to four images per second can be made, and an 8:1 or 10:1 carbon-fiber focused grid is used. Alternately a 10-centimeter air gap can be used. An 800-speed screen-film combination is also normal. The two standard cut-film changers are identified as AOT or Puck.

The AOT film changer is contained in a large cumbersome cabinet that is usually positioned on the floor under the patient couch (Figure 26-9).

The Puck film changer is much smaller and simpler than the AOT film changer. It is mounted on the image-

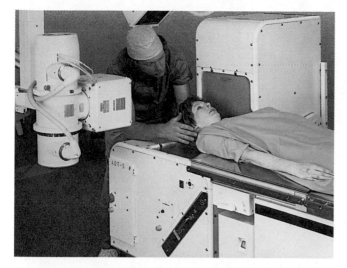

FIGURE 26-9 The AOT film changer may be positioned with difficulty for vertical or horizontal imaging. *(Courtesy Elema-Schonander.)*

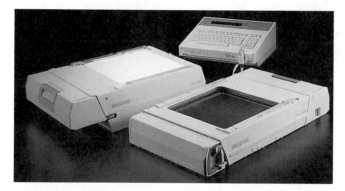

FIGURE 26-10 The Puck film changer can be mounted on the image intensifier and rotated into the x-ray beam or positioned on an independent stand during use. *(Courtesy Elema-Schonander.)*

intensifier tower and rotated into the x-ray beam for serial radiography (Figure 26-10).

Filming. After catheter placement during the angiointerventional procedure, a test injection is done under fluoroscopy before filming to check that the catheter tip is not wedged and is in the correct vessel. Injection rates of the automatic power injector are gauged by the test flow speed. A scout film is obtained by the radiographer to check positioning and exposure factors. Then the catheter is attached to the unit that injects the contrast media, the power injector. If subtraction films are needed, then the film and injection parameters include one exposure before the injection of contrast material. Exposures are made at the frame rate and injection sequence specific for the procedure. Rapid flow requires two to three frames per second, whereas delayed films may be included at 20 to 40 seconds after injection.

SUMMARY

Angiography refers to the many ways to image contrast-filled vessels. In 1953, Sven Ivan Seldinger described a method of arterial access that uses an 18-gauge hollow needle with a stylet. Using a guidewire and catheter, radiologists have access to the vascular network without surgery. The common femoral artery is most often used for arterial access in angiography.

Catheter-tip designs are illustrated in Figure 26-1, and each is used for access to specfic arteries. The contrast media used is generally nonionic, which reduces physiologic problems and adverse reactions in patients undergoing angiographic procedures. A complete medical, surgical, and allergic history of the patient is required before angiography. During the procedure the patient's vital signs must be carefully monitored. The most common risk to patients is continued bleeding at the puncture site. Most patients remain immobile during the 4 hours of postprocedure recovery.

Table 26-2 summarizes the specifications for a typical angiointerventional x-ray tube. It is designed for magnification, high resolution using a small focal spot, and the massive heat loads associated with serial radiography. The patient couch is a floating table top with a stepping capability to automatically allow imaging from abdomen to feet after a single injection of contrast media.

Cine cameras with 16- or 35-millimeter frames are used in cardiac catherization procedures. Serial changers or digital imaging are generally used for angiointerventional procedures. With both serial changers and digital imaging, power injection of contrast media and filming are synchronized to obtain the optimal visualization of the vessel of interest.

REVIEW QUESTIONS

1. Define arteriography and cardiac catherization.
2. Describe the Seldinger method for arterial access.
3. What is the most common artery used for arterial access in angiography?
4. Why is a guidewire used for arterial access in addition to catheters?
5. List four types of catheters and the selective vessels for which they are designed.
6. Name two reasons why the radiologist visits the patient before the angiointerventional procedure.
7. What is the most common problem patients encounter after the angiointerventional procedure?
8. Define thrombolysis and embolization.
9. What is the required heating capacity of the angiointerventional x-ray tube?

10. Name the titles and describe the duties of the team of personnel who work in the angiography suite.

11. List the focal-spot requirements for the angiointerventional x-ray tube. For what procedure is the small focal spot used?

12. What does it mean when the patient couch has a stepping capability?

13. Cinefluoroscopy is generally used for _____, and the serial changer or digital imaging is used for _____.

14. Name the frame rates for cine camera. Name the frame rates for the cut-film serial changer.

15. Discuss how subtraction films are obtained during filming of an angiointerventional procedure.

Additional Reading

Rosen RJ, Nosher J: *Angiography and interventional radiography,* St Louis, 1991, Mosby.

Wojtowycz M: *Handbook of angiography and interventional radiology,* ed 2, St Louis, 1991, Mosby.

27

Computer Science

OBJECTIVES

At the completion of this chapter the student will be able to:

1. Describe how a computer can be considered artificial intelligence
2. Discuss the early and modern history of computers and how the transistor led to the explosion of modern computer science
3. Explain the difference between a microcomputer, a minicomputer, and a mainframe computer
4. List and define the nine components of computer hardware
5. Define bit, byte, and word as used in computer terminology
6. Contrast the two classifications of computer programs—systems software and applications programs
7. List and explain the 10 main types of computer languages
8. Discuss the four computer processing methods

OUTLINE

Introduction to Computers

History of Computers
  Early history
  Modern computers

Anatomy of a Computer
  Hardware
  Secondary memory devices
  Software
  Computer languages
  Hexadecimal number system

Processing Methods

oday the word *computer* indicates the personal computer (PC) to most of us, but computer applications in diagnostic imaging departments are accelerating rapidly. The first large-scale computer application was computed tomographic scanning (CT). Magnetic resonance imaging and diagnostic ultrasound apply computer technology in the same way computers are used in CT. Computers now control x-ray generators and radiographic control panels, automatically setting radiographic and fluoroscopic technique for radiographers.

INTRODUCTION TO COMPUTERS

A computer is an electronic data processing machine that **computes, manipulates, makes decisions,** and **interacts** accurately and quickly. Computers provide **numerical computation** and **word manipulation.** The computer solves problems by accepting data and performing prescribed operations on the data as directed by a **stored program.** It then supplies the results of these operations to the user.

The computer has an extensive ability to make decisions. For instance, in the area of **artificial intelligence (AI)** the computer can make decisions based on conditions previously known, currently known, and expected. Almost anything definable can be decided automatically by a computer.

Finally, the computer is capable of interacting with the user. The interaction involves accepting data from the user and providing results to the user. Data can be entered by keyboard, scanner, or even voice. In addition, data already stored in the computer, such as a file containing patient data, can be entered automatically.

When a computer is performing operations on defined data without human input or intervention, the computer is said to be **batch processing** data. Depending on the amount of data involved and the operation, the computer could run by itself for weeks.

At the present time, computer applications are exploding at an incredibly fast rate. In addition to scientific, engineering, and business applications, the computer is becoming more familiar in everyday life. We know the computer is somehow involved in video games, automatic bank tellers, and highway toll booths. It may not be equally as obvious that computers now control things such as many supermarket checkouts, ticket reservation centers, industrial processes, touchtone phone answering services, traffic lights, and even automobile ignition systems. The widespread use of the personal computer has accelerated this explosion.

Computer applications in radiology are accelerating equally rapidly. The first large-scale computer application in radiology was computed tomographic (CT) scanning. Digital fluoroscopy and digital radiography are now routine. Magnetic resonance imaging and diagnostic ultrasound also use computer technology. X-ray generators are controlled by computers for even more automation and precision in setting radiographic and fluoroscopic technique. A radiographic operating console is controlled by a **microprocessor,** which is a computer on a chip. The microprocessor is able to interpret the examination input from the radiographer and logically select the proper mAs and kVp.

HISTORY OF COMPUTERS
Early History

The earliest calculating tool was the abacus (Figure 27-1). It was invented thousands of years ago in the Orient and is still used in some countries today. Further advancement in calculating tools did not occur until the seventeenth-century, when two mathematicians, Blaise Pascal and Gottfried Leibniz, built mechanical calculators using pegged wheels to automatically perform the four arithmetic functions—addition, subtraction, multiplication, and division. In 1842, Charles Babbage designed an analytical engine to perform general calcula-

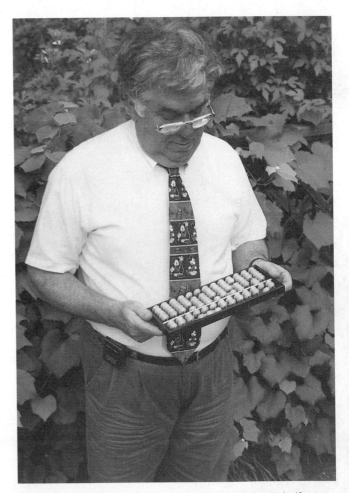

FIGURE 27-1 The abacus was the earliest calculating tool. *(Courtesy Robert J. Wilson.)*

tions automatically. Herman Hollerith designed a system to record census data in 1890. He stored information as holes on cards that were interpreted by machines with electrical sensors. It was Hollerith who started a company that eventually evolved into IBM. In 1939, John Atansoff and Clifford Berry designed and built the first electronic digital computer.

Modern Computers

The first general purpose modern computer was developed in 1944 at Harvard University. It was originally called the *Automatic Sequence Controlled Calculator (ASCC).* Now it is identified simply as the Mark I. It was an electromechanical device and was exceedingly slow and prone to malfunction.

The first general purpose electronic computer was developed in 1946 at the University of Pennsylvania by J. Presper Eckert and John Mauchly at a cost of $500,000. It was called *ENIAC* (electronic numerical integrator and calculator) and it contained over 18,000 vacuum tubes, which failed at an average of one every 7 minutes (Figure 27-2). Neither the Mark I nor the ENIAC had their instructions stored in a memory device.

In 1948, scientists led by William Shockley at the Bell Telephone Laboratories developed the **transistor,** which led to the creation of a smaller computer. It also made possible the development of the stored-program computer and thus the continuing explosion in computer science. The transistor allowed Eckert and Mauchly, under the Sperry-Rand Corporation, to develop **UNIVAC** (**universal automatic computer**), which appeared in 1951 as the first commercially successful general purpose stored-program electronic digital computer.

The word *computer* today identifies the **personal computer** (**PC**) to most of us (Figure 27-3). A PC is a **general purpose** computer, able to solve any solvable problem, but there are also **special-purpose** computers, which are designed for a particular singular task such as control of an assembly-line robot or an automobile ignition switch.

The computer used today is a **stored-program** electronic digital computer. The stored-program computers have their instructions (programs) and data stored in their memories. These stored-program computers are laid out so that the sequence of steps to be followed during any calculation is preestablished. **Electronic** implies that the computer is powered by electrical and electronic devices rather than by a mechanical device.

Finally, **digital computers** have largely replaced analog computers. The difference between analog and digital is illustrated in Figure 27-4, which shows two kinds of watches. An analog watch is mechanical and has hands that move continuously around a dial face. A digital watch contains a computer chip and indicates time with numbers.

Most calculators handle only arithmetic functions, whereas computers handle arithmetic and **logic functions.** Logic functions evaluate an intermediate result and perform subsequent computations, depending on that result. However, new technology has brought advanced calculators with graphing and programming abilities. Now calculators can execute logic functions, solve equations, draw lines, and transmit data to other calculators via cords or infrared beams.

Computers have undergone four generations of development distinguished by the technology of their electronic devices. First-generation computers were

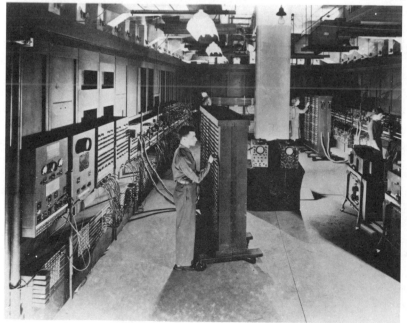

FIGURE 27-2 The ENIAC computer occupied an entire room. It was completed in 1946 and is recognized as the first all-electronic general-purpose digital computer. *(Courtesy Sperry-Rand Corporation.)*

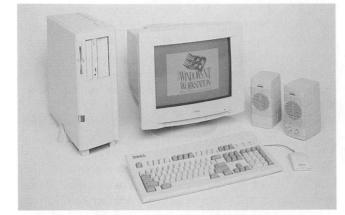

FIGURE 27-3 Today's personal computer has exceptional speed capacity and flexibility. There are numerous applications in radiology. *(Courtesy Dell Computer Corp.)*

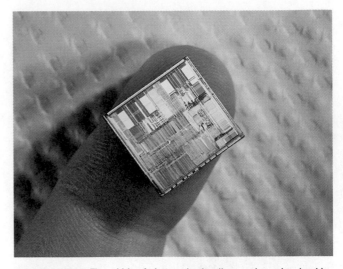

FIGURE 27-5 The width of the conductive lines and spacing in this microprocessor chip is 15 millimeters. *(Courtesy Intel.)*

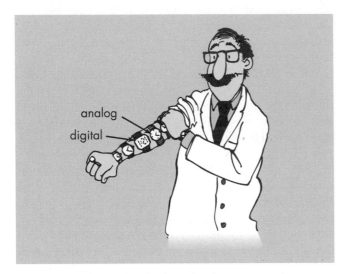

FIGURE 27-4 Two styles of wristwatches demonstrate analog versus digital.

vacuum-tube machines (1939-1958). Second-generation computers, which became generally available in 1958, were based on individually packaged **transistors.** The third-generation machines introduced in 1964 used integrated circuits (IC). **Integrated circuits** consist of many transistors and other electronic elements fused onto a **chip,** a tiny piece of semiconductor material, usually silicon. The fourth generation of computers, which first appeared in 1975, was an extension of the third generation and incorporated **large-scale integration (LSI),** now replaced by **very large-scale integration (VLSI),** which places hundreds of thousands of circuit elements on a chip less than 1 centimeter in size (Figure 27-5).

Today's computers come in basically three sizes. The **microcomputer** is the smallest. It appears as a personal computer (PC), a word processor, and a control for many industrial processes. The **minicomputer** is some-

what larger in capacity and flexibility. Most computer applications in radiology use a minicomputer. The **mainframe computer** is used for very large applications by organizations such as the U.S. Census Bureau. Microcomputers usually run with a single microprocessor, whereas minicomputers and mainframes use multiple microprocessors.

ANATOMY OF A COMPUTER

There are two principal parts to a computer (1) hardware and (2) software. Hardware and software each have have several components. The **hardware** is everything about the computer that is visible: the nuts, bolts, and chips of the system that form the central processing unit and the various input/output devices. The **software** is invisible. It consists of the computer programs that tell the hardware what to do and how to store data.

Hardware

CPU. The **central processing unit (CPU)** is built around a microprocessor. The CPU is the primary control center. In a PC the microprocessor is a single very large-scale integrated circuit on a silicon chip less than a centimeter on a side that contains hundreds of thousands of individual circuit elements. Figure 27-6 is a photomicrograph of the Pentium microprocessor produced by the Intel Corporation. It is an extremely powerful and fast microprocessor designed for high-performance, large, multi-user, multitask computer systems.

The CPU on this chip supervises all of the other components of the computer, performs the mathematical manipulations, and even stores information. Data is transferred to and from the CPU and other computer components along an electrical conductor called a *bus.* The CPU consists of a control unit, an arithmetic unit,

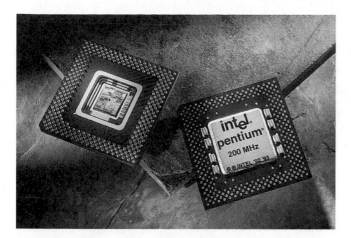

FIGURE 27-6 This Pentium microprocessor incorporates over one million transistors on a chip of silicon less than 1 centimeter on a side. *(Courtesy Intel.)*

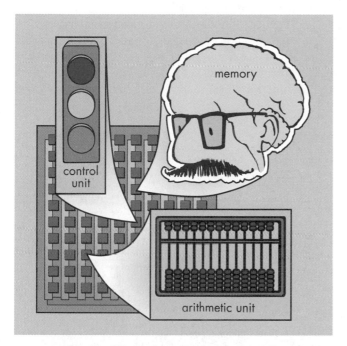

FIGURE 27-7 The CPU contains a control unit, an arithmetic unit, and sometimes memory.

and memory (Figure 27-7). Additional primary memory can be stored on separate chips.

Control unit. When data are entered into the computer through an **input device,** such as the keyboard or a disk, the **control unit** identifies the route of entry and directs the data to the arithmetic unit or to memory. Similarly, when a computation is completed, the control unit will transfer the results to the output device selected. The control unit is the computer's basic overseer in charge of interpreting the user's program instructions in the proper order. If a calculation is required, it passes data to the arithmetic unit. It also stores and retrieves

data from memory or from input/output devices. The speed of these tasks is determined by the frequency of an external electronic clock that synchronizes CPU operation with the rest of the computer. Clock frequencies of at least 10 MHz allow the computer to perform millions of simple operations per second. Most computers today run between 40 and 100 MHz. The fastest computer can perform ten billion calculations per second, and machines 10 and even 100 times faster are being designed.

Arithmetic unit. The arithmetic unit, sometimes referred to as an *authentic logic unit (ALU),* is that portion of the CPU that holds the numbers that are involved in the calculations, performs the logic and numeric calculations, and then temporarily holds the results until they can be transferred to memory. The speed of the arithmetic unit in performing these computations is also controlled by the external clock. In the arithmetic unit the clock synchronizes a very high-speed calculator that performs the four basic arithmetic functions and the logic functions.

Memory unit. The CPU contains two types of memory. It has **registers,** which store temporary information, and the **main memory,** where the programs and data are kept. Generally, the control unit extracts instructions and data from memory and transfers data between memory and various input and output devices. **Direct memory access (DMA)** controllers are available for many computers. These devices speed up the transfer of bulk data between main memory and external devices, bypassing the CPU itself.

A major change occured in computer technology in the mid-1970s. The magnetic core memory was changed to semiconductor memory. The **magnetic core** consisted of small magnetic dipoles that existed in one of two states, depending on the direction of the electric current passing through them. Compared with semiconductor memory, magnetic core memory was expensive and slow. The word *core,* however, still survives in computer terminology and is used to refer to primary memory even though primary memory now is based on semiconductors rather than magnetic loops.

Digital radiologic imaging owes its rapid development in part to semiconductor memory. **Semiconductor memory** consists of extremely small storage circuits etched on a silicon chip. The individual chips are arranged in groups to form a **memory module** complete with all interconnections to plug into the computer.

Semiconductor storage operates on the principle of a **flip-flop.** A switch is set in one of two states variously described as one or zero, A or B, "yes" or "no," "true" or "false," "set or reset," and "plus" or "minus." Each individual flip-flop stores one **bit** (**bi**nary digi**t**) of information.

Primary memory is available as **read-only memory (ROM)** and **random access memory (RAM).** The instructions in ROM are entered by the manufacturer and cannot be changed. The ROM usually contains the primary computer instructions, called *system programs.* These instructions get the computer going when it is first turned on. The ROM is also used extensively in single-application chips such as word processors, pocket calculators, and video games. Some types of ROM, erasable-programmable read-only memory (**EPROM**), have the capability of being erased when it is exposed to ultraviolet light. This procedure resets EPROM and allows it to be reprogrammed.

The RAM is sometimes called **read-write memory.** The RAM is used for storing computational instructions or data that might change from time to time. It is possible to both store data or instructions in RAM and to read what is stored without changing it. There are two principal types of RAM: (1) **static RAM (SCRAM)** and (2) **dynamic RAM (DRAM).** SCRAM retains its memory, even if power to the computer is lost. DRAM is structured in a parallel fashion, which increases computer speed.

All primary memory is **addressed.** Each memory location has a unique label identifying its position. Memory operates much like your home address, which allows you to receive mail that is uniquely yours. It allows the computer's CPU access to the data at specific spots in memory without disturbing the rest of memory.

A sequence of memory locations may contain steps of a computer program or a string of data. The CPU keeps track of the address in memory where the current program instructions are stored so that it can hop to other memory locations to read or write data and then return to the proper place in the program.

All information to be processed by the computer must pass through primary memory. It is most efficient to have sufficient primary memory to retain all the necessary data and instructions for processing. Most applications, however, require **secondary memory,** usually in the form of disks or tape.

In CT scanning, for instance, when contiguous transverse images are reconstructed in a coronal or sagittal plane, the images are sequentially routed from secondary memory to primary memory to the arithmetic unit of the CPU.

Input/output devices. The process of transferring information into primary memory is known as an *input operation.* The process of transferring the results of a computation from primary memory to storage or the user is known as an *output operation.* Input/output devices, commonly referred to as *I/O devices,* allow the user to communicate with the computer. In addition, I/O devices can provide secondary memory to handle more information than can be contained in primary memory at one time.

The I/O devices principally involved in computer applications in radiology are the keyboard, the video dis-

play terminal, the printer, the laser camera, and secondary memory devices. Figure 27-8 illustrates how the control unit behaves as an interface between these various I/O devices and primary memory. Because VLSI computers have become cheaper and more powerful, some I/O devices have evolved into very powerful data processing units in themselves. Some operate nearly independently with only minimum interaction with the control unit.

Video display terminal. The I/O device most familiar to the radiographer is the **video display terminal (VDT).** A VDT is found on every CT scanner, digital x-ray imager, and MR imager. A VDT consists of a keyboard and a **cathode-ray tube (CRT)** display, which looks like a television tube.

Terminal keyboards are nearly all electronic. The keys are switches. Each key depression produces a code, and the computer responds with a character on the screen of the CRT display. This is the usual method of data entry to the computer.

The keyboard resembles a conventional typewriter except that, in addition to the alphabetic key pad, there is usually a separate, calculator-type, 10-number key pad. There also are usually other key pads containing special-function keys, such as left, right, up, and down

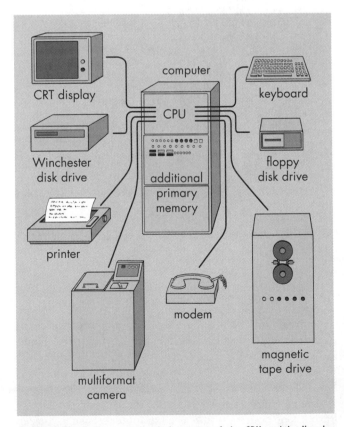

FIGURE 27-8 The control unit is a part of the CPU and is directly connected to additional primary memory and various input/output devices.

arrows, and function keys for use with a special operation, such as a radiographic examination.

For instance, digital fluoroscopy (see Chapter 28), uses special-function keys for masking, reregistration, and time-interval difference imaging. Optical scanners, trackballs, and electronic mice are also interactive input devices commonly used with VDTs.

VDTs may be designed for alphanumeric display and for graphic display. Alphanumeric display is the display normally encountered. It is a series of letters and numbers that conveys information. If graphic output is also available, one can display the results of numeric computations graphically. Virtually all radiographic terminals provide for alphanumeric and graphic output.

The characters needed for the display of text are generated by patterns of dots from a special ROM called a *character generator*. A typical VDT will display 24 lines of 80 characters each. Each character is produced by a matrix that typically consists of 63 dots (nine dots high by seven dots wide), where only the dots required to form a character are displayed (Figure 27-9). The characters on the CRT display and many printers are formed this way.

VDTs are either intelligent or nonintelligent devices. The intelligent terminal is also known as a *programmable*, or logic, terminal. This is the type used for most radiographic applications. It consists of a microprocessor with an associated memory that contains a program to direct the operation of the terminal, validate input, and direct communications with a larger computer.

The nonintelligent terminal must be connected directly to a computer. It behaves strictly as a passbox for the operator's input. It does not edit, compute, or perform any logic on its own.

Secondary Memory Devices

Magnetic disks. The principal medium for secondary memory is a magnetic disk. It is either rigid, like a phonograph record, or flexible. The former is usually called a *hard disk;* the latter is called a *floppy disk.* Floppy disks have been replaced by higher capacity hard disks and are no longer a part of new computers.

Hard disks are 5¼- or 3½-inch diameter and are housed in a rigid square plastic case. Data are stored on the disk in a series of concentric magnetic tracks. If they could be seen, the tracks would be similar in appearance to the grooves of a phonograph record. Most high-density 5¼-inch disks hold 1.6 MB, whereas most 3½-inch disks hold 2 MB of data. However, some hold anywhere from 4 to 21 MB and require a special drive.

Most disks are rigid plastic platters, coated on both sides with a recording material that can be magnetized. The data are recorded as binary digits and are accessible for reading or writing by positioning a read-write head on the disk. Both the top and bottom surfaces are used. For large amounts of data, a number of disks are stacked (Figure 27-10).

Hard disks are random access in nature. The data are grouped into fixed-length blocks, each of which is addressed. These blocks of data can each be read or written independently. Hard disks are frequently used in radiographic imaging procedures because of their large capacity and high speed as secondary memory devices. Some hard disks can hold 1 Gbyte or more of data and supply the data to the CPU in nanoseconds. This memory capacity is increasing as advances in technology lead to hard disks that can be used more efficiently.

Optical disks. The newest secondary memory device is the **laser disk,** or **optical disk.** This device stores digital data on a mirrored surface by modulating the reflective properties of the surface. A small laser is used to make the pits in the disk and later to read them. The principal advantage of the optical disk is storage capacity. Current optical disks can store several Gbytes (1 gigabyte = 10^{12} bytes), and higher capacity is coming.

Systems are currently being developed that use many optical disks in jukebox fashion. It is envisioned that in the all-digital imaging department of the future the optical disk jukebox will replace the film file room.

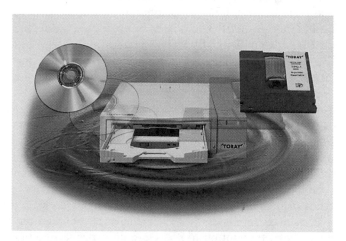

FIGURE 27-10 This disk drive reads all formats of optical compact discs and reads, erases, writes and rewrites to a 650MB optical cartridge. *(Courtesy Toray.)*

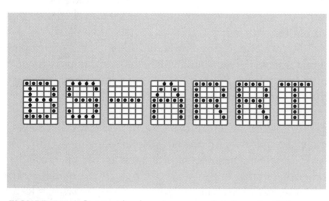

FIGURE 27-9 Dot matrix characters as produced on the VDT.

Today, optical disks are in use for read-only applications. They are called *CD-ROMs* (compact disk with read only memory). Whereas CDs are only commonly in use with ROM, **CD-Rs** (compact disk-recordables) have been developed for industrial use. They will be available in the future for consumer use. The **compact disc (CD)** enjoyed by audiophiles for its superior fidelity is an optical disk.

Magnetic tape. Magnetic tape is another secondary memory device. Since it is both the cheapest and slowest form of storage, it is used mainly for archiving patient images. The tapes come in various formats. The size of computer tape used most often in imaging departments is 0.5 inches (1.25 centimeters) wide and 2400 feet (720 meters) long and has nine magnetic data tracks. It can accommodate the records of dozens of patients.

Magnetic tape has a polyester base. It is coated on one side with iron oxide, which when magnetized is the recording medium. The tape is fed across the read-write heads. The write head produces a small magnetic field when an electric current is passed through it. The magnetic field is reversed when the direction of the current is reversed. The two binary digits, 0 and 1, thus are easily represented by changes in the current. When the magnetic field produced by the head comes in contact with the magnetic coating on the tape, it magnetizes a small spot on the coating. When a tape is to be read, this series of tiny magnetic fields moves rapidly past the read head. As each field comes in contact with the read head, it produces an electric current. The direction of the current depends on the direction of the field, and therefore the information originally recorded is retrieved. This entire process is based on electromagnetic induction (see Chapter 6). It is a little like the process that occurs in a transformer.

Laser camera. Hard-copy images from digital equipment are usually made with a laser camera. Instead of controlling the CRT, the computer output is used to modulate the intensity of a laser beam, which is directed onto single-emulsion film. The images are sharp, and the contrast is easily optimized. Digital image manipulation such as windowing, highlighting, and enhancing are possible. Laser camera images are characterized by a totally dark background.

Printers. Even though most imaging departments have as the final result a laser image, most computer applications output is in printed form. Printers are often available with radiographic equipment but are seldom used. Nevertheless, it is important to know the different types of printers that one might encounter.

Dot matrix printers are inexpensive and moderately fast. They can print up to 350 characters per second but the print quality is low. The dot matrix printer accompanies many micro- and minicomputers. Dot matrix printers form the characters with dots in the same way as CRTs. Earlier printers used a head containing nine pins, and later printers used as many as 24 pins. The pins punched an inked ribbon onto paper. Some printers use specially treated paper and heated pins. Such printers are called *thermal printers.* Common dot matrix printers in use today include **inkjets** and **bubblejets.** These offer economic monochrome and color printing abilities.

Laser printers have become the printers of choice for many users needing professional-quality printing. The technology uses an electrophotographic semiconductor laser to fuse special ink onto the paper. The digital information from the computer for each character is mapped onto a 300×300 dots-per-inch grid, which is then burned into the paper at temperatures of up to $200°$ C at 100 milliseconds per character.

The laser allows for great accuracy and speed, producing high-resolution graphics and text at speeds of up to 15 printed pages per minute on some systems. Furthermore, since the character style is stored in the digital memory of the printer and not the computer, the laser printer can print characters of virtually any style and language simply by programming the memory.

Color laser printers are available, in which colored wax is melted onto the paper by the laser. These printers are used to produce everything from colored brochures and posters to magazine and newspaper advertisements. The advent of **optical scanners** have also allowed printed materials, including photographs, to be scanned into a computer program, altered in any fashion, and reprinted with professional quality. Laser printers have given rise to the term *desktop publishing,* and many users now have access to superior printing quality at the same cost and ease of operation as a PC.

Modem. Data transmission between computers is routinely accomplished through the use of a **modem** (**modu**lator-**dem**odulator). The digital information to be passed from one system to another is first sent to the sending computer's modem, where it is converted into modulated analog signals, very similar to electromagnetic voice waves in a telephone system. The signals are then sent over the phone lines or a similar cabling system to the receiving computer, where they are demodulated back into digital signals to be used in the receiving computer.

The transmission is completed through the use of **terminal software,** through which the computer is turned into an intelligent terminal to be linked to another computer. The software ensures compatibility between systems for transmission speed, data type, and proper display of information on the screen. Some software even dials the phone and initiates a link automatically, as well as storing numbers and data as files for use by other programs. In this way, computers of any make can communicate with one another, as well as with microcomputers and minicomputers and mainframes. In this case the mainframe acts as the **host,** whereas the micro-computer logs on as a **remote terminal.**

Almost all modems today are of the **direct connection** kind. They replace the early acoustic coupling types, which required placing a telephone handset on a microphone or speaker base. The direct connect modem is interfaced directly between the computer and the phone line, sometimes having been built into the computer itself. Speeds for personal computer modems are usually between 1200 and 28,800 **baud,** or bits per second. A 300-baud modem takes about 6.5 seconds to transmit one page of text. Mainframe computers can transmit at over 96,000 baud, and can send **in parallel,** meaning multiple pages can be sent simultaneously. There are also facsimile (fax) modems that allow direct transmission and reception of fax documents from the computer to its printer without the need for a separate machine.

Software

All that has been described thus far regarding the computer has been hardware. Hardware refers to the fixed visible components of the system—the CPU, all I/O devices, and other auxiliary or peripheral devices. But these are only half of the computer. The other half is software. Software refers to the instructions written in a computer language that guide the computer through its designated operations.

Bits, bytes, and words. In computer language a single binary digit, 0 or 1, is called a *bit*. Depending on the microprocessor, a string of 8, 16, or 32 bits will be manipulated simultaneously. The computer will use as many bits as necessary to express a decimal digit, depending on how it is programmed. The 26 characters of the alphabet and other special characters are usually encoded by 8 bits. To **encode** is to translate from ordinary characters to computer-compatible characters or binary digits.

Bits are often grouped into bunches of eight called *bytes*. Computer capacity is expressed by the number of bytes that can be accommodated by computer memory. The most popular personal computers use 16- and 32-bit microprocessors with 1 to 40 megabytes (MB) of memory.

One kilobyte (kB) is equal to 1024 bytes. Note that kilo is not metric in computer use. Instead it represents 2^{10}, or 1024. The minicomputers used in radiology have capacities measured in megabytes, where $1 \text{ MB} = 1 \text{ kB} \times 1 \text{ kB} = 2^{10} \times 2^{10} = 2^{20} = 1,048,576$ bytes.

Question: How many bits can be stored on a 64-kB chip?

Answer:

$$\frac{1024 \text{ bytes}}{\text{kbytes}} \times 64 \text{ bytes} \times \frac{8 \text{ bits}}{\text{bytes}} = 2^{10} \times 2^6 \times 2^{19}$$

$$= 524,288 \text{ bits}$$

Depending on the computer configuration, two bytes usually constitute a **word.** In the case of a 16-bit microprocessor a word would be 16 consecutive bits of information that are interpreted and shuffled about the computer as a unit. Each word of data in memory has its own address.

Programs. The sequence of instructions developed by a software programmer is called a *computer program.* Computer programs are the software of the computer. It is useful to distinguish two classifications of computer programs (1) **systems software** and (2) **application programs.** Systems software consists of programs that make it easy for the user to operate a computer to its best advantage. Computer buffs describe good, efficient software as "user friendly." Application programs are those written in a higher-level language expressly to carry out some user function. Most computer programs are application programs.

System software. The computer program most closely related to the system hardware is the operating system. The **operating system** is that series of instructions that organizes the course of data through the computer to the solution of a particular problem. It makes the computer's resources available to application programs. Commands such as "run file" to begin a sequence or "save file" to store some information in secondary memory are typical of operating system commands.

This type of program is usually developed by the computer manufacturer and may be stored in ROM in the CPU. Since the CPU only recognizes instructions in binary or machine-language form, formulating the operating system is perhaps the most tedious of all computer programming.

Computers ultimately understand only zeros and ones. To save humans the task of writing programs in this form, other programs, called *assemblers, compilers,* and *interpreters,* have been written. These types of software provide a computer language to communicate between the language of the operating system and everyday language.

An **assembler** is a computer program that recognizes symbolic instructions such as "subtract (SUB)," "load (LD)," and "print (PT)" and translates them into the corresponding binary code. Assembly is the translation of a program written in symbolic, machine-oriented instructions into machine-language instructions.

Compilers and **interpreters** are computer programs that translate an application program from its high-level language, such as **BASIC, C++** or **Pascal,** into a form suitable for the assembler or into a form accepted directly by the CPU. Interpreters make program development easier because they are interactive. Compiled programs run faster because they create a separate machine-language program.

Application programs. Computer programs that are written by the computer manufacturer, a software manufacturer, or the users themselves to permit the computer to perform a specific task are called *application programs*. Examples are Lotus 1-2-3, Excel, and dBase. Application programs allow the user to print a mailing list, complete an income tax form, evaluate a financial statement, or reconstruct an image from an x-ray transmission pattern. They are written in one of many high-level computer languages and are then translated through an interpreter or compiler into a corresponding machine-language program that is subsequently executed by the computer.

The diagram in Figure 27-11 illustrates the flow of the software instructions from turning the computer on to completing a computation. When the computer is first turned on, nothing is in its memory except a program called a *bootstrap*. This is frozen permanently in ROM. When the computer is started, it automatically runs the bootstrap program, which is capable of transferring the other necessary programs off the disk and into the computer memory.

The bootstrap program loads the operating system into primary memory, which in turn controls all subsequent operations. A machine-language application program can likewise be copied from the disk into primary memory where the prescribed operations occur. After completion of the program, the results will be transferred from primary memory to an output device under the control of the operating system.

Computer Languages

Binary number system. Although the computer can accept and report alphabetic characters and numeric information in the decimal system, it operates in the binary system. In the decimal system (the system we normally use), 10 digits (0 to 9) are used. The word digit comes from the Latin for finger or toe. The origin of the decimal system is undoubtedly rooted in the fact that we have 10 fingers and 10 toes that simplify counting (Figure 27-12). The decimal system is a number system to the base ten. Other number systems have been formulated to many other base values. The duodecimal system, for instance, has 12 digits. It is used to describe the months of the year and the hours in a day and night. Computers operate on the simplest number system of all, the binary number system. It has only two digits—0 and 1.

When counting in the binary number system, one counts 0 to 1 and then counts over again (Table 27-1). Because there are only two digits, 0 and 1, the computer performs all operations by converting alphabetic characters, decimal values, and logic functions to binary values. Even the computer's instructions are stored in binary form. That way, although the binary numbers may become exceedingly long, computation can be handled by properly adjusting the thousands of flip-flop circuits in the computer. In the binary system, 0 is 0 and 1 is 1, but there the direct relationship with the decimal system ends. In fact, it ends at 0 because the 1 in binary notation comes from 2^0. Recall that any number raised to the zero power is 1, therefore 2^0 equals 1. In binary notation, the decimal number 2 is equal to 2^1 plus no 2^0. This is expressed as 10. The decimal number 3 is equal to 2^1 plus 2^0, or 11 in binary form; 4 is 2^2 plus no 2^1 plus no 2^0, or 100 in binary form. Each time it is necessary

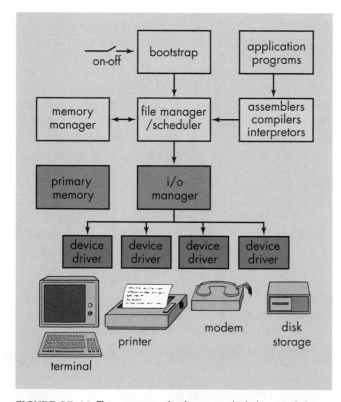

FIGURE 27-11 The sequences of software manipulations needed to complete an operation.

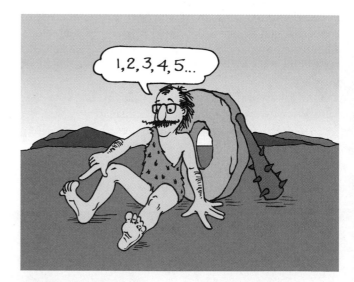

FIGURE 27-12 The origin of the decimal number system.

TABLE 27-1

Organization of the Binary Number System

Decimal Number	Binary Equivalent	Binary Number
0	0	0
1	2^0	1
2	$2^1 + 0$	10
3	$2^1 + 2^0$	11
4	$2^2 + 0 + 0$	100
5	$2^2 + 0 + 2^0$	101
6	$2^2 + 2^1 + 0$	110
7	$2^2 + 2^1 + 2^0$	111
8	$2^3 + 0 + 0 + 0$	1000
9	$2^3 + 0 + 0 + 2^0$	1001
10	$2^3 + 0 + 2^1 + 0$	1010
11	$2^3 + 0 + 2^1 + 2^0$	1011
12	$2^3 + 2^2 + 0 + 0$	1100
13	$2^3 + 2^2 + 0 + 2^0$	1101
14	$2^3 + 2^2 + 2^1 + 0$	1110
15	$2^3 + 2^2 + 2^1 + 2^0$	1111
16	$2^4 + 0 + 0 + 0 + 0$	10000

TABLE 27-2

Power-of-ten, Power-of-two, and Binary Notation

Power of Ten	Power of Two	Binary Notation
$10^0 = 1$	$2^0 = 1$	1
$10^1 = 10$	$2^1 = 2$	10
$10^2 = 100$	$2^2 = 4$	100
$10^3 = 1000$	$2^3 = 8$	1000
$10^4 = 10,000$	$2^4 = 16$	10000
$10^5 = 100,000$	$2^5 = 32$	100000
$10^6 = 1,000,000$	$2^6 = 64$	1000000
	$2^7 = 128$	10000000
	$2^8 = 256$	100000000
	$2^9 = 512$	1000000000
	$2^{10} = 1024$	10000000000

to raise 2 to an additional power to express a number, the number of binary digits increases by 1.

Just as we know the meaning of the powers of ten, it is necessary to recognize the powers of two. Power-of-two notation is used in radiologic imaging to describe image size, image dynamic range (shades of gray), and image storage capacity. Table 27-2 is a review of these power notations. Note the following similarity: in both power notations the number of zeros to the right of 1 equals the value of the exponent.

Question: Express the number 193 in binary form (refer to Table 27-2).

Answer: 193 falls between 2^7 and 2^8. Therefore it will be expressed as 1 followed by 7 binary digits. Simply add the decimal equivalents of each binary digit from left to right:

Yes $2^7 = 1 =$	128
Yes $2^6 = 1 =$	64
No $2^5 = 0 =$ No	32
No $2^4 = 0 =$ No	16
No $2^3 = 0 =$ No	8
No $2^2 = 0 =$ No	4
No $2^1 = 0 =$ No	2
Yes $2^0 = 1 =$	1
11000001 =	193

Digital radiologic images are made of discrete picture elements, **pixels,** arranged in a matrix (see Chapter 28). The size of the image is described in the binary system of numbers by power-of-2 equivalents. Most images are either 256×256 (2^8), 512×512 (2^9), 1024×1024 (2^{10}) or 2048×2048 (2^{11}). The 256×256 and 512×512 image matrices are particularly applicable to MRI and CT. The 1024×1024 and 2048×2048 matrices are used in digital fluoroscopy and digital radiography.

Hexadecimal Number System

The **hexadecimal number system** is used by assembly-level applications. As you have seen, assembly language acts as a midpoint between the computer's binary system and the user's human language instructions. The set of hexadecimal numbers is 0,1,2,3,4,5,6,7,8,9, A,B,C,D,E,F. Each of these symbols is used to represent a binary number, or more specifically, a set of 4 bits. Therefore, since it takes 8 bits to make a byte, a byte can be represented by two hexadecimal numbers. The set of hexadecimal numbers corresponds to the binary numbers for 0 to 15, as shown in Table 27-3.

High-level programming languages allow the programmer to write instructions in a form approaching human language, using words, symbols, and decimal numbers rather than the ones and zeros of machine language. An expanded list of the more popular programming languages is given in Table 27-4. Using one of these high-level languages, one can write a set of instructions that will be understood by the system software and be executed by the computer through its operating system.

FORTRAN. The oldest language for scientific, engineering, and mathematic problems is **FORTRAN** (formula translation). It was the prototype for today's algebraic languages, which are oriented toward computational procedures for solving mathematical and statistical problems. FORTRAN was developed in 1956 by IBM in conjunction with some major computer users.

BASIC. Developed at Dartmouth College in 1964 as a first language for students, BASIC (beginners all purpose symbolic instruction code) is an algebraic programming language. It is an easy-to-learn, interpreter-based language. Major applications of BASIC are with micro- and minicomputer systems and particularly with the popular personal computer. BASIC contains a powerful arithmetic facility, several editing features, a li-

TABLE 27-3

The Number System

The Number System

Decimal	Binary	Hexadecimal	Decimal	Binary	Hexadecimal
0	0000	0	8	1000	8
1	0001	1	9	1001	9
2	0010	2	10	1010	A
3	0011	3	11	1011	B
4	0100	4	12	1100	C
5	0101	5	13	1101	D
6	0110	6	14	1110	E
7	0111	7	15	1111	F

TABLE 27-4

Expanded List of Programming Languages

Language	Date Introduced	Description
FORTRAN	1956	First successful programming language; for solving engineering and science problems
COBOL	1959	Mini- and main-frame computer applications in business
ALGOL	1960	Especially useful in high-level mathematics
BASIC	1964	Most frequently used with micro- and minicomputers; science, engineering, and business applications
BCPL	1965	Developmental-stage language
B	1969	Developmental-stage language
C	1970	Combines the power of assembly language with the ease of use and portability of high-level language
Pascal	1971	High-level, general purpose language; used for teaching structured programming
Ada	1975	Based on Pascal; used by the U.S. Department of Defense
VisiCalc	1978	First electronic spreadsheet
C++	1980	Response to complexity of C; incorporates object-oriented programming methods
Quick BASIC	1985	Powerful high-level language with advanced user features
Visual C++	1992	Visual language programming methods; design environments
Visual BASIC	1993	Visual language programming methods; design environments; advanced user-friendly features

brary of common mathematical functions, and simple input and output procedures.

QuickBASIC. Microsoft developed BASIC into a powerful programming language that can be used for both commercial applications and quick, single-use programs. QuickBASIC's advanced features for editing, implementation, and decoding make it an attractive language for professional and amateur programmers.

COBOL. One high-level, procedure-oriented language designed for coding business data processing problems is COBOL (**common business oriented language**). A basic characteristic of business data processing is the existence of large files that are updated continuously. COBOL provides extensive file-handling, editing, and report-generating capabilities for the user.

Pascal. Pascal is a high-level, general-purpose programming language developed in 1971 by Nicklaus Wirth of the Federal Institute of Technology at Zürich, Switzerland. A general-purpose programming language is one that can be put to many different applications. Currently Pascal is the most popular programming language for teaching programming concepts, partly because its syntax is relatively easy to learn and closely resembles the English language in usage. Another reason for Pascal's popularity is that efficient Pascal compilers are available for almost all computers.

C, C++. C is considered by many to be the first modern programmer's language. It was designed, implemented and developed by real, working programmers, and it reflected the way they approached the job of programming. C is the result of a developmental process that started with an older language called *BCPL*, developed by Martin Richards. BCPL influenced Ken Thompson to invent a language called B. B led to the development of C, which was invented and first implemented by Dennis Ritchie in the 1970s. C is thought of as a middle-level language because it combines elements of high-level languages with the functionality of an assembler (low-level) language.

In response to the need to manage greater complexity, C++, developed by Bjarne Stroustrup in 1980, was initially called C with Classes. C++ contains the entire

C language, as well as many additions designed to support **Object-Oriented Programming (OOP)**. Once a program exceeds about 30,000 lines of code, it becomes so complex that it is difficult to grasp as one huge object. Therefore OOP is a method of dividing up parts of the program into groups, or objects, with related data and applications. In the same way that a book is broken up into chapters and subheadings to be more readable a program should be divided into a hierarchical structure of self-contained objects to be more understandable.

Today, C++ is the most widely used programming language for any common business or personal application. However, C++ is very much a work in progress, and improvements are still being made. Table 27-5 presents three sample programs to compute the sum of two numbers, A + B.

Visual C++, Visual Basic. Visual programming languages are the most recent languages and they are under continuing development. They are designed specifically for creating **Windows** applications. Although both Visual C++ and Visual Basic use their original respective programming language code structures, they both have one similar goal in mind—to create user-friendly Windows applications with minimal effort from the programmer. In theory the most inexperienced programmer should be able to create complex programs with visual languages. The idea is to have the programmer design the program in a design environment without ever really writing extensive code. Instead, the visual language creates the code to match the programmer's design.

Macros. Several new spreadsheet and word-processing applications offer built-in programming commands called *macros.* They work the same way as commands in programming languages, and they are used to carry out user-defined functions or a series of functions within the application. One application that offers a very good library of macro commands is EXCEL, a spreadsheet. The user can create a command to manipulate a series of data by performing a certain series of steps.

Macros can be written or they can be designed in a fashion similar to that of visual programming. This process of designing a macro is called *recording.* The programmer turns the macro recorder on, carries out the steps he wants the macro to carry out, and stops the recorder. The macro then knows exactly what the programmer wants implemented and can run the same series of steps over and over.

Other program languages have been developed for other purposes. LOGO is a language designed for children. Ada is the official language approved by the U.S. Department of Defense for software development. It is used principally for military applications and artificial intelligence.

PROCESSING METHODS

Regardless of the operating software or the application programs in use, the essential modes of computer processing are **batch, time-sharing, on-line,** and **real-time** systems. The modes often operate together as interactive systems when short response time between issuing a command and receiving a response is of major importance. Such processing methods are different from batch processing, which offers a relatively long turnaround time but aims at lowering computing costs. Many larger computer systems offer a choice of these processing methods.

Batch Processing

A batch operating system is the most widely used mode of processing with main-frame computers. The users submit the complete job, which includes the program, the data, and the control statements. After a relatively long time, tens of minutes to hours, the results are available. Normally the jobs in a batch are processed in sequence, one after the other. This method does not require the user to attend to the system once the batch has started. Batch processing can be handled by a remote job-entry, **RJE,** system in which users submit their batch jobs to a remote terminal connected to the computer by a cable or modem.

On-Line Systems

In an on-line system, certain transactions are processed immediately. In such a system the users have multiple-access terminals from which they may introduce one or a few of the transactions exclusively. The response comes within seconds. Examples of on-line systems include airline reservation systems, automatic bank tellers, and supermarket checkout systems.

Time-Sharing Systems

The goal of time-sharing systems is to provide the illusion of having the computer dedicated exclusively to each user. Several hundred users (the maximum number depending on the system) may simultaneously interact

TABLE 27-5

Three Sample Programs for Summing A & B

Pascal	QuickBASIC	C++
program sum;		main()
{calculates A + B}	'calculates A + B	//calculates A + B
var A,B,X: integer;	DEFINT A,B,X	{
begin		int A,B,X;
ReadLn(A);	INPUT A	cin>>A;
ReadLn(B);	INPUT B	cin>>B;
X: = A + B ;	X = A + B	X = A + B;
WriteLn(X)	PRINT X	cout<<X;
end.	END	return 0;}

with the computer. The time between the user's sign-on and sign-off is called a *session*. During a typical session, the user does the following:

1. Signs onto the system by presenting a password
2. Enters a program under the control of a text editor
3. Usually saves this program under an assigned name
4. Has the program compiled
5. Runs the program

While the program is being run, the user may interact with it. For example, the user may request the result of a partial execution of a program, or the computer may make a request of the user and then proceed based on the result. This type of system is in use in most large research-and-development institutions where multiple-user groups must be accommodated.

Real-Time Systems

Real-time systems are most often designed as special purpose operating systems to provide for fast management of the system hardware. This is the case in most radiologic imaging. The processing of the incoming data (e.g., from the detectors of a CT scanner) is completed in a matter of milliseconds or seconds at the most.

Real-time systems often use special-purpose, high-speed hardware to perform computationally intensive tasks such as image reconstruction and filtering. **Pipeline processors** work like an assembly line. Different parts of the data are processed by different parts of the processor at the same time. The data move through the processor ("down the pipe") and are fully processed by the time they reach the output. **Array processors** perform the same computations in parallel on many items of data at once.

SUMMARY

The word *computer* is used as an abbreviation for any general-purpose, stored-program electronic digital device. *General purpose* means the computer can solve any solvable problem. *Stored program* means the computer has instructions and data stored in its memory. *Electronic* means the computer is powered by electrical and electronic devices. *Digital* means that a computer chip controls the display on the screen.

The first stored-program computer was developed in 1948 by William Shockley at Bell Telephone Laboratories by using a transistor. The invention of the transistor led to the use of smaller devices and to the expansion in computer development and general use.

There are two principal parts of a computer—the hardware and the software. The hardware is the computer's nuts and bolts. The software is the computer's programs, which tell the hardware what to do. There are nine types of hardware—central processing unit (CPU), control unit, arithmetic unit, memory unit, input and output devices, video terminal display, secondary memory devices, printer, and modem. The basic parts of the software are the bits, bytes, and words. In computer language a single binary digit, either 0 or 1, is called a *bit*. Bits grouped in bunches of eight are called *bytes*. Computer memory is expressed in bytes or megabytes. A word is 2 bytes, depending on computer configuration.

The operating system and application programs are two types of software. The operating system is a series of instructions for organizing data through the computer. "Run file" or "save file" are typical operating system commands. Application programs are written by the software manufacturer to permit the computer to perform a particular task, for example, printing a mailing list.

Computers have a specific language to communicate commands within the software systems and programs. Computers operate on the simplest number system of all—the binary system. There are only two digits, 0 and 1. The computer performs all operations by converting alphabetic characters, decimal values, and logic functions into binary values. There are other computer languages allowing the programer to write instructions in a form approaching language. These are called *high-level programming languages*. Table 27-4 lists and describes many of the programing languages.

Regardless of the software in use, computers have essential processing methods. The computer can batch, time-share, be on-line, or operate in real-time.

REVIEW QUESTIONS

1. In what way can computers be considered an artificial intelligence?
2. Name three operations in diagnostic imaging departments that are computerized.
3. Name the earliest calculating tool invented in the Orient thousands of years ago?
4. The following code words abbreviate what titles: ASCC, ENIAC, and UNIVAC?
5. What is the difference between a calculator and a computer?
6. How did the invention of the transistor affect the computer industry?
7. Explain the difference between the microcomputer, the minicomputer, and the mainframe computer.
8. What are the two principal parts of a computer? Name distinguishing features of each.
9. List and define the nine parts of computer hardware.
10. Define bit, byte, and word as used in computer terminology.

11. Distinguish from each other the two classifications of computer programs: systems software and applications programs.

12. List and explain the 10 main types of computer languages.

13. What is the decimal value of the binary number 100110011? (First list the binary number, then compute each power of two.)

14. A memory chip is said to have 256 Mbytes of capacity. If each byte is 16 bits, what is the total bit capacity?

15. Commands such as run file or save file are part of the computer's _____ _____.

16. Define high-level computer language.

17. What computer language was the first modern programmers' language?

18. When the computer is first turned on, nothing is in its memory except a program called _____ _____.

19. List and define the four computer processing methods.

20. What type of computer is used by the U.S. Census Bureau?

Additional Readings

Delivering x-ray images on hospital computer networks, *MD Comput* 9(6):348, November-December 1992.

Hunter TB: The personal computer in the radiologist's office, *Appl Radiol* 20(8):33, August 1991.

Jones SA: Computer science for the non-wizard part 1, *Appl Radiol* 19(10):32, October 1990.

Jones SA: Computer science for the non-wizard part 2, *Appl Radiol* 20(2):32, February 1991.

Jones SA: Computer science for the non-wizard part 3, *Appl Radiol* 20(11):76, November 1991.

Jones SA: Computer science for the non-wizard part 4, *Appl Radiol* 21(9):45, September 1992.

Mixdorf MA, Goldsworthy RE: A history of computers and computerized imaging, *Radiol Technol* 67(4):291, March-April, 1996.

Turkanis RI: Computer networking: a specialization solution? *Appl Radiol* 21(8):43, August 1992.

28 Digital X-ray Imaging

OBJECTIVES

At the completion of this chapter the student will be able to:

1. Discuss the frequency of use of digital imaging in modern diagnostic imaging departments
2. Relate the research and development of digital imaging
3. Explain the characteristics of digital images, specifically image matrix and dynamic range
4. Describe the parts of a digital fluoroscopy system and their functions
5. Discuss the components and use of a digital radiography system
6. Explain the picture archiving and teleradiology systems used in diagnostic imaging departments

OUTLINE

Introduction to Digital Imaging
Historical Development of Digital Imaging
Image Characteristics
    Image matrix
    Dynamic range
Digital Fluoroscopy
    High-voltage generator
    Video system
    Charge-coupled device

Digital Radiography
    Scanned projection radiography
    X-ray tube-detector assembly
    Area beam and fan beam
    Computed radiography
Picture Archiving and Communication System
    Display system
    Network
    Storage system

igure 28-1 diagrams the imaging chain for conventional radiography. Figure 28-2 diagrams the components used in conventional fluoroscopy. These conventional systems have worked well for many years, providing increasingly better diagnostic images. However, they both have limitations. Static radiographic images require processing time that can delay the completion of the examination. Once an image is obtained, there is very little that can enhance the information content. When the examination is complete, the images are in the form of hard-copy film that must be cataloged and stored for future review.

Another and perhaps more severe limitation is the noise inherent in these images. Radiography and fluoroscopy both use area beams, that is, large rectangular beams of x-rays. The Compton-scattered portion of the remnant x-ray beam increases with increasing field size. That increases the noise of the image and severely degrades low-contrast resolution. The use of grids is only marginally helpful in improving this situation.

These limitations can be overcome somewhat by incorporating computer technology into diagnostic x-ray imaging. Computer technology is based on transforming the conventional analog images into digital form, processing the digital data, and displaying the images so they look like conventional images. Such data conversion and manipulation would not be possible if it were not for advanced computer technology.

■ ■ ■ ■ ■ ■ ■ ■ ■ ■ ■ ■ ■ ■ ■ ■ ■ ■ ■

INTRODUCTION TO DIGITAL IMAGING

Standard nomenclature for identifying the methods of obtaining digital images has not yet been uniformly adopted. Terms such as *digital vascular imaging (DVI)*,

digital subtraction angiography (DSA), *computed radiography (CR)*, *computed fluoroscopy, digital videoangiography, scan beam digital radiography*, and others are used.

In the following discussions, digital fluoroscopy (DF) is used to identify a digital x-ray imaging system that produces a series of dynamic images obtained with an **area x-ray beam** and an image intensifier. Digital radiography (DR) refers to the static images produced with either a **fan x-ray beam** intercepted by a linear array of radiation detectors or an area x-ray beam intercepted by a light-stimulated phosphor plate.

HISTORICAL DEVELOPMENT OF DIGITAL IMAGING

The development of digital radiologic imaging equipment was stalled until sufficient computer technology was available to process the large quantities of data generated. The microprocessor and semiconductor memory made this development possible and by 1980, digital imaging became a clinical reality.

Initial study, begun in the early 1970s, proceeded along two independent lines. The medical physics groups at the University of Wisconsin and the University of Arizona separately initiated studies of DF in the early 1970s. These studies were continued through the decade by the research-and-development groups of most x-ray equipment manufacturers. The approach was to use conventional fluoroscopic equipment and place a computer between the television camera and the television monitor. The video signal from the television camera was shunted through the computer, manipulated in various ways, and transmitted to the television monitor in a form ready for viewing.

The investigators of DF demonstrated that nearly instantaneous, high-contrast subtraction images could be obtained after intravenous injection. The two distinct advantages of DF over conventional fluoroscopy are (1) the speed of image acquisition and (2) the postprocessing image enhancement.

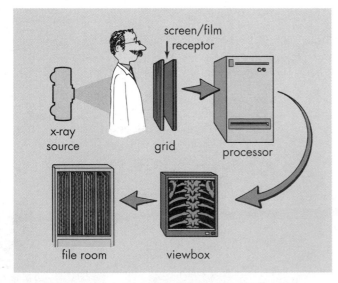

FIGURE 28-1 The imaging chain in conventional radiography.

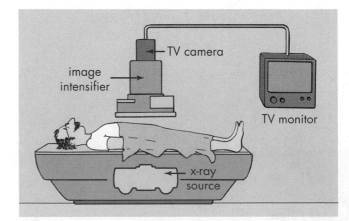

FIGURE 28-2 The imaging chain in conventional fluoroscopy.

DR also was developed by a number of different investigators. One approach, developed in the late 1970s to complement computed tomography, uses a narrow fan beam of x-rays that intercepts a linear array of radiation detectors. This is commonly referred to as *scanned projection radiography (SPR)*. The signal from each detector is computer manipulated to reconstruct an image. A second approach to DR was developed by Fuji also in the late 1970s and has been advanced and marketed by a number of x-ray companies. It is usually referred to as *computed radiography (CR)* and uses a light-stimulated phosphor as the image receptor. Although the image in digital x-ray techniques may appear as a conventional video or radiographic image, it is not. It is formed from individual image elements.

IMAGE CHARACTERISTICS

The image obtained in digital x-ray procedures is unlike the image in conventional fluoroscopy or radiography. With conventional imaging, x-rays form an image directly on the receptor. With digital techniques, x-rays form an electronic image on a radiation detector and are manipulated by a computer, temporarily stored in memory, and displayed as a **matrix** of intensities, each having a **dynamic range** of values.

Image Matrix

The term *image matrix* refers to a layout of cells in rows and columns. Each cell corresponds to a specific location in the image. The number in the cell represents the brightness or intensity at that location. Figure 28-3 shows a 10 by 10 matrix of cells, a 5 by 5 matrix of cells, and a 5 by 5 matrix of numbers in imaginary cells and the associated image (Figure 28-4). Each digital image consists of a matrix of cells that have various brightness levels on the video monitor. The brightness of a cell is determined by the computer-generated number stored in that cell.

Each cell of the image matrix is called a **pixel** (picture element). In digital x-ray imaging the value of the pixel determines pixel brightness. The value is relative and is used to provide subtraction images and to define the image contrast. In CT scanning the numerical value of each pixel is a CT number or **Hounsfield unit (HU)**. The value of the HU can be used to judge the composition of the tissue represented. In MRI, diagnostic ultrasound, and nuclear medicine the value of the pixel also has a relationship to the composition of the tissue imaged (Table 28-1).

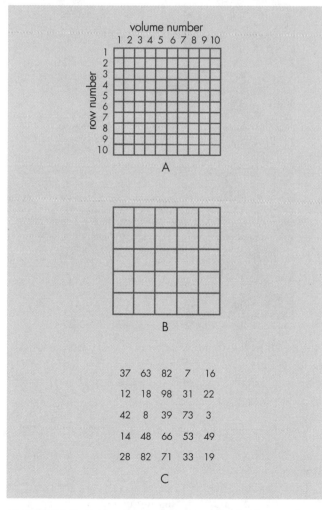

37 63 82 7   16

12 18 98 31 22

42 8   39 73 3

14 48 66 53 49

28 82 71 33 19

C

FIGURE 28-3 Matrix refers to an arrangement of columns and rows. Three matrices are shown. **A,** 10 by 10 matrix of cells. **B,** 5 by 5 matrix of cells. **C,** 5 by 5 matrix of numbers in imaginary cells.

TABLE 28-1	
Pixel Values as a Function of Tissue Characteristic for Imaging Modalities.	
Imaging Modality	**Tissue Characteristic**
Radiography or fluoroscopy	Atomic number, mass density
Computed tomography	Atomic number, mass density
Nuclear medicine	Radionuclide uptake
Diagnostic ultrasound	Interface reflectivity
Magnetic resonance	Spin density, spin relaxation

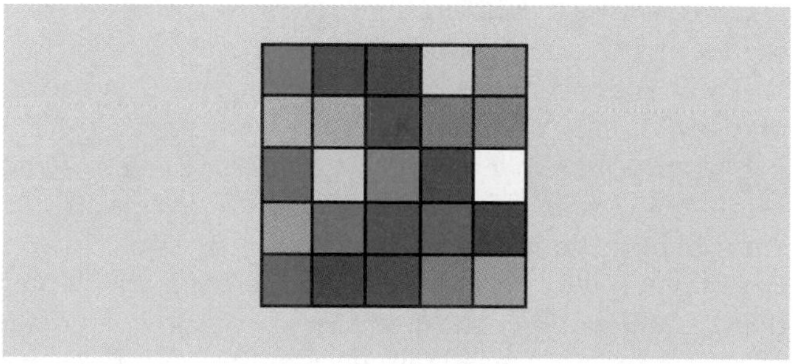

FIGURE 28-4 Associated image of the matrix in Figure 28-3.

The size of the image matrix is determined by characteristics of the imaging equipment and by the capacity of the computer. In addition, matrix size can usually be selected by the operator. Most digital x-ray imaging systems provide image matrix, or **fields of view (FOV)**, sizes of 512 by 512 and 1024 by 1024. For the same field of view, **spatial resolution** will be better with a larger image matrix.

Question: How many pixels are contained in an image matrix described as 256 by 256?

Answer: $256 \times 256 = 65,536$ pixels

A 1024 by 1024 image matrix is sometimes described as a 1000-line system. In DF the spatial resolution is determined both by the image matrix and by the size of the image intensifier. A rough estimate of the theoretical limits of spatial resolution can be obtained by dividing the size of the input phosphor of the image-intensifier tube by the matrix size.

Question: What is the pixel size of a 1000-line DF system operating in the 5-inch mode?

Answer: Five inches equals 127 mm. Therefore the size of each pixel is:

$$\frac{127 \text{ mm}}{1024 \text{ (image matrix)}} = 0.124 \text{ mm}$$

Figure 28-5 illustrates the influence of matrix size on image quality. A 64 by 64 image matrix appears definitely boxy. A 512 by 512 image is a good representation of the original analog image. However, a 1024 by 1024 image is nearly indistinguishable from the original.

Dynamic Range

An imaging system that could display only black or white would have a dynamic range of 2^1 or 2. Such an image would be very high contrast but would display very little information. Although actual value of each pixel is important, the range of values is extremely important in determining the final image.

The range of values over which a system can respond is called its *dynamic range*. Dynamic range in a digital system corresponds to the numerical range of each pixel. Visually, dynamic range refers to the number of shades of gray that can be represented.

The dynamic range of the human eye is approximately 2^5. This represents 32 shades of gray stretching from white to black. The dynamic range of the x-ray beam as it exits the patient is in excess of 2^{10}. Although we cannot visualize such a dynamic range, a computer with sufficient capacity can. The larger the dynamic range, the more gradual the gray scale representing the range from maximum x-ray intensity to minimum x-ray intensity will be. The greater the

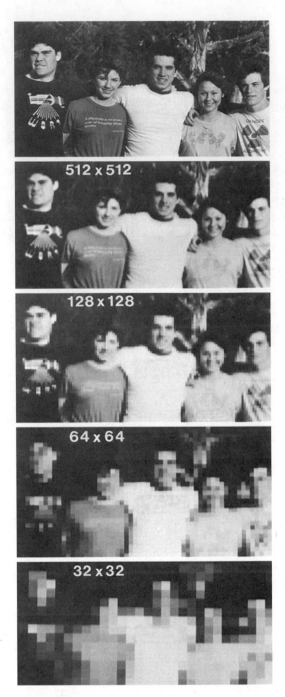

FIGURE 28-5 These Wisconsin radiography students posed to illustrate the loss of image resolution with decreasing matrix size. The 512 by 512 matrix is an acceptable rendition of the original. At a 32 by 32 matrix, the students became true blockheads.

dynamic range, therefore, the better the **contrast resolution.**

Digital x-ray imaging systems are characterized by their dynamic range and distinguished by the capacity of the computer and the software. Most use an 8-, 10-, or 12-bit range, meaning a 2^8, 2^{10}, or 2^{12} dynamic range. The electrical signal that characterizes the x-ray inten-

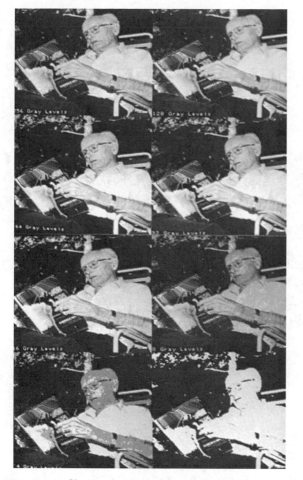

FIGURE 28-6 Photographs of this 34-year-old radiologist suffering from radiation-induced premature aging illustrate the meaning of dynamic range. The human eye can barely perceive the difference between 16 and 32 gray levels. The computer can accurately distinguish 256 gray levels and more.

sity of the image is converted into digital form. The digital information is displayed as an image matrix, each pixel of which is capable of a range of 2^8 (0 to 255), 2^{10} (0 to 1023), or 2^{12} (0 to 4095).

Figure 28-6 illustrates the effect of dynamic range on the image. Clearly a system with low dynamic range is high contrast but only over a limited portion of the image. High dynamic range allows for wide image latitude. The contrast of a **region of interest (ROI)** of the image can be electronically enhanced if the computer system has sufficient dynamic range.

Because some radiologists prefer not to diagnose from a CRT console, the radiographer is responsible for producing film images from the CRT of proper optical density and contrast. This is done by using the computer to postprocess an image through a technique called *windowing*.

A digital image with a ten-bit dynamic range will contain 1024 gray values; however, the human eye can see only about 30 such shades. The postprocessing com-

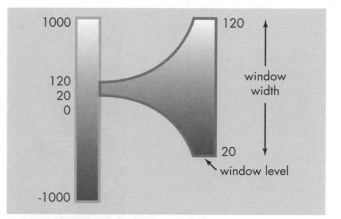

FIGURE 28-7 Windowing a digital image controls the image contrast and optical density. *(Courtesy Helen Schumpert.)*

puter is used to allow one to see only a window of the entire dynamic range.

The two characteristics of the window are **window level** and **window width** (Figure 28-7). Window level identifies the type of tissue to be imaged. For instance a CT window level of 50 will image abdominal tissue, whereas a window level of 750 will image lung tissue (Figure 28-8). Window width determines the gray-scale representation of that tissue. The wider the window width, the longer the gray scale will be. Narrow window widths produce high contrast (Figure 28-9).

DIGITAL FLUOROSCOPY

A DF examination is conducted in much the same manner as a conventional study. The equipment used looks the same, but such is not the case (Figure 28-10). A computer, two video monitors, and a complex operating console have been added.

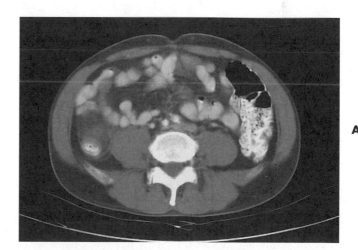

A

FIGURE 28-8 The selection of window level depends on the anatomy imaged. The abdomen **(A)** or soft tissue of the thorax **(B)** requires a low window level (level 50, width 500).

Continued.

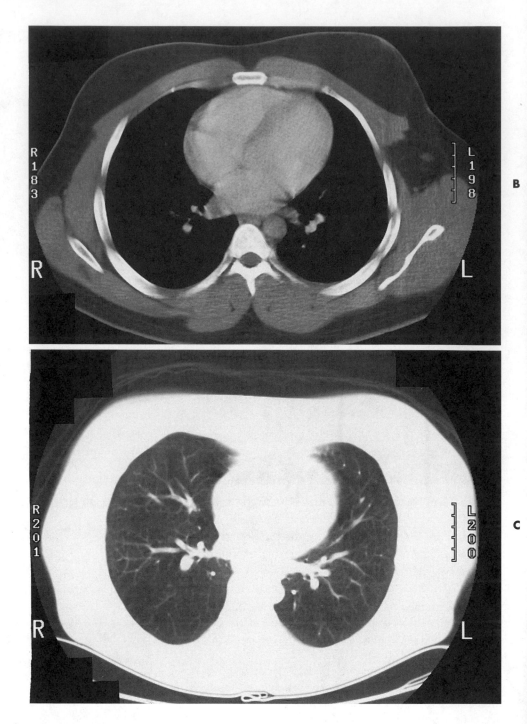

FIGURE 28-8, cont'd. *(Courtesy Helen Schumpert.)*

Figure 28-11 shows a representative digital fluoroscopic monitoring station, which displays the results of manipulation of the console. The operating console contains alphanumeric and function keys for entering patient data and for communicating with the computer. The operating console also contains special function keys for data acquisition, image display and image post-processing, such as histogram analysis or region of interest (ROI) manipulation. Three video screens are usually available: one for patient data, one for current image display, and one for subtracted image display.

High-Voltage Generator

During DF, the under-the-table x-ray tube actually operates in the radiographic mode. The tube current is measured in hundreds of mA instead of 5 mA or less as in conventional fluoroscopy. This is not a problem because the tube is not energized continuously. Images from DF are obtained in much the same fashion that rapid film changer images are obtained in angiointerventional procedures.

Image acquisition rates of one per second to 10 per second are common in many examinations. Since it re-

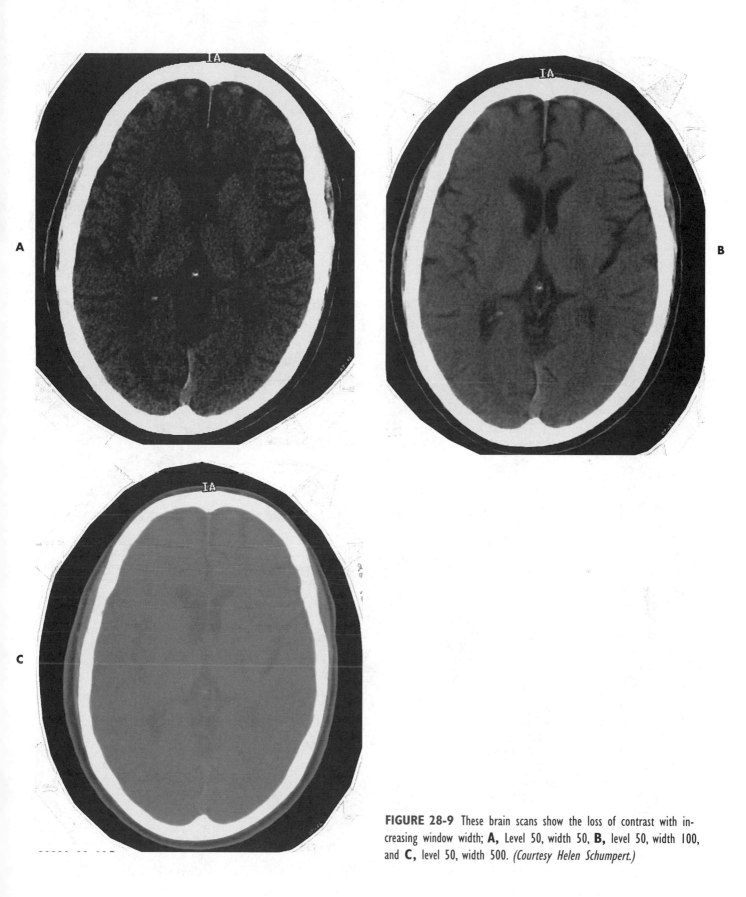

FIGURE 28-9 These brain scans show the loss of contrast with increasing window width; **A,** Level 50, width 50, **B,** level 50, width 100, and **C,** level 50, width 500. *(Courtesy Helen Schumpert.)*

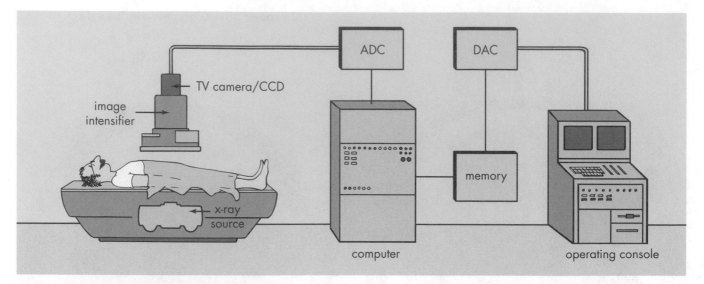

FIGURE 28-10 The components of a DF system.

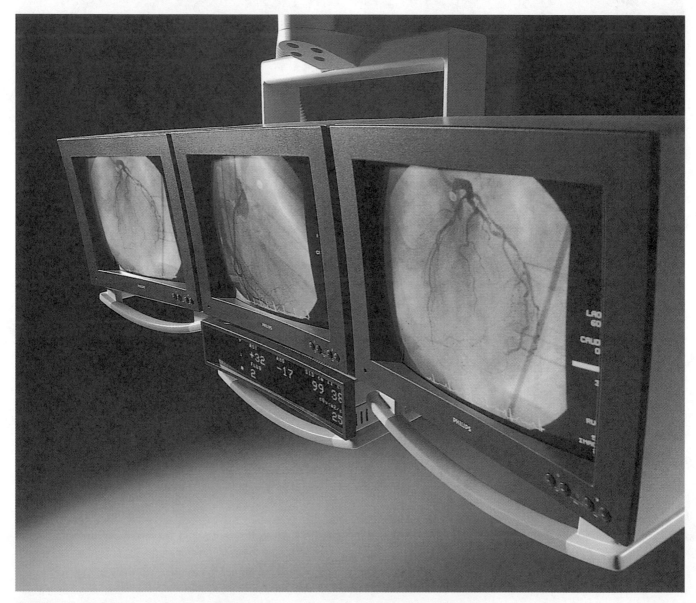

FIGURE 28-11 Monitoring station for a digital fluoroscopic system. (*Courtesy Philips Medical Systems.*)

quires 33 milliseconds to read one video frame, x-ray exposures longer than that can result in unnecessary patient dose. That is a theoretical limit, however, and longer exposures may be necessary to ensure low noise and good image quality.

Consequently the x-ray generator must be capable of switching on and off very rapidly. The time required for the x-ray tube to be switched on and reach the selected level of kVp and mA is called the **interrogation time.** The time required for the x-ray tube to be switched off is the **extinction time.** It is necessary that DF systems incorporate three-phase or high-frequency generators with interrogation and extinction times of approximately 1 millisecond.

Video System

The video system used in conventional fluoroscopy is usually a 525-line system. Such a system is adequate for DF, although higher spatial resolution can be obtained with 1000-line systems. Conventional video, however, has two limitations that restrict its application in digital techniques. First the interlaced mode of reading the target of the television camera can significantly degrade a digital image. Secondly the conventional television camera tubes are relatively noisy. They have a signal-to-noise (SNR) ratio of about 200:1, whereas an SNR ratio of 1000:1 is necessary for DF.

Interlace vs. progressive mode. In Chapter 25, the method by which a conventional television camera tube reads its target assembly was described. This was described as an interlace mode where two fields of $262\frac{1}{2}$ lines each were read in $\frac{1}{60}$ seconds (17 milliseconds) to form a 525-line video frame in $\frac{1}{30}$ s (33 milliseconds) as shown in Figure 25-15.

When reading the video signal in the progressive mode the electron beam of the television camera tube sweeps the target assembly continuously from top to bottom in 33 milliseconds (Figure 28-12). The video image is similarly formed on the television monitor. There is no interlace of one field with another, and this produces a sharper image with less flicker.

SNR. All electronic devices are inherently noisy. Because of heated filaments and voltage differences, there is always a very small electric current flowing in any circuit. This is called *background electronic noise.* It is similar to the noise on a radiograph in that it conveys no information and serves only to obscure the electronic signal.

Since conventional television camera tubes have an SNR of about 200:1, the maximum output signal will be 200 times greater than the background electronic noise. This is not sufficient for DF because the video signal is rarely at maximum and lower signals become even more lost in the noise. Especially when subtraction techniques are used, image contrast resolution will be severely degraded by a system with a low SNR.

Figure 28-13 illustrates the difference between the output of a 200:1 SNR television camera tube and a 1000:1 tube. At 200:1 the dynamic range is less than 2^8, and at 1000:1, it is about 2^{10}. The tube with a 1000:1 SNR ratio contains five times the useful information and is more compatible with computer-assisted image enhancement.

Charge-Coupled Device

Computer. Minicomputers are used in DF. The capacity of the computer is a most important factor in determining image quality, the manner and speed of image

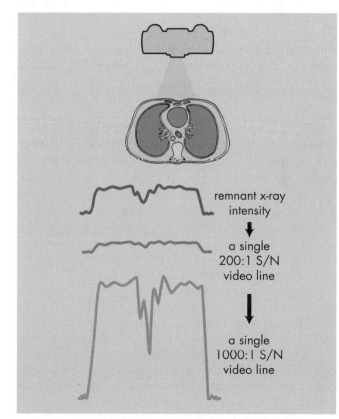

remnant x-ray intensity

a single 200:1 S/N video line

a single 1000:1 S/N video line

FIGURE 28-13 The information content of a video system with a high SNR is greatly enhanced. Shown here are a single video line through an object and the resulting signal at 200:1 and 1000:1 SNRs.

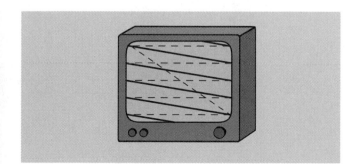

FIGURE 28-12 The progressive mode of reading a video signal.

acquisition, and image processing and manipulation. Important characteristics of a DF system that are computer controlled are the **image matrix size, the system dynamic range,** and the **image acquisition rate.**

The output signal from the television camera tube is transmitted by cable to an **analog-to-digital converter (ADC).** The ADC accepts the continuously varying television camera output signal (analog signal) and converts it to digital numbers.

To be compatible with the computer, the ADC must have the same dynamic range as the computer. An 8-bit ADC would convert the analog signal into values between 0 and 255. A 10-bit ADC would be more precise in that the analog-to-digital conversion would range from 0 to 2^{10}, or 0 to 1023.

The output of the ADC is then transferred to main memory and manipulated so that a digital image in matrix form is stored. The dynamic range of each pixel, the number of pixels, and the method of storage will determine the speed that the image can be acquired, processed, and transferred to an output device.

If image storage is in primary memory, which is usually the case, then data acquisition and transfer can be as rapid as 30 images per second. In general, if the image matrix is doubled (e.g., from 512 to 1024) the image acquisition rate will be reduced by a factor of four. A representative system might be capable of acquiring 30 images per second in the 512 by 512 matrix mode. However, if a higher spatial resolution image is required and the 1024 by 1024 mode is requested, then only eight images per second can be acquired. This limitation on data transfer is imposed by the time required to conduct such enormous quantities of data from one segment of memory to another.

Image formation. The principal advantages of DF examination are the image subtraction techniques that are possible and the ability to see vessels with a venous injection of contrast material. Unfortunately an area beam must be used. The associated scatter radiation reduces image contrast. Image contrast, however, can be enhanced electronically. Image contrast is obtained by subtraction techniques that provide for instantaneous viewing of the subtracted image, even during the passage of a bolus of contrast medium.

Temporal subtraction and **energy subtraction** are the two methods that receive attention in DF. Each has advantages and disadvantages as described in Table 28-2. Temporal subtraction techniques are most frequently used because the high-voltage generator has limitations in the energy subtraction mode. When the two techniques are combined, the process is called *hybrid subtraction.* Image contrast is enhanced still further by hybrid subtraction because of reduced patient motion between subtracted images.

Temporal subtraction. Temporal subtraction refers to a number of computer-assisted techniques whereby an image obtained at one time is subtracted from an image obtained at a later time. If, during the intervening period, contrast material was introduced into the vasculature, the subtracted image will contain only the vessels filled with the contrast material. Two methods are common—the **mask mode** and **time-interval difference mode.**

Mask mode. A typical mask mode procedure is diagramed in Figure 28-14. The patient is positioned under normal fluoroscopic control to ensure that the region of anatomy under investigation is within the field of view of the image intensifier. A power injector is armed and readied to deliver 30 to 50 milliliters of contrast material at the rate of approximately 15 to 20 milliliters per second through a venous entry. If an arterial entry is chosen, 10 to 25 milliliters of diluted contrast material

TABLE 28-2	
Comparison of Temporal and Energy Subtraction.	
Temporal Subtraction	**Energy Subtraction**
A single kVp is used	Rapid kVp switching is required
Normal x-ray beam filtration is adequate	X-ray beam filter switching is preferred
Contrast resolution of 1 millimeter at 1% is achieved	Higher x-ray intensity is required for comparable contrast resolution
Simple arithmetic image subtraction is necessary	Complex image subtraction is necessary
Motion artifacts are a problem	Motion artifacts are greatly reduced
Total subtraction of common structures is achieved	Some residual bone may survive subtraction
Subtraction possibilities are limited by the number of images	Many more types of subtraction images are possible

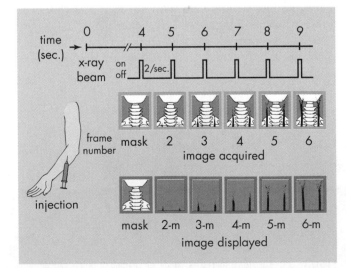

FIGURE 28-14 A schematic representation of mask-mode DF.

at 10 to 12 milliliters per second may be used. The imaging apparatus is changed from the fluoroscopic mode to the DF mode. This requires an increase in x-ray tube current of 20 to 100 times the fluoroscopic mode and the activation of a program of pulse image acquisition.

The injector is fired and, after a delay of 4 to 10 seconds, before the bolus of contrast medium reaches the anatomic site, an initial x-ray pulse exposure is made. The image obtained is stored in primary memory and displayed on video monitor A. This is the **mask image.**

This mask image is followed by a series of additional images that are stored in adjacent memory locations. While these subsequent images are being acquired, the mask image is subtracted from each and the result is stored in primary memory. At the same time the subtracted image is displayed on video monitor B. Figure 28-15 shows a preinjection mask, an unenhanced image after a venous injection, and an enhanced image obtained by subtracting the first from the second.

The subtracted images appear in real time and are then stored in memory. After the examination, each subtracted image can be recalled for closer examination.

As described here, each image was obtained from a 33-millisecond x-ray pulse. The time required for one video frame is 33 milliseconds. Because the video system is relatively slow to respond and the video noise may be high, several video frames (usually four or eight) may be added to the memory to make each image. This process is called *image integration*. Although the process improves contrast resolution, it also increases patient dose because more image frames are acquired.

In mask mode DF the imaging sequence after acquisition of the mask can be manually controlled or preprogrammed. If preprogrammed, the computer controls the data acquisition in accordance with the demands of the examination. For example, to evaluate carotid flow after a brachial vein injection, one could inject contrast material and, 2 seconds after injection, acquire a mask image. There then could follow another 2 second delay, followed by images obtained at the rate of two per second for 3 seconds, one per second for 5 seconds, and one every other second for 14 seconds. If the computer capacity for acquiring images is sufficient, any combination of multiple delays and varying image acquisition rates is possible.

Remasking. If, on subsequent examination, the initial mask image is inadequate because of patient motion, improper technique, or any other reason, later images may be used as the mask image. A typical examination may require a total of 30 images in addition to the mask image. If the intended mask image is technically inadequate and maximum contrast appears during the fifteenth image, one may obtain a better subtraction image by using image number five as the mask rather than image number one. One can even integrate several images (e.g., numbers four through eight) and use that composite image as the mask. Unacceptable mask images can be caused by noise, motion, and technical factors.

Time interval difference mode. Some examinations call for each subtracted image to be made from a different mask and follow-up frame. This is called *time interval difference (TID)* mode (Figure 28-16). A constant image-acquisition rate needs to be used for TID imaging. In a cardiac study, for example, image acquisition begins 5 seconds after injection at the rate of 15 images per second for 4 seconds. A total of 60 images will be obtained in such a study. These images are identified as frame numbers one through 30. Each image is stored in a separate memory address as it is acquired. If a time-interval difference of four images (268 milliseconds) is selected, the first image to appear will be that obtained when frame one is subtracted from frame five. The second image will contain the subtraction of frame two from frame six, the third will contain the subtraction of frame three from frame seven, and so on.

In real time the images observed convey the flow of the contrast medium dynamically. Subsequent closer examination of each TID image shows it to be relatively free of motion artifacts but with less contrast than mask-mode imaging. As a result, TID imaging is princi-

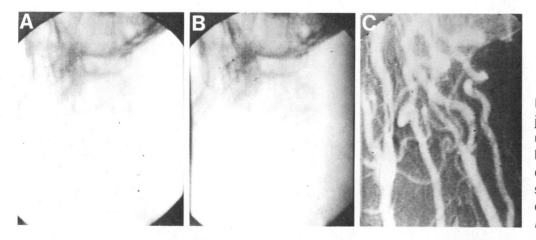

FIGURE 28-15 A, The preinjection mask. **B,** The postinjection unenhanced image. **C,** An enhanced subtration image produced when preinjection mask is subtracted from postinjection unchanged image. *(Courtesy Charles Mistretta.)*

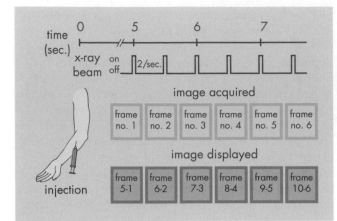

FIGURE 28-16 The manner in which sequentially obtained images are subtracted in a time-interval difference study is shown.

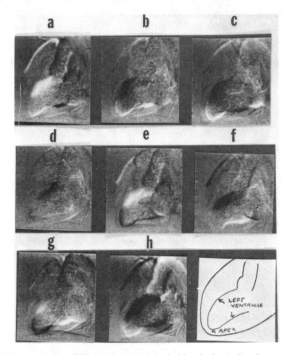

FIGURE 28-17 TID images showing dyskinesia in a dog heart. *(Courtesy Charles Mistretta.)*

pally applied in cardiac monitoring (Figure 28-17). These TID images of a dog heart show **dyskinetic** motion. In *h* the apex is expanding (white), whereas the rest of the left ventricular border is contracting (black). In a normal heart the whole border is either white or black.

Misregistration. If patient motion occurs between the mask image and a subsequent image, the subtracted image will contain **misregistration artifacts** (Figure 28-18). The same anatomy is not registered in the same pixel of the image matrix. This type of artifact can frequently be eliminated by **reregistration** of the mask, that is, by shifting the mask by one or more pixels so that **superimposition** of images is again obtained.

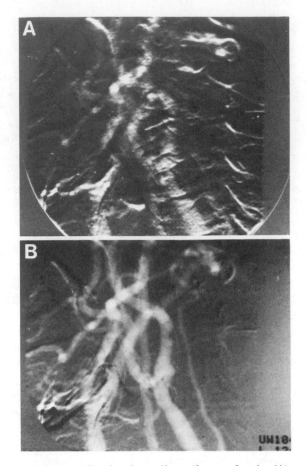

FIGURE 28-18 Misregistration artifacts. *(Courtesy Ben Arnold.)*

Reregistration can be a tedious process. Often, when one area of an image is reregistered, another area will become misregistered. This can be controlled on some systems by ROI reregistration. Most systems can reregister not only in increments of pixel widths but also down to one tenth of a pixel width.

Energy subtraction. Temporal subtraction techniques take advantage of changing contrast media during the time of the examination and require no special demands on the high-voltage generator. Energy subtraction uses two different x-ray beams alternately to provide a subtraction image resulting from differences in photoelectric interaction. The basis for this technique is similar to that described in Chapter 16 for rare-earth screens. It is based on the abrupt change in photoelectric absorption at the K edge of the contrast media compared with that for soft tissue and bone.

Figure 28-19 shows the probability of x-ray interaction with iodine, bone, and muscle as a function of x-ray energy. The probability of photoelectric absorption in all three decreases with increasing x-ray energy. At an energy of 33 keV, there is an abrupt increase in absorption in iodine and a modest decrease in soft tissue and bone.

This energy corresponds to the binding energy of the two K-shell electrons of iodine. When the incident x-ray

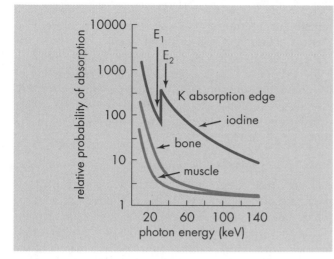

FIGURE 28-19 Photoelectric absorption in iodine, bone, and muscle.

energy is sufficient to overcome the K-shell electron binding energy of iodine, there is an abrupt and large increase in absorption. Graphically, this increase is known as the **K absorption edge.**

If x-ray beams of 32 and 34 keV could be alternately used, the difference in absorption in iodine would be enormous and the resulting subtraction images would have very high contrast. Such is not the case, however, since every x-ray beam contains a wide spectrum of energies.

Energy subtraction has the disadvantage of requiring an alternating x-ray beam of two different emission spectra. Two methods have been devised—(1) alternately pulsing the x-ray beam at 70 kVp and then 90 kVp and (2) introducing dissimilar metal filters into the x-ray beam alternately on a **fly wheel.**

Hybrid subtraction. Some DF systems are capable of combining temporal and energy subtraction techniques into what is called *hybrid subtraction* (Figure 28-20).

Image acquisition follows the mask mode procedure as previously described. However, the mask and each subsequent image are formed by an energy subtraction technique. If patient motion can be controlled, hybrid imaging can theoretically produce the highest-quality DF images.

DIGITAL RADIOGRAPHY

Digital radiography differs from conventional radiography in that the film is not the image receptor. Other types of radiation detectors are used that have an electrical output that is proportional to the radiation intensity. Initially this output signal may be in analog form, but it is converted to digital form. The image is then displayed on a video monitor after computer processing.

Scanned Projection Radiography

Perhaps the first clinical application of DR was developed by General Electric Medical Systems as a complement to CT (computed tomography). This has come to be known as scanned projection radiography (SPR). SPR involves the use of the existing CT gantry and computer to generate an image that looks surprisingly like a conventional radiograph (Figure 28-21).

This image is similar to a conventional radiographic image because there is superposition of tissues. It differs from a conventional image in that it is virtually free of scatter radiation and is digital in form. The reduced scatter radiation from **fan beam collimation** enhances radiographic contrast. The digital form of the image permits subtraction techniques as described for DF and provides for other types of image manipulation.

SPR with the reduction of scattered x-ray photons reduces image noise. Remember that Compton-scattered photons carry no useful information but simply contribute to the background noise. In any imaging system, noise covers up low-contrast anatomy. Consequently

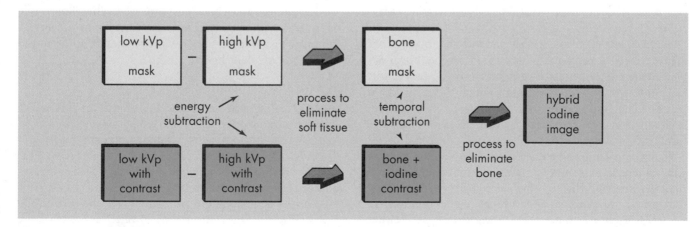

FIGURE 28-20 Hybrid subtraction involves temporal and energy subtraction techniques.

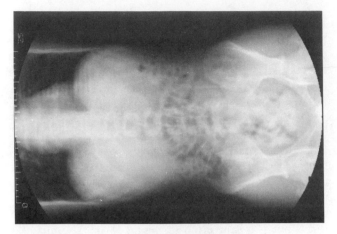

FIGURE 28-21 This computed radiograph is typical of scan projection radiographs obtained with CT scanners. *(Courtesy Larry Rothenberg.)*

the radiographic contrast is high and the detection of low-contrast anatomy is improved.

The principal disadvantage with SPR is its poor spatial resolution. Whereas a conventional screen-film system can image 100 μm objects, SPR can do no better than about 500 μm. Of course, this degree of resolution is adequate for most examinations.

The more detectors there are per degree of fan x-ray beam, the better the spatial resolution will be. Since gas-filled detectors can be packed more tightly, such a system will usually exhibit better resolution.

As the speed of **translation** is increased, fewer x-rays will be detected because the translation of the patient through the x-ray beam or the translation of the beam across the patient will decrease the resulting image quality, especially high- and low-contrast resolution.

The basic components of an SPR system is an x-ray beam shaped into a fan by collimators that confine the beam to 2 to 10 millimeter thickness through an arc of 30 to 45 degrees (Figure 28-22). There are two collimators. The prepatient collimators shape the beam, reduce scatter radiation, and control patient dose. The postpatient collimators further reduce scatter radiation.

After passing through the patient and postpatient collimators, the remnant x-rays are intercepted by a detector array. Each detector responds with a signal that is related to the body part through which the x-ray beam passed. The response of the total detector array therefore represents an attenuation profile of that body section.

To obtain enough profiles for a complete image, the source-detector assembly remains stationary and the patient is translated through the x-ray beam. Alternatively the patient may remain stationary while the source-detector assembly translates. During translation, either the x-ray beam is pulsed or the interrogation of the detector array is intermittent. The sequential profiles obtained during translation are computer processed to form an image resembling a radiograph.

SPR designs with patient translation are incorporated into most CT scanners. By proper positioning of the x-ray tube-detector array, one can obtain AP, PA, lateral, and oblique views. Dedicated DR systems use translation of the source-detector assembly across a stationary patient (Figure 28-23).

X-ray Tube-Detector Assembly

An x-ray tube used for DR must have a high heat capacity usually in excess of 1 MHu. The requirement for a high heat capacity occurs because of two characteristics of the system: (1) imaging time and (2) detector efficiency. One usually images 20 to 50 centimeters of the patient at a translation speed of 1 to 2 centimeters per second. The detectors may not be intrinsically as efficient as a screen-film receptor and, because of the precise beam collimation, few scattered photons reach the detectors. Consequently techniques of 500 to 2000 mAs are required.

There are presently two basic designs used in the detector array—(1) a gas-filled detector assembly and (2) scintillation detectors coupled to solid-state photodiodes. Similar designs are described in relation to CT (see Chapter 29).

The gas-filled detector array usually contains xenon under high pressure in many small chambers. Xenon is used because its high Z (53) results in high photoelectric absorption. The individual detector chamber can be made as small as 0.5 millimeter with an even smaller interspace.

The solid-state scintillation detector array incorporates individual crystal-photodiode assemblies. Such an array usually presents an active area to the x-ray beam of 5 by 20 millimeters with an interspace between detectors of 1 millimeter. This results in a limit to the number of detectors that can be incorporated. The scintillation crystal used is cadmium tungstate ($CdWO_4$), although bismuth germanate (BGO), cesium iodide (CsI), and sodium iodide (NaI) are also used. The photodiode is a semiconductor material, usually silicon or germanium, whose output signal is proportional to the intensity of the incident light.

Area Beam and Fan Beam

A principal limitation to the SPR mode of DR is the time required to obtain an image. In conventional radiography a latent image is produced in a matter of milliseconds. When a fan beam is used in digital radiography, several seconds may be required, which increases image blur because of patient motion.

The image acquisition time in DR can be reduced by decreasing the translation time in SPR or by using the area beam with an image receptor, as in conventional

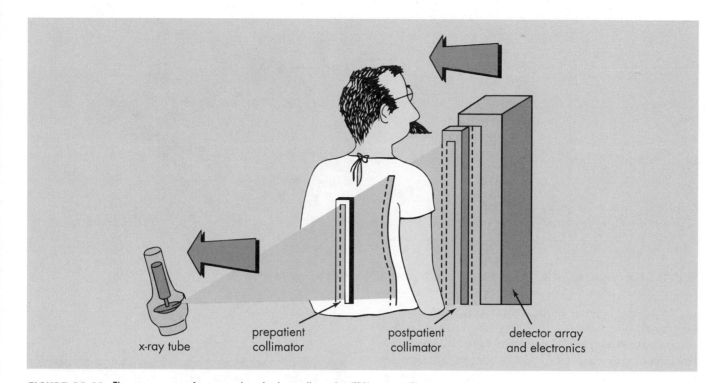

FIGURE 28-22 The components of a scanned projection radiography (SPR) system. The source detector assembly of the SPR system translates (moves) across the stationary patient as indicated by the large arrows. *(Courtesy Gary Barnes.)*

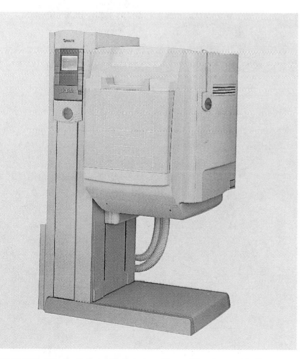

FIGURE 28-23 A dedicated digital radiographic chest unit incorporating a photostimulable phospor image receptor. *(Courtesy Fuji Medical Systems USA, Inc.)*

radiography. There is nothing special to providing an area beam. It is difficult, however, to fabricate an area image receptor that will retain the rapid response time required.

Two approaches are available. An assembly of solid-state detectors formed in a matrix fashion can be used. The electronics associated with the enormous number of detectors required is quite sophisticated and therefore expensive. The use of a charged-coupled device (CCD) was described in Chapter 26. The CCD was originally developed for military and space applications. Clearly it will become a component of future x-ray imaging systems.

Computed Radiography

Directly acquired digital radiographic images with a **photostimulable phosphor** are used as a plate-form solid-state image receptor. This process is shown schematically in Figure 28-24 and has been labeled computed radiography (CR).

The image receptor resembles a conventional radiographic intensifying screen and is exposed in a cassette with conventional x-ray equipment. It is composed of barium fluorohalide compounds, which are energized when exposed to x-rays. The sensitivity is approximately equal to a 200-speed screen-film combination and can be much greater when contrast resolution is sacrificed. The latent image consists of valence electrons stored in high-energy traps.

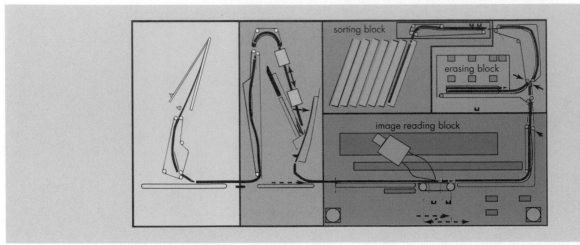

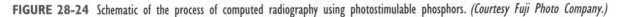

FIGURE 28-24 Schematic of the process of computed radiography using photostimulable phosphors. *(Courtesy Fuji Photo Company.)*

The latent image is made manifest by exposure to a very small beam from a high-intensity laser. The laser beam causes the trapped electrons to return to the valence band with the emission of blue light. This is **light-stimulated phosphorescence** as described in Chapter 16. The blue emission is viewed by an ultrasensitive photomultiplier tube. The electronic signal, which is the output of the photo-multiplier tube, is digitized and stored for subsequent display on a CRT or hard copy from a laser printer.

The spatial resolution of CR is not quite as good as conventional radiography, but the contrast resolution is better because of available image-postprocessing modes. The latitude of the system is exceptional, and for many examinations, patient dose is considerably less. CR promises to be important to future radiography because of its digital nature and reusable image receptor.

PICTURE ARCHIVING AND COMMUNICATION SYSTEM

Estimates of the present level of digitally acquired images from diagnostic imaging departments range up to 50%. Digital images come from nuclear medicine, digital ultrasound, DSA (digital subtraction angiography), CT, and MRI. Analog images (conventional radiographs) can be digitized by a device shown in Figure 28-25. Film digitizers are based on laser-beam technology.

All these digital images are still converted to film for interpretation and storage. A picture archiving and communication system (PACS), when fully implemented, will allow not only the acquisition but also the interpretation and storage of each medical image in digital form. With the conventional film filing and storage systems, projected efficiencies of time and money are enormous. The three principal components of a PACS are the display system, the network, and the storage system.

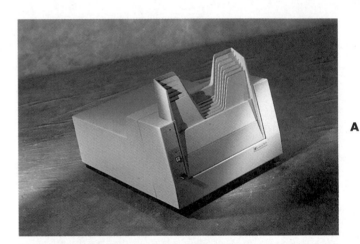

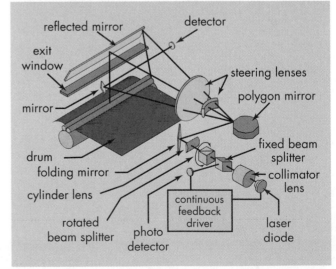

FIGURE 28-25 A, This device, called a *digitizer,* uses a laser beam to convert an analog radiograph into a digital image. **B,** Schematic of a digitizer. *(A, Courtesy Lumisys.)*

Display System

The heart of a PACS display system is the CRT monitor of a video workstation (Figure 28- 26). To truly replace film viewing, the CRTs must be high resolution, at least 2048 by 2048. Present image matrices used with most digitally acquired images range from 256 by 256 to 1024 by 1024, which is considerably less than that required to equal the spatial resolution of film. However, all PACS are equipped with a keyboard control for the various image-processing modes.

Some relaxation of the spatial resolution requirements of the workstation are allowed because of the electronic image-processing modes that are available. Image processing is possible because of the digital nature of the image and the interactive nature of the workstation. **Subtraction** of one image from another emphasizes vascular structures. **Edge enhancement** is effective for fractures and small, high-contrast objects. **Windowing** is useful for amplifying soft tissue differences. **Highlighting** can be effective in identifying diffuse nonfocal

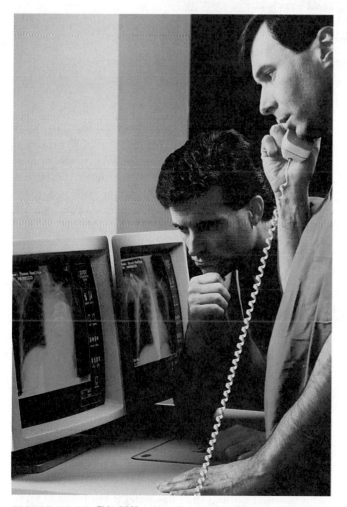

FIGURE 28-26 This PACS workstation supports filmless digital image transfer via network or compact disk. *(Courtesy Siemans Medical Systems.)*

disease. **Pan, scroll,** and **zoom** allow for careful visualization of precise regions of an image. To be truly effective, each of these image-processing modes must be quick and easy to use. This requires that each workstation be microprocessor controlled and interact with each imaging device and the central computer. To provide for such interaction, a **network** is required.

Network

Computer scientists use the term *network* to describe the manner in which many computers can be connected to interact with one another. In a business office, for instance, each secretary might have a microprocessor-based workstation, which is interfaced with a central office computer. Thus information can be transferred from one workstation to another or to and from the main computer memory.

In diagnostic imaging, in addition to secretarial workstations, the network may consist of various types of images, PACS workstations, remote PACS workstations, a departmental mainframe, and a hospital mainframe (Figure 28-27). Each of these devices is called a *node* of the network. Nodes are interconnected, usually by cable within a building, by telephone or CATV lines among buildings, and by microwave or satellite transmission to remote facilities.

The name *teleradiology* has been given to the process of remote transmission and viewing of images. To be adaptable to any radiographic equipment, The American College of Radiology (ACR), in cooperation with the National Electrical Manufacturers Association (NEMA), has produced a standard imaging and interface format.

The network begins operation at the imager where data are acquired in digital form. The images reconstructed from the data are then processed at the console of the imager or transmitted to a PACS workstation for processing. At any time, such images can be transferred to other nodes within or outside the hospital. Instead of running films up to surgery for viewing on a viewbox, one simply transfers the image electronically to the PACS workstation in surgery. When a radiologist is not immediately available for image interpretation, the image can be transferred to a PACS workstation in the radiologist's home. Essentially everywhere that film is required now, electronic images can be substituted. Time is essential when considering image manipulation and, therefore, very large and fast computers are required for this task.

These requirements are relaxed for the information management and database portion of PACS. Such lower-priority functions of PACS include message and mail utilities, calendar reporting, text data, and financial accounting and planning.

From the PACS workstation, any number of coded diagnostic reports can be initiated and transferred to a

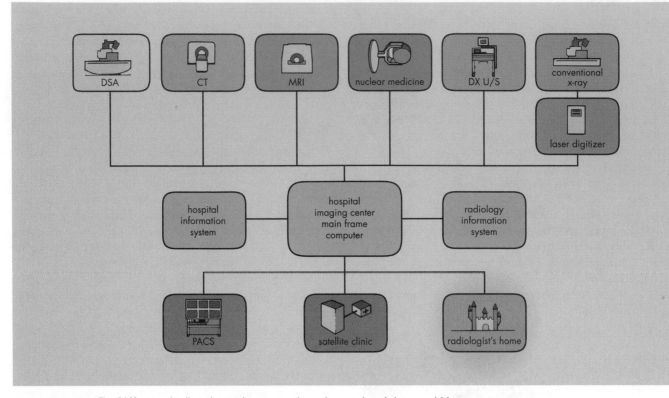

FIGURE 28-27 The PACS network allows interaction among the various modes of data acquisition, image processing, and image archiving.

secretarial workstation for report generation. The secretarial workstation in turn can communicate with the main hospital computer for patient identification, billing, accounting, and interaction with other departments. Similarly a secretarial workstation at the departmental reception desk can interact with a departmental computer for scheduling of patients, radiographers, and radiologists and for analysis of departmental statistics. Finally, at the completion of an examination, PACS allows for more efficient image archiving.

Storage System

One motivation for PACS is archiving. Often films are checked out from the file room and never returned. Many films disappear from jackets and many jackets also disappear. Finally films are often copied for clinicians. All of these problems are eliminated with PACS archiving. Just the cost of the hospital space to accommodate a film file is sufficient to justify PACS.

Question: How much computer capacity is required to store a single chest image having a 12-bit matrix and a 10-bit dynamic range?

Answer: This is a 4096 by 4096 matrix with 1024 shades of gray.

With PACS, a film room is replaced by a magnetic or optical memory device. The future of PACS, however, depends on the continuing development of the optical disk. Magnetic disk packs are available in configurations up to approximately 1000 megabytes or 1 gigabyte. Optical disks can accommodate 1 gigabyte on each side and, when positioned in a jukebox (Figure 28-28), will accommodate 100 gigabytes. An entire hospital file room is thereby accommodated by a storage device the size of a desk. Electronically, images can be recalled from this archival system to any workstation in seconds.

The acceptance of PACS in diagnostic imaging departments is slow in coming. Although image quality is equal to that of film in most instances, the cost is still high and the acceptance by radiologists and clinicians is slow. Even though diagnosis in many instances is presently made from a CRT, a radiologist still feels more secure with a hard copy. Undoubtedly, that will change with time.

SUMMARY

Conventional radiography has several limitations. First, images require processing time that can delay completion of an examination. Secondly, once images are obtained little can be done to enhance their information

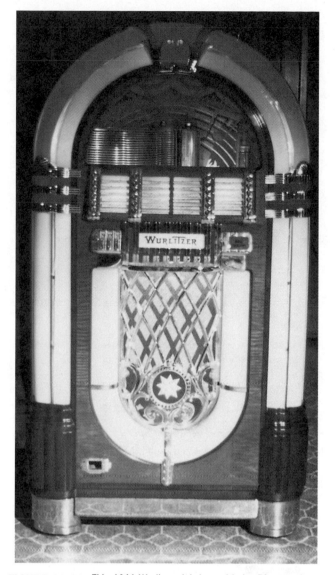

FIGURE 28-28 This 1946 Wurlitzer jukebox with its 78 rpm platters serves as a model for the optical disk jukebox of PACS. *(Courtesy Raymond Wilenzek.).*

content. Most important, however, is that noise is inherent in conventional radiography and fluoroscopy because of Compton-scattered radiation from the large rectangular x-ray beam.

Development of digital imaging equipment was stalled in the 1970s until the microprocessor and semiconductor memory systems were developed in the 1980s and were designed to process the large amount of data generated from this equipment. Digital images are displayed as a matrix of a dynamic range of gray values. Windowing allows the radiographer to postprocess the digital image for proper optical density and contrast.

Digital fluoroscopy has added a computer, two monitors, and a complex control panel to the conventional equipment. Interrogation and extinction time of 1 millisecond are the on-and-off selections of DF. The minicomputers in DF control the image matrix size, the system dynamic range, and the image acquisition rate. Eight to 30 images per second can be acquired with DF depending on the image matrix mode. A 512 by 512 matrix mode is capable of 30 images per second. If the higher matrix mode is required for improved spatial resolution, only eight images per second can be obtained.

Subtraction is a process of removing or masking all unnecessary anatomy from an image and enhancing only the anatomy of interest. With DF, subtraction is a computerized process accomplished by either temporal or energy subtraction.

Digital radiography collimation results in a fan-shaped beam to reduce scatter and enhance radiographic contrast. The primary disadvantage of DR is poor spatial resolution compared with film-screen radiography. The fan-shaped remnant beam is intercepted by a detector array, which is either a gas-filled detector or a solid-state scintillation detector. These devices are expensive. Another image receptor now in use is a solid-state plate. The barium-fluorohalide compounds are energized when exposed to x-rays. The latent image is made manifest by a high-intensity laser, which stimulates the electrons to phosphoresce-emitting light onto a photomultiplier tube. The photomultiplier forms an electronic signal that is digitized for display. The spatial resolution of the digitized image is not as good as film-screen images, but it does allow postprocessing modes.

Digital processing can be used in diagnostic imaging departments for picture archiving and communication systems (PACS). The file room can be replaced by a magnetic or optical memory device about the size of a desk. Teleradiology is a process of remote transmission of radiographs or digital images to workstations in other areas of the hospital or to radiologists off site.

Digital imaging techniques are applied to computer tomography (CT), diagnostic ultrasound, magnetic resonance imaging (MRI), digital fluoroscopy (DF), digital radiography (DR), picture achiving, and teleradiology in modern diagnostic imaging departments.

REVIEW QUESTIONS

1. List three uses of digital imaging at your clinical site.
2. What stalled the development of radiologic digital imaging until the 1980s?
3. Define image matrix. Explain what the dynamic range of values for digital imaging means.
4. What are the principal advantages of digital fluoroscopy over conventional fluoroscopy? What are the principal advantages of digital radiography over conventional radiography?

5. Using Table 28-1, name the tissue characteristics that determine the pixel brightness (Hounsfield number) of computed tomography.

6. For the same field of view (FOV), spatial resolution will be improved with a _____ image matrix.

7. How many pixels are contained in an image whose matrix size is 256 by 256?

8. The dynamic range of the human eye is approximately _____ or _____ shades of gray.

9. Define windowing and explain window level and window width.

10. Are the following statements true or false? Defend your answer.
    During DF, the x-ray tube is energized continuously. It frequently reaches thermal overload and patient dose is exceedingly high.

11. A digital image with a ten-bit dynamic range will contain how many gray values?

12. Describe the sequence of image acquisition in mask-mode fluoroscopy.

13. Describe the differences between a video system operating in the interlace mode and one operating in the progressive mode.

14. What is the reason that all electronic devices are inherently noisy?

15. Briefly describe the process of temporal subtraction and the process of energy subtraction. Using Table 28-2, contrast the advantages and disadvantages of the two processes.

16. In digital radiography, reduced scatter radiation from _____ _____ enhances radiographic contrast.

17. Briefly describe the process of recording an image with computed radiography.

18. List and describe the postprocessing image enhancements that can take place at the CRT monitor of the video workstation.

19. Define the computer network. List the possible nodes within the network.

20. _____ is the process of remote transmission and viewing of digital radiologic images.

Additional Reading

Beard DV, Hemminger BM, Denelsbeck KM, Johnston RE: How many screens does a CT workstation need? *J Digit Imaging* 7(2):69 May, 1994.

Bogucki TM: *Characteristics of a storage phostphor system for medical imaging,* Rochester NY: Eastman Kodak Company, July 1995.

Broussard CD: Documentation in the radiology department, *Images* 13(2):7 Summer, 1994.

Carey B, Kundel ML, Shile PE, Seshadri SB, Feingold ER: In situ evaluation of physician encounters with a PACS workstation in an MICU, *Appl Radiol* 22(12):31 December, 1993.

Choyke PL, Putnam BJ, Koby M, Mossy G, Feuerstein IM, Summers R: Morphing radiologic images: applications on a desktop computer, *Am J Roentgenol* 166(3):527 March, 1996.

Coons T: Teleradiology: the practice of radiology enters cyberspace, *Radiol Technol* 67(2):125 November-December, 1995.

Delivering x-ray images on hospital computer networks, *MD Comput* 9(6):348 November-December 1992.

Finlayson-Dutton G: The current state of PACS . . . picture archiving and communications systems, *Appl Radiol* 19(8)15 August, 1990.

Hendee WR, Youker JE: Teleradiology the maturation of a technology, *Appl Radiol* 21(7):13 July, 1992.

Hilsenrath P, Smith W, Franken FA Jr, Owen D, Chang P: Cost effectiveness of teleradiology for rural hospitals . . . including commentary by Crues JV III, *Appl Radiol* 21(12):54 December, 1992.

Kerr K, Staab EV, Loeffler W, Edeburn G, Geiger N: Selecting a radiology information system, *Appl Radiol* 23(7):27 July, 1994.

Khademi JA: Digital images and sound, *J Dent Educ* 60(1):41 January, 1996.

Kolodny GM: Getting started in PACS: The all-digital radiology department, *Appl Radiol* 22(4):50 April, 1993.

Mixdorf MA, Goldsworthy RE: A history of computers and computerized imaging, *Radiol Technol* 67(4):291 March-April, 1996.

Mullen JA: Selection of an affordable teleradiology system . . . including commentary by Crues JV III, *Appl Radiol* 21(10):22 October, 1992.

Nilsson M, Sjoberg S, Gladh T, Larsson R, Troedsson U: Digital image communication using a public digital telephone network, *Comput Methods Programs Biomed* 45:145 May, 1994.

Siegel E, Brown A: Preliminary impacts of PACS technology on radiology department operations, *Proc Annu Symp Comput Appl Med Care* 917, 1994.

Verhelle F, Van der Broeck R, Osteaux M: From archives to picture archiving and communications systems, *J Belge Radiol* 78(6):370 December, 1995.

Welch LS: Health effects of video display terminals, *J Am Acad Physician Assist* 4(5):395 July-August, 1991.

29 Computed Tomography

OBJECTIVES

At the completion of this chapter the student will be able to:

1. Name the individual who first demonstrated the process of CT
2. Discuss the concepts of transaxial tomography, translation, and reconstruction of images
3. List and describe the five generations of CT scanners
4. Relate the CT system components and their functions
5. Describe CT image characteristics of image matrix and CT numbers
6. Review image reconstruction
7. Discuss image quality as it relates to spatial resolution, contrast resolution, system noise, linearity, and spatial uniformity

OUTLINE

Historical Perspective
Principles of Operation
Operational Modes
  First-generation scanners
  Second-generation scanners
  Third-generation scanners
  Fourth-generation scanners
  Fifth-generation scanners
  Alternate scanners
System Components
  Gantry
  Collimation
  High-voltage generator
  Patient positioning and support couch
  Computer
Image Characteristics
  Image matrix
  CT numbers
Image Reconstruction
Image Quality
  Spatial resolution
  Contrast resolution
  System noise
  Linearity
  Spatial uniformity

The CT scanner is revolutionary. There is no ordinary image receptor, such as film or an image-intensifier tube. A collimated x-ray beam is directed on the patient, and the attenuated remnant radiation is measured by a detector whose response is transmitted to a computer. The computer analyzes the signal from the detector, reconstructs the image, and displays the image on a television monitor. The image can then be photographed for later evaluation and filing. The computer reconstruction of the cross-sectional anatomy is accomplished with mathematic equations (algorithms) adapted for computer processing.

At one time there were over 20 manufacturers of CT scanners. Now there are less than 10. The cost of these systems varies from approximately $400,000 to over $1 million. The difference in operating characteristics and image quality is far greater over the range of CT scanners than for a comparable top-to-bottom range of conventional radiographic equipment. It is important to perform a careful evaluation before purchasing a CT scanner because of the many features now available. As with conventional radiography, scheduled preventive maintenance on CT equipment is a must.

. . . .

HISTORICAL PERSPECTIVE

In the last 40 years no other advancement in x-ray apparatus has been as significant as the development of the computed tomography (CT) scanner. In the 1950s the components to construct a CT scanner were available to physicists and engineers. In the 1970s, Godfrey Hounsfield first demonstrated the process. Hounsfield was an engineer with EMI, Ltd., a British company. Both he and his company have received high acclaim. Alan Cormack, a physicist from Tufts University, shared the Nobel Prize in physics with Hounsfield in 1982. Cormack developed the mathematics used to reconstruct CT images.

PRINCIPLES OF OPERATION

When imaging the abdomen with conventional radiographic technique, the image is created directly on the film image receptor and is relatively low in contrast (Figure 29-1, *A*). The image is not as clear as one might expect because of superposition of all the anatomic structures within the abdomen. Scatter radiation further degrades the visibility of image detail.

Abdominal structures such as the kidneys are better seen when conventional tomography can be used (Figure 29-1, *B*). With **nephrotomography,** the renal outline is distinct because the overlying and underlying tissues are blurred. In addition, the contrast of the in-focus structures is enhanced. Even so, the image

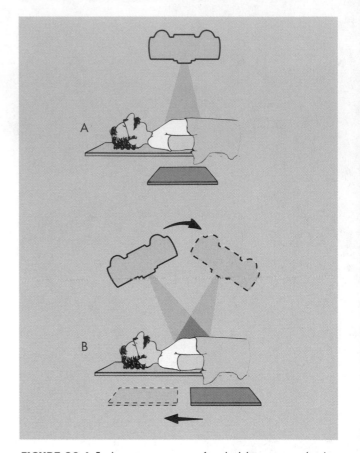

FIGURE 29-1 Equipment arrangement for obtaining a conventional radiograph, **A,** and a conventional tomograph, **B.**

is a poor representation of the the anatomic structure.

Conventional tomography results in an image that is parallel with the long axis of the body and results in sagittal and coronal images. A CT scan results in a **transverse (axial) image.** The image is perpendicular to the long axis of the body (Figure 29-2).

The way a CT scanner produces a cross-sectional image is complicated. The principles can be demonstrated looking at the simplest of CT systems. The simple CT consists of a finely collimated x-ray beam and a single detector (Figure 29-3). The x-ray source and detector are connected so that they move synchronously. When the source-detector assembly makes one sweep, or **translation,** across the patient, the internal structures of the body attenuate the x-ray beam according to their mass densities and atomic numbers as discussed in Chapter 13. The intensity of radiation detected varies according to this attenuation pattern and forms an intensity profile or **projection** (Figure 29-4). At the end of this translation the source-detector assembly returns to its starting position, and the entire assembly rotates and begins a second translation. During the second translation, the detector signal again is proportional to the

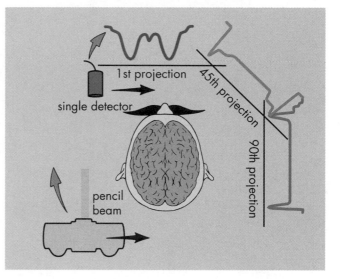

FIGURE 29-4 Each sweep of the source-detector assembly results in a projection that represents the attenuation pattern of the patient profile.

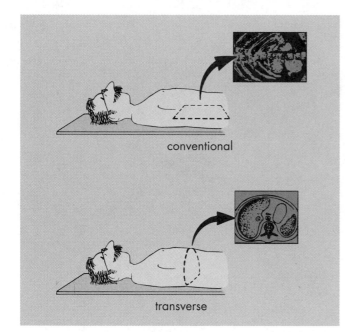

FIGURE 29-2 Conventional tomography results in an image that is parallel to the long axis of the body. A CT scan produces a transverse (axial) image.

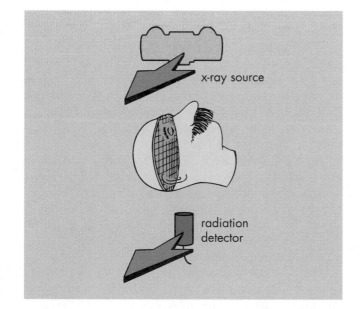

FIGURE 29-3 In its simplest form a CT scanner consists of an x-ray source emitting a finely collimated x-ray beam and a single detector, both moving synchronously in a translate-rotate mode.

x-ray beam attenuation of anatomic structures, and a second projection is scanned.

If this process is repeated many times, a large number of projections will be generated. These projections are not displayed visually but are stored in digital form in the computer. The computer processing of these projections involves the effective superposition of each projection to **reconstruct** an image of the anatomic structures in that slice. The superposition of the projections does not occur as one might imagine. The detector signal during each translation is registered in increments with values as high as 1000. The value for each increment is related to the x-ray attenuation coefficient of the total path through the tissue. Through the use of simultaneous equations, a matrix of values is obtained that represents the cross section of the anatomy scanned.

OPERATIONAL MODES

First-Generation Scanners

The previous description of a finely collimated x-ray beam, single-detector assembly translating across the patient and rotating between successive translations is characteristic of **first-generation CT scanners.** The original EMI scanner required 180 translations, each separated by a 1-degree rotation (Figure 29-5). It incorporated two detectors and split the finely collimated x-ray beam so that two contiguous slices could be imaged during each scan. The principal drawback to these units was that nearly 5 minutes was required to complete one scan.

Second-Generation Scanners

First-generation CT scanners can be considered a demonstration project. They demonstrated the feasibility of

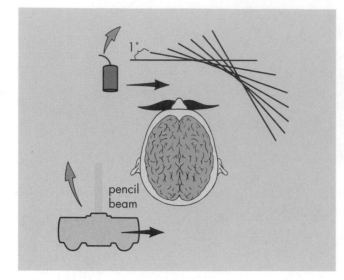

FIGURE 29-5 First-generation CT scanners used a pencil-sized x-ray beam and a single detector moving in the translate-rotate mode.

the functional marriage of the detector-source assembly, the mechanical gantry motion, and the computer to produce an image. **Second-generation scanners** were also of the translate-rotate type. These units incorporated the natural extension of the single detector to a multiple detector assembly intercepting a fan-shaped rather than a pencil-sized x-ray beam (Figure 29-6).

A disadvantage to the fan beam is the increased scatter radiation. This affects the final image in much the same way as it does in conventional radiography. The characteristic features of a second-generation CT scanner are shown in Figure 29-7.

The principal advantage of the second-generation CT scanner was speed. These scanners had 5 to 30 detectors in the detector assembly, and therefore shorter scan times were possible. Because of the multiple detector array, a single translation resulted in the same

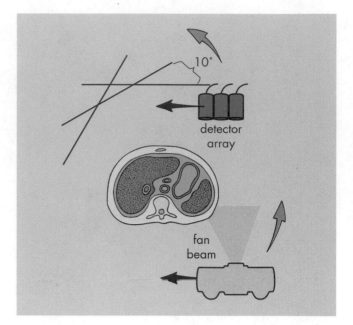

FIGURE 29-7 Second-generation scanners operated in the translate-rotate mode with a multiple detector array intercepting a fan-shaped x-ray beam.

number of data points as several translations with a first-generation CT scanner. Consequently, each translation was separated by rotation increments of 5 degrees or more. With a 10-degree rotation increment, only 18 translations would be required for a 180-degree scan.

Third-Generation Scanners

The principal limitation of second-generation CT scanners was examination time. Because of the complex mechanical motion of translate-rotate and the enormous mass involved in the scan gantry, most units were designed for scan times of 20 seconds or more. To overcome this limitation, **third-generation scanners** evolved in which the x-ray tube and detector array were rotated concentrically around the patient (Figure 29-8). As rotate-only units, third-generation scanners can produce an image in 1 second.

The third-generation CT scanner uses a curvilinear array containing many detectors and a fan beam. The number of detectors and the width of the fan beam, between 30 and 60 degrees, are both substantially larger than for second-generation scanners. In third-generation CT scanners the fan beam and detector array view the entire patient at all times.

The curvilinear detector array results in a constant source-to-detector path length, which is an advantage for good image reconstruction. This feature of the third-generation detector assembly also allows for better x-ray beam collimation to reduce the effect of scatter radiation. This type of collimation is called *predetector* or

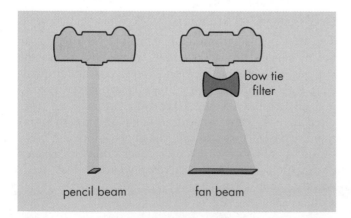

FIGURE 29-6 Two x-ray beam profiles used in CT scanning. With the fan beam, a bow-tie filter is sometimes used to equalize the radiation intensity reaching the detector array.

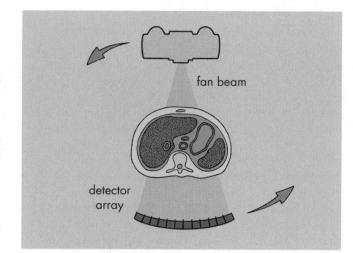

FIGURE 29-8 Third-generation CT scanners operate in the rotate-only mode with a fan x-ray beam-multiple detector array revolving concentrically around the patient.

postpatient collimation, and it functions much as a radiographic grid does in conventional radiographic examinations.

There is also **prepatient collimation** to restrict patient dose. Prepatient collimation also determines the thickness of the tissue slice that is imaged. **Slice thickness** is also called *sensitivity profile.* Figure 29-9 compares the detector assembly functions for second- and third-generation scanners.

One of the principal disadvantages of third-generation CT scanners is the occasional appearance of ring artifacts. These can occur for several reasons. Each detector views a separate **annulus** (ring) of anatomy (Figure 29-10). Should any single detector or bank of detectors malfunction, the resulting signal will result in a ring on the reconstructed image. Software-corrected image reconstruction algorithms minimize such artifacts.

Fourth-Generation Scanners

The **fourth-generation CT scanners** have a rotate-only motion. The x-ray source rotates but the detector assembly does not. Radiation detection is accomplished through a fixed circular array of detectors (Figure 29-11), which contains as many as 1000 individual elements. The x-ray beam is fan shaped with characteristics similar to those of third-generation fan beams. These units are capable of 1-second scanning times, can accommodate variable slice thickness through automatic prepatient collimation, and can provide the image manipulation capabilities of earlier scanners.

The fixed detector array of fourth-generation CT scanners does not result in a constant beam path from the source to all detectors, but it does allow each detector to be calibrated and its signal normalized during

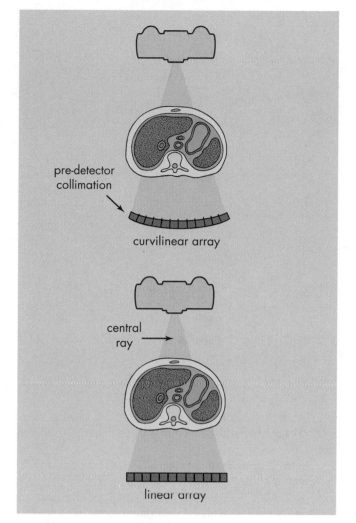

FIGURE 29-9 The linear detector array is characteristic of first- and second-generation CT scanners; the curvilinear array is used in third- and fourth-generation units.

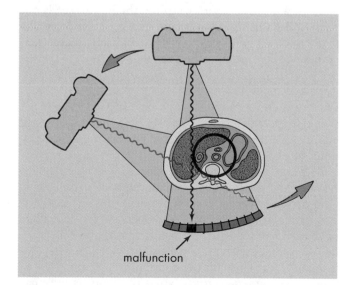

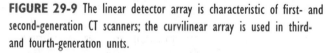

FIGURE 29-10 Ring artifacts can occur in third-generation scanners because each detector views an annulus of anatomy during each scan.

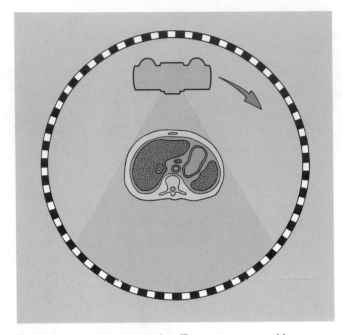

FIGURE 29-11 Fourth-generation CT scanners operate with a rotating x-ray source and stationary detectors.

each scan, as was possible with second-generation scanners. Fourth-generation scanners are generally free of ring artifacts.

The principal disadvantage of fourth-generation CT scanners is patient dose, which is somewhat higher than that with other types of scanners. The cost of these units may be somewhat higher also because of the large number of detectors and their associated electronics.

Although many attempts at image quality comparison have been conducted, no generalizations are possible, and a clear decision regarding the best image is not likely. Much of the final image quality depends on the mathematics of image reconstruction, and these techniques are continually being refined.

Fifth-Generation Scanners

There are continuing developments in CT scanner design that promise still further improvements in image quality at less patient dose. Some incorporate novel motions of either the x-ray tube or the detector array or both. Some involve patient motion as well.

Faster scanners have been developed, making cine CT possible. There is continuing development of reconstruction algorithms so that the operator can select one of several for a particular examination. **Slip-ring** technology is incorporated into spiral CT scanners (see Chapter 30). This allows continuous rotation of the x-ray tube and detectors. None of these designs has been acclaimed as fifth generation, but spiral CT is the leading candidate.

Alternate Scanners

Rotate-nutate. Toshiba produced a novel extension of fourth generation scanners. To maintain the x-ray source at the same distance from the patient as the detectors, the detector array **nutated** (wobbled) as the x-ray source rotated (Figure 29-12).

Electron beam CT (EBCT). This fundamentally different way to produce CT images was pioneered by Imatron for cardiac imaging. Currently, it is used to image all anatomy but is especially helpful when fast imaging is helpful. The EBCT consists of a **waveguide** to accelerate an electron beam onto a tungsten target through a bending magnet (Figure 29-13). Actually there are four tungsten targets so that four tissue slices are imaged at the same time. EBCT images are produced in as little as 100 milliseconds.

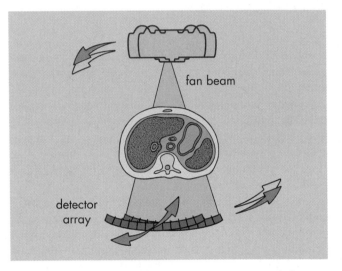

FIGURE 29-12 In this design the x-ray source rotates and the stationary detector array nutates.

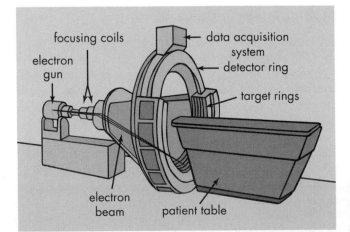

FIGURE 29-13 Electron beam CT has no moving parts in the gantry.

SYSTEM COMPONENTS

No matter which generation scanner is in use, there are three major components in the CT scanner—the gantry, the computer, and the operating console. Each of these major components has several subsystems (Figure 29-14).

Gantry

The gantry includes the x-ray tube, the detector array, the high-voltage generator, the patient support couch, and mechanical supports. These subsystems receive electronic commands from the operating console and transmit data to the computer for image production and analysis.

X-ray tube. X-ray tubes in CT scanning have special requirements. Although some operate at relatively low tube current, for many, the instantaneous power capacity must be high. The anode heating capacity must be at least 1 MHU, and some tubes designed specifically for CT have 4-MHU capacity.

High-speed rotors are used in most tubes for the best heat dissipation. Experience has shown that x-ray tube failure is a principal cause of CT scanner malfunction and the principal limitation on sequential scanning frequency.

Focal-spot size is also important in most designs, even though the CT scanner is not based on principles of direct geometric imaging. CT scanners designed for high spatial resolution imaging incorporate x-ray tubes with a small focal spot.

X-ray tubes are energized differently, depending on the CT scanner design. Rotate-only CT scanners operate with either a continuous or a pulsed x-ray beam. Continuous x-ray beams at tube currents up to 400 mA are produced during the entire rotation. Pulsed units produce x-ray beams at tube currents approaching 1000 mA with pulse widths from 1 to 5 milliseconds at pulse repetition rates of 60 Hz.

Detector assembly. Early CT scanners had one detector. Modern CT scanners use multiple detectors in an array numbering up to 2400 in two general classifications: (1) scintillation detectors and (2) gas detectors.

Scintillation detectors. Early scintillation detector arrays contained crystal photomultiplier tube assemblies. These detectors could not be packed very tightly together. They required a power supply for each photomultiplier tube. Consequently, they have been replaced by crystal-photodiode assemblies. Photodiodes are smaller and cheaper and do not require a power supply. They are also equally efficient as a CT radiation detector.

Sodium iodide (NaI) was the crystal used in the earliest scanners. This was quickly replaced by bismuth germanate ($Bi_4Ge_3O_12$ or BGO) and cesium iodide

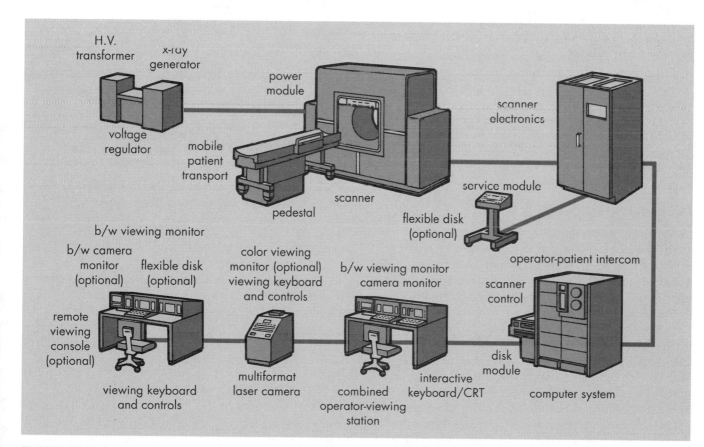

FIGURE 29-14 Components of a complete CT scanner system. *(Courtesy Picker International.)*

(CsI). Cadmium tungstate (CdWO₄) is the current crystal of choice.

The spacing of these detectors varies from one design to another, but generally one to eight detectors per centimeter or one to five detectors per degree are available. The concentration of scintillation detectors is an important characteristic of a CT scanner that affects the spatial resolution of the system.

Scintillation detectors have high x-ray detection efficiency. Approximately 90% of the x-rays incident on the detector are absorbed and contribute to the output signal. Unfortunately, it is not possible to pack the detectors so that the space between them is small. The detector interspace may occupy 50% of the total area intercepting the x-ray beam. Consequently the overall detection efficiency may be only 50%. Approximately 50% of the remnant x-rays exiting the patient contribute to patient dose without contributing to the image. This is diagramed in Figure 29-15, which shows a comparison between the scintillation detector array and the gas detector array.

Gas detectors. Gas-filled detectors are also used in CT scanners (Figure 29-16). They are constructed of a large metallic chamber with baffles spaced at approximately 1-millimeter intervals. The baffles are like grid strips and divide the large chamber into many small chambers. Each small chamber functions as a separate radiation detector. The entire detector array is hermetically sealed and filled under pressure with an inert gas with a high atomic number such as xenon or a xenon-krypton mixture. Ionization of the gas in each chamber is proportional to the radiation incident on the chamber and is detected in much the same way as the **ideal gas-filled detector** described in Chapter 39. However, the overall total detection efficiency is approximately 45%, which is similar to that for the scintillation detector array. All other characteristics being equal, therefore, patient dose is about the same for both types of detector arrays.

Collimation

Collimation is required during CT scanning for precisely the same reasons that it is required in conventional radiography. Proper collimation reduces patient dose by restricting the volume of tissue irradiated. More importantly it enhances image contrast by limiting scatter radiation.

In conventional radiography there is only one collimator, which is mounted on the tube housing. In CT scanning there are sometimes two collimators (Figure 29-17). One is mounted on the tube housing or adjacent to it. This collimator limits the area of the patient that intercepts the useful beam and thereby determines the slice thickness and patient dose. This prepatient collimator usually consists of several sections so that a nearly parallel x-ray beam results. Improperly adjusted

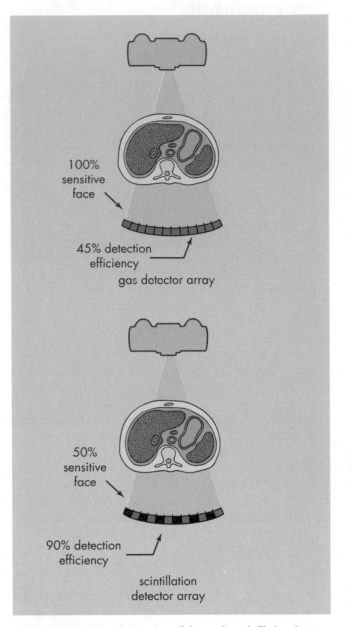

FIGURE 29-15 Overall detection efficiency of a scintillation detector array is approximately equal to that of the gas detector array.

prepatient collimators result in most of the unnecessary radiation dose during a CT scan.

The postpatient collimator restricts the x-ray field viewed by the detector array. This collimator reduces the scatter radiation incident on the detector and, when properly coupled with the prepatient collimator, helps define the slice thickness. The postpatient collimator does not influence patient dose.

High-Voltage Generator

All CT scanners operate on three-phase or high-frequency power. This accommodates the higher x-ray tube rotor speeds and the instantaneous power surges characteristic of pulsed systems. Some manufacturers

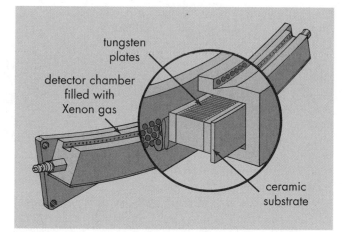

FIGURE 29-16 Gas-filled detector array features small detectors in high concentration with little interdetector dead space. *(Courtesy General Electric Medical Systems.)*

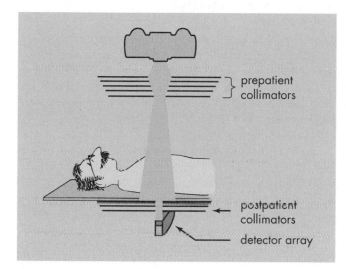

FIGURE 29-17 CT scanners incorporate both prepatient collimators and postpatient collimators.

conserve space by building the high-voltage generator into the gantry or even by mounting it on the rotating wheel of the gantry so that winding and unwinding a power cable is unnecessary.

Patient Positioning and Support Couch

The patient couch is one of the more important components of the CT scanner. In addition to supporting the patient comfortably, it must be constructed of low-Z material such as carbon fiber so that it does not interfere with x-ray beam transmission and patient imaging. It should be smoothly and accurately motor driven so that precise patient positioning is possible. This is particularly important during spiral CT. When positioning is not exact, the same tissue can be scanned twice or missed altogether. The patient couch should be capable

of automatic **indexing** so that the operator does not have to enter the examination room between each scan. Such a feature reduces the examination time required for each patient.

Computer

The computer is a unique subsystem of the CT scanner. Were it not for the ultra high-speed digital computer, CT scanning would not be possible. Depending on the image format, as many as 30,000 equations must be solved simultaneously; thus a large-capacity computer is required. Computer costs can easily run to one third the cost of the entire CT scan system, although such costs continue to fall.

Most computers require a special and controlled environment; consequently, many CT scan facilities must have an adjacent room dedicated to the computer. In the computer room, humidity must be maintained at less than 30% relative, and temperatures must be maintained below 20° C. Higher temperatures and humidity can contribute to computer failure.

At the heart of the computer used in CT are the microprocessor and primary memory. These determine the time between the end of a scan and the appearance of an image, which is called the *reconstruction time*. Reconstruction times of just a few seconds are now common. The efficiency of an examination is greatly influenced by reconstruction time, especially when a large number of slices are involved.

Many CT scanners use an **array processor** instead of a microprocessor for image reconstruction. The array processor does many calculations simultaneously. It is significantly faster than the microprocessor, and an image can be reconstructed in less than 1 second.

Control console. Many CT scanners are equipped with two consoles, one for the CT radiographer to operate the unit and one for the radiologist to view the image and manipulate its contrast, size, and general visual appearance. The operator's console contains meters and controls for selecting proper radiographic technique factors, for proper mechanical movement of the gantry and patient couch, and for computer commands that allow image reconstruction and transfer. The physician's viewing console accepts the reconstructed image from the operator's console and displays it for viewing and diagnosis.

Operator's console. A typical operator's console contains controls and monitors for the various technique factors (Figure 29-18). Operation is generally in excess of 100 kVp. The usual mA station will be 100 mA if the x-ray beam is continuous and several hundred mA if it is a pulsed beam. The **scan time** is often selectable and varies from 1 to 5 seconds. Subsecond CT scanners are available.

The thickness of the tissue slice to be imaged can also be adjusted. Nominal thicknesses are 1 to 10 millime-

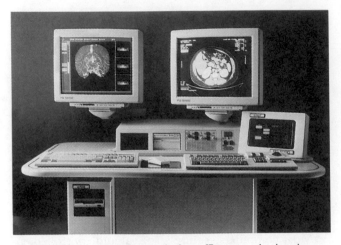

FIGURE 29-18 Operator's console for a CT scanner showing the various control functions. *(Courtesy Picker International.)*

ters, but some units provide slice thicknesses as small as 0.5 millimeters for high-resolution scanning. Slice thickness is selected from the console by automatic collimator adjustment. Controls are also provided for automatic movement and indexing of the patient support couch. This allows the operator to program for **contiguous slices,** for **intermittent slices,** or for **spiral scanning.**

The operating console usually has two television monitors. One is used by the operator to indicate patient data on the scan (hospital identification, name, patient number, age, and gender.) and to provide identification for each scan (scan number, technique, and couch position). The second monitor is used by the operator to view the resulting image before transferring it to either hard copy or the physician's viewing console.

Physician's viewing console. Smaller, less expensive CT systems may not have a physician's viewing console. If the workload is high and the system fully in use, however, a physician's viewing console is essential so that patient scans can be reviewed and reported without interfering with scanner operations. For maximum effectiveness, the physician's viewing console is supported by an independent computer. If the independent computer requires the main computer for image manipulation, viewing can be slowed during scanning because the scan mode takes precedence.

The console allows the physician to call up any previous image and manipulate images for maximum information. The manipulative controls provide for contrast and brightness adjustments, magnification techniques, region of interest (ROI) viewing, and use of on-line computer software packages. This software may include programs to generate CT number **histograms** along any preselected axis, computation of **mean** and **standard deviation** of CT values within an ROI, sub-

traction techniques, and **planar** and **volumetric quantitative analysis.** Reconstruction of images along coronal, sagittal, and oblique planes is also possible.

Image storage. There are a number of useful image storage formats. Current scanners store image data on either **magnetic tapes** or **disks.** If the disk format is used, data from a single patient are transferred to a single disk that can be stored in a jacket with other patient reports and films. If magnetic tape storage is used, data from many patients can be transferred to a single tape. Each tape will generally accommodate 150 scans, which is equivalent to five to ten patients.

For later viewing and filing, CT scan images are usually recorded on film in a laser camera. Typical cameras use 8×10 inch films and can provide one, two, four, or six images to a film. Naturally the more images per film, the smaller the image. Some cameras use 14×17 inch film and therefore provide a larger image format.

IMAGE CHARACTERISTICS
Image Matrix

The CT scan image format consists of many cells, each assigned a number and displayed as a density or brightness level on the video monitor. The original EMI format consisted of an 80 by 80 matrix for a total of 6400 individual cells of information. Current scanners provide matrices of 512 by 512, which results in 262,144 cells of information.

Each cell of information is a **pixel** (picture element), and the numerical information contained in each pixel is a CT number or **Hounsfield unit.** The pixel is a two-dimensional representation of a corresponding tissue volume (Figure 29-19). The tissue volume is known as a **voxel** (volume element), and it is determined by multiplying the pixel size by the thickness of the CT scan

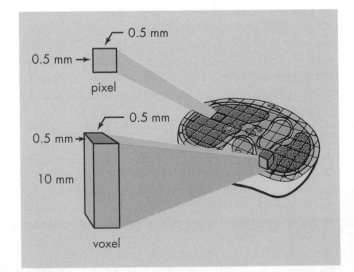

FIGURE 29-19 Each cell in a CT image matrix is a two-dimensional representation (pixel) of a volume of tissue (voxel).

slice. The diameter of the reconstructed image is called the **field of view (FOV)**. When the FOV is increased for a fixed matrix size, for example a 512 by 512 matrix, the size of each pixel is increased proportionately. When the matrix size is increased, for example from 512 by 512 to 1024 by 1024, pixel size is smaller.

Question: Compute the pixel size for the following characteristics of a CT scanner used for brain scans:

    a. Field of view 20 centimeters, 120 by 120 matrix

    b. Field of view 20 centimeters, 512 by 512 matrix

    c. Field of view 36 centimeters, 512 by 512 matrix

Answer:

$$\text{a.}\quad \frac{200\ \text{mm}}{120\ \text{pixels}} = 1.7\ \text{mm/pixel}$$

$$\text{b.}\quad \frac{200\ \text{mm}}{512\ \text{pixels}} = 0.4\ \text{mm/pixel}$$

$$\text{c.}\quad \frac{360\ \text{mm}}{512\ \text{pixels}} = 0.7\ \text{mm/pixel}$$

CT Numbers

Each pixel is displayed on the video monitor as a level of brightness and on the photographic image as a level of optical density. These levels correspond to a range of CT numbers from -1000 to $+1000$ for each pixel. A CT number of -1000 corresponds to air, and a CT number of $+1000$ corresponds to dense bone. A CT number of zero indicates water. Table 29-1 shows the CT values for various tissues along with respective x-ray **linear attenuation coefficients**.

The precise CT number of any given pixel is related to the x-ray attenuation coefficient of the tissue contained in the voxel. As discussed in Chapter 13 the de-

gree of x-ray attenuation is determined by the average energy of the x-ray beam and the effective atomic number of the absorber and is expressed by the attenuation coefficient.

The value of a CT number is given by:

$$\text{CT number} = k \times \frac{\mu_o - \mu_w}{\mu_w}$$

In the equation, μ_o is the x-ray attenuation coefficient of the pixel, μ_w is the x-ray attenuation coefficient of water, and k is a constant that determines the scale factor for the range of CT numbers.

This equation shows that the CT number for water is always zero. For the scanner to operate with precision, detector response must continuously be calibrated so that water is always represented by zero. When k is 1000, the CT numbers are Houndsfield Units (HUs).

Obviously there is an enormous amount of information wasted when the dynamic range of the image is 2000 but only 32 shades of gray are displayed on a video screen.

IMAGE RECONSTRUCTION

The projections acquired by each detector during a CT scan are stored in the memory of a very large computer. The image is reconstructed from these projections by a process called **filtered back projection**. Here the term **filter** refers to a mathematical function rather than an aluminum or other metal filter. This process is complicated, but a simple example helps explain how it works. Imagine a box with two holes cut in each side (Figure 29-20). The box is divided into four sections labeled a, b, c, and d, and there is a Texas-sized cockroach in section c. If the box is covered and someone looks through the four sets of holes, a way can be devised of determining precisely in which section the cockroach resides.

Let 1 represent the presence of the cockroach for each viewing. If two empty sections are seen through a

TABLE 29-1

CT Number for Various Tissues and X-ray Linear Attenuation Coefficients (cm⁻¹) at Three Operating kVp Levels

Tissue	Approximate CT Number	Linear Attenuation Coefficient (cm⁻¹)		
		100 kVp	125 kVp	150 kVp
Dense bone	1000	0.528	0.460	0.410
Muscle	50			
White matter	45	0.213	0.187	0.166
Gray matter	40	0.212	0.184	0.163
Blood	20	0.208	0.182	0.163
Cerebrospinal fluid	15	0.207	0.181	0.160
Water	0	0.206	0.180	0.160
Fat	−100	0.185	0.162	0.144
Lungs	−200			
Air	−1000	0.0004	0.0003	0.0002

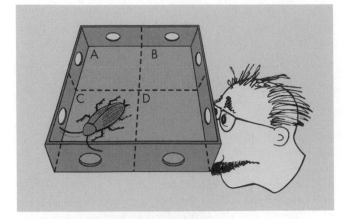

FIGURE 29-20 This four-pixel matrix demonstrates the method for reconstructing a CT image by back projection.

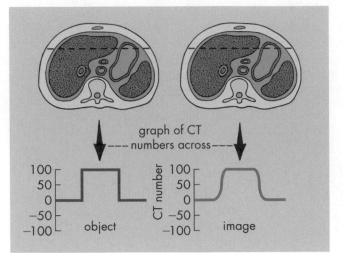

FIGURE 29-21 A CT scan of an object organ with distinct borders will result in an image with somewhat blurred borders. The actual CT number profile of the object would be abrupt, whereas that of the image would be smoothed.

hole, then obviously the cockroach is not there. The absence of the cockroach is indicated with a 0. The path being viewed in Figure 29-20 can be represented symbolically as: c + d = 1. Examining all possible paths shows the following:

$$a + b = 0$$
$$c + d = 1$$
$$a + c = 1$$
$$b + d = 0$$

Thus the solution is c = 1 and a, b, and d = 0.

In a CT scanner, there are not four sections (pixels) but rather over 250,000. Consequently the CT image reconstruction requires over 250,000 simultaneous equations.

IMAGE QUALITY

The image quality of conventional radiographs is expressed in terms of spatial resolution, contrast resolution, and noise. These characteristics are easy to describe but somewhat difficult to measure quantitatively.

Since CT images are composed of discrete pixel values that are then converted to film format, image quality is somewhat easier to quantify. There are a number of methods available for measuring CT image quality. There are four characteristics with numerical measurements. These are spatial resolution, contrast resolution, linearity, and noise.

Spatial Resolution

Scanning a regular geometric structure that has a sharp edge or interface, the image at the interface will be somewhat blurred (Figure 29-21). The degree of blurring is a measure of the spatial resolution of the system and is controlled by a number of factors. Since the im-

age of the interface is a visual rendition of pixel values, these values can be analyzed across the interface to arrive at a measure of spatial resolution.

Suppose the organ in Figure 29-21 were composed of material of a relatively high CT value (e.g., 100) and was immersed in water, which has a CT number of zero. This would be a relatively high-contrast interface. The CT numbers across the interface might have actual values such as those shown in the object graph in Figure 29-21.

Since, however, the image is somewhat blurred because of limitations of the CT scanner, the expected sharp edge of CT values is replaced with a smoothed range of CT values across the interface. This smoothing results in poor spatial resolution because of several features of the CT scanner. The larger the pixel size and the lower the subject contrast, the poorer the spatial resolution. The detector size and design of the prepatient and postpatient collimation affect the level of scatter radiation and influence spatial resolution by affecting the contrast of the system. Even x-ray tube focal-spot size influences spatial resolution in CT.

The ability of the CT scanner to reproduce with accuracy a high-contrast edge is expressed mathematically as the **edge response function (ERF)**. The measured edge response function can be transformed into another mathematical expression called the *modulation transfer function (MTF)*. The MTF and its graphic representation are most often cited to express the spatial resolution of a CT scanner.

Although the MTF is a rather complicated mathematical formulation, its meaning is not too difficult to represent. Consider, for instance, a series of bar patterns that are imaged by a CT scanner (Figure 29-22). One

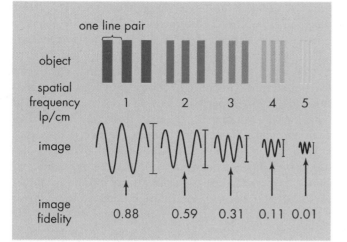

FIGURE 29-22 As a bar pattern of increasing spatial frequency is imaged, the fidelity of the image decreases. The tracing of density across the image reveals the loss of contrast.

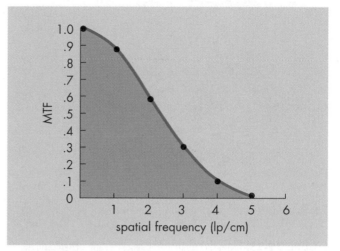

FIGURE 29-23 Modulation transfer function is a plot of the image fidelity versus spatial frequency. The six data points plotted here are from the analysis of Figure 29-22.

bar and its equal width interspace are called a *line pair (lp)*. The number of line pairs per unit length is called the *spatial frequency,* and for CT scanners it is expressed in line pairs per centimeter (lp/cm). A low spatial frequency represents large objects, and a high spatial frequency represents small objects.

The image obtained from the low-frequency bar pattern appears more like the object than the image from the high-frequency pattern. The loss in faithful reproduction with increasing spatial frequency occurs because of a number of limitations of the imaging system. Characteristics of the CT scanner that contribute to such image degradation are collimation, detector size and concentration, mechanical-electrical gantry control, and the reconstruction algorithm.

In simplistic terms the MTF is the ratio of the image to the object. If the image faithfully reproduced the object, the MTF of the CT scanner would have a value of 1. If the image were simply blank and contained no information whatsoever about the object, the CT scanner MTF would be equal to zero. Intermediate levels of fidelity result in intermediate MTF values.

In Figure 29-22, image fidelity is measured by the optical density along the axis of the image. At a spatial frequency of 1 lp/cm, for instance, the variation in optical density of the image is 0.88 times that of the object. At 4 lp/cm, it is only 0.1 or 10% that of the object. A graph of this ratio of image contrast to object contrast at each spatial frequency results in an MTF curve (Figure 29-23).

Figure 29-24 shows the MTF for two different CT scanners and illustrates how one should interpret such a curve. An MTF curve that extends farther to the right indicates higher spatial resolution, which means the imaging system is better able to reproduce very small

objects. Obviously MTF is a complex relationship, since it relates the imaging capacity of the system for various sized objects. Most CT scanners are judged by the spatial frequency at an MTF equal to 0.1, sometimes called the *limiting resolution*. As shown in Figure 29-24, scanner *A* has a 0.1 MTF at 5.2 lp/cm, whereas *B* can only manage 3.5 lp/cm. Therefore *A* has better spatial resolution than *B*.

Although CT scan resolution is most often expressed by the spatial frequency of the limiting resolution, it is easier to think in terms of the object size that can be reproduced. Figure 29-25 illustrates the relationship between spatial frequency and object size. The absolute object size that can be resolved by a scanner is equal to

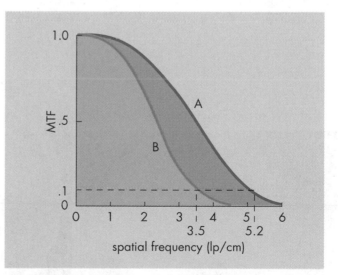

FIGURE 29-24 MTF curves for two representative CT scanners are shown. Scanner *A* will produce higher resolution images than scanner *B*.

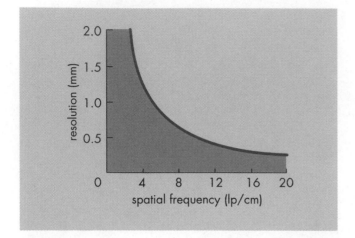

FIGURE 29-25. Increasing spatial frequency means better resolution of smaller objects.

one half the reciprocal of the spatial frequency at the limiting resolution.

Question: A CT scanner is said to be capable of 5 lp/cm resolution. What size object does this represent?

Answer: The reciprocal of 5 lp/cm = $(5 \text{ lp/cm})^{-1}$

$$= \frac{1}{5 \text{ lp/cm}}$$

$$= \frac{1 \text{ cm}}{5 \text{ lp}}$$

$$= \frac{10 \text{ mm}}{5 \text{ lp}}$$

$$= 2 \text{ mm/lp}$$

Since a line pair consists of a bar and an interspace of equal width, 2 mm/lp represents a 1-millimeter object

separated by a 1-millimeter interspace. The system resolution is therefore 1 millimeter.

Specially designed phantoms are necessary for evaluating CT scanner performance. Such phantoms are usually fabricated from plastic of different densities in various shapes and configurations. The important measures of scanner performance that can be evaluated with phantoms are **artifact generation,** contrast resolution, and spatial resolution. Figure 29-26, *A,* shows an anthropomorphic phantom designed to test the body mode of a CT scanner for artifacts. Figure 29-26, *B* shows a specially designed phantom containing an array of low-contrast holes and high-contrast bars to test both low- and high-contrast resolution with a single scan.

Contrast Resolution

The ability to distinguish material of one composition from another without regard for size or shape is called *contrast resolution.* This is an area in which the CT scanner excels. The absorption of x-rays in tissue is characterized by the x-ray linear attenuation coefficient. This coefficient, as we have seen, is a function of x-ray energy and the atomic number of the tissue. In CT scanning the amount of radiation penetrating the patient is determined also by the mass density of the body part.

Consider the situation outlined in Figure 29-27, which is a fat-muscle-bone structure. Not only are the atomic numbers somewhat different (Z = 6.8, 7.4, and 13.8), but the mass densities also are different (ρ = 0.91, 1.0, and 1.85). Although these differences are measurable, they are not imaged well in conventional radiography. The CT scanner is able to amplify these differences in subject contrast so that the image contrast is high. On computer reconstruction the range of CT numbers for these tissues will be approximately −100, 50, and 1000. This amplified contrast scale

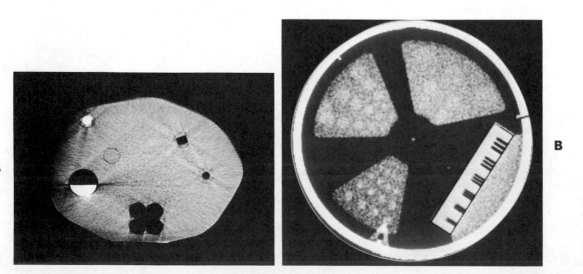

FIGURE 29-26
A, This anthropomorphic phantom for evaluating CT scan image quality contains objects simulating a barium-filled stomach, intestinal folds, a rib, and airways. **B,** This phantom is designed to measure both low-contrast resolution and high-contrast resolution. *(Courtesy Edwin C. McCullough, Mayo Clinic, Rochester, Minn.)*

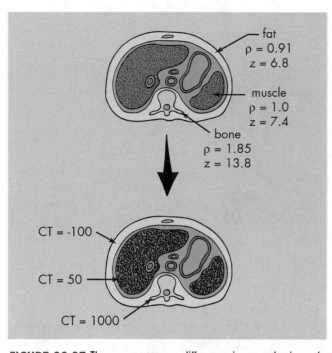

fat
$\rho = 0.91$
$z = 6.8$

muscle
$\rho = 1.0$
$z = 7.4$

bone
$\rho = 1.85$
$z = 13.8$

CT = -100

CT = 50

CT = 1000

FIGURE 29-27 There are not many differences in mass density and effective atomic number among tissues, but the differences are greatly amplified by the CT scanner.

allows the CT scanner to better resolve adjacent structures that are similar in composition.

The contrast resolution provided by CT scanners is considerably better than that available in conventional radiography principally because of the scatter radiation rejection of the fan-beam collimators. The ability to image low-contrast objects with a CT scanner, however, is limited by the size and uniformity of the object and by the noise of the system.

System Noise

If a homogenous medium such as water is scanned, each pixel should have a value of zero. Of course, this never occurs because the contrast resolution of the system is not perfect; therefore the CT numbers may average zero, but a range of values greater than or less than zero exists. A variation in CT numbers above or below the average value is the **noise** of the system. If all pixel values were the same, system noise would be zero. A larger variation of pixel values results in higher system noise.

Noise is defined as percent standard deviation of a large number of pixels obtained from a water bath scan. It should be clearly understood that system noise depends on many factors including the following:

1. kVp and filtration
2. Pixel size
3. Slice thickness
4. Detector efficiency
5. Patient dose

Ultimately it is patient dose, the number of x-rays used by the detector to produce the image, that controls noise. System noise is defined as follows:

$$Noise = \sqrt{\frac{\Sigma(x_i \times \overline{x})^2}{n - 1}}$$

In this equation, x_i is each CT value, $\overline{x}$ is the average of at least 100 values, and n is the number of CT values averaged. In statistics, noise is called a *standard deviation* and symbolized by σ.

Noise appears on the final image as graininess. Low-noise systems appear very smooth to the eye, and high-noise systems appear spotty or blotchy. The resolution of low-contrast objects is limited by the noise of a CT scanner.

System noise should be evaluated daily by scanning a 20-centimeter diameter water bath. All scanners have the ability to identify a region of interest (ROI) and compute the mean and standard deviation of CT numbers in that ROI. When the CT radiographer measures noise, the ROI must encompass at least 100 pixels. Such noise measurements should include five determinations—four on the periphery and one in the center to monitor the spatial uniformity.

Linearity

The CT scanner must be frequently calibrated so that water is consistently represented by CT number zero and other tissues by their appropriate CT value. A check calibration that can be made daily uses the five-pin performance phantom of the American Association of Physicists in Medicine (AAPM) (Figure 29-28). The five pins are each made of a different plastic material with known physical and x-ray absorption properties (Table 29-2).

After a scan of this phantom, the CT number for each pin should be recorded and its mean value and standard deviation plotted (Figure 29-29). The plot of CT number versus linear attenuation coefficient should be a straight line passing through CT number zero for water. A deviation from **linearity** is an indication of misalignment or malfunction of the CT scanner. A minor deviation would result in inaccurate CT number generation but would probably not significantly affect the visual image. Such a minor deviation, however, could affect quantitative CT analysis of tissue.

Spatial Uniformity

When imaging a uniform object such as a water bath with a CT scanner, each pixel should have the same value, since each pixel represents precisely the same object composition. Furthermore, if the CT scanner is properly adjusted, that value should be zero. Since the CT scanner is an extremely complicated electronic-mechanical device, however, such precision is not consistently possible. The CT value for water may drift from day to day or even from hour to hour.

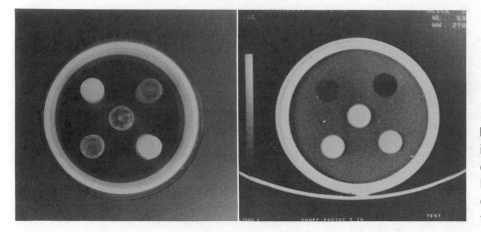

FIGURE 29-28 Photograph *(left)* and CT image *(right)* of the five-pin test phantom designed by the American Association of Physicists in Medicine. The attenuation coefficient for each pin is known precisely and the CT number computed.

TABLE 29-2

Characteristics of the Five-Pin AAPM Phantom

Material		Density (g/cm³)	Linear Attenuation Coefficient (cm⁻¹) at 60 keV	CT Number
Polyethylene	C_2H_4	0.94	0.185	−85
Polystyrene	C_8H_8	1.05	0.196	−10
Nylon	$C_6H_{11}NO$	1.15	0.222	100
Lexan	$C_{16}H_{14}O$	1.20	0.223	115
Plexiglas	$C_5H_8O_2$	1.19	0.229	130
Water	H_2O	1.00	0.206	0

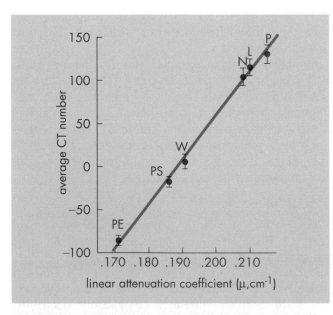

FIGURE 29-29 CT linearity is acceptable if a graph of average CT number versus the linear attenuation coefficient is a straight line.

At any time a water bath is scanned, the pixel values should be constant in all regions of the reconstructed image. Such a characteristic is called *spatial uniformity*. Testing for spatial uniformity can be done easily with an internal software package that allows the plotting of CT numbers along any axis of the image as a histogram or as a line graph. If all the values of the histogram or line graph are within two standard deviations of the mean value ($\pm 2\sigma$), the system is said to exhibit acceptable spatial uniformity. Because of x-ray beam hardening or reconstruction inadequacies, there may be either **cupping** of CT numbers in the middle of the scan field or a decrease at the periphery.

SUMMARY

The CT scanner is revolutionary because it does not record an image in a conventional way. The collimated x-ray beam is directed to the patient, the attenuated remnant beam is measured by a detector, the signal from the detector is measured by a computer, the image

TABLE 29-3

Synopsis of Five Operational Modes of CT Scanners

Operational Modes	Advantages	Disadvantages
First-generation scanner	Demonstration project; translate-rotate type; pencil beam	5 minutes to complete a scan; single detector assembly
Second-generation scanner	Multiple detector assembly; translate-rotate type; fan beam; increased speed	Increase scatter radiation
Third-generation scanner	Concentrically rotated around patient; 1-second scan time; curvilinear detectors; predetector and postdetector collimation	Ring artifacts
Fourth-generation scanner	Rotate-only motion; fixed circular array of detectors; automatic collimation; no ring artifacts	Increased patient dose; increased expense because of number of detectors
Fifth-generation scanner	Spiral scanning; faster examination time; decreased patient dose	

is reconstructed in the computer, and, finally the image is displayed on a television monitor. Five generations of scanners have been developed. The advantages and disadvantages of each development are listed in Table 29-3.

CT acquires transaxial images, which are slices of anatomy perpendicular to the long axis of the body (see Figure 29-2). The CT scanner's source-detector assembly translates or makes a sweep across the patient to acquire data. The internal structures of the body attenuate the x-ray beam according to their mass densities and atomic numbers. The resulting intensity profile or projection is repeated many times as the entire assembly rotates. All data from the projections are stored in digital form in the computer. Computer processing reconstructs the anatomic structures in each slice into an image.

The CT system components are similar in all scanners. There is the gantry, the x-ray tube, the detector assembly, collimation (prepatient and postpatient), the patient couch, and the computer. The resulting computer image is an electronic matrix of intensities. The matrix size is generally 512 by 512 individual cells or pixels. In each pixel is numerical information called a *CT number* or a *Hounsfield unit of intensity*. The pixel is a two-dimensional representation of a corresponding tissue volume. The voxel or volume element is determined by multiplying the pixel size by the thickness of the CT scan slice. A CT number of -1000 corresponds to air. A number of +1000 corresponds to dense bone. A CT number of zero indicates water.

Figure 29-20 illustrates a simplified version of the complex mathematics of image reconstruction. Image quality in CT is expressed in terms of spatial resolution, contrast resolution, and noise. The degree of blurring of high-contrast anatomic edges within the image is a measure of spatial resolution. Spatial resolution is translated into the mathematical expression called MTF (modulation transfer function) and the image fidelity is measured in line pairs per centimeter. Contrast resolution is

the ability of the CT image to distinguish anatomy of differing composition. Contrast resolution of the CT scanner excels because of limitation of scatter-radiation. The ability of the scanner to image low-contrast anatomy is limited by the noise of the system. System noise is determined by the number of x-rays used by the detector to produce the image. Noise appears as image graininess.

CT radiographers and physicists routinely check the CT scanner for malfunction and misalignment of collimation and detectors. Linearity and spatial uniformity tests are performed to examine the CT scanner for proper calibration.

■ ■ ■ ■ ■ ■ ■ ■ ■ ■ ■ ■ ■ ■ ■ ■ ■ ■ ■ ■

REVIEW QUESTIONS

1. Name the individual who first demonstrated the computed tomographic process in 1970.

2. Define the terms *axial, translation,* and *reconstruction*.

3. List the advantages and disadvantages of the five generations of CT scanners.

4. What are the components of the gantry portion of the CT scanner?

5. What are the special requirements of the x-ray tube used in CT scanning? What is the principal cause of CT scanner malfunction?

6. Discuss the spacing and concentration of scintillation detectors on the CT scanner.

7. Why is collimation as important in CT scanning as it is for conventional radiography?

8. Describe the two collimation devices used in CT scanning. Where are they placed? What is the importance of proper adjustment?

9. What material makes up the patient support couch? Define automatic indexing as it relates to the support couch.

10. Why must the CT computer be ultra-high speed and large capacity? The computer must be maintained under what environmental conditions?

11. What is the voxel size of a CT head scanner with a 320 by 320 matrix size, a 20-centimeter reconstruction diameter, and a 0.5-centimeter slice thickness?

12. What device controls the slice thickness of a CT scan?

13. What kVp level is generally used for CT scanning? What scan times are used?

14. The numerical information contained in each pixel is a(n) _____ or _____.

15. Referring to Table 29-1, a CT number of 20 relates to what tissue type?

16. Explain the mathematics of the computerized image reconstruction process.

17. What is the blurring of high-contrast interfaces called?

18. Refer to Figure 29-24. An MTF curve that extends farther to the right indicates _____ spatial resolution.

19. A CT scanner can resolve a 0.65-millimeter high-contrast object. How many lp/cm does this represent?

20. Define contrast resolution, system noise, linearity, and spatial uniformity.

Additional Reading

Advances in ultrafast computed tomography: 1995. An international symposium on electron beam tomography, Scottsdale, Arizona, October 6-8 1995, *Am J Card Imaging* 9:1 October, 1995.

Beard DV, Hemminger BM, Denelsbeck KM, Johnston RE: How many screens does a CT workstation need? *J Digit Imaging* 7(2):69 May, 1994.

Budzil RF Jr: Three-dimensional CT angiography, *Appl Radiol* March, 1993, 42-46.

Computed tomography, *Appl Radiol* 19(7):33 July, 1990.

Fishman EK, Ney DR, Scott WW Jr, Robertson DD: The role of CT with multiplaner reconstruction, *Appl Radiol* 21(11):36 November, 1992.

Kalbhen CL, Pierce KL: Fast CT scanning; applications of helical and electron-beam CT, *Appl Radiol* March, 1993, 47-51.

30

Spiral Computed Tomography

OBJECTIVES

At the completion of this chapter the student will be able to:

1. Explain the scan principles of interpolation, pitch ratio, and section sensitivity profile
2. Discuss the scanner design that makes spiral CT possible
3. Recognize the differences between conventional and spiral CT x-ray tubes
4. Describe the technique selection for spiral CT
5. Discuss the improvement of Z-axis spatial resolution with spiral CT
6. List the advantages and limitations of spiral CT

OUTLINE

Scan Principles
  Interpolation algorithms
  Spiral scan pitch ratio
  Section sensitivity profile
Scanner Design
  Slip-ring technology
  X-ray tube
  X-ray detectors
  High-voltage generator
Technique Selection
  Examination time
  Z-axis resolution
  Reconstruction

Image Characteristics
  Overlapping images
  Maximum intensity projection
  Shaded surface display
Advantages and Limitations of Spiral CT

n 1989, spiral computed tomography (CT) was introduced with great promise for advancement in the modality. The term *spiral,* or *helical,* was coined because it is the apparent motion of the x-ray tube during the scan. In some imaging departments, CT scanner use has declined in favor of magnetic resonance imaging (MRI). MRI was said to have all the advantages of CT with none of CT's limitations. However, the future of medicine is changing as fast as newspaper headlines. Cost containment and limited reimbursement for high-tech studies such as CT and MRI are part of the future of health care. For CT to grow or at least survive it had to provide more information than other imaging modalities in a cost-effective, time-efficient manner.

Spiral CT has emerged as a new and improved diagnostic tool. Spiral CT provides improved imaging of anatomy compromised by respiratory motion. Spiral CT is particularly good for the chest, abdomen, and pelvis. Spiral CT also has the ability to perform conventional transverse imaging for regions of the body where motion is not a problem such as the head, spine, and extremities.

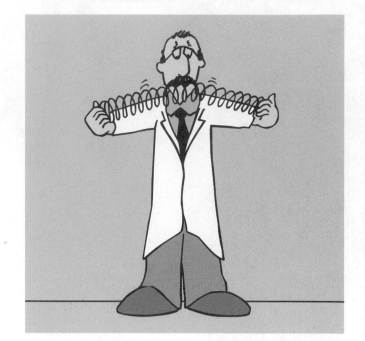

FIGURE 30-1 A slinky toy is a common example of a spiral.

SCAN PRINCIPLES

Even though the movement of a spiral CT seems to resemble the spirals of a slinky toy (Figure 30-1), the spiral CT scanning motion is not actually like a slinky toy. Figure 30-2 shows the difference.

When the examination begins, the x-ray tube rotates continuously without reversing. While the x-ray tube is rotating, the couch moves the patient through the plane of the rotating x-ray beam. With all spiral CT scans, data is collected continuously. This data can then be reconstructed at any desired z-axis position along the patient (Figure 30-3).

Interpolation Algorithms

The ability to reconstruct an image at any z-axis position is due to **interpolation.** Figure 30-4 presents a graphical representation of interpolation and **extrapolation.** If one wishes to estimate a value between two known values, that is interpolation. Estimating a value beyond the range of known values is extrapolation.

During spiral CT, image data is received continuously as shown by the data points of Figure 30-5, *A.* When an image is reconstructed as in Figure 30-5, *B,* the plane of the image does not contain enough data for reconstruction. Data must be estimated by interpolation.

Data interpolation is performed by a special computer program called an *interpolation algorithm.* The first interpolation algorithms used a 360-degree linear interpolation (Figure 30-6). Three hundred sixty degrees was used because the estimated image plane infor-

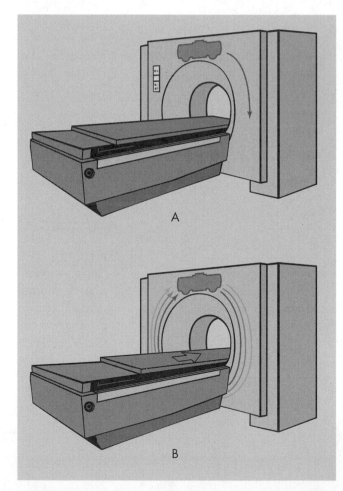

FIGURE 30-2 A, The movement of the x-ray tube is not a spiral. **B,** It just appears that way because the patient moves through the plane of rotation during the scan.

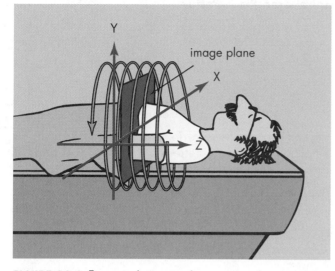

FIGURE 30-3 Transverse images can be reconstructed at any plane along the z-axis.

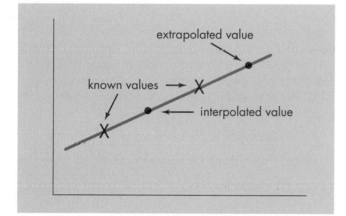

FIGURE 30-4 Interpolation estimates a value between two known values. Extrapolation estimates a value beyond known values.

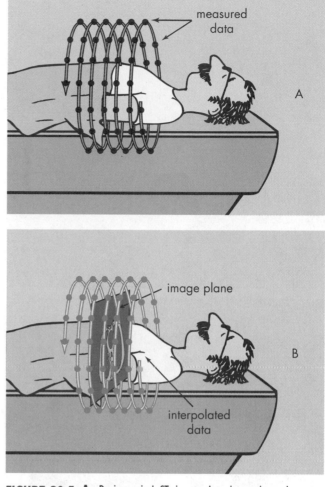

FIGURE 30-5 A, During spiral CT, image data is continuously sampled. **B,** Interpolation of data is performed to reconstruct the image in any transverse plane.

mation was interpolated from data 360 degrees apart in rotation. Linear was used because the algorithm assumed a straight-line relationship between the two known data points. The result is a transverse image nearly identical with that of a conventional CT.

When these images were formatted into **sagittal** and **coronal** views, prominent blurring was obvious compared with conventional CT reformatted views.

The solution to this problem is interpolation of values separated by 180 degrees (Figure 30-7). This results in improved Z-axis resolution and greatly improved reformatted sagittal and coronal views. The following two types of 180-degree algorithms have been developed: (1) **simple linear interpolation** and (2) **cubic-spline interpolation.** The disadvantage of the 180-degree interpolation algorithms is increased image noise compared with 360-degree interpolation algorithms.

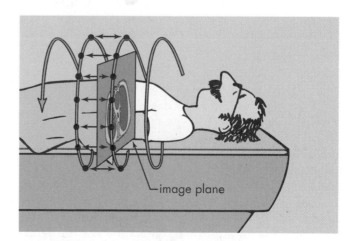

FIGURE 30-6 Interpolation between data points 360° apart was the earliest spiral CT reconstruction algorithm.

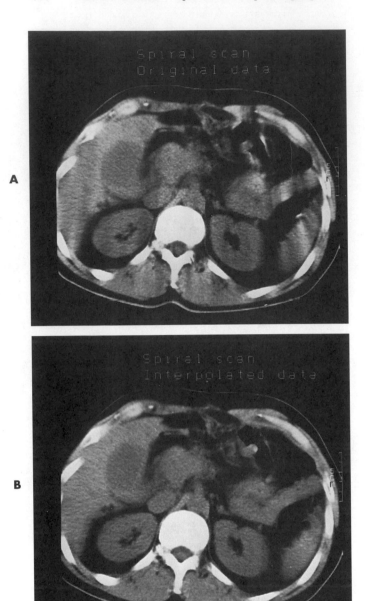

A

B

FIGURE 30-7 Z-interpolation is necessary in spiral CT. **A,** Image reconstruction directly from 360° segment will result in motion artifacts. **B,** Z-interpolation results in images free of such artifacts. *(Courtesy Will Kalander).*

Spiral Scan Pitch Ratio

Spiral scan pitch ratio, generally referred to as simple *pitch,* is the relationship between the patient couch movement and x-ray beam collimation.

$$\text{Pitch} = \frac{\text{Couch movement (mm/sec) per 360-degree rotation}}{\text{Collimation}}$$

Pitch is expressed as a ratio, 1:1, 1.5:1, or 2:1, for example. In most examinations a 1:1 pitch will result in the best image quality.

Question: During a 360-degree x-ray tube rotation the patient couch moves 8 millemeters. Section collimation is 5 millimeters. What is the pitch?

Answer:

$$\frac{8 \text{ mm}}{5 \text{ mm}} = 1.6:1$$

Increasing pitch above 1:1 increases the volume of tissue that can be imaged in a given time. The ability to image a larger volume of tissue in a single breathhold is the principle advantage to spiral CT. This is particularly helpful in CT angiography, radiation therapy treatment planning, and imaging uncooperative patients.

The relationship between the volume of tissue imaged and pitch is given as follows:

$$\text{Tissue imaged} = \text{Collimation} \times \text{Pitch} \times \text{Scan time}$$

Note that tissue imaged is a linear value along the z-axis but we think of it as the **volume of tissue imaged.** Table 30-1 shows this relationship for a fixed scan time and fixed section thickness.

Question: How much tissue will be imaged if collimation is set to 8 millimeters, scan time is 25 seconds, and the pitch is 1.5:1?

Answer: Tissue imaged = 8 mm × 25 s × 1.5

= 300 mm

= 30 cm

What if the gantry rotation time is not 360 degrees in 1 second? If the x-ray tube heat capacity is limited, slower

A 180-degree interpolation algorithm noise is not bothersome. However, the use of a cubic-spline interpolation algorithm can produce what is called a *breakup* artifact at high contrast interfaces such as bone-soft tissue. Linear interpolation at 180 degrees is preferred.

In addition to improved sagittal and coronal reformatted views, 180-degree interpolation algorithms allow imaging at a **pitch** greater than one.

TABLE 30-1				
Tissue Imaged with Changing Pitch				
Section thickness (mm)	10	10	10	10
Scan time (s)	30	30	30	30
Pitch	1:1	1.3:1	1.6:1	2:1
Tissue imaged (cm)	30	39	48	60

rotation may be necessary. In such a situation the equation on p. 398 becomes:

$$\text{Tissue imaged} = \frac{\text{Collimation} \times \text{pitch} \times \text{scan time}}{\text{Gantry rotation time}}$$

If the gantry rotation time is increased to 1.5 seconds, Table 30-1 is changed to Table 30-2.

Use of the above equation will allow the CT radiographer to compute the volume of tissue to be imaged before beginning the examination.

Question: How much tissue will be imaged with 5-millimeter collimation, a pitch of 1.6:1, and a 20-second scan time at a gantry rotation time of 2-second?

Answer:

$$\text{Tissue imaged} = \frac{5 \text{ mm} \times 1.6 \times 20 \text{ s}}{2 \text{ s}}$$

$$= 80 \text{ mm}$$

$$= 8 \text{ cm}$$

Section Sensitivity Profile

Consider the section sensitivity profile (SSP) of a 10-millimeter section obtained with a conventional CT scanner (Figure 30-8). If properly collimated, it will have a **full width at half maximum (FWHM)** of 10 millimeters. Some report SSP as full width at tenth maximum (FWTM). At a pitch of 1:1 the SSP is only approximately 10% wider than conventional CT (Figure 30-9). At a pitch of 2:1 the SSP is approximately 40% wider; but at a pitch of 3:1 the SSP soars.

In the same way that pitch influences SSP, so does the interpolation algorithm. The z-axis resolution is worse for a 360 degree interpolation algorithm compared with a 180-degree interpolation algorithm because the SSP is wider (Figure 30-10).

SCANNER DESIGN

Spiral CT was made possible by **slip-ring** technology. The results of shorter scan times and more tissue volume imaged without loss of image quality was also due

TABLE 30-2				
Tissue Imaged with Changing Pitch and a Gantry Rotation Time of 1.5 Seconds				
Section thickness (mm)	10	10	10	10
Scan time (s)	30	30	30	30
Gantry rotation time (s)	1.5	1.5	1.5	1.5
Pitch	1:1	1.3:1	1.6:1	2:1
Tissue imaged (cm)	20	26	32	40

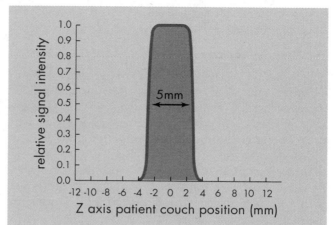

FIGURE 30-8 The section sensitivity profile for a conventional CT scanner is nearly a square at the edge of the x-ray beam.

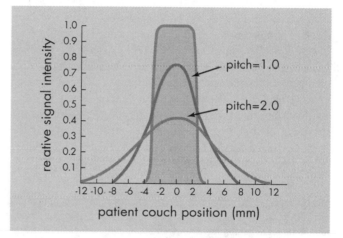

FIGURE 30-9 The section sensitivity profile for spiral CT widens as pitch is increased.

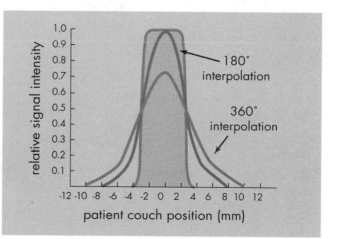

FIGURE 30-10 The section sensitivity profile is wider for 360 degree interpolation than 180 degree interpolation.

to improvements in the x-ray tube, the high voltage section, and the detector array.

Slip-Ring Technology

Slip rings are electromechanical devices that conduct electricity and electric signals through rings and brushes across a rotating surface onto a fixed surface. One surface will be a smooth ring and the other a ring with brushes that sweep the smooth ring. Spiral CT is made possible by the use of slip-ring technology, which allows the gantry to rotate continuously without interruption. Remember, conventional CT scanning is performed with a pause between each gantry rotation. During the pause the patient couch is moved and the gantry may be rewound to a starting position.

In a slip-ring gantry system, power and electric signals are transmitted through stationary rings within the gantry that make continuous rotation possible and eliminating the need for electrical cables. There are two slip-ring designs in spiral CT scanners, the **disk** and the **cylinder**. The disk design incorporates concentric conductive rings in the plane of rotation. The cylindrical design has the conductive rings lying parallel to the axis of rotation forming a cylinder. The brushes that transmit power to the gantry components glide in contact grooves on the stationary slip ring. Composite brushes made of conductive material (e.g., silver-graphite alloy) are used as a sliding contact. The rings should last the life of the scanner. The brushes have to be replaced every year or so during normal maintenance.

There are usually three slip rings on a gantry. One provides high-voltage power to the x-ray tube and high-voltage generator. A second provides low-voltage power to control systems on the rotating gantry. The third slip ring transfers digital data from the rotating detector array in the case of a third-generation scanner.

The design of the high-voltage slip ring differs among manufacturers. One approach generates the high voltage off the gantry. In this design the slip ring must be sealed to insulate the transfer of up to 150 kVp. Another approach transfers a low voltage onto the rotating gantry, where it is increased to the desired kVp. This requires that invertors and transformers be designed to produce that high power but that are also compact enough to fit on the rotating gantry. Intermediate between these two approaches are hybrid designs. Figure 30-11 shows how compact a rotating gantry must be.

X-ray Tube

In conventional CT the x-ray tube is energized for one rotation, usually 1 second, every 6 to 10 seconds. This allows the tube to cool between scans. Spiral CT places a considerable thermal demand on the x-ray tube. The x-ray tube is energized for up to 30 seconds continuously.

Because of the continuous rotation and energization of the x-ray tube for longer exposure times, higher power levels must be sustained. Most systems use an x-ray tube with two focal spots. The small spot is used for high-resolution examinations, and the large spot is

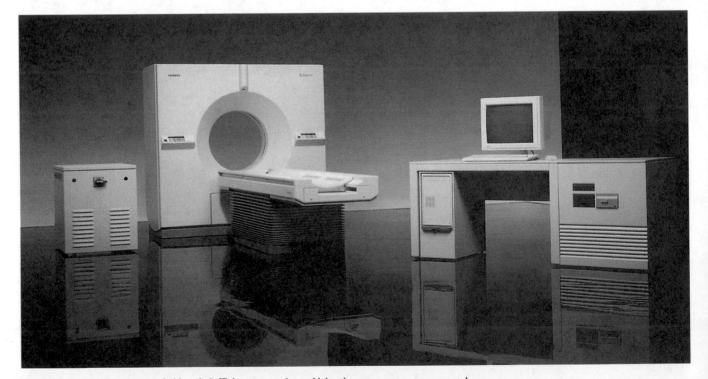

FIGURE 30-11 The gantry of this spiral CT image contains a high-voltage generator, an x-ray tube, a detector array, and assorted control systems. *(Courtesy Siemens Medical Systems, Inc.)*

used for high-technique studies of large anatomy. High heat capacity and high cooling rates are trademarks of x-ray tubes designed for spiral CT.

Spiral CT x-ray tubes are very large. They have anode heat storage capacity of 5 MHU or more. Less than 3 MHU is unacceptable. Spiral CT x-ray tubes have anode cooling rates of 1 MHU per minute.

The limiting characteristics of spiral CT scanners are the focal-spot design and the rate of heat dissipation. The small focal spot must be a well-engineered design. Manufacturers design **focal-spot cooling algorithms** to predict the focal spots thermal state and to adjust mA accordingly.

The x-ray tube in Figure 30-12 is designed especially for spiral CT. This x-ray tube is expected to last for at least 50,000 exposures, which is the approximate x-ray tube life for conventional CT.

X-ray Detectors

The efficiency of the x-ray detector array reduces patient dose, allows faster scan times, and improves image quality by increasing signal-to-noise ratio. Detector ar-

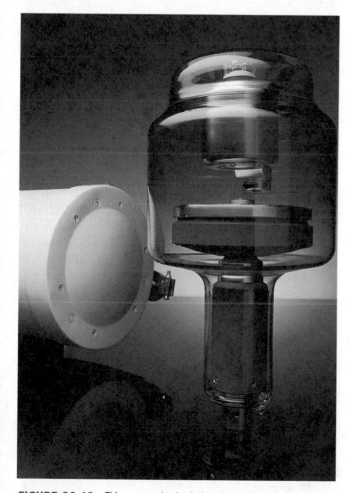

FIGURE 30-12. This x-ray tube is designed especially for spiral CT. It has a 15-centimeter diameter disk, which is 5 centimeters thick with an anode heat capacity of 1.8 MHV. *(Courtesy Varion Interay.)*

ray design is especially critical for spiral CT. The overall efficiency for solid-state arrays is approximately 80%, whereas that for gas-filled detectors is approximately 60%. Consequently solid state is the preferred detector array.

High-Voltage Generator

The design constraints placed on the high-voltage generator are the same as those for the x-ray tube. In a properly designed spiral CT scanner the two should be matched to maximum capacity. Approximately 50-kW power is necessary.

Designing such a high-voltage generator to fit onto the rotating gantry was indeed a challenge. Designing the insulated high-voltage slip rings was equally challenging. Both design requirements have been adequately met.

TECHNIQUE SELECTION

The radiologist and CT radiographer have more decisions to make and more work to do for spiral CT. The principal advantage to spiral CT is the ability to image a large volume of anatomy in one breathhold. However, the patient's ability at breathholding determines the scan parameters selected.

The volume of tissue imaged is determined by the examination time, couch travel, pitch, and collimation. Additionally, rotation time, reconstruction algorithm, reconstruction interval, and skip scan delay must be selected.

Examination Time

Most spiral CT scanners can image up to 60 seconds continuously. Most patients can breathhold 40 seconds. Some can breathhold only 20 seconds. Therefore, if one requires 45 seconds of imaging as shown in Figure 30-13, *A,* it may be necessary to skip scan as in Figure 30-13, *B* with a 10-second interscan delay to allow the patient to breathe.

Z-axis Resolution

Depending on the spatial resolution requirements of the examination, the Z-axis resolution must be specified by technique selection. Transverse resolution is determined by the reconstruction matrix. Longitudinal (Z-axis) resolution is determined by several technique factors that must be preselected.

When the required Z-axis resolution is high, thin-section collimation will be selected. High z-axis resolution also requires selection of low pitch, slow couch motion, and 180-degree interpolation reconstruction.

Examinations requiring high Z-axis resolution are those attempting to image small structures such as lung calcifications and contrast-filled arteries as in CT angiography. Normal resolution would be required for imaging organs such as liver, spleen, and kidneys. Table

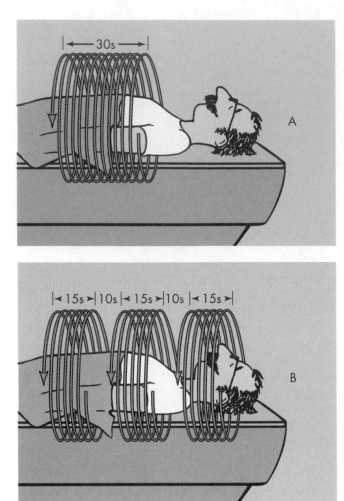

FIGURE 30-13 A, Most spiral CT examinations can be completed in a single breathhold. **B,** When patient breathing is limited, a skip-scan technique must be selected.

	Lung Nodules	Renal Parenchyma
TABLE 30-3		
Representative Technique Factors for Imaging Lung Nodules and Renal Parenchyma		
Slice thickness (mm)	2 mm	10 mm
Pitch	1:1	2:1
Couch movement (mm)	2 mm	5 mm
Gantry rotation (s)	1.0	1.5

30-3 provides representative technique factors for a high-resolution and normal-resolution spiral CT examination.

To be sure to cover the required anatomy a chart such as that shown in Table 30-3 should be constructed. The number in each box shows the length of anatomy to be imaged. A different table would be assembled for each scan time.

Reconstruction

For high-resolution imaging, 180-degree interpolation is required. Transverse images, longitudinally reformatted images, or both may be required. If a longitudinally reformatted image is required, one may choose from shaded volume display, shaded surface display, or **CT angiography.**

IMAGE CHARACTERISTICS

Image quality in spiral CT is measured by spatial resolution and contrast resolution, which is comparable with conventional CT. Since the number of detectors, detector spacing, and number of projections in the scan plane are generally the same as that in conventional CT, **inplane resolution** is the same.

However, although the SSP is worse in spiral CT there can be notable improvement in the Z-axis spatial resolution because there are no gaps in the data and image reconstruction can be made at any position along the Z-axis. Reconstructed images can even overlap.

Overlapping Images

Consider the calcified lung nodule in Figure 30-14. With conventional CT, the nodule may be missed if it lies at a section interface. By overlapping the transverse-image reconstruction, the nodule can be brought into the midsection with an accompanying improvement in contrast resolution.

In addition to overlapping transverse images for improved contrast resolution, spiral CT excels in three-dimensional **multiplanar reformation (MPR).** Transverse images are stacked to form a three-dimensional data set that can be rendered as an image in several ways. The following three-dimensional MPR algorithms are most frequently used: (1) **maximum intensity projection (MIP),** (2) **shaded surface display (SSD)** and (3) **shaded volume display (SVD).**

Maximum Intensity Projection

MIP reconstructs an image by selecting the highest value pixels along any arbitrary line through the data set and exhibiting only those pixels (Figure 30-15). MIP images are widely used in CT angiography (CTA) because they can be reconstructed very fast.

Only approximately 10% of the three-dimensional data points are used. The result can be a very high contrast three-dimensional image of contrast-filled vessels (Figure 30-16). On most computer workstations the image can be rotated to show striking three-dimensional features.

MIP is the simplest form of three-dimensional imaging. It provides excellent differentiation of vasculature

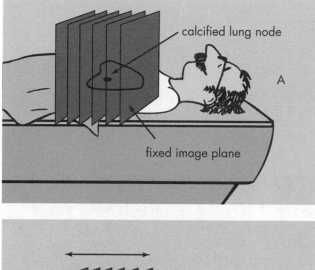

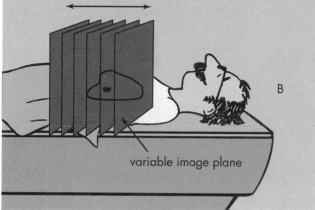

FIGURE 30-14 **A,** A very small structure such as this lung nodule will be poorly imaged by conventional CT if the nodule is at the section interface. **B,** With spiral CT a 50% overlap can be performed in reconstruction to improve the contrast resolution.

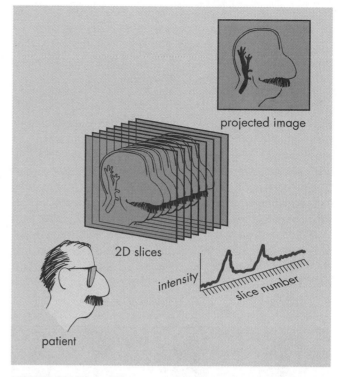

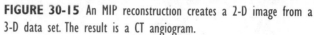

FIGURE 30-15 An MIP reconstruction creates a 2-D image from a 3-D data set. The result is a CT angiogram.

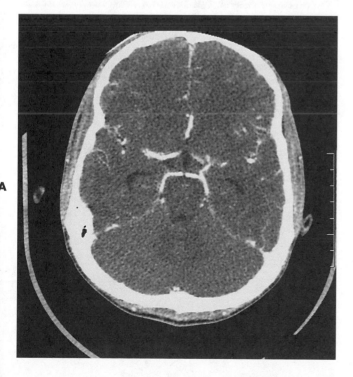

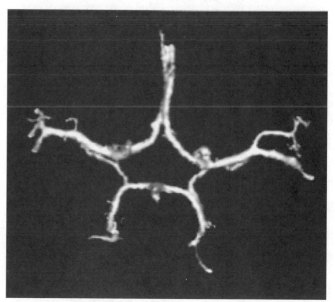

FIGURE 30-16 **A,** Contrast-enhanced transverse CT image through the circle of Willis. **B,** Corresponding 3-D MIP image reconstructed from 2 mm slices. *(Courtesy James Leffler.)*

from surrounding tissue but lacks vessel depth since superimposed vessels are not displayed. This is accommodated somewhat by image rotation. Small vessels that pass obliquely through a voxel may not be imaged because of **partial volume averaging.**

Shaded Surface Display

SSD is a computer-aided technique borrowed from computer-aided design and manufacturing applications. It was initially applied to bone imaging (Figure 30-17). SSD identifies a narrow range of values as belonging to the object to be imaged and displays that range. The range displayed appears as an organ surface that is determined by operator-selected values.

The computer capacity required for SSD is comparatively modest. Surface boundaries can be made very distinctive; the image appears very three dimensional (Figure 30-18).

SSD does appear somewhat shallow in depth because structures inside or behind the surface are not shown. SSD is very sensitive to the operator-selected pixel range, which can make imaging of actual anatomic structures difficult.

ADVANTAGES AND LIMITATIONS OF SPIRAL CT

The advantages and limitations of spiral CT are summarized in Table 30-4.

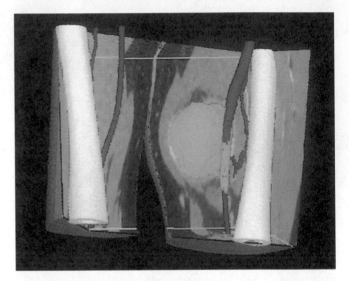

FIGURE 30-18 Shaded surface image of a femoral artery after AV fistula and stent graft insertion, which shows a pseudoaneurysm. *(Courtesy Elscint.)*

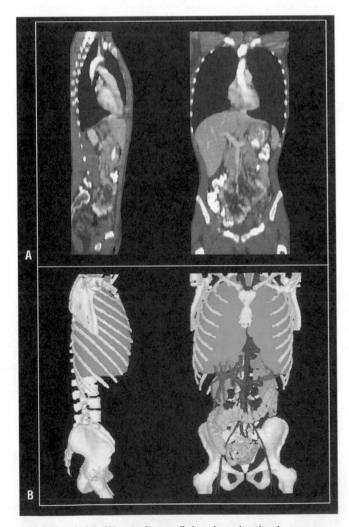

FIGURE 30-17 SSD was first applied to bone imaging in trauma patients. **A,** The rapid scanned projection radiographs were followed by **B,** sagittal and coronal reconstructions of a spiral CT examination. *(Courtesy Elscint.)*

TABLE 30-4	
Features of Spiral CT	
Advantages	**How/Why**
No motion artifacts	Removes respiratory misregistration
Improved lesion detection	Reconstructs at arbitrary intervals
Reduced partial volume	Reconstructs at overlapping intervals
	Reconstructs smaller than scan interval
Optimized IV contrast	Data obtained during peak of enhancement
	Reduced volume of contrast agent
Multiplanar images	Higher quality reconstruction
Improved patient throughput	Reduced scanning time
Limitations	
Increased image noise	Need bigger x-ray tubes
Reduced/-axis resolution	Increases with pitch
Increased processing time	More data, more images

SUMMARY

Spiral CT has the following three advantages over conventional CT: (1) there are no motion artifacts, (2) there is reduced scanning time, and (3) there is reduced partial volume, which means reconstruction occurs at overlapping intervals. These improvements allow CT to compete with the resolution and versatility of MRI. Spiral CT has emerged as a new and improved diagnostic tool.

When the examination begins, the x-ray tube rotates continuously and the patient couch moves through the plane of the rotating beam. This data is then reconstructed at any desired z-axis position. The ability to reconstruct images in the z-axis position is due to interpolation, which estimates unknown values between two known values. Data interpolation is performed by a special computer program called *interpolation algorithm*. Linear (straight-line relationship between two data points) interpolation at 180 degrees (data 180 degrees apart in rotation) is preferred to reduce artifacts, blurring, and noise. A 180-degree interpolation allows imaging at a pitch greater than one.

Spiral scan pitch ratio is the relationship between the patient couch movement and the x-ray beam collimation. Most 1:1 pitch ratios will result in the best image quality. Increasing the pitch above 1:1 increases the volume of tissue that can be imaged at a given time. The relationship between volume and pitch is given in the equation on p. 398. The equation on p. 398 allows the CT radiographer to compute the volume of tissue to be imaged before the beginning of the examination.

Spiral CT is made possible by slip-ring technology. Slip rings are electromechanical devices that conduct electricity and electric signals through rings and brushes across a rotating surface onto a fixed surface. One surface is a smooth ring and the other surface is a ring with brushes that sweep the smooth ring. This slip-ring technology allows the gantry to rotate continuously without restarting. Because of the continuous rotation and the need for the x-ray tube to be energized for longer periods, high power levels are required in the spiral CT x-ray tube. The spiral CT x-ray tubes are very large with a heat storage capacity of 5 MHU and cooling rates of 1 MHU per minute. Opposite the tube, solid-state detector arrays are preferred with an overall efficiency of 80%.

The radiologist and CT radiographer determine scan parameters. The volume of tissue imaged is determined by examination time, couch travel, pitch, and collimation. In addition, rotation time, reconstruction algorithm, reconstruction interval, and skip scan delay must be selected.

The image characteristics of spiral CT are noteworthy. There is improvement in z-axis spatial resolution because there are no gaps in data and image reconstruction. Reconstructed images can even overlap. In addition, spiral CT excels in three-dimensional multiplanar reformation (MPR).

The limitations of spiral CT are insignificant compared with the advantages, but they include the need for bigger and costlier x-ray tubes and the increased processing time with the accumulation of more data and images.

REVIEW QUESTIONS

1. What is one advantage of CT examinations over MRI examinations?
2. Define interpolation. Discuss the special computer program called the *interpolation algorithm*.
3. Explain the term *linear interpolation at 180 degrees*.
4. Write the formula for the spiral scan pitch ratio.
5. Using Table 30-1, what is the amount of tissue imaged with section thickness of 10 millimeters, scan time of 30 seconds, and pitch of 1.6:1?
6. Write the formula for tissue imaged that includes scan time and gantry rotation time.
7. When imaging 40 centimeters of tissue in 25 seconds with a slice thickness of 8 millimeters, what would be the pitch if the gantry rotation time is 1.5 seconds?
8. Explain why slip-ring technology contributed to the development of spiral CT.
9. What special characteristics are required of the spiral CT x-ray tube?
10. Why is the solid-state detector array preferred over the gas-filled detector?
11. The volume of tissue imaged in spiral CT is determined by which technique selections?
12. Which examinations require high z-axis resolution?
13. Define multiplanar reformation (MPR).
14. Discuss the concept of maximum intensity projection (MIP).
15. List the advantages and limitations of spiral CT scanning.

Additional Reading

Advances in ultrafast computed tomography: An international symposium on electron beam tomography, Scottsdale, Arizona, *Am J Card Imaging* 9:1 October, 1995.

Beard DV, Hemminger BM, Denelsbeck KM, Johnston RE: How many screens does a CT workstation need? *J Digit Imaging* 7(2):69 May, 1994.

Budzil RF Jr: Three-dimensional CT angiography, *Appl Radiol* March, 1993, 42-46.

Fishman EK, Ney DR, Scott WW Jr, Robertson DD: The role of CT with multiplaner reconstruction, *Appl Radiol* 21(11):36, November, 1992.

Kalbhen CL, Pierce KL: Fast CT scanning; applications of helical and electron-beam CT, *Appl Radiol* March, 1993, 47-51.

Quality Assurance and Quality Control

OBJECTIVES

At the completion of this chapter the student will be able to:

1. Define quality assurance and quality control
2. List a quality assurance model used in hospitals
3. Name the three steps of quality control
4. State the quality control program schedule for radiographic systems in a diagnostic imaging department
5. List and describe the ten quality control tests for radiographic systems
6. Discuss the three quality control processes for fluoroscopy
7. Explain the quality control process for conventional tomography
8. Name and describe the eight parts of CT quality control
9. Discuss radiographic processor quality control

OUTLINE

Quality Assurance
   Definition of quality assurance
   Quality assurance systems
Quality Control
   Definition of quality control
   Three steps of quality control
Radiographic Quality Control
   Quality control program
   Filtration
   Collimation
   Focal-spot size
   Kilovolts peak calibration
   Exposure timer accuracy
   Exposure linearity
   Exposure reproducibility
   Radiographic intensifying screens
   Protective apparel
   Film illuminators

Fluoroscopy Quality Control
   Exposure rate
   Spot-film exposures
   Automatic exposure systems
Conventional Tomographic Quality Control
Computed Tomography Quality Control
   Noise and uniformity
   Linearity
   Spatial resolution
   Contrast resolution
   Slice thickness
   Couch incrementation
   Laser localizer
   Patient dose
Processor Quality Control
   Processor cleaning
   Processor maintenance
   Processor monitoring

Today every field of medicine and every hospital department develops and conducts programs that ensure the quality of patient care and management. Diagnostic imaging departments are leaders in promoting quality patient care and management programs. There are two areas of activity designed to make certain that patients receive the benefit of the best possible diagnosis, at the lowest level of radiation dose, and at the lowest possible cost. These areas of quality management are called *quality assurance (QA)* and *quality control (QC)*. Both programs rely heavily on proper record keeping.

■ ■ ■ ■ ■ ■ ■ ■ ■ ■ ■ ■ ■ ■ ■ ■ ■ ■ ■

QUALITY ASSURANCE
Definition of Quality Assurance

Quality assurance (QA) deals with people. A QA program in diagnostic imaging monitors patients from scheduling, to reception, to patient preparation for examinations, to patients' relationships with radiographers, to patients' belongings being stored safely, and more. The imaging team of radiographers and managers are concerned about patient waiting time, about patient education, and about whether the patient follows up appropriately with his or her physician to receive examination results.

QA also involves image interpretation. The patient's disease or condition must agree with the radiologist's diagnosis. If there is a variance, steps are taken to improve the situation in the future. A study may be done to examine the process. This is called *outcome analysis*. A committee studies if the report of the diagnosis was promptly prepared, distributed, and filed for subsequent evaluation or if the clinician or patient was informed of examination results in a timely fashion. All of these QA activities are principally the responsibility of the radiologists and the management team.

Quality Assurance Systems

Hospitals and clinics often adopt quality assurance models for management to implement. The Joint Commission on Accreditation of Healthcare Organizations promotes "The Ten-Step Monitoring and Evaluation Process." This quality assurance process identifies a problem with patient care and uses the following ten-step process for resolution: 1) assign responsibility, 2) delineate scope of care, 3) identify aspects of care, 4) identify outcomes affecting the aspects of care, 5) establish limits to the scope of assessment, 6) collect and organize data, 7) evaluate care when outcomes are reached, 8) take action to improve care, 9) assess and document actions, and 10) communicate information to organization-wide QA programs. To make sure a health care organization has a commitment to providing high-quality services and care to patients, accreditating agencies have encouraged adoption of quality assurance models.

QUALITY CONTROL
Definition of Quality Control

Quality control (QC) monitors radiology instrumentation and equipment. A program of QC is designed to ensure that the radiologist is provided with an optimal image resulting from good equipment performance. QC begins with the x-ray equipment used to produce the image and it continues with the routine evaluation of the image processing facilities. It concludes with an analysis of each image to identify artifacts and their causes and to minimize the occurrence of retakes.

QC is a team effort, but it is principally the responsibility of the medical physicist. In private offices, clinics, and hospitals the medical physicist is a consultant and will establish the QC program and oversee its implementation at a frequency determined by the activity of the institution. In a large medical center where the medical physicist is a member of the professional staff the physicist will perform many of the routine activities and supervise other activities. With the help of the QC radiographer and the radiologic engineers, the medical physicist will see that all necessary measurements and observations are performed.

In addition to optimal image quality, there are other reasons for conducting a QC program in diagnostic imaging. QC records are important if a patient or employee is involved in a legal case. Some insurance carriers pay for services only from facilities with an approved QC program. The Joint Commission on Accreditation of Healthcare Organizations (JCAHO) will not grant approval to facilities that do not develop a QC program. Most states, through their Department of Health and with guidance from the Council of Radiation Control Program Directors (CRCPD), require QC by regulation.

Three Steps of Quality Control

Three steps are involved in a QC program: (1) **acceptance testing**, (2) **routine performance evaluation**, and (3) **error correction**. Each new piece of radiologic apparatus, whether x-ray equipment or processing equipment, should be acceptance tested before clinical application. The acceptance test is done by a medical physicist or a radiologic engineer. The acceptance test is designed to show that the equipment is performing within the manufacturer's specifications. With use, all equipment deteriorates and may malfunction. Periodic evaluation and maintanance of equipment performance is required. On most systems, annual evaluation is satisfactory unless there has been a replacement of a major component like the x-ray tube.

RADIOGRAPHIC QUALITY CONTROL
Quality Control Program

Organizations such as the American College of Medical Physics (ACMP) and the American Association of Physicists in Medicine (AAPM) have developed guide-

TABLE 31-1

Elements of a Quality Control Program for Radiographic Systems

Measurement	Frequency*	Tolerance
Filtration	Annually	≥2.5 mm aluminum
Collimation	Semiannually	±2% SID
Focal-spot size	Annually	±50%
kVp calibration	Annually	±4 kVp
Exposure timer accuracy	Annually	±5% > 10 ms ±20% ≤ 10 ms
Exposure linearity	Annually	±10%
Exposure reproducibility	Annually	±5%

*Evaluation should follow any major equipment modification.

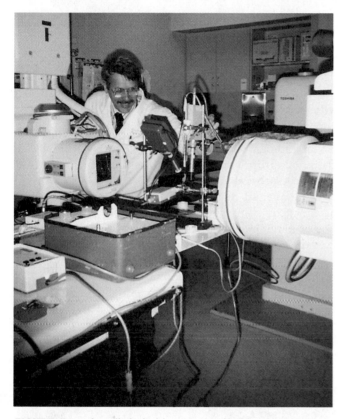

FIGURE 31-1 A medical physicist preparing for QC measurements. *(Courtesy Louis Wagner.)*

lines for QC programs in radiography, as well as other imaging modalities. Table 31-1 presents the essentials of a radiography program, the recommended frequency of evaluation, and the tolerance limit for each assessment. Figure 31-1 shows a medical physicist preparing **dosimetry** equipment for QC measurements.

Filtration

Perhaps the most important patient-protection characteristic of a radiographic unit is x-ray beam filtration. State statutes require that general-purpose radiographic units have a minimum total filtration of 2.5-millimeters aluminum. It is normally not possible to measure filtration directly, so one resorts to a measurement of the half-value layer (HVL) of the x-ray beam as described in Chapter 12. The measured HVL must meet or exceed that value shown in Table 31-2 for the total filtration to be considered adequate. This determination of filtration should be made annually or at any time after a change in the x-ray tube or tube housing.

Collimation

It is essential to radiation protection that the x-ray field coincide with the light field of the variable aperture light-localizing collimator. If these fields are misaligned, intended anatomy will be missed and unintended anatomy irradiated.

Determination of adequate collimation can be done with any of a number of test tools designed for that purpose (Figure 31-2). During such assessment, the misalignment must not exceed ±2% of the source-to-image receptor distance (SID).

TABLE 31-2

Required Minimum HVL as a Function of kVp

Operating kVp	Minimum HVL (mm Al)
30	0.3
40	0.4
50	1.2
60	1.3
70	2.1
80	2.3
90	2.5
100	2.7
120	3.2
140	3.8

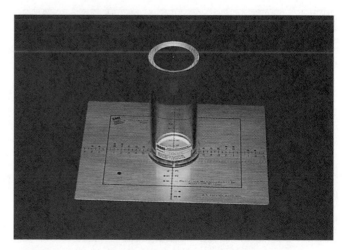

FIGURE 31-2 A test tool for monitoring x-ray beam, light-field coincidence. *(Courtesy Gammex RMI.)*

Most systems today are equipped with **positive beam-limiting collimators (PBL).** These devices are automatic collimators that sense the size of the image receptor and adjust the collimating shutters to that size. Since different sizes of image receptors must be accommodated, the PBL function must be evaluated for all possible receptor sizes. With a PBL collimator the x-ray beam must not be larger than the image receptor except in the override mode.

Distance and centering indicators must be accurate to within 2% and 1% of the SID respectively. The distance indicator can be checked simply with a tape measure. The location of the focal spot will be marked on the x-ray tube housing. Centering is checked visually for the light field and with markers for the exposure field.

Focal-Spot Size

The spatial resolution of a radiographic imaging system is principally determined by the focal-spot size of the x-ray tube. When new equipment or a replacement x-ray tube is installed, a measurement of focal-spot size must be made. The **pinhole camera,** the **star pattern,** and the **slit camera** are used to make measurements (Figure 31-3).

The pinhole camera is difficult to use and requires excessive exposure time. The star pattern is easy to use but has significant limitations for focal-spot sizes less than 0.3 millimeter. The standard for measurement of effective focal-spot size is the slit camera.

The fabrication of an x-ray tube is an exceptionally complex process. Specification of focal-spot size depends not only on the geometry of the tube but also on the focusing of the electron beam. Consequently, vendors and manufacturers are permitted a substantial variance from their advertised focal-spot sizes (Table 31-3).

TABLE 31-3

Permitted Variation in Advertised Focal-Spot Size

Advertised Size (mm)	Maximum Permitted Focal-spot Dimension Width (mm) × Length (mm)
0.05	0.075 × 0.075
0.10	0.15 × 0.15
0.20	0.30 × 0.30
0.30	0.45 × 0.65
0.40	0.60 × 0.85
0.50	0.75 × 1.10
0.60	0.90 × 1.30
0.80	1.20 × 1.60
1.00	1.40 × 2.00
1.20	1.70 × 2.40
1.60	2.10 × 3.10

Focal-spot size should be evaluated annually or at any time that an x-ray tube is replaced.

Kilovolts Peak Calibration

Kilovolts peak (kVp) is selected for every examination by the radiographer. The radiographic technical factors require appropriate kVp; therefore the x-ray generator should be properly calibrated.

A number of methods are available to evaluate the accuracy of kVp. Today, most medical physicists use one of a number of devices based on **filtered ion chambers** or **filtered photo diodes** (Figure 31-4). Other methods using **voltage diodes** and **oscilloscopes** are more accurate but require an exceptional amount of time.

The kVp calibration should be evaluated annually or at any time there has been a significant change in high-voltage generator components. A variation of 2 or 3 kVp will measurably affect patient dose and image optical density. A variation of 4 or 5 kVp is necessary to

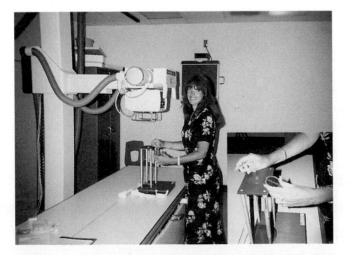

FIGURE 31-3 The pinhole camera, star pattern, and slit camera may be used to measure focal-spot size. *(Courtesy Teresa Rice.)*

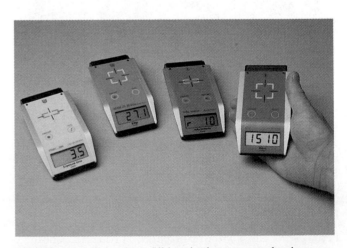

FIGURE 31-4 High voltage (kVp) and other generator functions can be evaluated with compact test devices. *(Courtesy Radical Corp.)*

affect radiographic contrast. The test measurement of kVp should be within ±4 kVp of the actual kVp.

Exposure Timer Accuracy

Exposure time is operator selectable on most radiographic consoles. Although many high-capacity radiographic systems are phototimed or mAs controlled, exposure time is still the responsibility of the radiographer of many operating consoles. This parameter is particularly responsible for patient dose and image optical density.

There are a number of ways to assess exposure timer accuracy. The **spinning top** is sufficiently effective with single-phase radiographic equipment, and the **synchronous spinning top** may be used with three-phase and high-frequency equipment. Most medical physicists, however, use one of several commercially available products that measure exposure time based on the acquisition time of radiation by any ion chamber or photodiode assembly.

The accuracy of the exposure timer should be assessed annually or more frequently if there has been a major change or repair to a component of the operating console or the high-voltage generator. Exposure timer accuracy should be within ±5% of the indicated time for exposure times greater than 10 milliseconds. An accuracy of ±20% is acceptable for exposure times of 10 milliseconds or less.

Phototimers must also be evaluated. These devices are common and designed to provide a constant image optical density regardless of tissue thickness, composition, or failure of the reciprocity law (see Chapter 19). Phototimed systems are evaluated by exposing an image receptor through various thicknesses of aluminum or acrylic. Regardless of the material thickness and the absolute exposure time, the optical density of the processed image should be constant.

Insertion of a lead filter allows one to adequately assess the functioning of the backup timer. If the photo timer fails, the backup timer should terminate the exposure at 6 seconds or 600 mAs, whichever occurs first.

Exposure Linearity

Many combinations of mA and exposure time produce the same mAs. The ability of a radiographic unit to produce a constant radiation output for multiple combinations of mA and exposure time is called *exposure linearity.*

Exposure linearity is determined by using a precision radiation dosimeter to measure radiation intensity at various combinations of mA and exposure time. Suppose, for example, that one were to choose 10 mAs for evaluation of the combinations of mA and exposure time shown in Table 31-4. Each of these combinations would be energized, and radiation measurements would

TABLE 31-4
Exposure Time and mA Combinations Equal to 10 mAs

Exposure Time (ms)	mA
1000	10
400	25
200	50
100	100
50	200
25	400
13	800
10	1000
8	1200

be made. When evaluated in this fashion, the radiation output for adjacent mA stations should be within ±10%. Exposure linearity should be evaluated annually or after any significant change or repair of the operating console or high-voltage generator.

This method of assessing exposure linearity will be flawed if the exposure timer is inaccurate. Consequently, most would hold exposure time constant and vary only the mA. Under these conditions the value of mR/mAs should be within ±10% between adjacent mA stations.

Question: The following data is obtained to evaluate exposure linearity. Are the mA stations correctly calibrated?

Exposure Time	mA	mR
100 ms	50	29
100 ms	100	61
100 ms	200	109
100 ms	400	236

Answer:

mA	mR/mAs	% Difference
50	5.8	
100	6.1	> +5.2 OK
200	5.5	> +9.7 OK
400	5.9	> +7.3 OK

Exposure Reproducibility

When selecting the proper kVp, mA, and exposure time for a given examination, the radiographer expects the image optical density and contrast to be optimal. If any or all of these technique factors are changed and then returned to the previous value, precisely the same radiation exposure should occur. The radiation exposure should be **reproducible.**

Two accepted ways are available to evaluate exposure reproducibility. Both rely on a precision radiation dosimeter. First, one can make a series of at least three exposures at the same technique factors, changing the technique controls between each exposure. If the result is not reproducible, it is usually so because of error in the kVp control. Second, one can select a combination of technique factors and hold them constant for a series of 10 exposures. There are mathematical formulas that allow the determination of reproducibility in both instances. They basically require that the output radiation intensity not vary by more than ±5%.

Radiographic Intensifying Screens

Intensifying screens require periodic attention to minimize the appearance of artifacts. Screens should be cleaned with a soft, lint-free cloth and a cleaning solution provided by the manufacturer. The frequency of cleaning will depend on the workload in the department, but it should certainly not be less than once every other month.

Screen-film contact should be evaluated once or twice a year. This is done by radiographing a wire-mesh pattern and analyzing the image for areas of blur. Should blur appear, the felt or foam pressure pad under the screen should be replaced. If that does not correct the problem, replace the cassette.

Protective Apparel

All protective aprons, gloves, and gonadal shields should be radiographed or fluoroscoped annually for defects. If there are cracks, tears, or holes, the apparel may require replacement.

Film Illuminators

Photometric analysis of viewbox illumination should be conducted annually. This is done by measuring light intensity at several areas of the illuminator with an instrument called a *photometer* (Figure 31-5). This intensity should not vary by more than ±10%. If a bulb requires replacement, all bulbs should be replaced in that illuminator and matched to the type of bulb in adjacent illuminators.

FLUOROSCOPY QUALITY CONTROL

Fluoroscopic procedures result in the highest individual patient doses. The **entrance skin dose** for an adult will average 3 to 5 rad per minute (30 to 50 mGy per minute) during fluoroscopy and will result in an average skin dose of up to 10 rad for most fluoroscopic examinations. Patient doses can be minimized through the perfomance of proper QC measurements. Some measurements may be required more frequently after significant changes in the operating console or high-voltage generator.

Exposure rate

Federal law and most state statutes require that under normal operation the entrance skin exposure (ESE) rate shall not excceed 10 R per minute (100 mGy per minute). For angiointerventional procedure the fluoro-

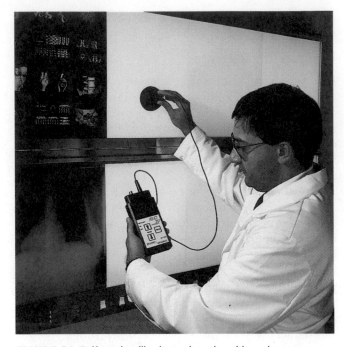

FIGURE 31-5 Measuring illuminator intensity with a photometer. *(Courtesy Graseky Optronics.)*

scope may be equipped with a high level control that will allow an ESE up to 20 R per minute (200 mGy per minute).

Measurements should be made with an accurate radiation dosimeter to ensure that these levels are not exceeded. Lucite, aluminum, copper, and lead filters will be required to determine the adequacy of any automatic brightness stabilization (ABS) system.

Spot-film Exposures

There are two types of spot-film devices, both of which must be evaluated for radiation exposure. Proper exposure of the **cassette spot film** depends on the kVp, mAs, and sensitivity characteristics of the screen-film combination. Entrance skin exposures for such a spot-film device vary widely (Table 31-5). The values reported in Table 31-5 were obtained with a 10:1 grid using a 300-speed image receptor. Nongrid exposures will be approximately half of the values reported here.

TABLE 31-5	
Entrance Skin Exposure with Cassette-Loaded Spot Films	
kVp	ESE (mR)
60	450
70	270
80	170
90	150
100	130

The use of photofluorospot images is more routine. These images use less film, require less personnel interaction, and are produced with a lower patient dose.

In addition to the factors that affect cassette spot films, photofluorospot images depend on characteristics of the image intensifier, particularly the diameter of the input phosphor. Photofluorospot images are recorded on film from the image of the output phosphor of an image-intensifier tube. Table 31-6 shows representative entrance skin exposure for two input phosphor sizes and no grid. They are substantially lower than those with cassette spot films.

As the active area of the input phosphor of the image-intensifier tube is increased, patient dose is decreased in approximate proportion to the diameter of the input phosphor. Use of a grid during photofluorospot imaging will approximately double ESE.

Question: A photofluorospot image is made at 80 kVp in the 15-centimeter mode without a grid, as seen in Table 31-6. The measured ESE is 50 mR. What would be the expected ESE if the 25-centimeter mode was used?

Answer:
$$x \div 50 = 15 \div 25$$
$$x = 50 \left(\frac{15}{25} \right)$$
$$= 30 \text{ mrad}$$

Automatic Exposure Systems

All fluoroscopes are equipped with some sort of automatic brightness stabilization (ABS), automatic brightness control (ABC), or automatic exposure control (AEC). Each system functions like the phototimer of a radiographic unit, producing constant image brightness on the video monitor regardless of the thickness or composition of the anatomy under examination. These systems are prone to deteriorate or fail with use. They should be evaluated at least annually.

Such evaluation is conducted by determining that the radiation exposure to the input phosphor of the image-intensifier tube is constant regardless of the thickness of the patient. With a test phantom in place, the image brightness on the video monitor should not change perceptibly when various thicknesses of patient-stimulating material are inserted in the beam. A measurement of the input exposure rate to the image-intensifier tube is made and should be in the range of 10 to 40 μR per second (0.1 to 0.4 μGy per second).

CONVENTIONAL TOMOGRAPHIC QUALITY CONTROL

In addition to the QC tests and measurements performed on radiographic systems, several additional measurements are required for those systems that can also perform conventional tomography.

Precise performance standards do not exist for conventional tomography. QC measurements are designed to ensure that the established characteristics remain constant.

Patient exposure should be measured for the most frequent type of tomographic examinations. Table 31-7 is a sample of the results from a three-phase system and six tomographic examinations.

The geometric characteristics of a tomogram can be evaluated with any of a number of phantoms designed for this use. Agreement between the indicated section level and the measured level should be within ±5 millimeters. When incrementing from one tomographic section to the next, the section level should be accurate to within ±2 millimeters. Constancy of ±1 millimeter from one QC evaluation to the next should be achieved. Section uniformity is evaluated by imaging a hole in a lead sheet. The optical density of the image tracing of the hole should be uniform with no perceptible variations, no gaps, and no overlaps (Figure 31-6).

COMPUTED TOMOGRAPHY QUALITY CONTROL

Computed tomography (CT) scanners are subject to all the misalignment, miscalibration, and malfunction difficulties of conventional x-ray units. They have the additional complexities of the multimotional gantry, the interactive console, and the computer. Each of these subsystems increases the risk of drift and instability that could result in degradation of image quality. Conse-

TABLE 31-6

Entrance Skin Exposure with Photo-fluorospot Imagers

kVp	ESE (mR)	
	15 cm II	*25 cm II*
60	90	50
70	65	35
80	50	30
90	40	25
100	30	20

TABLE 31-7

Exposure Technique and Entrance Skin Exposure During Conventional Tomographic Examination

Examination	Technique (kVp/mAs)	ESE (mR)
Temporomandibular joint	90/300	2300
Cervical spine	76/200	1300
Thoracic and lumbar spine	78/250	1700
Chest	110/8	75
Intravenous pyelogram	70/300	1800
Nephrotomogram	74/350	2200

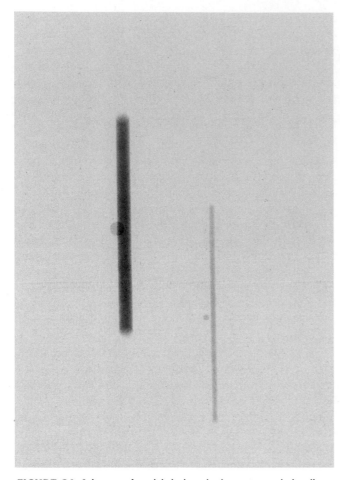

FIGURE 31-6 Images of a pinhole in a lead attenuator during linear tomography. The larger pinhole image shows modest staggering motion resulting in variation in optical density. *(Courtesy Sharon Glaze.)*

TABLE 31-8		
Elements of a QC Program for Computed Tomography		

Measurement	Frequency*	Tolerance
Noise	Weekly	±10 HU
Uniformity	Weekly	±10 HU
Linearity	Semiannually	+
Spatial resolution	Semiannually	20%
Contrast resolution	Semiannually	5 mm at 0.5%
Slice thickness	Semiannually	≥5 mm, 1 mm; <5 mm, 0.5 mm
Couch incrementation	Semiannually	±2 mm
Laser localizer	Semiannually	±1 mm
Patient dose	Annually	†
Dose profile	Annually	±10 %

*Evaluation should follow any major equipment modification.

†Within manufacturer's specifications.

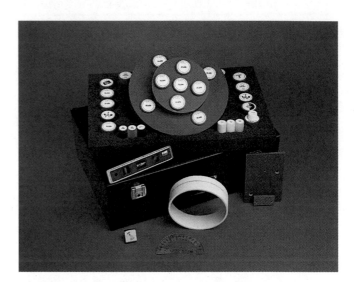

FIGURE 31-7 This CT phantom is used to evaluate noise, spatial resolution, contrast resolution, slice thickness, linearity, and uniformity. *(Courtesy Gammex RMI.)*

quently a dedicated QC program is essential for each CT scanner. Such a program includes daily, weekly, monthly, and annual measurements and observations, in addition to the ongoing **preventive maintenance program.**

Table 31-8 identifies the measurements and the scheduled times for adequate CT scanner QC program. Figure 31-7 shows the phantom for CT measurements. The measurements specified for an annual evaluation should also be conducted on all new equipment and on all equipment that has had a component replaced or repaired.

Noise and Uniformity

A 20-centimeter **waterbath** should be imaged weekly, and the average value for water should be within ±10 HU of 0. Furthermore the uniformity across the image should not vary by more than ±10 HU from center to periphery. Finally the noise as determined by the built-in computational algorithm should not exceed ±10 HU. Nearly all CT scanners easily meet these performance specifications unless there is a major malfunction. If, however, a system is used for **quantitative CT,** then tighter specifications may be appropriate. When performing this assessment, one should change one or more of the following: the CT scan parameters, the slice thickness, the reconstruction diameter, and the reconstruction algorithm.

Linearity

The assessment of linearity is performed with an image of the AAPM five-pin insert. Analysis of the values of the five pins should show a linear relationship among the Hounsfield units and also shows the electron density. The **coefficient of correlation** for this linear relationship should equal or exceed 0.96% (or two standard deviations). This feature of the QC program should be conducted semiannually.

Spatial Resolution

Monitoring spatial resolution is the most important component of the QC program. Ensuring constant spatial resolution ensures that not only the detector array and reconstruction electronics are performing properly but also that the mechanical components are performing properly as well.

Spatial resolution is assessed by imaging an edge to get edge-response function (ERF). These functions are then mathematically transformed to obtain the modulation-transfer function (MTF). This process, however, requires considerable time and attention. Most medical physicists find it acceptable to image a bar pattern or hole pattern. Spatial resolution should be assessed on a semiannual basis and should be within the manufacturer's specifications.

Contrast Resolution

Computed tomography has superior contrast resolution. The performance specifications of the various CT scanners differ from one manufacturer to another and form one model to another, depending on the design of the scanner. All scanners should be capable of resolving 5-millimeter objects at 0.5% contrast.

Contrast resolution should be assessed seminannually. It is done with any one of a number of low-contrast

phantoms with the built-in analytical schemes available on all CT scanners (Figure 31-8).

Slice Thickness

Slice thickness (**sensitivity profile**) is measured using a specially designed phantom that incorporates a ramp, a spiral, or a step wedge. This assessment should be performed semiannually. The slice thickness should be within 1 millimeter of the intended slice thickness for a thickness of 5 millimeters or greater. For less than a 5 millimeter intended slice thickness, the acceptable tolerance is 0.5 millimeter.

Couch Incrementation

With the automatic maneuvering of the patient through the CT gantry, it is essential that the patient couch position be precise. This evaluation should be done monthly. The measurement is simple to perform and can be done during a clinical examination. When the patient is on the couch, note the position of the couch at the beginning and at the end of the examination using tape and a straightedge on the couch rails. Compare this with the intended couch movement. It should be within ±2 millimeters.

Laser Localizer

On most CT imagers, internal and external laser localizing lights are used for patient positioning. The accuracy of these lasers can be determined with any number of specially designed phantoms. Their accuracy should be assessed at least semiannually, and this will usually be done at the same time as the evaluation of couch incrementation.

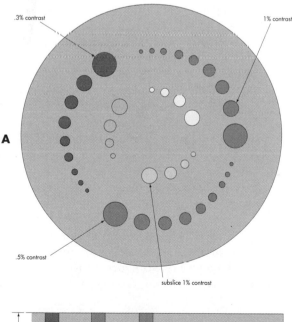

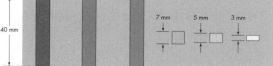

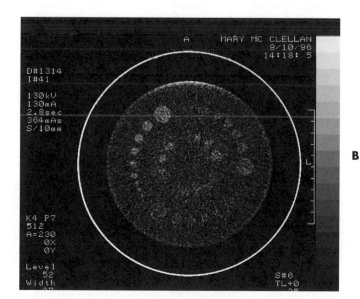

FIGURE 31-8 A low contrast CT phantom, **(A)** and its image, **(B)**. The phantom is designed especially for special CT. *(Courtesy The Phantom Laboratory.)*

Patient Dose

No maximum levels are specified for the permissible dose to a patient in CT. Furthermore, dose will vary considerably according to the scan parameters. High-resolution scanning requires more dose. Still, when a fixed technique is used, patient dose should not vary by more than ±10% from one assessment to the next. Such assessment should be made on a semiannual basis or after replacement of the x-ray tube.

Patient dose can be monitored with specially designed ionization chambers or thermoluminescent dosimeters. It is not only necessary to measure patient dose but also **dose profile** for the most common slice thickness. Figure 31-9 illustrates these measurements in progress.

PROCESSOR QUALITY CONTROL

QC in any activity refers to the routine and special procedures developed to ensure that the final product is of consistently high quality. QC in diagnostic radiology requires a planned, continuous program of evaluation and surveillance of radiologic equipment and procedures. When applied to automatic processing, such a program involves periodic cleaning, system maintenance, and daily monitoring. Table 31-9 lists the scheduled processor monitoring program to maintain QC.

Processor Cleaning

The first automatic processor had a processing time of 7 minutes. Soon this was shortened to 3 minutes by what are known as **double-capacity (DC) processors.** A further reduction in processing time was made with the **fast-access (FA) system,** which is today's popular 90-second processor.

Such a processor can handle up to 500 films per hour, but to do so it requires a high concentration of process-

TABLE 31-9		
Quality Control Program for Radiographic Processor		
Activity	Procedure or Item	Schedule
Processor cleaning		
	Cross-over racks	Daily
	Entire rack assembly and processing tanks	Weekly
Scheduled maintenance		
	Observation of belts, pulleys, and gears	Weekly
	Lubrication	Weekly or monthly
Processor monitoring	Planned parts replacement	Regularly
	Check developer temperature	Daily
	Check wash water temperature	Daily
	Check replenishment tanks	Daily
	Sensitometry and densitometry	Daily

ing chemistry, a high development temperature (95° F [35° C]), and a developer immersion time of 22 seconds. The wash water temperature should be 87° F (30.5° C). Earlier automatic processors were supplied with hot and cold water, so the primary control of wash temperature was through a mixing valve. Nearly all current processors are supplied with only cold water. Temperature control is maintained with a thermostatically controlled heater.

This rapid activity carried on at high temperature with concentrated chemistry tends to wear and corrode the mechanism of the transport system and contaminate the chemistry with processing sludge. A deposit of sludge and debris on the rollers can severely affect film quality. Any sludge or debris causes artifacts on film. As a result, the processor must be completely cleaned weekly. The cross-over racks that are easily removeable can be cleaned daily to prevent sludge buildup. Cleaning the cross-over racks daily helps prevent films from being hung-up on the rollers, which causes a film jam. Proper records of cleaning should be an up-to-date listing of the following: (1) work performed, (2) date of cleaning, and (3) initials of radiographer or maintenance personnel.

The weekly cleaning procedure is rather simple. The transport and cross-over racks are removed and washed. The processing tanks are then rinsed and cleaned. This takes no more than a few minutes and pays great dividends in reduced processor wear and the consistent pro-

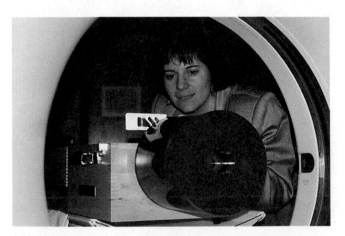

FIGURE 31-9 Medical physics evaluation of CT performance requires a number of measurements using specially designed test objects. *(Courtesy Cynthia McCollough.)*

duction of high-quality radiographs that are free of artifacts.

Processor Maintenance

As with any electromechanical device, preventive maintenance is a must. If equipment is not properly maintained, when least expected or when the workload is the heaviest, the processor will malfunction. There are three types of maintenance programs that should be a part of the QC program for an automatic processor.

Scheduled maintenance refers to those procedures that are performed on a routine basis, usually weekly or monthly. Such maintenance includes (1) observation of all moving parts for wear; adjustment of all belts, pulleys, and gears and (2) lubrication to minimize wear. When lubricating a processor, it is especially important to keep the lubricant off of your hands, thereby keeping it away from film and rollers and, of course, out of processor chemistry.

Preventive maintenance is a planned program of parts replacement at regular intervals. Preventive maintenance requires that a part be replaced before its failure. With such a program, unexpected downtime should not occur.

Nonscheduled maintenance is, of course, the worst kind. A failure in the system that necessitates processor repair is a nonscheduled event. A proper program of scheduled maintenance and preventive maintenance will ensure that nonscheduled maintenance is kept to a minimum.

Processor Monitoring

At least once per day the operation of the processor should be observed and certain measurements recorded. The temperature of the developer and wash water should be noted. The developer and fixer replenishment rates should be observed and recorded.

The replenishment tanks should be checked to determine if the floating lids are properly positioned and if fresh chemistry is needed. It is often appropriate to check the pH and specific gravity of the developer and fixer solutions. Residual hypo should be determined.

A sensitometric strip should be fed through the processor. Appropriate measurements of fog, speed, and contrast is then determined and recorded. Most film manufacturers will provide representatives to assist a department in conducting a program of processer QC. The written record of the results of such a program is critically important. It is important to observe daily and monthly trends. The processor must be checked by the QC radiographer before the daily work schedule begins. The processor monitoring described in Chapter 24 for the mammography processor can be applied to all other processors in the department.

SUMMARY

In diagnostic imaging, quality assurance involves assessment and evaluation of patient care. Quality control is the measurement and testing of radiographic equipment. Both processes ensure that the radiologist is provided with an optimal image for proper diagnosis. The QA/QC team includes radiographers, management and secretarial personnel, the film manufacturer's representative, the medical physicist, radiologic engineers, and radiologists. For many hospitals and clinics, JCAHO will not accredit the facility unless proper QA and QC programs are evident.

The three steps of QC are (1) acceptance testing, (2) routine performance evaluation, and (3) error correction. Table 31-1 lists guidelines for radiographic equipment QC as determined by the two national organizations of medical physicists.

Radiographic QC tests filtration, collimation, focal-spot size, kVp, timers, linearity, and reproducibility. Filtration is required by state statutes as a total filtration of 2.5-millimeters aluminum. Collimation misalignment must not exceed above or below 2% of the SID. Table 31-3 shows the allowable focal-spot variations. Kilovoltage calibration can vary only by 4 kVp to be within acceptable limts. Exposure timer accuracy must be within 5% of the indicated time of exposure at times greater than 10 milliseconds. Phototimer systems are also tested, and the backup timer should terminate the exposure at 6 seconds or at 600 mAs, whichever comes first. Linearity is the ability of a radiographic unit to produce constant radiation output. The mA stations are evaluated for radiation output, and linearity of mA must be within 10% of stated values. Reproducibility tests the precision of output of the same radiation values exposure after exposure. Radiation output should not vary more than 5%. Intensifying screens are evaluated regularly for cleanliness and film-screen contact. All lead apparel is checked for cracks, tears, and holes. Finally, viewboxes or film illuminators are examined for intensity and cleanliness. The individual bulbs should not vary more than 10% in intensity.

Because fluoroscopy has the highest patient dose of all x-ray procedures, fluoroscopic equipment is tested regularly for exposure rate. Under federal law the entrance skin exposure shall not exceed 10 R per minute.

Conventional tomography slice section level is evaluated regularly. The precision of the tomographic section should be within 5 millimeters of the indicated section level.

Each of the subsystems of computed tomography (CT) is regularly checked for misalignment and miscalibration. Table 31-8 lists the measurement, frequency of evaluation, and tolerance levels for CT equipment systems.

Radiographic processor QC is essential for optimal film quality. Table 31-9 states the three major activities, the number of subsystems and items that are checked regularly, and the frequency of evaluation of the radiographic processor. Sensitometry and densitometry are important daily functions of the QC radiographer and are discussed in detail in Chapter 24 on mammographic QC.

REVIEW QUESTIONS

1. Define quality assurance and quality control. Give examples of each process.

2. List and explain the theory behind the JCAHO QA program used in hospitals.

3. Discuss the three steps of quality control for radiographic equipment.

4. Name the people on the diagnostic imaging QC team.

5. Using Table 31-1, state the parts of the radiographic equipment that is tested regularly and indicate the tolerance specifications for each measurement.

6. How is filtration measured in radiographic equipment?

7. Why is it important to have proper alignment of collimation? What are the misalignment limitations?

8. Describe the testing being done in Figure 31-5.

9. The indicated kVp should fall within _____ of the actual tested kVp.

10. What are the three QC tools used to measure focal-spot size?

11. _____ is the parameter particularly responsible for errors in patient dose and image optical density.

12. The backup timer of a phototimed system should terminate the exposure at _____ seconds or at _____ mAs.

13. Define linearity. Define reproducibility. What are the allowed variations of each?

14. What test is performed on intensifying screen and cassettes to check that there is proper screen-film contact?

15. What product(s) are used to clean intensifying screens?

16. How often should lead apparel be checked for integrity of the lead?

17. What is the average skin dose during a fluoroscopic examination?

18. Describe the process of monitoring the spatial resolution in a CT scanner.

19. List and briefly describe the eight parts of CT quality control.

20. What is the importance of preventive maintenance for a radiographic processor?

Suggested Readings

Archibald DI: Quality assurance: a personal commitment—a professional responsibility, *Can J Med Radiat Technol* 23(1):11 March, 1992.

David G, Prince SC: Improved calibrations using personal computers, *Radiol Technol* 63(1):32 September-October, 1991.

Farria DM, Dassett LW, Kimme-Smith C, DeBruhl N: Mammography quality assurance from A to Z, *Radiographics* 14(2):371 March, 1994.

Juran D: Achieving sustained quantifiable results in an interdepartmental quality improvement project, *JT Comm J Qual Improve* 20(3):105, 1994.

Keats TE: Quality assurance in diagnostic radiology, *Appl Radiol* 22(8):8 August, 1993.

Mintz AP, Spiro AH, Crues JV III: Practicing radiology in a managed-care world, *Appl Radiol* 22(2):65 February, 1993.

Pirtle OL: X-ray machine calibration: a study of failure rates, *Radiol Technol* 65(5):291, May-June, 1994.

Tan KM: Quality assurance by any other name: redux . . . impassioned editorial on quality assurance by Dr. Kenneth R. Kattan, *Appl Radiol* December, 23(12):8 1994.

Worrell JA, Price RR, Partain CL, Kessler RM, James AE Jr: Academic quality assurance in the radiology department, *Appl Radiol* 20(5):25 May, 1991.

32 Film Artifacts

OBJECTIVES

At the completion of this chapter the student will be able to:

1. Visually identify artifacts on the radiographs shown in this chapter, including pi lines, guide-shoe marks, chemistry fog, wet-pressure sensitization, kinking, and static
2. List and discuss the three categories of artifacts
3. Explain the derivation of exposure artifacts
4. Describe the types of artifacts caused by processor problems
5. Discuss how improper handling and storage of film can cause artifacts

OUTLINE

Definition of Film Artifacts
Exposure Artifacts
Processing Artifacts
   Dirty rollers
   Chemical fog
   Roller marks
   Wet-pressure sensitization

Handling and Storage Artifacts
   Light or radiation fog
   Kink marks
   Static
   Hypo retention

F or student radiographers, one of the most interesting areas of radiographic study is the identification of film artifacts. Most schools have an extensive film file of artifacts from pi lines to necklaces on chest x-ray films. At the clinical sites, students are eager to assess a film with artifacts to determine the derivation. However, artifacts need to be prevented. Identification of the artifact and its cause is critical for quality control (QC). It is important for every radiographer to be alert to artifacts and their derivations so that QC personnel and managers can be informed. The cause of the artifact must be removed to prevent the same problem in subsequent radiographs. Finally, records of artifacts must be kept to indicate trends; for example, if sludge artifacts show up more than once before processor cleaning, consider cleaning the processor more frequently.

DEFINITION OF FILM ARTIFACTS

An artifact is any optical density on a radiograph that is not caused by the superimposition of anatomy in the primary x-ray beam. Artifacts, therefore, are undesirable densities or blemishes on a radiograph. They can interfere with the radiologist's diagnosis by limiting the entire view of the image. Artifacts can be controlled when their causes are identified. There are generally three radiographic time periods in which artifacts occur: (1) during the radiographic exposure, (2) during the processing of the film, and (3) when the film is being handled and stored either before or after processing.

EXPOSURE ARTIFACTS

Exposure artifacts are associated with the manner in which the radiographer conducts the examination. Incorrect screen-film match, poor screen-film contact, warped cassettes, and improper positioning of the grid can all lead to artifacts. Improper patient position, patient motion, double exposure, and incorrect radiographic technique can result in very poor images that some would call artifacts. These examples of poor technique have been shown to result in the largest number of repeat examinations. Exposure artifacts are usually easy to detect and correct.

Improper preparation of the patient can lead to disturbing artifacts as represented by the jewelery, eyeglasses, and other artifacts in Figure 32-1, *A, B, C,* and *D.* Proper patient preparation easily corrects these artifacts.

A radiograph with patient motion appears unsharp or blurred. The patient may have moved or may not have breathed according to the radiographer's instructions. It is important to communicate clear instructions to the patient to encourage cooperation. Postioning errors cause artifacts on the film. If the patient is placed under the tube when the tube is not centered to the table or Bucky tray, cut-off artifacts will occur. Artifacts occur if the wrong film is loaded into a cassette. If high contrast single-emulsion mammography film is loaded into a radiographic cassette, an unexpected film will be the result. Cassettes that have not been checked for proper screen-film contact cause a smoothness in the area of poor contact, which obscures detail and is considered an artifact. When radiographers mix-up cassettes, double exposures can occur. Warped cassettes cause geometric artifacts, for example, foreshortening of a long bone. Chapter 18 discussed the many artifacts caused by improper positioning of grids.

PROCESSING ARTIFACTS

During processing, any number of artifacts can be produced. Most are pressure types of artifacts caused by the transport system of the processor.

Dirty Rollers

Dirty or warped rollers can cause **emulsion pickoff** and **gelatin buildup,** which results in **sludge** deposits on the film. These artifacts usually appear as sharp areas of either increased or reduced optical density. Occasionally, particles of sludge are transported through the processor and are actually dried on the film in the dryer.

Chemical Fog

Improper or inadequate processing chemistry can result in a chemical fog called a *dichroic stain.* The dichroic stain appears as a curtain effect on the radiograph (Figure 32-2). **Chemical fog** looks like light or radiation fog and is usually a uniform, dull gray. Dichroic stain is a term generally applied to all chemical stains. *Dichroic* means two colors. The chemical stains seen on a radiograph can appear yellow, green, blue, or purple. In slow processors the chemistry may not be properly squeezed from the film, and it either runs down the leading edge of the film or runs up the trailing edge. Both are called a *curtain effect.*

Roller Marks

Guide-shoe marks occur when the guide shoes in the turn-around assembly of the processor are sprung or improperly positioned. The ridges in the guide shoes press against the film, sensitize it, and leave a characteristic mark. Guide-shoe marks can be found on the leading edge or the trailing edge of the film.

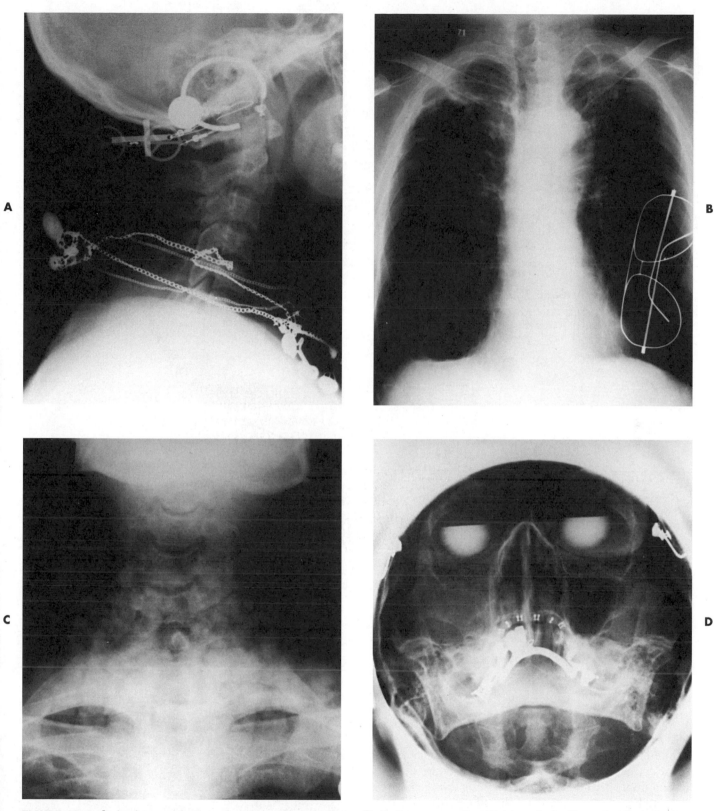

FIGURE 32-1 A, Jewelry remaining on patient during x-ray examination. **B,** Eyeglasses were radiographed in patient's shirt pocket. **C,** An ice bag under the neck was not removed before AP cervical spine examination. **D,** This Waters view was properly coned, but the bifocals, earrings, and dental apparatus should have been removed. *(Courtesy Paul Laudicina.)*

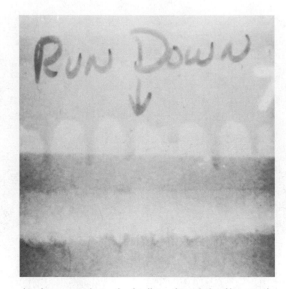

FIGURE 32-2 Excess chemistry runs down the leading edge of the film, creating a curtain effect. *(Courtesy William McKinney.)*

Pi lines occur at 3.1416-inch (π) intervals because of dirt or a chemical stain on a roller. Since the rollers are 1 inch in diameter, 3.1416 inches represent one revolution of a roller. Figure 32-3 is an example of pi lines and guide-shoe marks appearing on the same film.

Wet-pressure Sensitization

Wet-pressure sensitization is a common artifact produced in the developer tank (Figure 32-4). Irregular or dirty rollers cause pressure during development and produce small circular patterns of increased optical density.

HANDLING AND STORAGE ARTIFACTS
Light or Radiation Fog

White-light leaks in the darkroom or within the cassette causes streak-like densities on the film. If the safelight has an improper filter, if the safelight is too bright, or if the safelight is too close to the film-processing tray, fog artifacts can show up on the film. Films left in the x-ray room during an exposure can become fogged by radiation exposure. Radiation fog and light fog look alike.

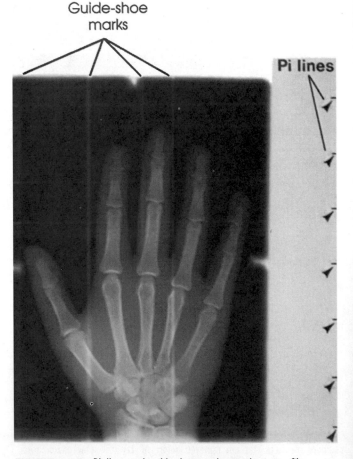

FIGURE 32-3 Pi lines and guide-shoe marks on the same film. *(Courtesy William Hendee, Medical College of Wisconsin.)*

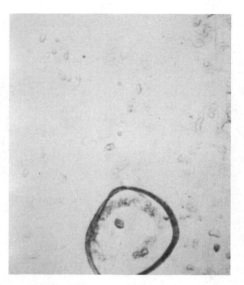

FIGURE 32-4 Wet-pressure sensitization caused by a dirty processor. *(Courtesy William McKinney.)*

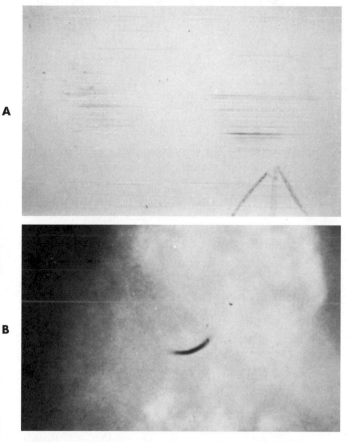

A

B

FIGURE 32-5 Preprocessing pressure artifacts can appear as scratches caused by heavy finger pressure on the feed tray and as kink marks caused by kinking of the film. **A,** Scratches. **B,** Kink marks. *(Courtesy William McKinney.)*

Kink Marks

Characteristic artifacts can be caused by improper handling or storage either before or after processing. Rough handling before processing can cause scratches and kink marks, such as those shown in Figure 32-5. Although the kink mark may appear as a fingernail mark, it is not. It is caused by the kinking or abrupt bending of film.

Static

Static is probably the most obvious artifact. It is caused by the buildup of electrons in the emulsion and is most noticeable during the winter or during periods of extremely low humidity. The following are three kinds of distinct patterns of static: (1) crown, (2) tree, and (3) smudge. Tree static and smudge static are illustrated in Figure 32-6.

Hypo Retention

A yellowish stain slowly appearing on the radiograph after storage time indicates a problem with hypo retention from the fixer. If thiosulfate from the fixer solution remains after washing, silver sulfide slowly builds up, appearing yellow in the stored radiograph.

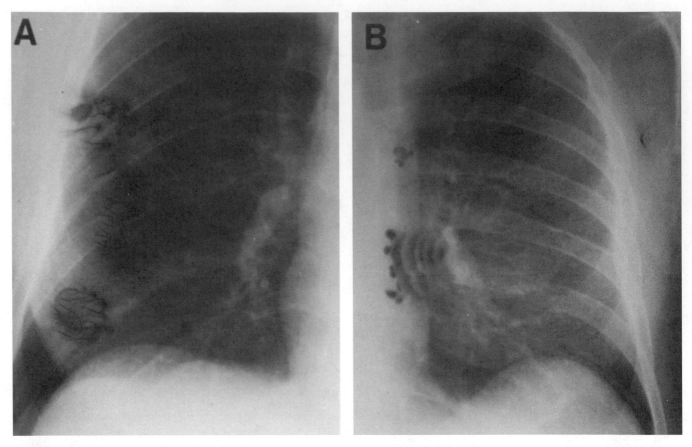

FIGURE 32-6 A, Tree static. **B,** Smudge static. These are the two most common types of static artifacts. (*Courtesy Joel Gray.*)

■ ■ ■ ■ ■ ■ ■ ■ ■ ■ ■ ■ ■ ■
SUMMARY

An artifact is an undesirable optical density that appears on the radiograph. The following are three time periods in which artifacts occur: (1) during the radiographic exposure, (2) during the processing of the film, and (3) when the film is being handled and stored either before or after processing.

Exposure artifacts result from the radiographer conducting the examination. They include patient motion, positioning errors, wrong screen-film combinations, double exposures, and improper grid positioning.

Processing artifacts are mostly pressure types of blemishes on the film emulsion caused by the roller-transport system in the processor. They include sludge from dirty rollers, chemical fog, roller marks, and wet-pressure sensitization.

Storage and handling film artifacts include light or radiation fog, kink marks, static artifacts, and yellowing of stored film from residual fixer (thiosulfate).

■ ■ ■ ■ ■ ■ ■ ■ ■ ■ ■ ■ ■ ■
REVIEW QUESTIONS

1. Why is it important for radiographers to be alert to film artifacts?

2. What is the reason records must be kept when artifacts are seen by the QC radiographer?

3. Refer to Figures 32-2 through 32-6. Cover up the figure legends and identify the name and cause of the artifact demonstrated in the radiograph.

4. Define the term *artifact*.

5. List the three time periods in diagnostic imaging in which artifacts tend to occur.

6. Name three examples of exposure artifacts.

7. How would a radiographer correct a blurred radiograph if it was due to patient motion?

8. What is the reason double exposures occur?

9. Name three types of processing artifacts.

10. Define dichroic stain.

11. How do guide-shoe marks occur?

12. Explain what 3.1416 inches has to do with pi lines.

13. Describe the cause of wet-pressure sensitization marks.

14. Explain three ways fog can occur on a radiograph.

15. Abrupt bending of the unprocessed film causes _____.

16. What is the cause of a static artifact on the processed radiograph?

17. List the three kinds of static artifact patterns.

18. Hypo retention on the films in storage causes _____ to appear on the film?

Additional Reading

Widmer JH, Lillit RF, Jaskulski SM, Haus AG: *Identifying and correcting processing artifacts,* Rochester, NY, 1995, Eastman Kodak.

PART V

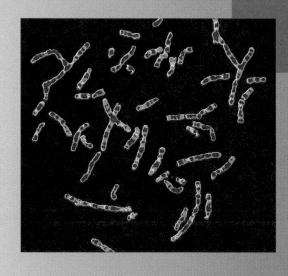

PREGNANT?

or you think you might be...

**tell your doctor
before getting
an x-ray or
prescription**

Distributed by the Food and Drug Administration and the American College of Obstetricians and Gynecologists
DEPARTMENT OF HEALTH, EDUCATION, AND WELFARE • PUBLIC HEALTH SERVICE SERVICE
FOOD AND DRUG ADMINISTRATION, ROCKVILLE, MD 20857
HEW PUBLICATIONS NO. (FDA) 78-1045

RADIATION PROTECTION

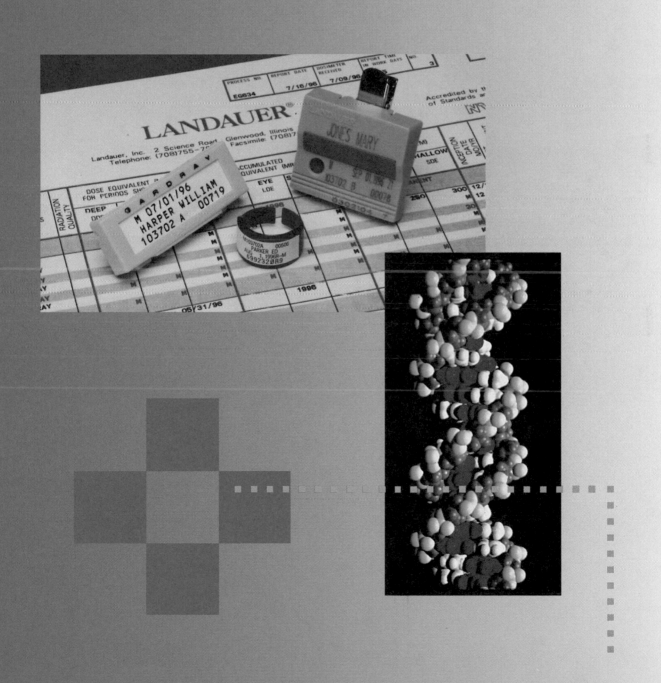

33

Human Biology

OBJECTIVES

At the completion of this chapter the student will be able to:

1. Discuss the cell theory of human biology
2. List and describe the molecular composition of the human body
3. Explain the parts and function of the human cell
4. Describe the processes of mitosis and meiosis
5. Evaluate the radiosensitivity of tissues and organs

OUTLINE

Human Response to Ionizing
    Radiation
Composition of the Body
    Cell theory
Molecular composition
Human cell
Tissues and organs

It is known that x-rays can be harmful. However, there is a growing body of evidence supporting **radiation hormesis.** Radiation hormesis suggests that low levels of radiation, less than approximately 5 rad (50 mGy), provide a protective effect by stimulating molecular repair mechanisms in the human body.

There is no doubt that the benefits derived from the diagnostic application of x-rays in medicine are enormous. It is the job of the radiographer, the radiologist, and the medical physicist to produce high-quality x-ray images with a minimum of radiation exposure. This approach results in the highest benefit with the lowest risk to patients and radiation workers.

This chapter examines the concepts of human biology. Assuming any radiation exposure is potentially harmful, this chapter also discusses the known radiosensitivity of tissues, organs, and cells.

HUMAN RESPONSE TO IONIZING RADIATION

The effects of x-rays on humans are the result of interactions at atomic levels (see Chapter 12). These atomic interactions take the form of ionization or excitation of orbital electrons and result in the deposition of energy in tissue. The deposited energy can result in a molecular change, the consequences of which can be measurable if significant damage results.

When an atom is ionized, its chemical-binding properties change. If the atom is a constituent of a large molecule, the ionization may result in breakage of the molecule or relocation of the atom within the molecule. The abnormal molecule may in time function improperly or cease to function, which can result in serious impairment or death of the cell.

This process is reversible. At each stage of radiation damage it is possible to recover. Ionized atoms can become neutral again by attracting a free electron. Molecules can be mended by repair enzymes. Cells and tissues can regenerate and recover from the radiation injury. If the radiation response occurs within minutes or days after the radiation exposure, it is classified as an immediate or **early effect of radiation.** On the other hand, if the human injury is not observable for many months or years, it is termed *a delayed* or *late effect of radiation.*

The box summarizes the possible early and late human responses to radiation exposure. In addition, many other radiation responses have been experimentally observed in animals. Most of the human responses have been observed after rather large radiation doses, but caution suggests that even small doses are harmful.

Table 33-1 lists some of the human population groups in which many of these radiation responses have been detected.

Human Responses to Ionizing Radiation

Early effects of radiation on humans

Acute radiation syndrome
   Hematologic syndrome
   Gastrointestinal syndrome
   Central nervous system syndrome
Local tissue damage
   Skin
   Gonads
   Extremities
Hematologic depression
Cytogenetic damage

Late effects of radiation on humans

Leukemia
Other malignant disease
   Bone cancer
   Lung cancer
   Breast cancer
Local tissue damage
   Skin
   Gonads
   Eyes
Life span shortening
Genetically significant dose

Effects of fetal irradiation

Prenatal death
Neonatal death
Congenital malformation
Childhood malignancy
Diminished growth and development

TABLE 33-1

Human Populations in Which Radiation Effects Have Been Observed

Population	Effect Observed
American radiologists	Leukemia, life-span shortening
Atomic bomb survivors	Malignant disease
Radiation accident victims	Acute lethality
Marshall Islanders	Thyroid cancer
Uranium miners	Lung cancer
Radium watch-dial painters	Bone cancer
^{131}I patients	Thyroid cancer
Children treated for enlarged thymus	Thyroid cancer
Ankylosing spondylitis patients	Leukemia
Thorotrast patients	Liver cancer
Irradiation in utero	Childhood malignancy
Volunteer convicts	Fertility impairment
Cyclotron workers	Cataracts

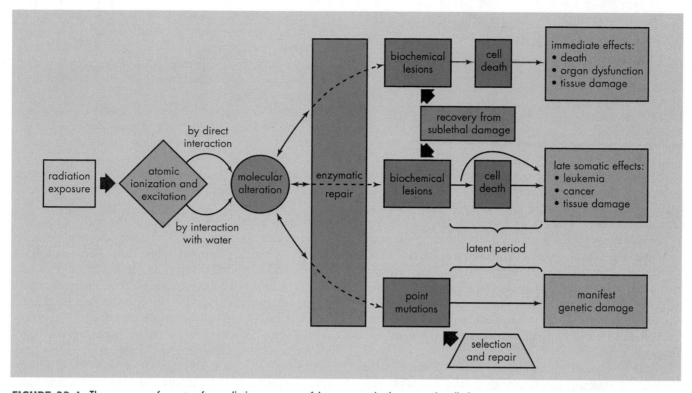

FIGURE 33-1 The sequence of events after radiation exposure of humans can lead to several radiation responses. At nearly every step, mechanisms for recovery and repair are available.

Radiobiology is the study of the effects of ionizing radiation on biologic tissue. The ultimate goal of radiobiologic research is the accurate description of the effects of radiation on humans so that radiation can be used more safely in diagnosis and more effectively in therapy. Figure 33 1 illustrates the sequence of events in human tissue after radiation exposure.

COMPOSITION OF THE BODY
Cell Theory

The composition of the human body has its basis in atoms. Radiation interacts at this atomic level. The atomic composition of the body determines the character and degree of the radiation interaction, and the molecular and tissue composition defines the nature of the radiation injury. The box in the next column summarizes the atomic composition of the body and illustrates that over 85% of the body is hydrogen and oxygen.

Radiation interaction at the atomic level results in molecular change, and molecular change can produce a cell abnormal in growth and metabolism. In 1665, Robert Hooke, the English schoolmaster, first named the **cell** as the biologic building block. Shortly thereafter, in 1673, Anton van Leeuwenhoek accurately described a living cell based on his microscopic observations. It was more than 100 years later, however, in 1838, that Schneider and Schwann showed conclusively that all

Atomic Composition of the Body
60% hydrogen
25.7% oxygen
10.7% carbon
2.4% nitrogen
0.2% calcium
0.1% phosphorus
0.1% sulfur
0.8% trace elements

plants and animals contain cells as their basic functional units. This is the beginning of the **cell theory.**

The most significant milestone in recent studies of the living cell was the Watson and Crick description in 1953 of the molecular structure of deoxyribonucleic acid (DNA), which is the genetic substance of the cell.

Molecular Composition

There are five principal types of molecules in the body (see the box on p. 432). Four of these molecules are **macromolecules**—(1) proteins, (2) lipids (fats), (3) carbohydrates (sugars and starches), and (4) nucleic acids. A macromolecule is a very large molecule, which sometimes consists of hundreds of thousands of atoms. Proteins, lipids, and carbohydrates are the principal classes

Molecular Composition of the Body

80% water
15% protein
2% lipids
1% carbohydrates
1% nucleic acid
1% other

of **organic molecules.** An organic molecule is life supporting and contains carbon. One of the rarest molecules, DNA, a nucleic acid concentrated in the nucleus of a cell, is considered to be the most critical and **radiosensitive** molecule.

Water is the most abundant molecule in the body and also the simplest. Water, however, plays a particularly important role in delivering energy to the **target molecule,** thereby contributing to radiation effects. In addition to water and the macromolecules, there are some trace elements and inorganic salts that are essential to proper metabolism.

Water. The most abundant molecular constituent of the body is water. It consists of two atoms of hydrogen and one atom of oxygen (H_2O) and constitutes approximately 80% of human substance. Humans are basically a structured aqueous suspension. The water molecules exist both in the free and bound states. They may be dissociated or bound to other molecules. Water molecules provide some form and shape, assist in maintaining body temperature, and enter into some biochemical reactions.

During vigorous exercise, body water is lost through perspiration to stabilize temperature and respiration, and it must be replaced to maintain **homeostasis** (the constancy of the internal environment of the human body). Water and carbon dioxide are end products in the **catabolism** (breaking down into smaller units) of macromolecules. **Anabolism,** the production of large molecules from small, and catabolism are collectively termed *metabolism.*

Proteins. Approximately 15% of the molecular composition of the body is protein. Proteins are long-chain macromolecules that consist of a linear sequence of **amino acids** connected by **peptide bonds.** There are twenty-two amino acids used in protein production, or **protein synthesis.** The linear sequence, or arrangement, of these amino acids determines the precise function of the protein molecule.

Figure 33-2 shows the general chemical form of a protein molecule. The generalized formula for a protein is $C_nH_nO_nN_nT_n$, where the subscript n refers to the number of atoms of each element in the molecule. T represents trace elements. In general, 50% of the mass of a protein molecule is carbon, 20% oxygen, 17% nitrogen, 7% hydrogen, and 6% other elements.

Proteins have a variety of uses in the body. They provide structure and support. Muscles are very high in protein content. Proteins also function as enzymes, hormones, and antibodies. **Enzymes** are molecules that are necessary in small quantities to allow a biochemical reaction to continue, but they do not directly enter into the reaction. **Hormones** are molecules that exercise regulatory control over some body functions such as growth and development. Hormones are produced and secreted by the **endocrine glands,** which are pituitary, adrenal, thyroid, and parathyroid glands, and the pancreas and gonads. **Antibodies** constitute a primary defense mechanism of the body against infection and disease. The molecular configuration of an antibody may be precise for attacking a particular type of invasive or infectious agent, the **antigen.**

Lipids. Lipids are organic macromolecules composed solely of carbon, hydrogen, and oxygen. They have the general formulation $C_nH_nO_n$. Structurally, lipids have the form shown in Figure 33-3. This structure distinguishes them from carbohydrates. In general, lipids are composed of two kinds of smaller molecules, **glycerol** and **fatty acid.** Each lipid molecule is composed of one molecule of glycerol and three molecules of fatty acid.

Lipids are present in all tissues of the body and are the structural components of cell membranes. Lipids often are concentrated just under the skin and serve as a thermal insulator from the environment. Polar bears, for instance, have a particularly thick layer of subcutaneous fat (blubber) as a means of protection from the

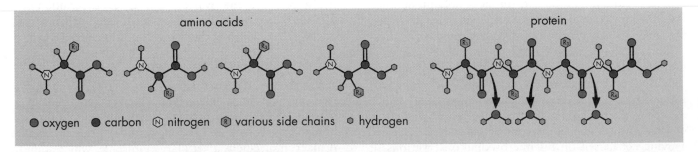

FIGURE 33-2 Proteins consist of amino acids linked by peptide bonds. To create the peptide bond, a molecule of water must be removed.

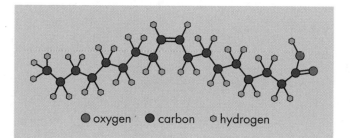

FIGURE 33-3 Structural configuration of a lipid is represented by the following, which is a molecule of oleic acid: $CH_3(CH_2)_7CH = CH(CH_2)_7COOH$.

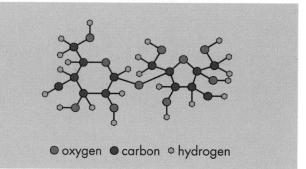

FIGURE 33-4 Carbohydrates are structurally different from lipids, even though their composition is similar. This is a molecule of sucrose, or ordinary table sugar: $(C_{12}H_{22}O_{11})$.

cold. Lipids also serve as fuel for the body by providing energy stores. It is more difficult, however, to extract energy from lipids than from the other major fuel source, carbohydrates.

Carbohydrates. Carbohydrates, like lipids, are composed solely of carbon, hydrogen, and oxygen, but their structure is different (Figure 33-4). This structural difference determines the contribution of the carbohydrate molecule to body biochemistry. The ratio of the number of hydrogen atoms to oxygen atoms in a carbohydrate molecule is 2:1, as in water. A large fraction of this molecule consists of these atoms. Consequently, carbohydrates are considered to be watered, or **hydrated,** carbons. Hence their name, carbo-hydrate.

Carbohydrates are also called *saccharides.* **Monosaccharides** and **disaccharides** are sugars. The chemical formula for glucose, a simple sugar, is $C_6H_{12}O_6$. These molecules are relatively small. **Polysaccharides** are large and include plant **starches** and animal **glycogen.** The chemical formula for a polysaccharide is $(C_6H_{10}O_5)_n$, where n is the number of simple sugar molecules in the macromolecule.

The chief function of carbohydrates in the body is to provide fuel for cell metabolism. To a lesser extent, some carbohydrates are incorporated into the structure of cells and tissues to provide shape and stability. The human polysaccharide, glycogen, is stored in the tissues of the body and used as fuel only when the simple sugar, glucose, is not present in adequate quantities. Glucose is the ultimate molecule that fuels the body. Lipids can be catabolized into glucose for energy but only with great difficulty. Polysaccharides are much more readily transformed into glucose.

Nucleic acids. There are two principal nucleic acids in human metabolism: (1) **DNA** and (2) **ribonucleic acid (RNA).** Located principally in the nucleus of the cell, DNA serves as the command or control molecule for cell function. The DNA contains all the hereditary information representing a cell and, of course, if the cell is a **germ cell,** all the hereditary information of the whole individual.

RNA is found in the **nucleus** and outside the nucleus in the **cytoplasm.** There are two types—**messenger RNA (mRNA)** and **transfer RNA (tRNA).** They are distinguished according to their biochemical functions. These molecules are involved in the growth and development of the cell through a number of biochemical pathways, notably **protein synthesis.**

The nucleic acids are very large and extremely complex macromolecules. Figure 33-5 shows the structural composition of DNA and the manner in which the component molecules are joined. DNA consists of a backbone composed of alternating segments of deoxyribose (a sugar) and phosphate. For each deoxyribose-phosphate conjugate formed, a molecule of water is removed.

Attached to each deoxyribose molecule is one of four different nitrogen-containing or nitrogenous organic bases—**adenine, guanine, thymine,** or **cytosine.** Adenine and guanine are **purines.** Thymine and cytosine are **pyrimidines.**

The base-sugar-phosphate combination is called a **nucleotide,** and the nucleotides are strung together in one long-chain macromolecule. Human DNA exists as two of these long chains attached together in ladder fashion (Figure 33-6). The side rails of the ladder are the alternating sugar-phosphate molecules, and the rungs of the ladder consist of bases joined together by hydrogen bonds.

To complete the picture, the ladder is twisted about an imaginary axis like a spring. This produces a molecule having the **double-helix** configuration (Figure 33-7). The sequence of base bonding is limited to adenines bonded to thymines and cytosines bonded to guanines. No other base-bonding combinations are possible.

RNA resembles DNA structurally. The sugar component is ribose rather than deoxyribose, and uracil replaces thymine as a base component. In contrast, RNA forms a single spiral, not a double helix.

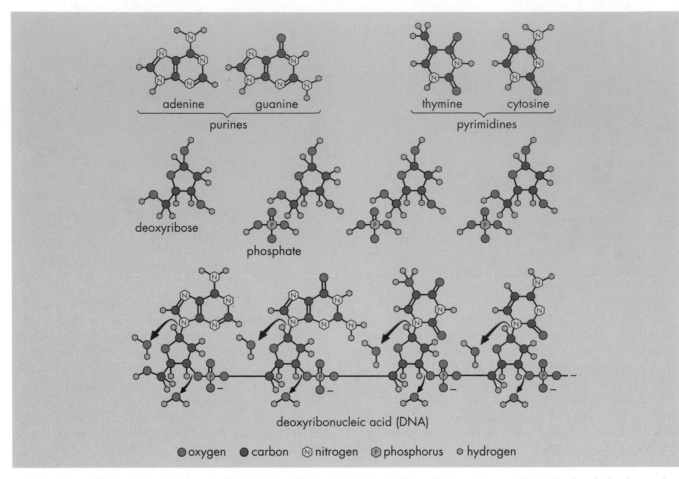

adenine   guanine

purines

thymine   cytosine

pyrimidines

deoxyribose

phosphate

deoxyribonucleic acid (DNA)

● oxygen   ● carbon   Ⓝ nitrogen   Ⓟ phosphorus   ○ hydrogen

FIGURE 33-5 DNA is the control center for life. A single molecule consists of a backbone of alternating sugar (deoxyribose) and phosphate molecules. Each sugar molecule has one of the four organic bases attached to it.

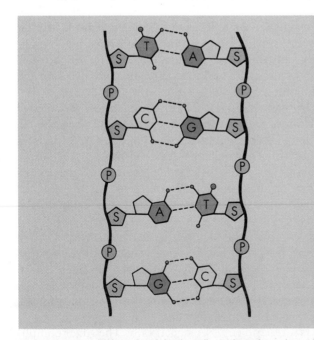

FIGURE 33-6 DNA, as found in the cell, consists of two long chains of alternating sugar and phosphate molecules fashioned like the side rails of a ladder with five pairs of bases as the rungs.

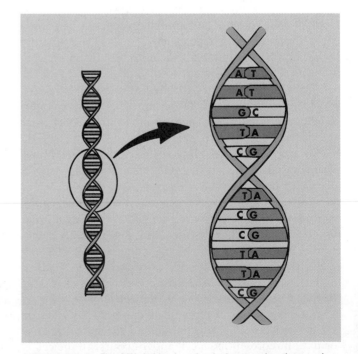

FIGURE 33-7 The DNA ladder is twisted about an imaginary axis to form a double helix.

Human Cell

The principal molecular components of the human body are made up of intricate cellular structures. The structures of the cell are assembled in much the same way as the parts of an automobile. This assembly ensures proper growth, development, and function of the cell. Figure 33-8 is a cutaway view of a human cell with its principal parts labeled.

The two major segments of the cell are the **nucleus** and the cytoplasm. The principal molecular component of the nucleus is DNA, which is the genetic material of the cell. The nucleus also contains some RNA, protein, and water. Most of the RNA is contained in a rounded structure, the **nucleolus**. The nucleolus is often attached to the nuclear membrane, which is a double-walled structure that at some locations is connected to the **endoplasmic reticulum**. The nature of this connection controls the passage of molecules, particularly RNA, from nucleus to cytoplasm.

The cytoplasm makes up the bulk of the cell and contains all the molecular components in great quantity, except DNA. Found in the cytoplasm are a number of intracellular structures. The endoplasmic reticulum is a channel or series of channels that allows the nucleus to communicate with the cytoplasm.

The large bean-shaped structures are **mitochondria**. Macromolecules are digested in the mitochondria to produce energy for the cell. The mitochondria are therefore called the *workhorses of the cell.*

The small dotlike structures are **ribosomes**. Ribosomes are the site of protein synthesis and therefore are essential to normal cellular function.

The small pealike sacs are **lysosomes**. The lysosomes contain enzymes capable of digesting cellular fragments and, in some situations, the cell itself. Lysosomes are helpful in the control of intracellular contaminants.

All these structures, including the cell itself, are surrounded by membranes. These membranes consist principally of lipid-protein complexes that selectively allow small molecules and water to diffuse from one side to the other. These cellular membranes, of course, also provide structure and form for the cell and its components.

When one irradiates the critical macromolecular cellular components by themselves, a dose of approximately 1 Mrad (10 kGy) is required to produce a measurable change in any physical characteristic of the molecule. When such a molecule is incorporated into the apparatus of a living cell, only a few rad are necessary to produce a measurable biologic response. The dose necessary to produce lethality in some single-cell organisms such as bacteria is measured in kilorad, whereas human cells can be killed with a dose of less than 100 rad (1 Gy).

A number of experiments have been conducted to show that the nucleus is much more sensitive to the effects of radiation than is the cytoplasm. Such experiments are conducted with either precise microbeams of electrons that can be focused and directed to a particular cell part or through the incorporation of the radioactive isotopes ^{3}H and ^{14}C into cellular molecules that localize exclusively either in the cytoplasm or in the nucleus.

Cell function. Every human cell has a specific function in supporting the total body. In addition to its specialized function, each cell to some extent performs the function of absorbing through the cell membrane all molecular nutrients. These nutrients are used in the production of energy and molecular synthesis. If the molecular synthesis is damaged by radiation exposure, the cell may malfunction and die.

Protein synthesis is a good example of a most important and critical cellular function necessary for survival (Figure 33-9). DNA, located in the nucleus, contains a molecular code that identifies what proteins that

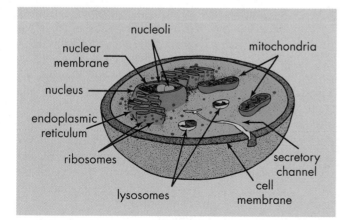

FIGURE 33-8 Schematic view of a human cell that shows the principal structural components.

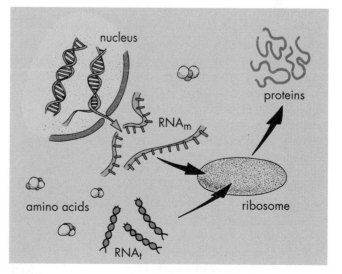

FIGURE 33-9 Protein synthesis is a complex process and involves many different molecules and cellular structures.

cell will make. This code is determined by the sequence of base pairs adenine-thymine and cytosine-guanine. A series of three base pairs called a *codon* identifies one of the 22 human amino acids available for protein synthesis.

This genetic message is transferred in the nucleus to a molecule of messenger RNA (mRNA). The mRNA leaves the nucleus by way of the endoplasmic reticulum and makes its way to a ribosome, where the genetic message is transferred to yet another RNA molecule called *transfer RNA (tRNA)*.

The tRNA searches the cytoplasm for the amino acids for which it is coded. It attaches to the amino acid and carries it to the ribosome, where it is joined with other amino acids in sequence by peptide bonds to form the required protein molecule.

Interference with any phase of this procedure for protein synthesis could result in damage to the cell. Radiation interaction with the molecule having primary control over protein synthesis, DNA, produces a response interaction with other molecules involved in protein synthesis.

Cell proliferation. Although many thousands of rad are necessary to produce physically measurable disruption of macromolecules, single ionizing events at a particularly sensitive site of a critical target molecule are thought to be capable of disrupting cell proliferation. **Cell proliferation** is the act of a single cell or group of cells reproducing and multiplying in number. This increase in number of cells by reproduction is a result of the process of **cell division,** a mechanism that results in twice the number of cells.

Two general types of cells exist in the human body, **somatic cells** and **genetic cells.** The genetic cells are the **oogonium** of the female and the **spermatogonium** of the male. All other cells of the body are somatic cells. When somatic cells undergo proliferation, or cell division, they undergo mitosis. Genetic cells undergo **meiosis.**

Mitosis. The cell cycle is seen differently by the cell biologist than by the geneticist (Figure 33-10). Each cycle includes the various states of cell growth, development, and division. The geneticist considers only two phases of the cell cycle: **mitosis (M)** and **interphase.** Mitosis, the division phase, is characterized by four subphases: **prophase, metaphase, anaphase,** and **telophase.** The portion of the cell cycle between mitotic events is termed *interphase.* Interphase is the period of growth of the cell between divisions.

The cell biologist usually identifies four phases of the cell cycle: M, G_1, S, and G_2. These phases of the cell cycle are characterized by the structure of the chromosomes, which contain the genetic material DNA. The **gap** in cell growth between M and S is G_1. It is termed the *pre-DNA synthesis phase.*

The DNA synthesis phase is S. During this period, each DNA molecule is replicated into two identical

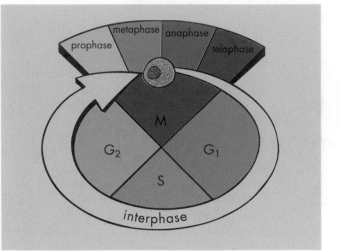

FIGURE 33-10 As the cell progresses through one growth cycle, several phases are observed. The cell biologist and the geneticist identify each phase differently.

daughter DNA molecules. The chromosome is transformed from a structure with two chromatids attached to a centromere to a structure with four chromatids attached to centromere (Figure 33-11). The result is two pairs of homologous chromatids, that is, chromatids having precisely the same DNA content and structure. The G_2 phase is the post-DNA synthesis gap of cell growth.

During interphase, the chromosomes are not visible; however, during mitosis, the DNA slowly takes the form of the chromosome. Figure 33-12 shows the process of mitosis schematically. During prophase, the nucleus swells and the DNA becomes more prominent and begins to take structural form. At metaphase the chromosomes appear and are lined up along the equator of the nucleus. It is during metaphase that mitosis can be stopped and chromosomes studied carefully under the microscope. Radiation-induced chromosome damage is analyzed during metaphase.

Anaphase is characterized by each chromosome splitting at the centromere so that a centromere and two chromatids are connected by a fiber to the poles of the nucleus. These poles are called *spindles,* and the fibers are called *spindle fibers.* The number of chromatids per centromere has been reduced by half, and these newly formed chromosomes migrate slowly toward the nuclear spindle.

The final segment of mitosis, **telophase,** is characterized by the disappearance of the structural chromosomes into a mass of DNA and the closing off of the nuclear membrane like a dumbbell into two nuclei. At the same time the cytoplasm is divided into two equal parts, each accompanying one of the new nuclei.

Cell division is now complete. The two daughter cells appear precisely as the parent and contain exactly the same genetic material.

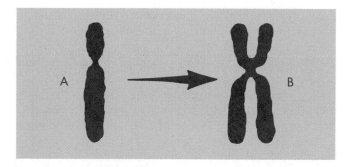

FIGURE 33-11 During the synthesis portion of interphase, the chromosomes replicate from a two-chromatid structure (**A**) to a four-chromatid structure (**B**).

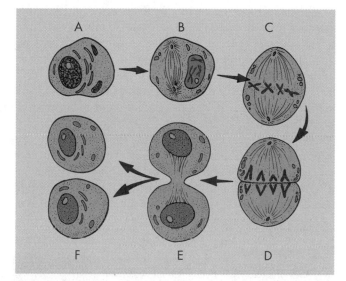

FIGURE 33-12 Mitosis is the phase of the cell cycle during which the chromosomes become visible, divide, and migrate to daughter cells. **A**, Interphase. **B**, Prophase. **C**, Metaphase. **D**, Anaphase. **E**, Telophase. **F**, Interphase.

Meiosis. Changes in genetic material can occur during the division process of genetic cells, which is called meiosis. The primary genetic cells, the germ cells, begin with the same number of chromosomes as somatic cells, 23 pairs (46 chromosomes), but for a germ cell to be capable of marriage with another germ cell, its complement of chromosomes must be reduced by half to 23 so that, following conception and the union of two germ cells, the daughter cells will contain 46 chromosomes. This process of **reduction division** of germ cells is meiosis (Figure 33-13).

The primary germ cell begins meiosis with 46 chromosomes, appearing as a somatic cell having completed G_2 phase. It then progresses through the phases of mitosis into two daughter cells, each containing 46 chromosomes of two chromatids each. The names of the subphases of meiosis and mitosis are the same.

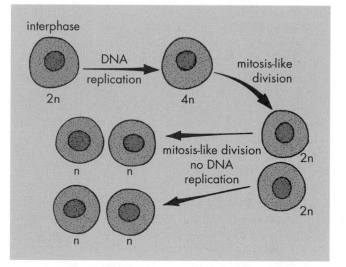

FIGURE 33-13 Meiosis is the process of reduction and division, and it occurs only in germ cells. n is the number of similar chromosomes.

Each of the daughter cells of this first division now progresses through a second division in which all the cellular material is divided, including the chromosomes; however, the second division is not accompanied by an S phase, and therefore there is no replication of DNA and consequently no duplication of the chromosomes. The resulting granddaughter cells contain only 23 chromosomes each.

Each parent has undergone two division processes, resulting in four daughter cells. During the second division, there is some exchange of chromosomal material among chromatids by a process called *crossing over.* Crossing over results in changes in genetic constitution and changes in inheritable traits.

Tissues and Organs

During the development and maturation of a human from the two united germ cells, a number of different types of cells evolve. Collections of cells of similar structure and function form **tissues**. Table 33-2 is a breakdown of the composition of the body according to its tissue constituents.

TABLE 33-2	
Tissue Composition of the Body	
Tissue	**Abundance**
Muscle	43.9%
Fat	14%
Organs	12%
Skeleton	10%
Blood	7.7%
Bone marrow	4.2%
Subcutaneous tissue	5.8%
Skin	2.9%

These tissues in turn are bound together in precise fashion to form **organs**. The tissues and the organs of the body serve as discrete units with specific functional responsibilities. Some tissues and organs will combine into an overall integrated organization known as an *organ system*.

The principal organ systems of the body are the nervous system, the digestive system, the endocrine system, and the reproductive system. The effects of radiation that appear at the whole-body level result from damage to these organ systems, which in turn are a result of radiation injury to the cells of that system.

The cells of a tissue system are identified by their rate of proliferation and their stage of development. Immature cells are called *undifferentiated cells, precursor cells,* or *stem cells.* As a cell matures through growth and proliferation, it can pass through various stages of differentiation into a fully functional and mature cell.

The sensitivity of the cell to radiation is determined to some degree by its state of maturity and its functional role. Generally speaking, immature cells are more sensitive to radiation than mature cells. Table 33-3 is a list of a number of different types of cells in the body according to their degree of radiosensitivity.

The tissues and organs of the body consist of both stem cells and mature cells. There are several types of tissue that can be classified according to structural or functional features. These features influence the degree of radiosensitivity of the tissue.

Epithelium is the covering tissue, and it lines all exposed surfaces of the body, both exterior and interior. Epithelium covers the skin, the blood vessels, the abdominal and chest cavities, and the gastrointestinal tract.

Connective and **supporting tissues** are high in protein and are composed principally of fibers that usually have a high degree of elasticity. Connective tissue binds tissues and organs together. Bone and cartilage are examples of connective tissue.

Muscle is a special type of tissue that is capable of contracting. It is found throughout the body and also is high in protein content.

Nervous tissue is also called *conductive tissue* and consists of specialized cells called **neurons** that have long, thin extensions from the cell to distant parts of the body. Nervous tissue is the avenue through which electrical impulses are transmitted throughout the body for control and response.

When these various types of tissue are combined to form an organ, they are identified according to two parts of the organ. The **parenchymal** part contains tissues that are representative of that particular organ, whereas the **stromal** part is composed of connective tissue and vasculature that provides structure to the organ.

When considering the early effects of radiation exposure of high dose levels, it is organ damage that ultimately results in observable effects. The various organs of the body exhibit a wide range of sensitivity to radiation. This radiosensitivity is determined by (1) the function of the organ in the body, (2) the rate at which cells mature in the organ, and (3) the inherent radiosensitivity of the cell type.

A precise knowledge of these various organ radiosensitivities is unnecessary; however, knowledge of the general levels of radiosensitivity (Table 33-4) is helpful in understanding the effects of **whole-body radiation exposure** and, in particular, the **acute radiation syndrome.**

TABLE 33-3
Response to Radiation is Related to Cell Type

Radiosensitivity	Cell Type
High	Lymphocytes
	Spermatogonia
	Erythroblasts
	Intestinal crypt cells
Intermediate	Endothelial cells
	Osteoblasts
	Spermatids
	Fibroblasts
Low	Muscle cells
	Nerve cells

TABLE 33-4
The Relative Radiosensitivity of Tissues and Organs Based on Clinical Radiotherapy

Level of Radiosensitivity (Rad)*	Tissue or Organ	Effects
High: 200 to 1000	Lymphoid tissue	Atrophy
	Bone marrow	Hypoplasia
	Gonads	Atrophy
Intermediate: 1000 to 1500	Skin	Erythema
	Gastrointestinal tract	Ulcer
	Cornea	Cataract
	Growing bone	Growth arrest
	Kidney	Nephrosclerosis
	Liver	Ascites
	Thyroid	Atrophy
Low: >5000	Muscle	Fibrosis
	Brain	Necrosis
	Spinal	Transection

*The minimum dose delivered at the rate of approximately 200 rad per day that will produce a response.

■ ■ ■ ■ ■ ■ ■ ■ ■ ■ ■ ■ ■ ■ ■ ■ ■ ■ ■

SUMMARY

After a radiation exposure, the human body responds in predictable ways. Radiobiology is the study of the effects of ionizing radiation on biologic tissue. Table 33-1 lists the types of damage that result from an exposure incident. If a response occurs within minutes or days of exposure, it is called an *early effect of radiation*. If the injury is not observable for months or years, it is termed a *late effect of radiation exposure*.

The cell theory describes the cell as the basic functional unit of all plants and animals. Radiobiology studies radiation effects on the cellular and molecular level. On the molecular level, the body is mostly composed of water, protein, lipids, carbohydrates, and nucleic acid. The two important nucleic acids in human metabolism are DNA and RNA. DNA contains all the hereditary information in the cell. If the cell is a genetic cell or germ cell, the DNA contains the hereditary information of the whole individual. DNA is a macromolecule made up of two long chains of base-sugar-phosphate combinations twisted in a double-helix configuration.

Figure 33-8 is a cut-away view of the human cell with the cellular components labeled. Cellular function consists of protein synthesis and cell division. Mitosis is the growth, development, and division of cells. *Meiosis* is the term for the division of genetic cells.

Cells of similar structure bind together to form tissue. Tissue binds together to form organs. An overall integrated organization of tissue and organs is called an *organ system*. The principal systems of the body are the nervous, digestive, endocrine, and reproductive systems. Table 33-4 lists the radiosensitivity of various tissues and organ systems. Reproductive cells are highly radiosensitive, whereas nerve cells are less radiosensitive.

■ ■ ■ ■ ■ ■ ■ ■ ■ ■ ■ ■ ■ ■ ■ ■ ■ ■ ■

REVIEW QUESTIONS

1. What is the term to describe the concept that states low levels of radiation (less than 5 rad) provide a protective effect by stimulating the molecular repair mechanism of the human body?

2. The effects of x-rays on humans are the result of interactions at the _____ level.

3. How does ionizing radiation affect an atom? How does ionizing radiation affect an atom within a large molecule?

4. Define early effect and late effect of radiation exposure.

5. List five parts of the human population in which radiation effects have been observed? What are the radiation effects on these populations?

6. Who first named the cell as the building block of biologic tissue?

7. Who described the molecular structure of DNA in 1953?

8. Explain the following statement: Humans are basically a structured aqueous suspension.

9. Define homeostasis.

10. What is the function of proteins in the human body?

11. What is the chief function of carbohydrates in the body?

12. For what words are DNA and RNA abbreviations?

13. The two major segments of the cell are _____ and _____.

14. The principal molecular component of the nucleus is _____, the genetic material of the cell.

15. Define the endoplasmic reticulum.

16. What dosage of radiation is required to produce a measurable physical change in a macromolecule?

17. List the stages of cell division in a somatic cell.

18. List the stages of cell reduction division in a germ cell.

19. What cell type has the highest radiosensitivity?

20. What type of tissue has the lowest radiosensitivity?

Additional Readings

Alters S: *Biology: Understanding Life,* ed 2, St Louis, 1995, Mosby.

Gottfried SS: *Human Biology,* St Louis, 1994, Mosby.

Mannino JA: *Human Biology,* St Louis, 1995, Mosby.

34

Fundamental Principles of Radiobiology

OBJECTIVES

At the completion of this chapter the student will be able to:

1. State the Law of Bergonie and Tribondeau
2. List and describe the physical factors that affect the degree of tissue damage in relation to radiation exposure
3. Name and discuss the biologic factors that affect the degree of tissue damage in relation to radiation exposure
4. Explain dose-response relationships
5. List the four types of dose-response relationships

OUTLINE

Law of Bergonie and Tribondeau
Physical Factors Affecting
    Radiosensitivity
    Linear energy transfer
    Relative biologic effectiveness
    Fractionation and protraction
Biologic Factors Affecting
    Radiosensitivity
    Oxygen effect
    Age
    Gender
    Recovery
    Chemical agents

Radiation Dose-response
    Relationships
    Linear dose-response relationships
    Nonlinear dose-response
        relationships
    Constructing a dose-response
        relationship
    Linear, quadratic dose-response
        relationships

Certain tissues are more sensitive than others to radiation exposure and damage. Reproductive cells are sensitive compared with nerve cells. This and other radiobiologic concepts were detailed in 1906 by two French scientists.

There are physical factors and biologic factors that affect radiosensitivity in biologic tissue. Most of this study comes from interest in radiation therapy; however, radiographers should be alert to the effects of the accumulation of low-dose radiation exposure.

The study of radiobiology has expanded in the atomic age. The object of study in modern times is the establishment of radiation dose-response relationships. A dose-response relationship is a graph that cites the relationship between the radiation dose and the observed tissue response.

■ ■ ■ ■ ■ ■ ■ ■ ■ ■ ■ ■ ■ ■ ■ ■ ■ ■ ■

LAW OF BERGONIE AND TRIBONDEAU

In 1906, two French scientists, Bergonie and Tribondeau, theorized and observed that radiosensitivity was a function of the metabolic state of the tissue being irradiated. This has come to be known as the *Law of Bergonie and Tribondeau* and has been verified many times. Basically the law states that the radiosensitivity of living tissue varies as follows:

1. Stem cells are radiosensitive. The more mature a cell is, the more resistant to radiation it is.
2. The younger the tissues and organs are, the more radiosensitive they are.
3. When the level of metabolic activity is high, radiosensitivity is also high.
4. As the proliferation rate for cells and the growth rate for tissues increase, the radiosensitivity increases also.

This law is of interest principally as a historical note in the development of radiobiology. It has found some application in radiotherapy. In diagnostic imaging, it serves to remind us that the fetus is considerably more sensitive to radiation exposure than the child or the mature adult.

PHYSICAL FACTORS AFFECTING RADIOSENSITIVITY

When irradiating a biologic medium, the response (tissue damage) is determined principally by the amount of energy deposited per unit mass: the dose in rad (Gy). Even under controlled experimental conditions, however, when equal doses are delivered to equal specimens, the response may not be the same because of other modifying factors. There are a number of physical factors that affect the degree of radiation response.

Linear Energy Transfer

The **linear energy transfer (LET)** is a measure of the rate at which energy is transferred from ionizing radiation to soft tissue. LET has units of keV of energy transferred per micrometer of track length in soft tissue (keV/μm).

The ability of ionizing radiation to produce a biologic response increases as the LET of radiation increases. Table 34-1 lists the approximate LET of various types of ionizing radiation. The LET of diagnostic x-rays is about 3 keV/μm, which is relatively low among all radiations.

Relative Biologic Effectiveness

As the LET of radiation increases, the ability to produce biologic damage also increases. This relative effect is quantitatively described by the **relative biologic effectiveness (RBE)**. The RBE is defined as follows:

$$RBE = \frac{\text{Dose of standard radiation necessary to produce a given effect}}{\text{Dose of test radiation necessary to produce the same effect}}$$

The standard radiation, by convention, is orthovoltage x-radiation in the 200 to 250 kVp range. Diagnostic x-rays have an RBE of 1. Radiations with lower LET than diagnostic x-rays have an RBE less than 1, whereas radiations with higher LET have a higher RBE. Figure 34-1 shows the relationship between RBE and LET and identifies some of the more common types of radiation. The maximum value of the RBE is approximately 3.

Question: In a hypothetical situation, if mice are irradiated with 250 kVp x-rays, 640 rad (6.4 Gy) are necessary to produce death. If similar mice are irradiated with fast neutrons, only 210 rad (2.1 Gy) are needed. What is the RBE for the fast neutrons?

Answer:

$$RBE = \frac{650 \text{ rad}}{210 \text{ rad}}$$
$$= 3.1$$

TABLE 34-1

The LET of Various Radiations

Type of Radiation	LET (keV/μm)
25 MeV x-rays	0.2
Cobalt 60 gamma rays	0.25
1 MeV electrons	0.3
Diagnostic x-rays	3
10 MeV protons	4
Fast neutrons	50
5 MeV alpha particles	100
Heavy nuclei	1000

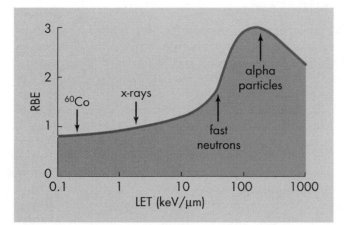

FIGURE 34-1 As LET increases, RBE increases also, but a maximum value is reached beyond which the RBE can increase no further.

Fractionation and Protraction

If a dose of radiation is delivered over a long period of time rather than quickly, the effect of that dose is less. Stated differently, if the time of irradiation is lengthened, a higher dose is required to produce the same effect. This lengthening of time can be accomplished in two ways.

If the dose is delivered continuously but at a lower dose rate, it is said to be **protracted**. Six hundred rad (6 Gy) delivered in 3 minutes (200 rad/min [2 Gy/min]) is lethal for a mouse. When 600 rad is delivered at the rate of 1 rad/hr (10 mGy/hr) for a total time of 600 hours, however, the mouse will survive. Dose protraction causes less effect because of the lower dose rate and the longer irradiation time.

If the 600 rad dose is delivered at the same dose rate, 200 rad per minute but in 12 equal fractions of 50 rad (500 mGy), each separated by 24 hours, the mouse will survive. In this situation the dose is said to be **fractionated**. Dose fractionation causes less effect because tissue repair and recovery occur between doses. Dose fractionation is used routinely in radiation oncology when radiating tumors.

BIOLOGIC FACTORS AFFECTING RADIOSENSITIVITY

In addition to these physical factors, there are a number of biologic conditions that alter the radiation response of biologic tissue. Some of these factors have to do with the inherent state of the host, such as age, gender, and metabolic rate. Other factors are related to artificially introduced modifiers of the biologic system.

Oxygen Effect

Biologic tissue is more sensitive to radiation when irradiated in the oxygenated, or **aerobic**, state than when irradiated under **anoxic** (without oxygen) or **hypoxic**

(low-oxygen) conditions. This characteristic of biologic tissue is called the *oxygen effect* and is described numerically by the **oxygen enhancement ratio (OER)**. The OER is calculated as follows:

$$OER = \frac{\text{Dose necessary under anoxic conditions to produce a given effect}}{\text{Dose necessary under aerobic conditions to produce the same effect}}$$

Generally the irradiation of tissue is conducted under conditions of full oxygenation. **Hyperbaric** (high-pressure) oxygen has been used in radiation therapy in an attempt to increase the radiosensitivity of nodular, avascular tumors, which are less radiosensitive than tumors with an adequate blood supply.

Question: When experimental mouse mammary carcinomas are clamped and irradiated under hypoxic conditions, the tumor control dose is 10,600 rad (106 Gy). When the tumors are not clamped and are irradiated under aerobic conditions, the tumor control dose is 4050 rad (40.5 Gy). What is the OER for this system?

Answer:

$$OER = \frac{10,600}{4050}$$

$$= 2.6$$

The OER is LET dependent (Figure 34-2). The OER is greatest for low-LET radiation, which has a maximum of approximately 3; the OER decreases to approximately 1 for high-LET radiation.

Age

The age of a biologic structure affects its radiosensitivity. The response of humans is characteristic of this age-

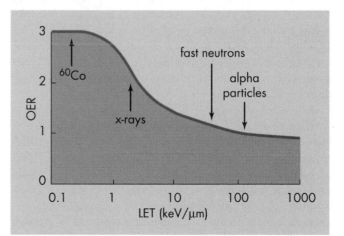

FIGURE 34-2 The OER is high for low-LET radiation and decreases in value as the LET increases.

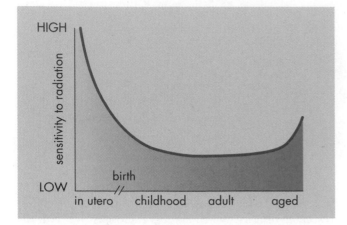

FIGURE 34-3 Radiosensitivity varies with age. Experiments with animals have shown that the very young and the very old are more sensitive to radiation.

related radiosensitivity (Figure 34-3). Humans are most sensitive before birth. The sensitivity then decreases until adulthood, which is when humans are most resistant to radiation-induced effects. In old age, humans again become somewhat more radiosensitive.

Gender

Many experiments have been conducted to determine which gender is more resistant to the effects of radiation. The results are not all in agreement nor are they conclusive; however, taken together, the indication is that the female can sustain approximately 5% to 10% more radiation than the male.

Recovery

It has been shown without question from experiments **in vitro** that human cells are capable of recovering from radiation damage. If the radiation dose is not sufficient to kill the cell before its next division (**interphase death**), then given sufficient time the cell will recover from **sublethal radiation damage.**

This intracellular recovery is due to a repair mechanism inherent in the biochemistry of the cell. Some types of cells have greater capacity for repair of sublethal damage than others.

At the whole-body level this recovery from radiation damage is assisted through **repopulation** by the surviving cells. If a tissue or organ receives a sufficient radiation dose, it responds by shrinking in size. This is called *atrophy* and occurs because some cells die, disintegrate, and are carried away as waste products. If a sufficient number of cells sustain only sublethal damage and survive, they may proliferate and repopulate the irradiated tissue or organ. The combined processes of repair and repopulation contribute to recovery from radiation damage.

Chemical Agents

Some chemicals can modify the response of cells, tissues, and organs to radiation. For the chemical agents to be effective, they generally must be present at the time of irradiation. Postirradiation application will not usually alter the degree of response.

Radiosensitizers are agents that enhance the effect of radiation. Some examples are halogenated pyrimidines, methotrexate, actinomycin D, hydroxyurea, and vitamin K. The halogenated pyrimidines become incorporated into the DNA of the cell and cause the radiation effects on that molecule to be amplified. All the radiosensitizers have an **effectiveness ratio** up to 2. That is, if 90% of a cell culture is killed by 200 rad (2 Gy) then, in the presence of a sensitizing agent, only 100 rad (1 Gy) will be required for the same percent lethality.

Radioprotectors are compounds with molecules containing a sulfhydryl group (sulfur and hydrogen bound together) such as cysteine and cysteamine. Hundreds of others have been tested and found effective to within a ratio of approximately 2. For example, if 600 rad (6 Gy) is a lethal dose to a mouse, then in the presence of a radioprotective agent 1200 rad (12 Gy) would be required to produce lethality. Radioprotective agents have not found human application because, to be effective, they must be administered in toxic levels. Thus the protective agent can be worse than the radiation.

RADIATION DOSE-RESPONSE RELATIONSHIPS

Radiobiology is a relatively new science. Although some scientists worked with animals to observe the effects of radiation within a few years after the discovery of x-rays, these studies were not experimentally sound nor were their results applied. Interest in radiobiology increased enormously, however, during the 1940s with the advent of the atomic age.

The object of nearly all radiobiologic research is the establishment of radiation dose-response relationships. A dose-response relationship is a mathematical relationship between different radiation doses and the magnitude of the observed response.

Radiation dose-response relationships have two important applications in radiology. First, these experimentally determined relationships are used to design therapeutic treatment routines for patients with cancer. Second, radiobiologic studies have been designed to provide information on the effects of low-dose irradiation. These studies and the dose-response relationships obtained are the basis for the radiation control activities. Radiation control is of significance to diagnostic imaging.

Linear Dose-Response Relationships

Every radiation dose-response relationship has two characteristics. It is either **linear** or **nonlinear,** and it is either **threshold** or **nonthreshold.** These characteristics can be described mathematically. The various radiation dose-response relationships are illustrated on the following graphs.

Figure 34-4 shows examples of the simplest type. The linear dose-response relationship is so called because the response is directly proportional to the dose. When the radiation dose is doubled, the response to radiation is likewise doubled.

Dose-response relationships A and B intersect the dose axis at zero or below (see Figure 34-4). A and B relationships are therefore **linear, nonthreshold.** In a nonthreshold dose-response relationship, any dose, regardless of its size, is expected to produce a response. At zero dose, relationship A exhibits a measurable response, R_A. The level R_A is called the *ambient,* or natural, response level and indicates the type of response (cancer for instance) that occurs even without a radiation exposure.

Dose-response relationships C and D are identified as **linear, threshold** because they intercept the dose axis at some value greater than zero. The threshold doses for C and D are D_C and D_D, respectively. At doses below these values, no response would be expected. Relationship D has a steeper slope than C and, therefore, above the threshold dose, any increment of dose will produce a larger response if that response follows relationship D rather than C.

Nonlinear Dose-Response Relationships

All other radiation dose-response relationships are defined as nonlinear (Figure 34-5). Curves A and B are **nonlinear, nonthreshold.** Curve A shows that a large response will result from very little radiation dose. At high dose levels the radiation is not so efficient, since an incremental dose at high levels results in less rela-

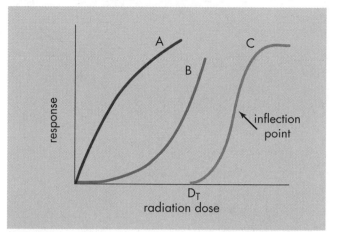

FIGURE 34-5 Nonlinear dose-response relationships can assume several shapes.

tive damage than the same incremental dose at low levels.

The dose-response relationship represented by curve B is just the opposite. Incremental doses in the low-dose range result in very little response. At high doses, however, the same increment of dose will produce a much larger response.

Curve C is a **nonlinear, threshold** relationship. At doses below D_C no response will be measured. As the dose is increased above D_C, it becomes increasingly effective per increment of dose until it reaches the dose corresponding to the inflection point of the curve. Above this level, incremental doses become less effective. Relationship C is sometimes called an *S-type,* or **sigmoid-type,** dose-response relationship.

These general types of radiation dose-response relationships are referred to in discussing the forms of human radiation injury. Diagnostic x-ray imaging is almost exclusively concerned with the late effects of radiation exposure and therefore with linear, nonthreshold dose-response relationships. For completeness, however, Chapter 36 contains a brief discussion of early radiation damage.

Constructing a Dose-Response Relationship

Determining the radiation dose-response relationship for a whole-body response is complex. It is very difficult to determine the degree of response, even that of early effects, because the number of experimental animals that can be used is relatively small. It is nearly impossible to measure low-dose, late effects, and that is the area of greatest interest to diagnostic imaging.

Therefore scientists resort to irradiating a limited number of animals to very large doses of radiation in hopes of observing a statistically significant response. Figure 34-6 shows the results of such an experiment in which four groups of animals were irradiated at different doses. The observations on each group results in an

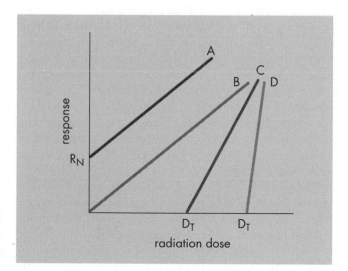

FIGURE 34-4 Linear dose-response relationships *A* and *B* are nonthreshold types; *C* and *D* are threshold types.

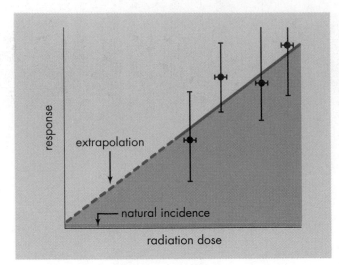

FIGURE 34-6 A dose-response relationship is produced by extrapolating high-dose experimental data to low doses.

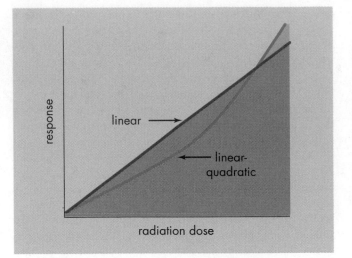

FIGURE 34-7 The linear, quadratic dose-response relationship applies to low-dose, low-LET, late radiation effects.

ordered pair of data: (1) a dose and (2) the associated biologic response.

The error bars in each ordered pair indicate the confidence associated with each data point. The error bars on the dose measurements are very narrow; one radiation dose can be measured very accurately. The error bars on the response, however, are very wide because of biologic variability and the limited number of observations at each dose.

The principal interest in diagnostic imaging is to estimate the response at very low radiation doses. Since this cannot be done directly, scientists **extrapolate** the dose-response relationship from the high-dose, known region into the low-dose, unknown region. This invariably results in a **linear, nonthreshold** dose-response relationship. Such an extrapolation, however, may not be correct because of the many qualifying conditions on the experiment.

Linear, Quadratic Dose-Response Relationship

In 1980 the Committee on the Biological Effects of Ionizing Radiations (BEIR) of the National Academy of Sciences completed an exhaustive study of scientific data bearing on the effects of low doses of low-LET radiation. These findings are directly applicable to diagnostic imaging.

The committee's conclusion at that time stated that effects follow a **linear, quadratic dose-response relationship** (Figure 34-7). The essence of its finding is that the linear, nonthreshold relationship overestimates the risk associated with diagnostic radiation.

In 1990, with an additional 10 years of human data to apply, the BEIR committee revised its radiation risk estimates and adopted the linear, nonthreshold dose-response relationship as most appropriate. Consequently, research scientists and medical physicists use

the **linear, nonthreshold** model for establishing radiation protection guidance that reflects a safe approach.

SUMMARY

In 1906, two French scientists first theorized that radiosensitivity was a function of the metabolic state of tissue being irradiated. Their theories have been found to be true. The Law of Bergonie and Tribondeau states the following: (1) stem cells are radiosensitive, mature cells are less so, (2) young tissue is more radiosensitive than older tissue, (3) high metabolic activity is radiosensitive, and (4) increases in proliferation and growth rates of cells makes them more radiosensitive.

There are physical and biologic factors affecting radiosensitivity of tissue. The physical factors are the LET (rate at which energy is transferred from radiation to soft tissue), RBE (as LET increases, the damage to tissue increases), fractionation (dose delivered over a long time), and protraction (a lower dose delivered continuously). The biologic factors affecting radiosensitivity are the oxygen effect (aerobic state of tissue is more radiosensitive), the age-related effect (human fetus is most sensitive to radiation than adults), and the recovery effect (intracellular recovery is due to the inherent repair biochemistry of the cell). Some chemicals can modify the response of cells. They are called *radiosensitizers* and *radioprotectors*.

Radiobiology research concentrates on radiation dose-response relationships. A radiation dose-response relationship is the relationship between different doses and the magnitude of the observed response. In linear dose-response relationships the response is directly proportional to the dose. In nonlinear dose-response relationships, varied responses are produced from varied doses. The threshold dose-response (greater than 0 on the dose axis) is the level below which there is no response. The nonthreshold dose-response (0 or below on the dose axis) relationship means that any dose is expected to produce a response. For establishing radiation protection guidelines for diagnostic imaging, the linear, nonthreshold model is used.

REVIEW QUESTIONS

1. Name the French scientists who theorized about the radiosensitivity of human tissue. State the law that bears their names.

2. The response of radiated biologic tissue is determined principally by _____.

3. Linear energy transfer is the measure of _____.

4. The LET for diagnostic x-rays is _____ (refer to Table 34-1).

5. Define RBE. Write the RBE formula.

6. Give examples of fractionated and protracted doses.

7. When is high pressure (hyperbaric) oxygen used in radiation therapy?

8. Write the OER formula. Define the oxygen effect.

9. How does age of the host affect the radiosensitivity of the tissue?

10. Define in vitro.

11. When an organ is radiated and shrinks in size, this is called _____.

12. Agents that enhance the effect of radiation are called _____.

13. Name three agents that enhance the effect of radiation.

14. Name three radioprotective agents.

15. Are radioprotective agents used for human application? Why or why not?

16. Define the radiation dose-response relationship.

17. In a linear dose-response relationship _____.

18. What occurs in a nonlinear dose-response relationship?

19. Define threshold and nonthreshold dose-response relationships.

20. Explain why the linear, nonthreshold dose-response relationship is used as a model for diagnostic imaging radiation protection guidelines?

Additional Reading

Beer JZ, Dean CJ, Lett JT: In memoriam Peter Alexander (1922-1993) and the genesis of modern cellular radiation biology, *Radiat Res* 143(3):352 September, 1995.

Dowd SB: The practice of radiobiology in the radiologic sciences, *Radiol Technol* 66(1):25 September-October, 1994.

Elking MM: Enhanced risks of cancer from protected exposures to x- or gamma-rays: a radiobiological model of radiation-induced breast cancer, *Br J Cancer* 73(2):133 January, 1996.

Fienendegen LE, Loken MK, Booz J, Muhlensiepen H, Sondhaus CA, Bond VP: Cellular mechanisms of protection and their consequences for cell system responses, *Stem Cells* 13:7 May, 1995.

Gray LH, Mottram JC, Read J, Spear FG: Some experiments upon the biological effects of fast neutrons, *Br J Radiol* 68(809):H101 May, 1995.

35

Molecular and Cellular Radiobiology

OBJECTIVES

At the completion of this chapter the student will be able to:

1. Discuss the three effects of in vitro irradiation of macromolecules
2. Explain the radiation effects on DNA macromolecules
3. Write the formulas and discuss the radiolysis of water
4. Relate the effects of in vivo irradiation
5. Describe the principles of the target theory of radiobiology
6. Discuss the cell survival kinetics of human cells in the radiobiology laboratory

OUTLINE

Irradiation of Macromolecules
Main-chain scission
Cross-linking
Point lesions
Macromolecular synthesis
Radiation effects on DNA
Radiolysis of Water
Direct and Indirect Effect

Target Theory
Cell Survival Kinetics
Single-target, single-hit model
Multitarget, single-hit model
Recovery
Cell cycle effects
LET, RBE, and OER

ven though the initial interaction between radiation and tissue occurs at the atomic level, it is believed that observable human radiation injury results from change at the molecular level. The occurance of molecular lesions is categorized into effects on macromolecules and effects on water. Irradiation of macromolecules and the radiolysis of water is discussed in this chapter. Since the human body is an aqueous solution containing 80% water molecules, radiation interaction with water is the principal radiation interaction in the body.

IRRADIATION OF MACROMOLECULES

The results of irradiation of macromolecules differ from those of irradiation of water. When macromolecules are irradiated **in vitro,** that is, outside the body or outside the cell, a larger radiation dose is required to produce a measurable effect than with **in vivo** irradiation. This demonstrates that molecules are considerably more radiosensitive in their natural state. When macromolecules are irradiated in solution in vitro, the following three major effects occur: (1) **main-chain scission,** (2) **cross-linking,** and (3) **point lesions** (Figure 35-1).

Main-chain Scission

Main-chain scission is the breakage of the thread or backbone of the long-chain macromolecule. The result is the reduction of a long, single molecule into many smaller molecules, each of which may still be macromolecular in nature. Main-chain scission not only reduces the size of the macromolecule but also the **viscosity** of the solution. A viscous solution is one that is very thick and slow to flow, such as cold maple syrup. Tap water, on the other hand, has a low viscosity. Measurements of viscosity are used to determine the degree of main-chain scission.

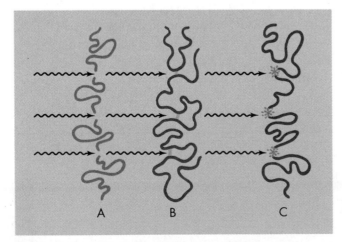

FIGURE 35-1 The results of irradiation of macromolecules. **A,** Main-chain scission. **B,** Cross-linking. **C,** Point lesions.

Cross-linking

Some macromolecules have small, spurlike molecules extending off the main chain. Others produce them as a consequence of irradiation. After irradiation, these side structures can behave as though they had a sticky substance on the end, and they will attach to a neighboring macromolecule or to another segment of the same molecule. This process is called *cross-linking*. Radiation-induced molecular cross-linking increases the viscosity of a macromolecular solution.

Point Lesions

Radiation interaction with macromolecules can result in disruption of single chemical bonds, which produces **point lesions** in a molecule. Such point lesions are not detectable by current analytic techniques, but they can result in a minor modification of the molecule, which can in turn cause it to malfunction in the cell. At low radiation doses, point lesions are considered to be the cellular radiation damage process, which results in the late radiation effects observed at the whole-body level.

Laboratory experiments have shown that all these types of radiation effects on macromolecules are reversible through intracellular repair and recovery.

Macromolecular Synthesis

Modern molecular biology has developed a generalized scheme for the function of a normal human cell. Molecular nutrients are brought to the cell and diffused through the cell membrane, where they are broken down (**catabolized**) into smaller molecular units with an accompanying release of energy. This energy is expended in several ways, but one of the more important ways is in the construction, or **synthesis,** of macromolecules from smaller molecules (**anabolism**). The synthesis of proteins and nucleic acids is critical to the survival of the cell and to cell reproduction.

In Chapter 33 the scheme of protein synthesis and its dependence on nucleic acids are described. Proteins are manufactured by **translation** of the genetic code from tRNA, which in turn is **transferred** from mRNA. The information carried by the mRNA is in turn **transcribed** from the DNA. This chain of events is shown schematically in Figure 35-2.

Radiation damage to any of these macromolecules may result in cell death or late effects. Proteins occurring abundantly are continuously synthesized throughout the cell cycle. Furthermore, multiple copies of specific protein molecules are always present in the cell. Consequently, proteins are less radiosensitive than the nucleic acids.

Similarly, multiple copies of both types of RNA molecules are present in the cell, although RNA molecules are not as abundant as protein molecules. On the other hand, the DNA molecule, with its unique assembly of

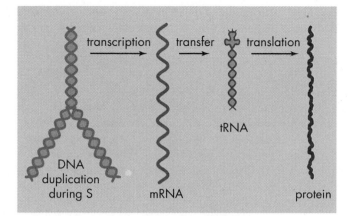

FIGURE 35-2 The genetic code of DNA is transcribed by mRNA and transferred to tRNA, which translates it into a protein.

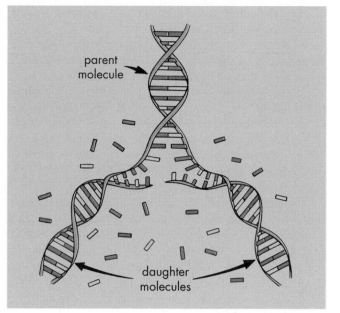

FIGURE 35-3 During S phase, the DNA separates like a zipper and two daughter DNA molecules are formed, each alike and each a replicate of the parent molecule.

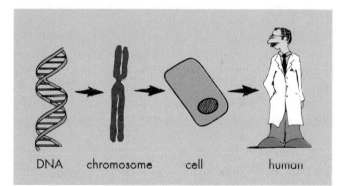

FIGURE 35-4 DNA is the most important molecule subject to radiation damage. It forms chromosomes and controls cell and human growth and development.

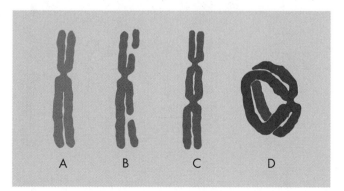

FIGURE 35-5 Normal and radiation-damaged human chromosomes. **A,** Normal. **B,** Terminal deletion. **C,** Dicentric formation. **D,** Ring formation.

bases, is not so abundant. Therefore DNA is the most radiosensitive of these macromolecules.

DNA is synthesized somewhat differently than proteins. During the G_1 portion of interphase, the deoxyribose, phosphate, and base molecules accumulate in the nucleus. These molecules combine to form one large molecule that, during the S portion of interphase, is attached to an existing single chain of DNA (Figure 35-3). During G_1, the molecular DNA is in the familiar double-helix form. As the cell moves into S phase, the ladder begins to open up in the middle of each rung, much like a zipper. At this point the DNA consists of only a single chain, and there is no pairing of bases. This state does not exist long, however, because the combined base-sugar-phosphate molecule attaches to the single strand DNA sequence as determined by the permitted base pairing. Consequently, where there was one double-helix DNA molecule, there are two similar molecules, each a duplicate of the original. In G_2, there is twice as much DNA as in G_1. The parent DNA is said to be replicated into two duplicate DNA daughter molecules.

Radiation Effects on DNA

Deoxyribonucleic acid is the most important molecule in the human body because it contains the genetic information for each cell. Each cell has a nucleus containing DNA complexed with other molecules in the form of chromosomes. The chromosomes therefore control the growth and development of the cell, which in turn determine the characteristics of the individual (Figure 35-4).

If radiation damage to the DNA is sufficiently severe, visible chromosome aberrations may be detected. Figure 35-5 is a representation of a normal chromosome and several distinct types of chromosome aberrations. Radiation-induced **chromosome aberrations,** or **cytogenetic damage,** is discussed more completely in Chapter 36.

The DNA molecule can be damaged without the production of a visible chromosome aberration. Although such damage is reversible, it can lead to cell death. If enough cells of the same type respond similarly, then a particular tissue or organ can be destroyed.

Damage to the DNA can also result in abnormal metabolic activity. The uncontrolled rapid proliferation of cells is the principal characteristic of radiation-induced malignant disease. If the damage to the DNA occurs in a germ cell, it is possible that the response to the radiation exposure will not be observed until the following generation or even later.

The chromosome contains miles of DNA, and therefore when a visible aberration does appear, it signifies a considerable amount of radiation damage. Unobserved damage to the DNA is also responsible for responses at the cell and whole-body level. The types of damage that can occur in the DNA molecule fall into the following categories, which were previously discussed for macromolecules:

1. Main-chain scission with only one side rail severed
2. Main-chain scission with both side rails severed
3. Main-chain scission and subsequent cross-linking
4. Rung breakage causing a separation of bases
5. A change or loss of a base

Damage types 1 through 4 are diagrammed schematically in Figure 35-6. Although each of these effects results in a structural change in the DNA molecule, they are all reversible. In some of these types of damage the sequence of bases can be altered, and therefore the triplet code of codons may not remain intact.

The fifth type of damage, the change or loss of a base, also destroys the triplet code and may not be reversible. This type of radiation damage is a molecular lesion of the DNA and causes genetic mutation.

These molecular lesions are called *point mutations* and can be of either minor or major importance to the cell. One critical consequence of such point mutations is the transfer of the incorrect genetic code to one of the two daughter cells. This sequence of events is shown in Figure 35-7.

In summary, there are the following three principal observable effects resulting from irradiation of DNA: (1) cell death, (2) malignant disease, and (3) genetic damage. The latter two effects at the molecular level conform to the linear, nonthreshold dose-response relationship (any dose is expected to produce a tissue or cellular response).

RADIOLYSIS OF WATER

Since the human body is an aqueous solution containing approximately 80% water molecules, irradiation of water represents the principal radiation interaction in the body. When water is irradiated, it dissociates into other molecular products. This dissociation action is termed the **radiolysis of water** (Figure 35-8).

When an atom of water (H_2O) is irradiated, it is ionized and dissociates into two ions (an ion pair) as shown by the following equation:

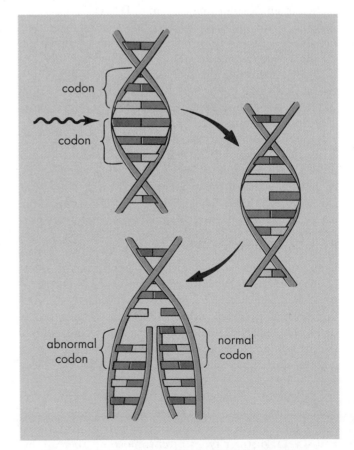

FIGURE 35-7 Point mutation results in the change or loss of a base, which creates an abnormal codon. This is therefore a genetic mutation that is passed to one of the daughter cells.

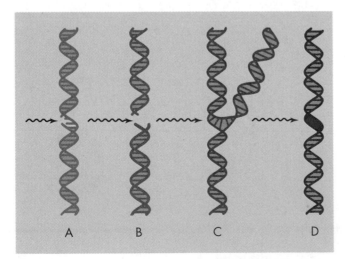

FIGURE 35-6 Types of damage that can occur in DNA. **A,** One side rail severed. **B,** Both side rails severed. **C,** Cross-linking. **D,** Rung breakage.

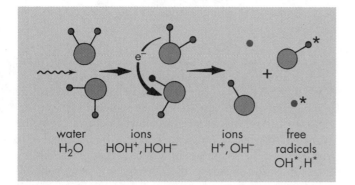

FIGURE 35-8 Radiolysis of water results in the formation of ions and free radicals.

$$H_2O + \Uparrow \to HOH^+ + e^-$$

After this initial ionization, a number of reactions can happen. First the ion pair may rejoin into a stable water molecule. In this case, no damage occurs. Second, if these ions do not rejoin, it is then possible for the negative ion (the electron) to attach to another water molecule by the following reaction and produce yet a third type of ion:

$$H_2O + e^- \to HOH^-$$

The HOH^+ and HOH^- ions are relatively unstable and can dissociate into still smaller molecules as follows:

$$HOH^+ \to H^+ + OH^*$$
$$HOH^- \to OH^- + H^*$$

The final result of the radiolysis of water is the formation of an ion pair, H^+ and OH^-, and two free radicals, H^* and OH^*. The ions can recombine, and therefore no biologic damage would occur. These types of ions are not unusual. Many molecules in aqueous solution exist in a loosely ionized state because of their structure. Salt (NaCl), for instance, easily dissociates into Na^+ and Cl^- ions. Even in the absence of radiation, water can dissociate into H^+ and OH^- ions.

The free radicals are another story. A free radical is an uncharged molecule containing a single unpaired electron in the valence or outermost shell. This causes them to be highly reactive. Free radicals are unstable and therefore exist with a lifetime of less than 1 millisecond. During that time, however, they are capable of diffusion through the cell and interaction at a distant site. Free radicals contain excess energy that can be transferred to other molecules to disrupt bonds and produce point lesions at some distance from the initial ionizing event.

The H^* and OH^* molecules are not the only free radicals that are produced during the radiolysis of water. The OH^* free radical can join with a similar mole-

cule and form hydrogen peroxide by the following equation:

$$OH^* + OH^* \to H_2O_2$$

Hydrogen peroxide is poisonous to the cell and therefore acts as a toxic agent.

The H^* free radical can interact with molecular oxygen if it is present to form the hydroperoxyl radical:

$$H^* + O_2 \to HO^*_2$$

The hydroperoxyl radical, along with hydrogen peroxide, is considered to be the principal damaging product after the radiolysis of water. Hydrogen peroxide can also be formed by interaction of two hydroperoxyl radicals:

$$HO^*_2 + HO^*_2 \to H_2O_2 + O_2$$

Some organic molecules, symbolized as RH, can become reactive free radicals as follows:

$$RH + \Uparrow \to RH^* \to H^* + R^*$$

When oxygen is present, yet another species of free radical is possible:

$$R^* + O_2 \to RO^*_2$$

DIRECT AND INDIRECT EFFECT

When biologic material is irradiated in vivo, the harmful effects of irradiation occur because of damage to a particularly sensitive molecule such as DNA. If the initial ionizing event occurs on that molecule, the effect is said to be direct. Evidence for the direct effect of radiation comes from in vitro experiments in which various molecules are irradiated in solution. The effect is produced by ionization of the target molecule.

On the other hand, if the initial ionizing event occurs on a distant, noncritical molecule that transfers the energy of ionization to the target molecule, the **indirect effect** has occurred. Free radicals, with their excess energy of reaction, are the intermediate molecules. They migrate to the target molecule and transfer their energy, which results in damage to that target molecule.

It is not possible to identify whether the damage to the target molecule resulted from direct or indirect effect. Since the human body is 80% water, however, it follows that the principal action of radiation on humans is indirect. Most would agree that more than 95% of the effects of irradiation in vivo occur via indirect effect. When oxygen is present, as in living tissue, the indirect effects are amplified because of the additional types of free radicals that are formed.

TARGET THEORY

The cell contains many species of molecules, most of which exist in overabundance. Radiation damage to such molecules probably would not result in noticeable injury to the cell because additional similar molecules would be available to continue to support the cell. On the other hand, there are some molecules in the cell that are necessary for normal cell function. These molecules are not in abundant supply, and, in fact, there may be only one such molecule. Radiation damage to such a molecule could affect the cell severely, since there would be no similar molecules available as substitutes.

This concept of a sensitive key molecule is the basis for the **target theory.** According to target theory, for a cell to die after radiation exposure, its target molecule must be inactivated (Figure 35-9). There is considerable experimental evidence in support of the target theory that suggests overwhelmingly that the key molecular target is the DNA. Originally, target theory was used to represent cell lethality. It can be used equally well, however, to describe nonlethal radiation-induced cell abnormalities.

In target theory the target is considered to be an area of the cell occupied by the target molecule or by a sensitive site on the target molecule. This area changes position with time because of intracellular molecular movement.

The interaction between radiation and cellular components is random. In addition, interaction with the target molecule is a random event. Its sensitivity to radiation occurs simply because of its vital function in the cell.

When an interaction does occur between radiation and the target, a hit is said to have occurred. Radiation interaction with molecules other than the target molecule can also result in a hit. Hits occur through both the direct and the indirect effect. It is not possible to distinguish between a direct and an indirect hit.

When a hit occurs through indirect effect, the size of the target appears considerably larger because of the mobility of the free radicals. This increased target size contributes to the importance of the indirect effect of radiation.

Figure 35-10 illustrates some of the consequences of using target theory to explain the relationships among LET, the oxygen effect, and direct versus indirect effect. With low-LET radiation, in the absence of oxygen, the probability of a hit on the target molecule is low because of the relatively large distances between ionizing events. If oxygen is present, reactive free radicals are formed and the volume of effectiveness surrounding each ionization is enlarged. Consequently the probability of a hit is increased.

With the use of high-LET radiation, the distance between ionizations is so close that the probability of a hit by direct effect is high, possibly higher than that for the low-LET, indirect effect. When oxygen is added to the system and high-LET radiation is used, the effect of the radiation may not be increased. The added sphere of influence for each ionizing event, although somewhat larger, will not result in additional hits, since the maximum number of hits has already been produced by direct effect with the high-LET radiation.

CELL SURVIVAL KINETICS

Early radiation experiments at the cell level were conducted with simple cells such as bacteria. It was not until the middle 1950s that laboratory techniques were developed to allow the growth and manipulation of human cells in vitro. These techniques required the development of an artificial growth medium that would nourish a human cell. Now cells can be grown in tubes, flasks, Petri dishes, or nearly any type of laboratory container.

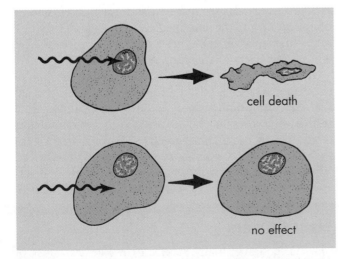

FIGURE 35-9 According to target theory, cell death occurs only if the target molecule is inactivated.

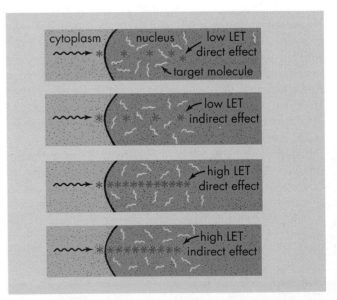

FIGURE 35-10 In the presence of oxygen the indirect effect is amplified and the volume of action for low-LET radiation is enlarged. The effective volume of action for high-LET radiation remains unchanged, since maximum injury will have been inflicted by direct effect.

One technique for measuring the lethal effects of radiation on cells is shown in Figure 35-11. If normal cells are planted individually in a Petri dish and incubated for 10 to 14 days, they divide many times and produce a visible **colony** consisting of as many as 1000 cells. This is **cloning.** After irradiation of such single cells, some will not survive, and therefore fewer colonies are formed. The higher the radiation dose, the fewer colonies formed. This allows the lethal effects of radiation to be determined by observing cell survival.

Using a mathematic extension of target theory, two models of cell survival result. The models are the radiation dose-response relationships for the cell. The **single-target, single-hit** model applies to biologic targets such as enzymes, viruses, and simple cells like bacteria. The **multitarget, single-hit** model applies to more complicated biologic systems such as human cells. The following discussion concerns the equation of these models. The mathematics of these models is relatively unimportant but is given here for the interested student.

Single-Target, Single-Hit Model

Consider for a moment the situation illustrated in Figure 35-12. A large concrete runway containing 100 squares is shown in the rain. A square is considered wet when one or more raindrops have fallen on it. When the first drop falls on the pavement, 1 of the 100 squares will be wet. When the second drop falls, it will probably fall on a dry square and not the one already wet. Consequently, two out of 100 squares will be wet. When the third raindrop falls, there will probably be three wet and 97 dry squares. As the number of raindrops increases, however, it will become more probable that a given square will be hit by two or more drops.

Because the raindrops are falling **randomly,** the probability that a square will become wet is governed by a statistical law called the ***Poisson distribution.*** According to this law, when the number of raindrops is equal to the number of squares (100 in this case), 63% of the squares will be wet and 37% of the squares will be dry. If the raindrops had fallen **uniformly,** all 100 squares would become wet with 100 raindrops.

Obviously, many of the 63 squares in this example have been hit twice and even more. When the number of raindrops equals twice the number of squares, then 0.37×0.37, or 14, squares will be dry. After 300 raindrops, only five squares will remain dry. A graph of the number of dry squares as a function of the number of raindrops is shown in Figure 35-13. If the number of squares exposed to the rain were large or unknown, the scale on the right, expressed in percent, would be used.

Like raindrops, radiation interacts randomly with matter. The wet squares analogy can be extended to the irradiation of a large number of biologic specimens, for example, 1000 bacteria. The bacteria presumably contains a single sensitive site, or **target,** that must be inactivated for the cell to die. As the 1000 cells are irradiated with increasing increments of dose, more cells will be killed (Figure 35-14). Just as with the wet squares, however, as the dose increases, some cells will suffer two or more hits. All hits per target in excess of one represent wasted radiation dose, since the bacteria had already been killed by the first hit. Remember, a hit is not simply an ionizing event but rather an inactivating ionization in the target molecule.

When the radiation dose reaches a level sufficient to kill 63% of the cells (37% survival), it is called D_{37}. If there were no wasted hits, that is, uniform interaction, D_{37} is the dose that would be sufficient to kill 100% of

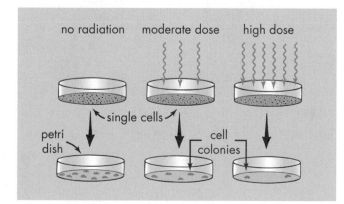

FIGURE 35-11 When single cells are planted in a Petri dish, they grow into visible colonies. Fewer colonies develop if the cells are irradiated.

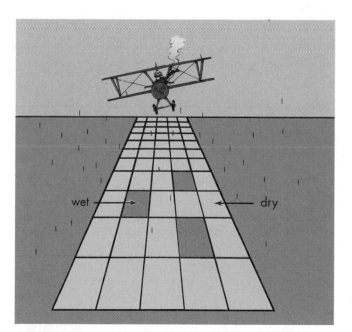

FIGURE 35-12 When rain falls on a dry pavement consisting of a large number of squares, the number of squares that remains dry decreases exponentially as the number of raindrops increases.

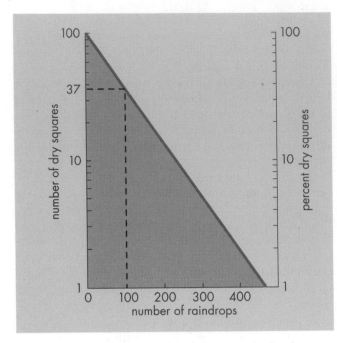

FIGURE 35-13 When the number of dry squares is plotted on semilog paper as a function of the number of raindrops, a straight line results because after a few drops some squares will be hit more than once.

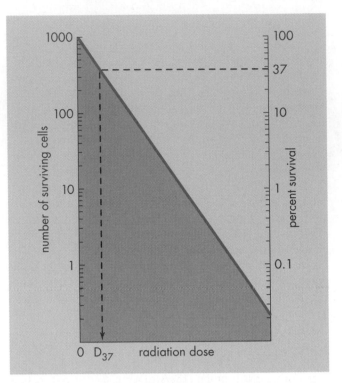

FIGURE 35-14 Dose-response relationship after the irradiation of 1000 cells with graded doses of radiation is exponential. D_{37} is that dose that results in 37% survival.

the cells. After a dose equal to $2 \times D_{37}$, 14% of the cells would survive, and so on. D_{37} is a measure of the radiosensitivity of the biologic specimen. A low D_{37} represents a highly radiosensitive specimen, and a high D_{37} represents radioresistance.

The equation that describes the dose-response relationship represented by the graph in Figure 35-14 is as follows:

$$S = N/N_o = e^{-D/D_{37}}$$

S is the surviving fraction, N is the number of cells surviving a dose D, N_0 is the initial number of cells, and D_{37} is a constant dose related to the cell radiosensitivity. The equation is the single-target, single-hit model of radiation-induced lethality.

Multitarget, Single-Hit Model

Returning to the wet squares analogy, suppose that each pavement square were divided into two equal parts (Figure 35-15). By definition, each half must now be hit with a raindrop for the square to be considered wet. The first few raindrops will probably hit only one half of any given square, and therefore, after a very light rain, no squares may be wet. Many raindrops must fall before any single square suffers a hit in both halves so that it can be considered wet. This represents a **threshold phenomenon**, since, according to our definition, a number of raindrops can fall and all squares will remain dry.

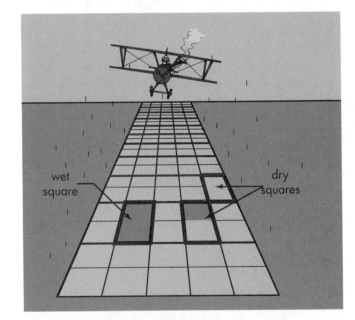

FIGURE 35-15 If each pavement square has two equal parts, each will have to be hit for the square to be considered wet.

As the number of raindrops increases, the point will be reached when some squares will have both halves hit and therefore be considered wet. This portion of the curve is represented by region A in Figure 35-16. When a large number of raindrops has fallen, region C will be reached, and every square will have at least one half

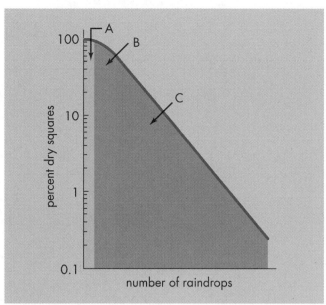

FIGURE 35-16 When a square contains two equal parts, both of which have to be hit to be considered wet, three regions of the graphic relationship can be identified.

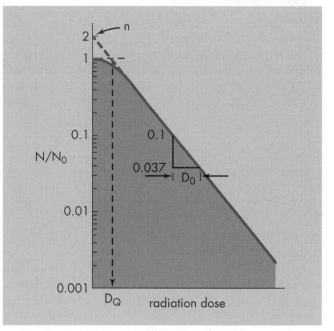

FIGURE 35-17 The multitarget, single-hit model of cell survival is characteristic of human cells containing two targets.

wet. When this occurs, each additional raindrop will produce a wet square. In region C the relation between number of raindrops and wet squares is that described by the single-target, single-hit model. The intermediate region B is the region of accumulation of hits.

Complex biologic specimens such as human cells are thought to have more than a single critical target. Suppose that the human cell has two targets, each of which has to be inactivated for the cell to die. This would be analogous to the square having two halves, each of which had to be hit by rain for it to be considered wet. Figure 35-17 is a graph of single-cell survival for human cells having two targets.

At very low radiation doses there will be nearly 100% cell survival. As the radiation dose increases, fewer cells will survive because more will have sustained a hit in both target molecules. At some higher radiation dose, all cells will have sustained at least one hit in one of its two targets. All cells that survive this dose will have one target hit, and therefore at all higher doses the dose-response relationship would appear as the single-target, single-hit model.

The model of cell survival just described is the **multitarget, single-hit** model. The equation of this model is as follows:

$$S = N/N_0 = 1 - (1 - e^{-D/D_0})n$$

S is the surviving fraction, N is the number of cells surviving a dose D, N_0 is the initial number of cells, D_0 is the dose necessary to reduce survival by 37% in the straight-line portion of the graph, and n is the **extrapolation number.**

The D_0 is called the **mean lethal dose,** and it is a constant related to the radiosensitivity of the cell. It is equal to D_{37} in the linear portion of the curve and therefore represents the dose that would result in one hit per target in the straight-line portion of the graph if no radiation were wasted. As with D_{37} of the single target, single-hit model, a large D_0 indicates a radioresistant cell line, and a small D_0 is characteristic of radiosensitive cells.

The extrapolation number is also called the *target number.* When this type of experiment was first conducted with human cells, the observed extrapolation number was 2. That result agreed with the hypothesis that similar regions on two homologous chromosomes (an identical pair) had to be inactivated to produce cell death. Since chromosomes come in pairs, the experimental results confirmed the hypothesis.

Subsequent experiments, however, have resulted in extrapolation numbers ranging from 2 to 12, and therefore the precise meaning of n is unknown. The D_Q is called the *threshold dose.* It is a measure of the width of the shoulder of the multitarget, single-hit model and is related to the capacity of the cell to recover from sublethal damage. A large D_Q indicates that the cell can readily recover. Table 35-1 lists reported values for D_0 and D_Q for various experimental cell lines.

Recovery

The shoulder of the graph of the multitarget, single-hit model shows that for mammalian cells some damage must be accumulated before the cell dies. This accumulated damage is termed *sublethal damage.* The wider

TABLE 35-1

The Reported Mean Lethal Dose (D_0) and
Threshold Dose (D_Q) for Various Experimental
Mammalian Cell Lines

Cell Type	D_0 (Rad)	D_Q (Rad)
Mouse oocytes	91	62
Mouse skin	135	350
Human bone marrow	137	100
Human fibroblasts	150	160
Mouse spermatogonia	180	270
Chinese hamster ovary	200	210
Human lymphocytes	400	100

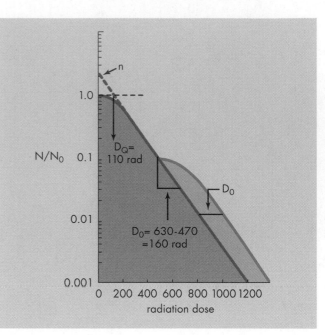

FIGURE 35-18 Split-dose technique results in a second cell survival curve with the precise characteristics of the first displaced along the dose axis by D_Q.

the shoulder, the more sublethal damage that can be sustained and the higher the value of D_Q.

Figure 35-18 demonstrates the results of a **split-dose technique** designed to describe the capacity of a cell to recover from sublethal damage. This illustration shows a rather typical human cell survival curve with $D_0 = 160$ rad (1.6 Gy), $D_Q = 110$ rad (1.1 Gy), and n = 2. If one takes those cells that survive any large dose (e.g., 470 rad [4.7 Gy]) and reincubates them in a growth medium, they will grow into another large population.

This new population of cells can then be used to perform a second cell survival experiment. When the cells that survived the first dose are subsequently subjected to additional incremental radiation doses, a second dose-response curve will be generated that has precisely the same shape as the first. The extrapolation number is the same, the mean lethal dose is the same, and it is separated along the dose axis from the first dose-response curve by D_Q. The time between such split doses must be at least as long as the cell generation time for full recovery to occur.

Such experiments show that cells that survive an initial radiation insult exhibit precisely the same characteristics as nonirradiated cells, and therefore they have fully recovered from the sublethal damage produced by the initial irradiation. Consequently, D_Q is not only a measure of the capacity to accumulate sublethal damage but also a measure of the ability of the cell to recover from sublethal damage.

Question: From Figure 35-18, estimate the overall surviving fraction for a cell receiving a split dose of 400 rad followed by 400 rad (4 Gy).

Answer: At a dose of 400 rad approximately 0.15 of the cells survive. Therefore, at a split dose of 400 rad and 400 rad, the surviving fraction should equal $0.15 \times 0.15 = 0.023$. The total dose is 800 rad (8 Gy), and the surviving fraction on the split-dose curve at 800 rad should equal 0.023 and it does. Had the 800 rad been delivered at one time, the surviving fraction would have been 0.012, as shown by the single-dose curve of Figure 35-18.

Cell Cycle Effects

When human cells replicate by mitosis, the average time from one mitosis to another is called the *cell cycle time* or the *generation time*. Most human cells that are in a state of normal proliferation have generation times of 10 to 20 hours. Some specialized cells have generation times extending to hundreds of hours, and some cells, such as neurons (nerve cells), do not normally proliferate. Longer generation times usually result from a lengthening of the G_1 phase of the cell cycle.

Techniques are now available for taking a randomly growing population of cells that are uniformly distributed in position throughout the cell cycle and **synchronizing** them. A population of synchronized cells can then be subdivided into smaller populations and irradiated sequentially as they pass through the phases of the cell cycle.

Figure 35-19 is representative of results that are obtained from human fibroblasts. The fraction of cells surviving a given dose can vary by a factor of ten from the most sensitive to the most resistant phase of the cell cycle. This pattern of change in radiosensitivity as a function of phase in the cell cycle is known as the *age-response function*. It varies from cell type to cell type, but the results illustrated in Figure 35-19 are characteristic of most human cells. Cells in mitosis are always most sensitive. The fraction of surviving cells will be the lowest in this phase. The next most sensitive phase of the cell cycle occurs at the G_1-S transition. The most resistant portion of the cell cycle occurs in late S phase.

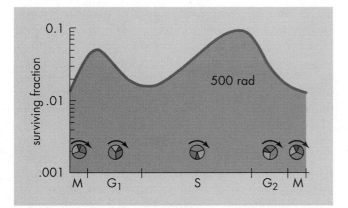

FIGURE 35-19 Age-response function for human fibroblasts. Such cells are most radiosensitive during mitosis and most radioresistant during the late S.

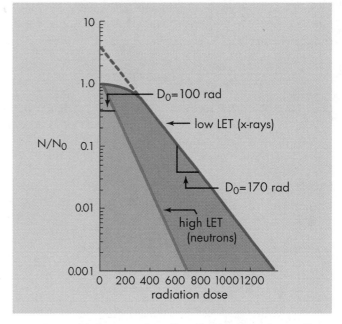

FIGURE 35-20 Representative cell survival curves for human fibroblasts after exposure to 200 kVp x-rays and 14 MeV neutrons.

LET, RBE, AND OER

Mammalian cell survival experiments have been used extensively to measure the effects of various types of radiation and to determine the magnitude of various dose-modifying factors such as oxygen. Since the mean lethal dose, D_0, is related to radiosensitivity, the ratio of D_0 for one condition of irradiation compared with another will be a measure of the effectiveness of the dose modifier, whether it is physical or biologic.

If the same cell type is irradiated by two different radiations under identical physical and biologic conditions, results may appear as in Figure 35-20. At the very high-LET values (as with alpha particles and neutrons), even with mammalian cells, the cell survival kinetics follow the single-target, single-hit model. With low-LET radiation (x-rays) the multitarget, single-hit model is representative. The mean lethal dose after low-LET irradiation is always greater than that after high-LET irradiation. If the low-LET D_0 is representative of x-rays, then the ratio of these D_0s will equal the RBE for the high-LET radiation.

$$RBE = \frac{D_0 \text{ (standard radiation)}}{D_0 \text{ (test radiation) to produce the same effect}}$$

Question: Figure 35-20 shows the radiation dose-response relationship to human fibroblasts exposed to x-rays and to 14 MeV neutrons. The D_0 after radiation is 170 rad (1.7 Gy); the D_0 for neutron irradiation is 100 rad. What is the RBE of 14 MeV neutrons relative to x-ray?

Answer: $RBE = \dfrac{170 \text{ rad}}{100 \text{ rad}}$

$= 1.7$

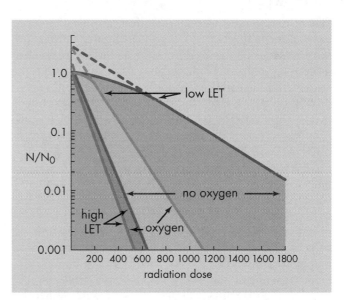

FIGURE 35-21 Cell survival curves for human cells irradiated in the presence and absence of oxygen with high- and low-LET radiation.

The most completely studied dose modifier is oxygen. In the presence of oxygen the effect of low-LET radiation is maximal. When hypoxic or anoxic cells are exposed, a considerably higher dose is required to produce a given effect. When high-LET radiation is used, there is little difference between the response of oxygenated cells and anoxic cells. Figure 35-21 shows typical cell survival curves for each of these combinations of LET and oxygen.

Such experiments are designed to measure the magnitude of the oxygen effect. The OER determined from single cell survival experiments is defined as follows:

$$OER = \frac{D_0 \text{ (anoxic)}}{D_0 \text{ (oxygenated)}} \text{ to produce the same effect}$$

Question: With reference to Figure 35-21, what is the estimated OER for human cells exposed to low-LET radiation and to high-LET radiation?

Answer: Low-LET, no oxygen $D_0 = 340$ rad

Low-LET, oxygen $D_0 = 140$ rad

$$OER = \frac{340 \text{ rad}}{140 \text{ rad}} = 2.4$$

High-LET, no oxygen, $D_0 = 90$ rad

High-LET, oxygen $D_0 = 70$

$$OER = \frac{90}{70} = 1.3$$

SUMMARY

When macromolecules in solution are irradiated in vitro, three major effects occur: (1) Main-chain scission, the breakage of the backbone of a long-chain macromolecule, occurs. (2) Side sections of the macromolecule attach to a neighboring macromolecule and cross-linking occurs. (3) Disruption of single chemical bonds in a macromolecule by irradiation cause point lesions. All these types of damage are reversible through intracellular repair and recovery.

DNA with its unique assembly of bases is not abundant in the cell. As a result, DNA is the most radiosensitive of all macromolecules. Chromosome aberrations or abnormal metabolic activity can result from DNA irradiation and damage. There are three observable effects of DNA irradiation: cell death, malignant disease, and genetic damage.

Because the human body is 80% water, irradiation of water is the principal interaction in the body. When radiated, water dissociates into free radicals that are highly reactive. Free radicals are capable of diffusion through the cell and can cause point lesions at some distance from the ionizing event. The initial ionizing event is said to be a direct effect. If the ionizing event occurs and transfers the energy of ionization to a distant target molecule, the indirect effect has occurred.

The concept of a sensitive key molecule in a cell is the basis for the target theory. For a cell to die after radiation exposure, according to the target theory, the target molecule must be inactivated.

After radiation exposure, two models of cell survival result. The models are derived from human cell colony growth experiments in laboratories. Because radiation reacts randomly with matter, according to the Poisson Distribution law, these complex models of cell survival have been developed to explain dose-response relationships. The single-target, single-hit model is used mostly for simple cells such as bacteria. The single-target, single-hit model is the mathematical description of radiation-induced lethality. The multitarget, single-hit model states that at low radiation doses there is 100% cell survival. However, at higher doses, the relationship becomes a single-hit, single-target (lethal dose) model. Experiments in cell recovery show that cells have the ability to recover from sublethal radiation damage. Finally, experiments also show that cells in mitosis are most sensitive to radiation damage; however, within the cell cycle, the most resistant portion occurs in the late S phase.

REVIEW QUESTIONS

1. Contrast the terms *in vivo* and *in vitro*.

2. List the effects of irradiation of macromolecules in solution in vitro. Explain each molecular damage process.

3. How is solution viscosity used to determine the degree of radiation macromolecular damage?

4. At low radiation doses, _____ _____ are considered to result in late radiation effects at the whole body level.

5. Define catabolism and anabolism.

6. In what phase does the DNA ladder open up in the middle of each rung and consist of only a single chain?

7. Name the three principal observable effects of DNA irradiation.

8. Differentiate between transcription, transfer, and translation when applied to molecular genetics.

9. Draw a diagram illustrating the point mutations of DNA that transfer the incorrect genetic code to one of the two daughter cells.

10. The human body is an aqueous solution containing approximately _____ water.

11. Write the formula for the radiolysis of water in which the atom of water is ionized and dissociates into two ions.

12. Define free radical. What is the reactive state of free radicals within the cell?

13. If the initial ionizing event occurs on a molecule, the effect is said to be _____.

14. If the initial ionizing event occurs on a distant, noncritical molecule and the energy of ionization has transferred to the target molecule, an _____ _____ has occurred.

15. Discuss the target theory of radiobiology.

16. Using the target theory, discuss the relationships among LET, the oxygen effect, and direct/indirect effect.

17. Scientists can isolate human cells in the laboratory by planting individual cells that divide many times and produce a visible _____, consisting of as many as 1000 cells.

18. Explain the Poisson Distribution statistical law. State the radiobiologic concept that the Poisson Distribution law supports.

19. Write the equation for the single-target, single-hit model of dose-response relationships.

20. Write the equation for the multitarget, single-hit model of dose-response relationships.

Additional Reading

Dowd SB: The practice of radiobiology in the radiologic sciences, *Radiol Technol* 66(1):25 September-October, 1994.

Elking MM: Enhanced risks of cancer from protected exposures to x- or gamma-rays: a radiobiological model of radiation-induced breast cancer, *Br J Cancer* 73(2):133 January, 1996.

Fienendegen LE, Loken MK, Booz J, Muhlensiepen H, Sondhaus CA, Bond VP: Cellular mechanisms of protection and their consequences for cell system responses, *Stem Cells* 13:7 May, 1995.

Hahnfeldt P, Hlatky L: Resensitization due to redistribution of cells in the phases of the cell cycle during abitrary radiation protocals, *Radiat Res* 145(2):134 February, 1996.

36 Early Effects of Radiation

OBJECTIVES

At the completion of this chapter the student will be able to:

1. Describe the three syndromes that follow an acute radiation incident
2. Identify the two stages leading to acute radiation lethality
3. Define $LD_{50/30}$
4. Discuss local tissue damage as a result of localized irradiation
5. Explain the early effects of acute radiation syndrome to the hemopoietic system
6. Review the cytogenetic effects of acute radiation syndrome

OUTLINE

Acute Radiation Lethality
    Prodromal syndrome, latent period, and manifest illness
    Hematologic syndrome
    Gastrointestinal (GI) syndrome
    Central nervous system (CNS) syndrome
    $LD_{50/30}$
Local Tissue Damage
    Effects on skin
    Effects on gonads

Hematologic Effects
    Hemopoietic system
    Hemopoietic cell survival
Cytogenetic Effects
    Normal karotype
    Single-hit chromosome aberrations
    Multihit chromosome aberrations
    Kinetics of chromosome aberration

To produce a radiation response in humans in days or weeks, the dose must be substantial. These early effects of radiation exposure are never encountered in diagnostic radiology today. Many years ago, however, early effects were the principal responses observed in radiologists, radiographers, and even some patients involved in diagnostic x-ray examinations.

For a radiographer in practice during the 1920s and the 1930s, it would not have been unusual to visit the hematology laboratory once a week for a routine blood examination. Before the introduction of personnel radiation monitors, the only monitoring performed on x-ray and radium workers was a periodic blood examination. The examination included total cell counts and a white cell (leukocyte) differential count. Most institutions had a radiation safety regulation such that, if the leukocytes were depressed by greater than 25% of normal level, the employee was either given time off or assigned to nonradiation activities until the count returned to normal. What was not entirely understood at this time was that the minimum whole-body dose necessary to produce a measurable hematologic depression was approximately 25 rad (250 mGy). These workers were being heavily irradiated by today's standards.

- - - - - - - - - - - - - - - - - -

ACUTE RADIATION LETHALITY

Early effects have been studied completely with animals in the laboratory. There is some data available from observations on humans. Table 36-1 lists the principal early effects of radiation exposure on humans, as well as the minimum radiation dose for each effect.

Death is, of course, the most devastating human response to radiation exposure. No cases of death after diagnostic x-ray exposure have been recorded, although some early x-ray pioneers died from the **late effects** of x-ray exposure. In each of these cases, however, the total radiation dose was extremely high by today's standards.

TABLE 36-1		
The Principal Early Effects of Radiation Exposure on Humans and the Approximate Minimum Radiation Dose Necessary to Produce Them		
Effect	Anatomic Site	Minimum Dose (Rad)
Death	Whole body	100
Hematologic depression	Whole body	25
Skin erythema	Small field	300
Epilation	Small field	300
Chromosome aberration	Whole body	5
Gonadal dysfunction	Local tissue	10

Acute radiation-induced human lethality is only of academic interest in diagnostic radiology. Diagnostic x-ray beams are neither sufficiently intense nor sufficiently large to cause death. Diagnostic x-ray beams result in partial-body exposure.

Some accidental exposures of persons in the nuclear weapons and nuclear energy fields have resulted in immediate death, but the number of such accidents has been small considering the length of the atomic age. The unfortunate incident at Chernobyl in April 1986 is the one notable exception. After Chernobyl, 30 people died of acute radiation syndrome, and a number of late effects are expected. No one died or was even seriously exposed in the March 1979 incident at the nuclear power reactor at Three-Mile Island. Employment in the nuclear industry is still considered a safe occupation.

The sequence of events after high-level radiation exposure that leads to death within days or weeks is called **acute radiation syndrome.** There are, in fact, three separate syndromes that are dose related and that follow a rather distinct course of events. These syndromes are called (1) *hematologic death,* (2) *gastrointestinal (GI) death,* and (3) *central nervous system (CNS) death.*

Prodromal Syndrome, Latent Period, and Manifest Illness

In addition to the three lethal syndromes, there are three other stages of acute radiation lethality. The **prodromal syndrome** consists of acute clinical symptoms that occur within hours of the exposure and continue for up to a day or two. After the prodromal syndrome, there may be a **latent period,** during which time the subject is free of visible effects.

The clinical signs and symptoms of the **manifest illness stage** of acute radiation lethality can be classified into the following three principal groups: hematologic, gastrointestinal, and neuromuscular. The hematologic signs relate to changes in the cells of the peripheral blood. Red cells (erythrocytes), white cells (leukocytes), and platelets (thrombocytes) are reduced in number in the blood after exposure. The gastrointestinal symptoms are nausea, vomiting and diarrhea, anorexia, intestinal cramps, dehydration, and weight loss. Neuromuscular symptoms are listlessness, apathy, sweating, fever, headache, and hypertension.

At radiation doses above approximately 100 rad delivered to the total body, the signs and symptoms of radiation sickness may appear within a matter of minutes to hours. The symptoms of this early radiation sickness most often take the form of nausea, vomiting, diarrhea, and a reduction in the white cells of the peripheral blood (**leukopenia**). This immediate radiation sickness is the prodromal syndrome.

The prodromal syndrome may last from a few hours to a couple of days. The severity of the symptoms is dose related, and at doses in excess of 1000 rad (10 Gy) the symptoms can be rather violent. At still higher doses the duration of the prodromal syndrome becomes shorter, until it is difficult to separate the prodromal syndrome from the stage of manifest illness.

After the period of initial radiation sickness, there is a period of apparent well-being. In the latent period, there is no sign of radiation sickness. The latent period will extend from hours or less (at doses in excess of 5000 rad) to weeks (at doses from 100 to 500 rad). The latent period is sometimes mistakenly thought to indicate the early recovery from a moderate radiation dose. It may be quite different, however, giving no indication of the extensive radiation response yet to follow. The prodromal syndrome and the latent period lead to the manifestation of the illness that results in hematologic, GI, and CNS syndromes.

Hematologic Syndrome

Radiation doses in the range of approximately 200 to 1000 rad produce the **hematologic syndrome.** The subject initially experiences mild symptoms of the prodromal syndrome, which appear in a matter of a few hours and may persist for several days. The latent period that follows can extend as long as 4 weeks and is characterized by a general feeling of well-being. There are no obvious signs of illness, although the number of cells in the peripheral blood decline during this time.

The period of manifest illness is characterized by possible vomiting, mild diarrhea, malaise, lethargy, and fever. Hematologic syndrome is characterized by a reduction in numbers of white cells, red cells, and platelets in the circulating blood. Each of these types of cells follows rather characteristic patterns of cell depletion. If the dose is not lethal, recovery begins in 2 to 4 weeks, but it may take as long as 6 months for full recovery.

If the radiation injury is sufficiently severe, the reduction in blood cells will continue unchecked until the body's defense against infection is nil. Just before death, hemorrhage and dehydration may be pronounced. Death occurs because of generalized infection, electrolyte imbalance, and dehydration.

The dose necessary to produce a given syndrome and the mean survival time are the principal quantitative measures of human radiation lethality (Table 36-2). Although ranges of effective dose and resulting mean survival times are given, it should be clear that there is rarely a precise difference in the dose and time-related sequence of events associated with each syndrome. At very high radiation doses the latent period disappears altogether. At very low radiation doses there may be no prodromal syndrome and consequently no associated latent period.

Gastrointestinal (GI) Syndrome

After radiation doses extending from approximately 1000 to 5000 rad (10 to 50 Gy), the **gastrointestinal (GI) syndrome** occurs. The prodromal symptoms of vomiting and diarrhea occur within hours of exposure and persist for hours to as long as a day. A latent period of 3 to 5 days follows, during which time no symptoms are present.

The manifest illness stage begins with a second wave of nausea and vomiting, followed by diarrhea. The individual experiences a loss of appetite (**anorexia**) and may become lethargic. Diarrhea persists and increases in severity, leading to loose and then watery and bloody stools. Supportive therapy is unable to prevent the rapid progression of symptoms that ultimately leads to death within 4 to 10 days of exposure.

Death occurs principally because of severe damage to the cells lining the intestines. These cells are normally in a rapid state of proliferation and are continuously being replaced by new cells. The turnover time for this cell renewal system in a normal individual is 3 to 5 days. Radiation exposure kills the most sensitive cells, the stem cells, and this controls the length of time until death. When the intestinal lining is completely denuded of functional cells, there is uncontrolled passage of fluids across the intestinal membrane, a severe destruction of electrolyte balance, and conditions promoting infection.

At doses consistent with the GI syndrome, damage to the hematologic system will also occur. The cell renewal system of the blood takes a longer time of development into mature cells from the stem cell population, and

TABLE 36-2

Summary of Acute Radiation Lethality

Stage	Dose (Rad)	Mean Survival Time (Days)	Clinical Signs and Symptoms
Prodromal	>100	—	Nausea, vomiting, diarrhea
Latent	100-10,000	—	None
Hematologic	200-1000	10-60	Nausea, vomiting, diarrhea, anemia, leukopenia, hemorrhage, fever, infection
Gastrointestinal	1000-5000	4-10	Same as hematologic, electrolyte imbalance, lethargy, fatigue, shock
Central nervous system	>5000	0-3	Same as GI, ataxia, edema, vasculitis, meningitis

therefore sufficient time is not provided for maximum hematologic effects to occur. There will be measurable and even severe hematologic changes accompanying death.

Central Nervous System (CNS) Syndrome

After a radiation dose in excess of approximately 5000 rad (50 Gy), a series of signs and symptoms occur that lead to death within a matter of hours to 3 days. First, there is an onset of severe nausea and vomiting, usually within a few minutes of exposure. During this time, the individual may become extremely nervous and confused, complain of a burning sensation in the skin, and may lose vision and perhaps consciousness within the first hour. This may be followed by a latent period lasting up to 12 hours, during which time the earlier symptoms subside or disappear.

After the latent period is the period of manifest illness, when the symptoms of the prodromal stage return more severely. The person becomes disoriented, loses muscle coordination, has difficulty breathing, may go into convulsive seizures, experiences loss of equilibrium, **ataxia,** and lethargy, lapses into a coma, and dies.

Regardless of the medical attention given the patient, the symptoms of manifest illness appear rather suddenly and always with extreme severity. At radiation doses sufficiently high to produce central nervous system effects, the outcome has always been death within a few days of exposure.

The cause of death in CNS syndrome is apparently the elevated fluid content of the brain, which results in increased intracranial pressure, inflammatory changes in the blood vessels of the brain (**vasculitis**), and inflammation of the meninges (**meningitis**).

At doses sufficient to produce CNS damage, damage to all other organs of the body would be equally as severe. The classical radiation-induced changes in the gastrointestinal tract and the hematologic system cannot occur because sufficient time between exposure and death is not available for their appearance.

The clinical signs and symptoms of each are outlined in Table 36-2. Table 36-2 also shows that death resulting from CNS syndrome requires radiation doses in excess of 5000 rad (50 Gy) and results in death within hours. Death resulting from hematologic and GI syndromes follow lower exposures and require a long time for death to occur.

LD$_{50/30}$

If one irradiates experimental groups of animals with varying doses of radiation, for example, 100 to 1000 rad (1 to 10 Gy), a plot of the percentage of animals that die as a function of the radiation dose would appear as in Figure 36-1. This figure illustrates the radiation dose-response relationship for acute human lethality. It is a threshold relationship and nonlinear. At the

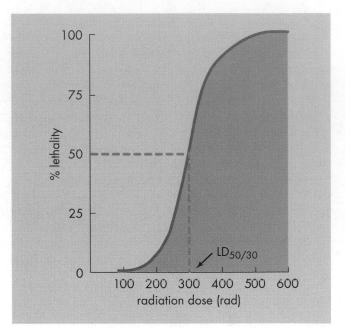

FIGURE 36-1 Radiation-induced death in humans follows a nonlinear, threshold dose-response relationship.

lower dose of approximately 100 rad (1 Gy), no one is expected to die, whereas above approximately 600 rad (6 Gy), all those so irradiated would die unless vigorous medical support was available. Above 1000 rad (10 Gy) even vigorous medical support will not prevent death.

If death is to occur, it will usually happen within 30 days of exposure. Acute radiation lethality is measured quantitatively by the LD$_{50/30}$. The LD$_{50/30}$ is the dose of radiation to the whole body that will result in death within 30 days to 50% of the subjects so irradiated. The LD$_{50/30}$ for humans is estimated to be approximately 300 rad (3 Gy). With clinical support humans can tolerate much higher doses, the maximum is reported to be 850 rad (8.5 Gy). Table 36-3 lists values of LD$_{50/30}$ for various experimental species and humans.

Sometimes additional measures of acute lethality are identified. LD$_{10/30}$ and LD$_{90/30}$ indicate a dose resulting in 10% lethality or 90% lethality within 30 days, respectively. LD$_{50/60}$ is the lethal dose to 50% when the observed survival time is extended for 60 days. Normally, this is not much different from the LD$_{50/30}$.

Question: From Figure 36-1, estimate the radiation dose that will produce 25% lethality in humans within 30 days.

Answer First, draw a horizontal line from the 25% level on the y-axis until it intersects the S curve. Now drop a vertical line from this point to the x-axis. This intersection with the x-axis occurs at the LD$_{25/30}$, which is approximately 250 rad (2.5 Gy).

TABLE 36-3

LD$_{50/30}$ for Various Species After Whole-body X-radiation

Species	LD$_{50/30}$ (Rad)
Pig	250
Dog	275
Human	300
Guinea pig	425
Monkey	475
Opossum	510
Mouse	620
Goldfish	700
Hamster	700
Rat	710
Rabbit	725
Gerbil	1050
Turtle	1500
Armadillo	2000
Newt	3000

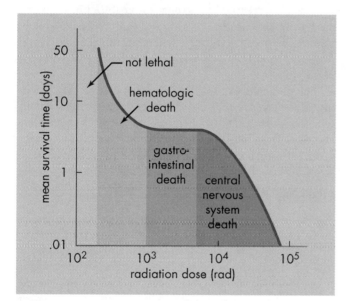

FIGURE 36-2 Mean survival time after radiation exposure shows three distinct regions. If death is due to hematologic or CNS effects, the mean survival time will depend on the dose. If GI effects cause death, it occurs in approximately 4 days.

As the whole-body radiation dose increases, the average time between exposure and death decreases. This time is known as the *mean survival time*. A plot of radiation dose versus mean survival time is shown in Figure 36-2. There are three distinct regions to this plot, and they are associated with the three radiation syndromes.

As the radiation dose increases from 200 to 1000 rad (2 to 10 Gy), the mean survival time decreases from approximately 60 to 4 days, and this region is consistent with death resulting from the hematologic syndrome.

Mean survival time is dose dependent with the hematologic syndrome. In the dose range associated with the GI syndrome, however, the mean survival time remains relatively constant at 4 days. With larger doses, those associated with the CNS syndrome, the mean survival time is again dose dependent, varying from approximately 3 days to a matter of hours.

LOCAL TISSUE DAMAGE

When only part of the body is irradiated, compared with whole-body irradiation, a higher dose is needed to produce a response. Every organ and tissue of the body can be affected by partial-body irradiation. The effect is cell death, resulting in a shrinkage, or reduction in size (**atrophy**), of the tissue or organ. This can lead to a total nonfunction of that tissue or organ or it can be followed by recovery.

There are many examples of local tissue damage immediately after radiation exposure. In fact, if the dose is high enough, there will be a response in any tissue. The manner in which local tissues respond depends on their intrinsic radiosensitivity and the kinetics of cell proliferation and maturation. Examples of local tissues that can be affected immediately are the skin, the gonads, and bone marrow.

Effects on Skin

Normal skin consists of three layers—an outer layer (the epidermis), an intermediate layer of connective tissue (the dermis), and a subcutaneous layer of fat and connective tissue. There are additional accessory structures in the skin, such as hair follicles, sweat glands, and sensory receptors. All the cell layers and the accessory structures participate in the response to radiation exposure.

The skin, like the lining of the intestine, represents a continuing cell renewal system, only at a much slower rate than that experienced by intestinal cells. Almost 50% of the cells lining the intestine are replaced every day, whereas the skin cells are replaced at the rate of only 2% per day. The outer skin layer, the epidermis, consists of several layers of cells, and the lowest layer is made up of **basal cells**. The basal cells are the **stem cells** that mature as they slowly migrate to the surface of the epidermis. Once these cells arrive on the surface as mature cells, they are slowly lost and have to be replaced by new cells from the basal layer. It is damage to these basal cells that results in the earliest manifestation of radiation injury to the skin.

Before the advent of cobalt teletherapy, the limitations of radiation therapy with **orthovoltage x-rays** (200 to 300 kVp x-rays) were determined by the tolerance of the patient's skin. The object of x-ray therapy is to deposit x-ray energy in the tumor while sparing the surrounding normal tissue. Since the x-rays must pass through the skin to reach the tumor, the skin was often necessarily subjected to higher radiation doses than the tumor. The resultant skin damage was **erythema** (a sunburnlike reddening of the skin), followed by **desquamation** (ulceration and denudation of the skin), which often required that the therapy be interrupted.

After a single dose of 300 to 1000 rad (3 to 10 Gy), an initial mild erythema may occur within the first or second day. This first wave of erythema then subsides, only to be followed by a second wave that reaches maximum intensity in about 2 weeks. At higher doses, this second wave of erythema is followed by a moist desquamation, which in turn may lead to a dry desquamation. Moist desquamation is known as *clinical tolerance* for radiation therapy.

In the clinical situation, radiation exposure of the skin is delivered in a fractionated scheme, usually approximately 200 rad per day (2 Gy per day), 5 days a week. To assist the radiotherapist in planning patient treatments, isoeffect curves have been generated that accurately project the dose necessary to produce a skin erythema or clinical tolerance after a prescribed treatment routine (Figure 36-3).

Erythema was perhaps the first observed biologic response to radiation exposure. Many of the early x-ray pioneers, including Roentgen, suffered radiation-induced skin burns. One of the hazards to the patient during the early years of radiology was radiation-induced erythema. During those years, x-ray tube potentials were so low that it was usually necessary to position the tube very close to the patient's skin, and 10- to 15-minute exposures were required to obtain a suitable radiograph. Often the patient would return several days later suffering from an x-ray burn.

These skin effects follow a nonlinear, threshold dose-response relationship similar to that described for radiation-induced lethality. Small doses of radiation do not cause erythema. Extremely high doses of radiation cause erythema in all persons so irradiated. Whether intermediate radiation doses produce erythema depends on the individual's radiosensitivity, the dose rate, and the size of the skin field irradiated. Analysis of persons irradiated therapeutically with superficial x-rays has shown that the **skin erythema dose** required to affect 50% of persons so irradiated (SED_{50}) is about 600 rad (6 Gy).

Before the definition of the roentgen and the development of accurate radiation measuring apparatus, the skin was observed and its response to radiation used in formulating radiation protection practices. The unit used was the SED_{50}, and permissible radiation exposures were specified in fractions of SED_{50}.

Another response of the skin to radiation exposure is **epilation,** or loss of hair. For many years soft x-rays (10 to 20 kVp), called *grenz rays,* were used as the treatment of choice for skin diseases such as ringworm. Ringworm of the scalp, not uncommon in children, was successfully treated by grenz radiation, but unfortunately the patient's hair would fall out for weeks or even months. In some instances, where an unnecessarily high dose of grenz rays was used, the epilation was permanent.

The response of the skin to x-rays is currently receiving more attention because of the higher radiation intensities allowed—20 R/min—and the longer fluoroscopy times required for angiointerventional procedures. Injuries have been reported and steps are being taken to better control such exposures.

Effects on Gonads

The human gonads are critically important target organs. As an example of local tissue effects, they are particularly sensitive to radiation. Responses to doses as low as 10 rad have been observed. Since these organs produce the germ cells that control fertility and heredity, their response to radiation has been studied extensively.

Much of what is known in the area of both the type of radiation response and dose-response relationships has been derived from numerous animal experiments. Some significant data are also available from human populations as well. Radiotherapy patients, radiation accident victims, and volunteer convicts have all provided data to allow a rather complete description of the response of the gonads to radiation.

The cells of the testes, the male gonads, and the ovaries, the female gonads, respond differently to radiation because of differences in progression of the germ cells from the stem cell phase to the mature cell. Figure 36-4 illustrates this progression, indicating the most radiosensitive phase of cell maturation.

Germ cells are produced by both ovaries and testes, but they develop from the stem cell phase to the mature

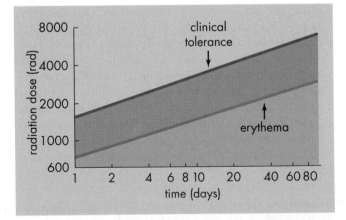

FIGURE 36-3 These isoeffect curves show the relationship between the number of daily fractions and the total radiation dose that will produce erythema or moist desquamation. As the fractionation of the dose increases, so will the total dose required.

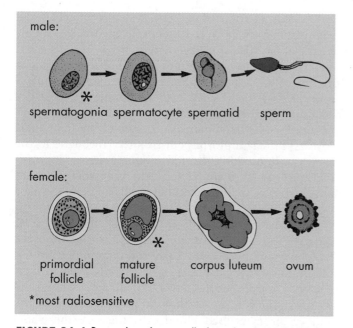

male:

spermatogonia   spermatocyte   spermatid   sperm

female:

primordial   mature   corpus luteum   ovum
follicle   follicle

*most radiosensitive

FIGURE 36-4 Progression of germ cells from the stem cell phase to the mature cell.

cell phase at different rates and at different times. This process of development is called **gametogenesis.** The stem cells of the ovaries are the **oogonia,** and they multiply in number only during fetal life. The oogonia reach a maximum number of about 7 million during midpregnancy and then begin to decline because of spontaneous degeneration.

During late fetal life many **primordial follicles** grow to encapsulate the oogonia, which become **oocytes.** These follicle-containing oocytes remain in a suspended state of growth until puberty. In prepuberty the number of oocytes has been reduced to only several hundred thousand. Commencing at puberty, the follicles rupture with regularity, ejecting a mature germ cell, the **ovum.** There will be only 400 to 500 such ova available for fertilization (number of years of menstruation times thirteen per year).

The germ cells of the testes are continually being produced from stem cells progressively through a number of stages to maturity, and, like the ovaries, the testes provide a sustaining cell renewal system. The male stem cell is the **spermatogonia,** which matures into the **spermatocyte.** The spermatocyte in turn multiplies and develops into a spermatid, which finally differentiates into the functionally mature germ cell, the **spermatozoa,** or **sperm.** The maturation process from stem cell to spermatozoa requires 3 to 5 weeks.

Ovaries. Irradiation of the ovaries early in life will cause a reduction in their size (atrophy) because of germ cell death. After puberty such irradiation also causes a suppression and delay of menstruation. The most radiosensitive cell in female gametogenesis is the oocyte in the mature follicle.

Radiation effects on the ovaries are somewhat age dependent. At the fetal stage and early childhood the ovaries are especially radiosensitive. They decline in sensitivity, reaching a minimum in the 20- to 30-year age range and then increase continually with age. Doses as low as 10 rad (100 mGy) in the mature female may result in the delay or suppression of menstruation. A dose of approximately 200 rad (2 Gy) produces a pronounced temporary sterility; approximately 500 rad (5 Gy) to the ovaries is necessary to produce permanent sterility.

In addition to the destruction of fertility, irradiation of the ovaries of experimental animals has been shown to produce genetic mutations. Even moderate doses such as 25 to 50 rad (250 to 500 mGy) have been associated with measurable increases in genetic mutations. There is also some evidence to indicate that oocytes surviving such a modest dose are capable of repairing some genetic damage as they mature into ova. On the basis of those data, some radiation scientists advise women to abstain from procreation for a period of several months after ovarian doses in excess of 10 rad (100 mGy). The object is to minimize the possibility of genetic mutations in offspring.

Testes. The testes, like the ovaries, atrophy after high doses of radiation. Data on testicular damage have been gathered from observations of volunteer convicts and radiotherapy patients treated for testicular carcinoma in one testis while the other was shielded. Many investigators have recorded normal infants fathered by such patients whose remaining functioning testis received a radiation dose between 50 and 300 rad (0.5 and 3 Gy). Nevertheless, procreation at any time after such testicular irradiation is not advised.

The spermatogonial stem cells are the most sensitive phase in the gametogenesis of the spermatozoa. After irradiation of the testes, the maturing cells, spermatocytes, and spermatids are relatively radioresistant and continue to mature. Consequently, there is no significant reduction in spermatozoa until several weeks after exposure, and therefore fertility continues during this time. At this time the irradiated spermatogonia would have developed into mature spermtaozoa had they survived.

Radiation doses as low as 10 rad (100 mGy) can result in a reduction in the number of spermatozoa (Table 36-4). With increasing dose the depletion of spermatozoa becomes greater and extends over a longer period of time. A dose of 200 rad (2 Gy) produces temporary infertility, which will commence approximately 2 months after irradiation and persist for up to 12 months. A dose of 500 rad (5 Gy) to the testes produces permanent sterility.

Since male gametogenesis is a self-renewing system, there is some evidence to suggest that genetic mutations induced in surviving postspermatogonial cells represent the most hazardous mutations. Consequently, after tes-

TABLE 36-4

Response of Testes to Radiation

Dose (Rad)	Response
10	Minimal aspermia
200	Temporary infertility
500	Sterility

ticular irradiation of doses above approximately 10 rad (100 mGy), the male should refrain from procreation for 2 to 4 months until all cells in the spermatogonial and postspermatogonial stages at the time of irradiation have matured and disappeared. This will reduce but probably not eliminate any increase in genetic mutations because of the persistence of the stem cell. Evidence from animal experiments suggests that there is some repair of genetic mutations even when the stem cell is irradiated.

HEMATOLOGIC EFFECTS
Hemopoietic System

The hemopoietic system consists of bone marrow, circulating blood, and lymphoid tissue. Lymphoid tissues are the lymph nodes, spleen, and thymus. The principal effect of radiation on this system is the depression of the number of blood cells in the peripheral circulation. The time- and dose-related effects on the various types of circulating blood cells are determined by the normal growth and maturation of these cells.

All cells of the hemopoietic system apparently develop from a single type of stem cell (Figure 36-5). This stem cell is called a *pluripotential stem cell* because it has the ability to develop into several different types of mature cells. Although the spleen and thymus manufacture one type of leukocyte (the lymphocyte), most circulating blood cells, including lymphocytes, are manufactured in the bone marrow. In a child the bone marrow is rather uniformly distributed throughout the skeleton. In an adult the active bone marrow responsible for producing circulating cells is restricted to flat bones, such as the ribs, sternum, and skull, and the ends of long bones.

From the single pluripotential stem cell a number of cell types are produced, but principally these are the **lymphocytes** (those involved in the immune response), the **granulocytes** (scavenger type of cells used to fight bacteria), **thrombocytes** (also called platelets and involved in the clotting of blood to prevent hemorrhage), and **erythrocytes** (red blood cells that are the transportation agents for oxygen). These cell lines develop at different rates in the bone marrow and are released to the peripheral blood as mature cells. While in the bone marrow, the cells proliferate in number, differentiate in function, and mature. The developing granulocytes and erythrocytes spend about 8 to 10 days in the bone marrow. Thrombocytes have a lifetime of about 5 days in the bone marrow. Lymphocytes are produced over varying times and have varying lifetimes in the peripheral blood. Some are thought to have lives measured in

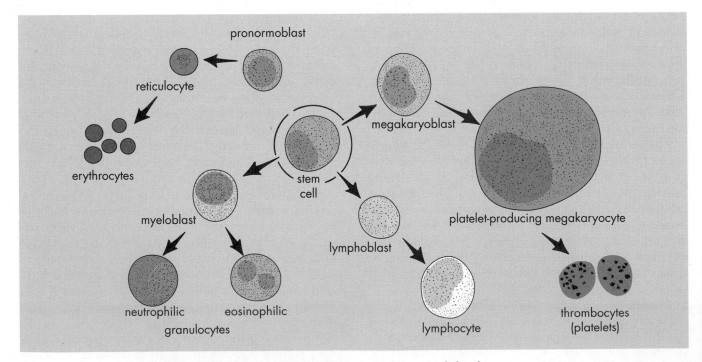

FIGURE 36-5 Four principal types of blood cells—lymphocytes, granulocytes, erythrocytes, and thrombocytes—develop and mature from a single pluripotential stem cell.

terms of hours and others in terms of years. In the peripheral blood the granulocytes have a lifetime of only a couple of days. Thrombocytes have a lifetime of approximately 1 week, and erythrocytes a life span of nearly 4 months.

The hemopoietic system, therefore, is another example of a cell renewal system. The effect of radiation on this system is determined by the normal cell growth and development.

Hemopoietic Cell Survival

The principal response of the hemopoietic system to radiation exposure is a decrease in the number of all types of blood cells in the circulating peripheral blood. Lethal injury to the precursor cells causes the depletion of these mature circulating cells.

Figure 36-6 shows the radiation response of three of the four principal circulating cells. Examples are given for low, moderate, and high radiation doses. The degree of cell depletion increases with increasing dose. These figures are the results of observations on experimental animals, radiotherapy patients, and the few radiation accident victims.

After exposure, the first cells to become affected are the lymphocytes. These cells are reduced in number (**lymphopenia**) within minutes or hours after exposure. They are very slow to recover. The lymphocytes and the spermatogonia are considered the most radiosensitive cells in the body. Because their response is so immediate, the radiation effect is apparently a direct one on the lymphocytes themselves, rather than on the precursor cells.

Granulocytes experience a rapid rise in number (**granulocytosis**), followed first by a rapid decrease and then a slower decrease in number (**granulocytopenia**). If the radiation dose is moderate, then approximately 15 to 20 days after irradiation an abortive rise in granulocyte count may occur. Minimum granulocyte levels are reached approximately 30 days after irradiation. If recovery is to occur, return to normal will take approximately 2 months.

The depletion of platelets (**thrombocytopenia**) after irradiation develops more slowly, again because of the longer time required for the more sensitive precursor cells to reach maturity. Thrombocytes reach a minimum in about 30 days and exhibit recovery in about 2 months, similar to the response kinetics of granulocytes.

The erythrocytes are less sensitive than the other blood cells. This occurs apparently because of the very long lifetime they experience in the peripheral blood. Injury of these cells is not apparent for a matter of weeks. Total recovery may take 6 months to a year.

CYTOGENETIC EFFECTS

Cytogenetics is the study of the genetics of cells, in particular, cell chromosomes. When a cell is irradiated, damage to its chromosomes can occur and this damage takes several characteristic forms.

A technique developed in the early 1950s contributed enormously to human genetic analysis and radiation genetics. The technique calls for a culture of human cells to be prepared and treated so that the chromosomes of each cell can be easily observed and studied. This has re-

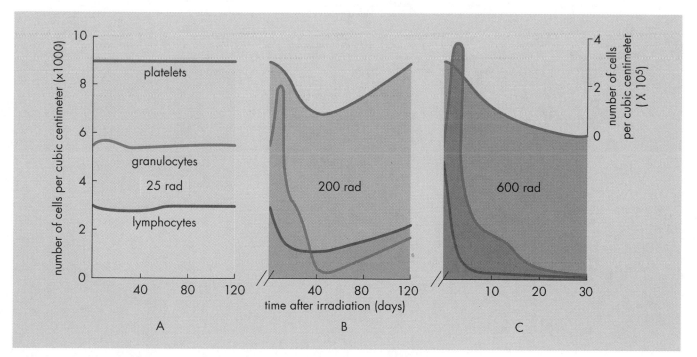

FIGURE 36-6 These graphs show the response of the major circulating blood cells to radiation after different approximate doses. **A,** 25 rad. **B,** 200 rad. **C,** 600 rad.

sulted in many observations on human radiation-induced chromosome damage. Figure 36-7 is a photomicrograph of the chromosomes of a human cancer cell after radiation therapy. The many chromosome aberrations seen represent a high degree of damage. Radiation cytogenetic studies have shown that nearly every type of chromosome aberration can be radiation induced and that some may be specific to radiation. The rate of induction of chromosome aberrations is related in a complex way to the radiation dose, but in every case, it is apparently of the **nonthreshold form.**

Attempts to measure chromosome aberrations in patients after diagnostic radiographic examination have been largely unsuccessful. Some studies involving higher-dose fluoroscopic special procedures have shown the presence of radiation-induced chromosome aberrations soon after the examination.

High doses of radiation, without question, cause chromosome aberrations. Low doses, no doubt, do also, but it is difficult technically to observe aberrations at doses that are less than approximately 5 rad (50 mGy). An even more difficult task is the identification of the link between radiation-induced chromosome aberrations and latent illness or disease.

When the body is irradiated, all cells can suffer cytogenetic damage. Such damage is classified here as an early response to radiation because, if the cell survives, the damage will be manifested during the next mitosis after the radiation exposure. Human peripheral lymphocytes are most often used for cytogenetic analysis, and these lymphocytes do not move into mitosis until stimulated in vitro by an appropriate laboratory technique.

Cytogenetic damage to the stem cells will be sustained immediately but may not be manifested for the considerable time required for that stem cell to reach maturity as a circulating lymphocyte. Consequently, although chromosome damage is produced at the time of irradiation, it can be months and even years before the damage is measured. For this reason some workers who were irradiated in industrial accidents 20 years ago continue to show chromosome abnormalities in their circulating lymphocytes.

Normal Karyotype

The human chromosome consists of many long strings of DNA mixed with a protein and folded back on itself many times. A normal chromosome was shown in Figure 33-11 as it would appear in the G_1 phase of the cell cycle, when only two chromatids are present, and in the G_2 phase of the cell cycle after DNA replication. The chromosome structure of four chromatids represented

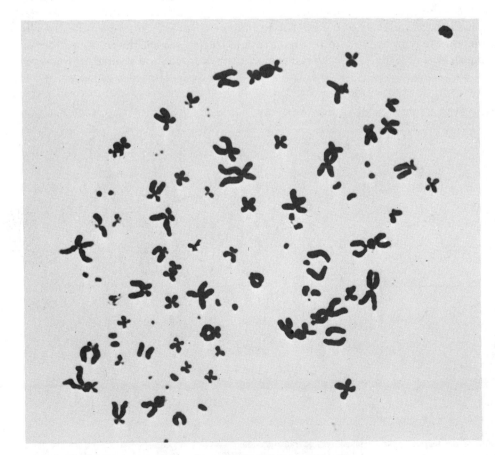

FIGURE 36-7 Chromosome damage in an irradiated human cancer cell.

for the G_2 phase is that which is visualized in the metaphase portion of mitosis.

For certain types of cytogenetic analyses of the chromosomes, photographs are taken and enlarged so that each individual chromosome can be cut out like a paper doll and paired with its sister into a chromosome map, which is called a *karyotype* (Figure 36-8). There are 22 pairs of **autosomes** and one pair of **sex chromosomes**, which are the X chromosome from the female and the Y chromosome from the male.

Structural radiation damage to individual chromosomes can be visualized without constructing a karyotype. These are the single- and double-hit chromosome aberrations. Reciprocal translocations generally require a karyotype for detection. Point genetic mutations are undetectable even with karyotype construction.

Single-Hit Chromosome Aberrations

When radiation interacts with chromosomes, the interaction can occur through direct or indirect effect. In either mode, these interactions result in a **hit**. The hit, however, is somewhat different from the hit described previously in radiation interaction with DNA. The DNA hit results in an invisible disruption of the molecular structure of the DNA. A chromosome hit, on the other hand, produces a visible derangement of the chromosome. This indicates that such a hit has disrupted many molecular bonds and severed many chains of DNA. A chromosome hit represents severe damage to the DNA.

Single-hit effects produced by radiation during the G_1 phase of the cell cycle are shown in Figure 36-9. The breakage of a chromatid is called *chromatid deletion*.

During S phase, both the remaining chromosome and the deletion are replicated. The chromosome aberration visualized at metaphase consists of a normal-looking chromosome with material missing from the ends of two sister chromatids and two acentric fragments (without a centromere). These fragments are called *isochromatids.*

Chromosome aberrations could also be produced by single-hit events during the G_2 phase of the cell cycle (Figure 36-9). The probability of ionizing radiation passing through sister chromatids to produce isochromatids is low. Usually the radiation produces a chromatid deletion in only one arm of the chromosome. The result is a chromosome with an arm that is obviously missing genetic material and a chromatid fragment.

Multihit Chromosome Aberrations

It is possible that a single chromosome will sustain more than one hit. Multihit aberrations are not uncommon (Figure 36-10). In the G_1 phase of the cell cycle, ring chromosomes are produced if the two hits occur on the same chromosome. Dicentrics are produced when adjacent chromosomes each suffer one hit and recombine as shown. The mechanism for the joining of chromatids depends on the quality of **stickiness** that appears at the site of the severed chromosome.

In the G_2 phase of the cell cycle, similar aberrations can be produced; however, such aberrations again require that (1) either the same chromosome be hit two or more times or (2) adjacent chromosomes be hit and joined together. These are rare.

Reciprocal translocations. The multihit chromosome aberrations previously described represent rather severe

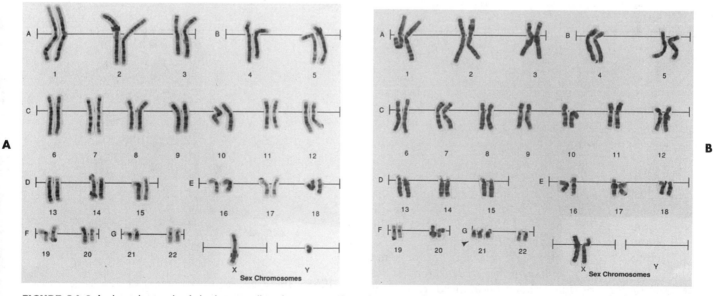

FIGURE 36-8 A photomicrograph of the human cell nucleus at metaphase shows each chromosome distinctly. The karyotype is made from the photograph by cutting and pasting **A,** male **B,** female. *(Courtesy Carolyn Caskey.)*

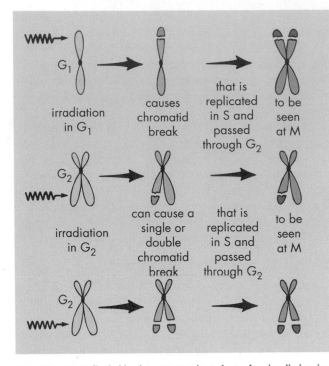

FIGURE 36-9 Single-hit chromosome aberrations after irradiation in G_1 and G_2. The aberrations are visualized and recorded at M.

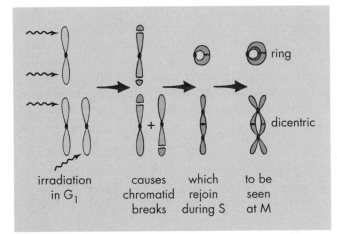

FIGURE 36-10 Multihit chromosome aberrations after irradiation in G_1 phase result in ring and dicentic chromosomes in addition to chromatid fragments. Similar aberrations can be produced by irradiation during G_2, but they are rarer.

damage to the cell. At mitosis the acentric fragments will either be lost or be attracted to only one of the daughter cells, since they are unattached to a spindle fiber. Consequently, one or both of the daughter cells will be missing considerable genetic material.

Reciprocal translocations are multihit chromosome aberrations that require karyotypic analysis for the detection (Figure 36-11). Radiation-induced reciprocal translocations result in no loss of genetic material, simply a rearrangement of the genes. Consequently, all or

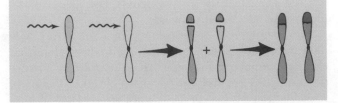

FIGURE 36-11 Radiation-induced reciprocal translocations are multihit chromosome aberrations that require karyotypic analysis for detection.

nearly all genetic codes are available; they simply may be organized in an incorrect sequence.

Kinetics of Chromosome Aberration

At very low doses of radiation, only single-hit types of aberrations are observed. When the radiation dose exceeds perhaps 100 rad (1 Gy), the frequency of multihit aberrations increases more rapidly. Figure 36-12 shows the general dose-response relationship for production of single- and multihit aberrations. Single-hit aberrations are produced with a **linear, nonthreshold** dose-response relationship. Multihit aberrations are produced after a **nonlinear, nonthreshold** relationship. These relationships have been determined experimentally by a number of investigators. The approximate equations for each of these relationships are as follows:

$$\text{Single hit: } Y = a + bD$$

$$\text{Multihit: } Y = a + bD + cD^2$$

Y is the number of single- or multihit chromosome aberrations, a is the naturally occurring frequency of

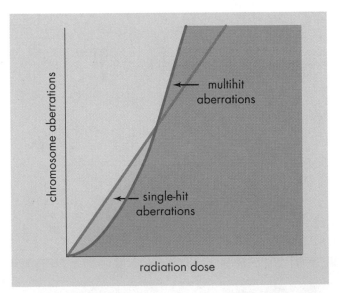

FIGURE 36-12 Dose-response relationship for single-hit aberrations is linear, nonthreshold, whereas that for multihit aberrations is nonlinear, nonthreshold.

chromosome aberrations, and b and c are coefficients of damage for single- and multihit aberrations. The variable, radiation dose, is represented by D.

Some laboratories use cytogenetic analysis as a biologic radiation dosimeter. The multihit aberrations are considered to be the most significant in terms of latent human damage. If the radiation dose is unknown yet not life threatening, the approximate chromosome aberration frequency will be two single-hit aberrations per rad per 1000 cells and one multihit aberration per 10 rad per 1000 cells. This approximation holds through a total dose of perhaps 200 rad.

SUMMARY

After an exposure to a massive dose of radiation (100 to 5000 rad) there can be a response in humans within a few days to a few weeks. This immediate response is called an *early effect of radiation exposure*. The sequence of events after high-level radiation exposure that leads to death within days or weeks is called *acute radiation syndrome* or *acute radiation lethality*. The sequence of events are hematologic syndrome, gastrointestinal (GI) syndrome, and central nervous system (CNS) syndrome. The syndromes are dose related. Death resulting from CNS syndrome requires doses in excess of 5000 rad. In addition to the three lethal syndromes, there are two stages of radiation lethality: (1) prodromal syndrome and (2) manifest illness. Within the prodromal stage there may be a latent period in which the subject is free of visible effects. Table 36-2 summarizes the causes and effects of acute radiation lethality.

$LD_{50/30}$ is the dose of radiation to the whole body in which 50% of the subjects will die within 30 days. For humans, this dose is estimated at approximately 300 rad. As radiation doses increase the time between exposure and death decreases. This time between exposure and death is termed the *mean survival time*.

When only part of the body is irradiated, higher doses are tolerated. The generalized effect is cell death that results in shrinkage or atrophy. Examples of local damage are the effects on the skin, gonads, and bone marrow. The first manifestation of radiation injury to the skin is damage to the basal cells. Located in the lowest layer of the epidermis, the basal cells are the stem cells that mature as they migrate to the surface of the skin. Resulting skin damage is erythema, desquamation, or epilation. Analysis of superficial x-ray therapy has shown that there is a skin dose affecting 50% of subjects with erythema. The skin erythema dose or SED_{50} is 600 rad. The gonads are particularly sensitive to radiation. Irradiation of the ovaries early in life will cause organ atrophy because of germ-cell death. The oocyte in the mature follicle is the most radiosensitive cell during the reproductive cycle. Radiation sensitivity in the female is age-dependent. The fetus and young girls are especially radiosensitive. Sensitivity then declines until the twenties and thirties when it gradually increases with age. Radiation doses can delay or suppress menstruation in a mature female. Radiation doses to the male testes can result in a reduction of spermatozoa. A dose of 200 rad produces temporary infertility. A dose of 500 rad to the testes produces permanent sterility. In the male as in the female, stem-cell development is the most radiosensitive phase. The hemopoietic system consists of bone marrow, circulating blood, and lymphoid tissue. The principal effect of radiation on this system is a depression of the number of blood cells in the peripheral circulation. In the hemopoietic system the pluripotential stem cells develop into several different mature cells, including lymphocytes, granulocytes, thrombocytes, and erythrocytes. Radiation exposure decreases the number of all precursor cells, which reduces the number of mature cells in the circulating blood. Lymphocytes and spermatogonia are considered the most radiosensitive cells in the body.

The study of chromosome damage from radiation exposure is called cytogenetics. Chromosome damage takes on the following different forms: (1) chromatid deletion, (2) ring chromosome aberration, and (3) reciprocal translocations.

REVIEW QUESTIONS

1. Define acute radiation syndrome. What was the result of acute radiation syndrome for thirty people after the Chernobyl nuclear power plant accident in 1986?

2. Using Table 36-1, what is the minimum dose in rad that results in reddening of the skin?

3. Radiation doses of greater than _____ rad results in CNS damage and death in hours.

4. Anorexia is the clinical sign of which syndrome of acute radiation lethality?

5. The time during which the subject is free of visible effects is called the _____ _____.

6. Explain the prodromal syndrome.

7. The clinical signs and symptoms of the manifest illness stage of acute radiation lethality can be classified into what three groups?

8. Which stage of acute radiation syndrome simulates recovery?

9. What causes death in the hematologic syndrome?

10. What doses of radiation result in the gastrointestinal syndrome? What is the length of the latent period?

11. What is the reason death occurs with the GI syndrome?

12. Identify the cause of death from the CNS syndrome and the three resulting conditions.

13. Define LD$_{50/30}$.

14. What radiation dose-response relationship is illustrated for LD$_{50/30}$ by Figure 36-1?

15. What is the LD$_{50/30}$ for the human (Table 36-3)? What is the human SED$_{50}$?

16. What species is most radioresistant on Table 36-3?

17. Describe the stages of gametogenesis in the male and female. Identify the most radiosensitive phases.

18. What cells mature from pluripotential stem cells?

19. Discuss the maturation of basal cells in the epidermis.

20. What two cells are the most radiosensitive cells in the human body?

Additional Readings

Baranov AE, Guskova AK, Nadejina NM, Nugis V: Chernobyl experience: biological indicators of exposure to ionizing radiation, *Stem Cells* 13:69 May, 1995.

Fienendegen LE, Loken MK, Booz J, Muhlensiepen H, Sondhaus CA, Bond VP: Cellular mechanisms of protection and their consequences for cell system responses, *Stem Cells* 13:7 May, 1995.

Katz R: Dose, *J Radiat Res* 137(3):410 March, 1994.

37

Late Effects of Radiation

OBJECTIVES

At the completion of this chapter the student will be able to:

1. Define late effects of radiation exposure and identify the radiation dose needed to produce late effects
2. Discuss the results of epidemiologic studies of persons exposed to radiation
3. List the local tissue effects of low dose radiation to the skin, chromosomes, and the cornea of the eye
4. Discuss the risks of life-span shortening to radiographers and radiologists
5. Explain the estimates of radiation risk
6. Analyze the radiation-induced malignancies of leukemia and cancer
7. Review the risks of low-dose radiation to fertility and pregnancy

OUTLINE

Epidemiologic Studies
Local Tissue Effects
  Skin
  Chromosomes
  Cataracts
Life-span Shortening
  Risks to radiographers
  Risks to radiologists
Risk Estimates
  Relative risk
  Excess risk
  Absolute risk

Radiation-induced Malignancy
  Leukemia
  Cancer
Total Risk of Malignancy
  Three-Mile Island
  BEIR committee
Radiation and Pregnancy
  Effects on fertility
  Irradiation in utero
  Genetic effects

arly effects of radiation exposure are produced by high radiation doses. Late effects of radiation exposure are the result of low doses delivered over a long time period. The radiation exposures experienced by personnel in diagnostic imaging are low dose and low LET. In addition, the exposures in diagnostic imaging are delivered intermittently over long periods of time.

The principal late effects of low-dose radiation over long periods of time are radiation-induced malignancy and genetic effects. Life-span shortening and effects on local tissues have also been reported as late effects, but these are not considered significant. Radiation protection guides are based on the suspected or observed late effects of radiation and on an assumed linear, nonthreshold dose-response relationship.

Late effects are organ, tissue, and cellular damage that occur after low doses of radiation are delivered to a subject over long periods of time. The most important late effects are radiation-induced malignancy and genetic effects. Radiation protection guides in diagnostic imaging are based on the observed late effects of low-dose radiation exposure. Low-dose radiation and late effects present a linear, nonthreshold dose-response relationship.

EPIDEMIOLOGIC STUDIES

Studies of large numbers of people exposed to toxic substances require statistical manipulation of data. These studies are called *epidemiologic studies* and are required when the number of persons responding is small. Epidemiologic studies of people exposed to radiation are difficult because (1) the dose is usually not known but is presumed to be low, and (2) the frequency of response is very low. Consequently the results of radiation epidemiologic studies do not carry the statistical accuracy that observations of early radiation effects do.

Table 37-1 illustrates the difficulty of the problem. It shows the minimum number of persons that must be observed as a function of radiation dose to definitely link an increase in the incidence of leukemia with the radiation dose in question.

LOCAL TISSUE EFFECTS
Skin

In addition to the acute effects of erythema and desquamation and late developing carcinoma, chronic irradiation of the skin can result in severe nonmalignant changes. Early radiologists who performed fluoroscopic examinations without protective gloves developed a very callused, discolored, and weathered appearance to the skin of their hands and forearms. In addition, the skin would be very tight and brittle and sometimes severely crack or flake. The dose necessary to produce such an effect is very high.

Chromosomes

Irradiation of blood-forming organs can produce hematologic depression as an early response or leukemia as a late response. Chromosome damage in the circulating lymphocytes can be produced as both an early and a late response.

The types and frequency of chromosome aberrations have previously been described, but even a low dose of radiation can produce chromosome aberrations that may not be apparent until many years after the radiation exposure. For example, individuals irradiated accidentally with rather high radiation doses continue to show chromosome abnormalities in their peripheral lymphocytes as long as 20 years afterward. This presumably occurs because of radiation damage to the lymphocytic stem cells. These cells may not be stimulated into replication and maturation for many years.

Cataracts

In 1932, E.O. Lawrence of the University of California developed the first **cyclotron,** a 5-inch diameter machine capable of accelerating charged particles to very high energies. These charged particles are used as "bullets" and are shot at the nuclei of target atoms in the study of nuclear structure. By 1940, every university physics department of any worth had built its own cyclotron and was engaged in what has come to be called *high-energy physics.*

The modern cyclotron is used principally to produce radionuclides for use in nuclear medicine (Figure 37-1). The largest particle accelerator in the world was to be constructed near Waxahachie, Texas (Figure 37-2). This superconducting supercollider, nicknamed SuperClyde, measures 50 miles around.

Early machines were usually located in one room, and a beam of high-energy particles would be extracted through a tube and steered and focused by electromagnets onto the target material in the adjacent room. At that time, sophisticated electronic equipment was not

TABLE 37-1

Minimum Population Sample Required to Show that the Given Radiation Dose Significantly Elevated the Incidence of Leukemia

Dose (Rad)	Required Sample Size (Number of People)
5	6,000,000
10	1,600,000
15	750,000
20	500,000
50	100,000

available for controlling this high-energy beam. The cyclotron physicists used a tool of the radiologist, the fluorescent screen, to aid in locating the high-energy beam. Unfortunately, in so doing, the physicists would receive high-radiation exposures to the lens of the eye because they had to look directly into the beam.

In 1949 the first paper reporting cataracts in cyclotron physicists was presented. By 1960, several hundred such cases of radiation-induced cataracts had been reported. This was particularly tragic, since there were few high-energy physicists.

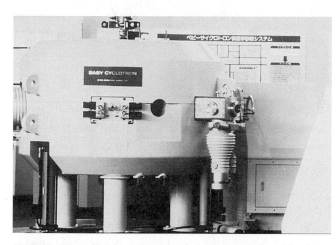

FIGURE 37-1 Modern cyclotron used to produce radionuclides for nuclear medicine applications. *(Courtesy Positron Corporation.)*

On the basis of these observations and animal experimentation, several conclusions can be drawn regarding radiation-induced cataracts. The radiosensitivity of the lens of the eye is age dependent. The older the individual, the greater the radiation effect and the shorter the latent period. Latent periods varying from 5 to 30 years have been observed in humans, and the average latent period is approximately 15 years. High-LET radiation, such as neutrons, has a high RBE for the production of cataracts.

The dose-response relationship for radiation-induced cataracts is apparently threshold, nonlinear. If the local tissue dose is high enough, in excess of approximately 1000 rad (10 Gy), nearly 100% of those who are irradiated develop cataracts. The precise level of the threshold dose is difficult to assess. Most investigators would suggest that the threshold after an acute x-ray exposure is approximately 200 rad (2 Gy). The threshold after fractionated exposure, such as that in diagnostic imaging, is probably in excess of 1000 rad (10 Gy).

Occupational exposures to the lens of the eye are too low to require protective lens shields for radiographers or radiologists. It is nearly impossible for a medical radiation worker to reach the threshold dose. However, the radiation administered to patients undergoing head and neck examination by either fluoroscopy or computed tomography can be significant. In computed to-

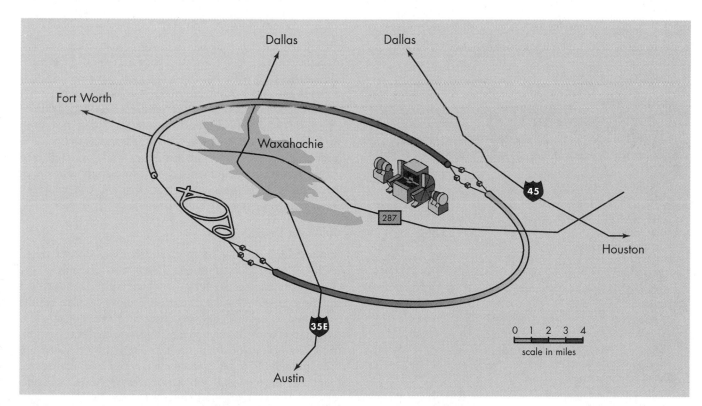

FIGURE 37-2 The superconducting supercollider will be the world's largest particle accelerator when completed in 1997.

mography the lens dose can be 5 rad per slice. In this situation, however, usually no more than one or two slices intersect the lens. In either case, protective lens shields are not normally required.

LIFE-SPAN SHORTENING
Risks to Radiographers

There have been many experiments conducted with animals after both acute and chronic irradiation that show that irradiated animals die young. Figure 37-3 is redrawn from several such representative experiments. The graph shows that the relationship between life-span shortening and dose is apparently linear, nonthreshold. When all the animal data are considered collectively and a meaningful extrapolation to humans is attempted, it is concluded that, at worst, humans can expect a reduced life span of 10 days for every rad.

Review the data presented in Table 37-2, which was compiled by Bernard L. Cohen of the University of Pittsburgh and extrapolated from various statistical sources of mortality. The expected loss of life in days is given as a function of occupation, disease, or other conditions. As one can see, the most grievous risk is being male rather than female. Whereas the average life shortening caused by occupational accidents is 74 days, that for radiation workers is only 12 days. It can be concluded that radiography is a safe occupation.

One investigator has evaluated the death records of radiographers who operated field x-ray machines during World War II. These machines were poorly designed and inadequately shielded so that the radiographers received higher than normal exposures. About 7000 radi-

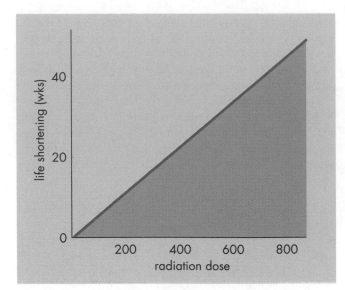

FIGURE 37-3 In chronically irradiated animals the extent of life shortening appears linear, nonthreshold. This graph shows the representative results of several such experiments with mice.

ographers have been studied and no radiation effects have been observed.

An investigation of health effects from radiation exposure of American radiographers is currently underway. This is a mail survey covering many work-related conditions of approximately 150,000 subjects that will take many years to complete. Early reports show no effects.

This radiation-induced life-span shortening is nonspecific, that is, there are no characteristic disease entities associated with it, and it does not include late malignant effects. Radiation-induced life-span shortening simply means accelerated premature aging and death.

Observations on human populations have not been totally convincing. No life-span shortening has been observed in the atomic bomb survivors, and some received rather substantial radiation doses. Life-span shortening in watch-dial painters, x-ray patients, and other human radiation populations does not exist.

Risks to Radiologists

One population that has been rather extensively studied is the American radiologist. Such a study has many shortcomings, not the least of which is the fact that it is retrospective in nature. Figure 37-4 shows the results obtained when the age at death for radiologists was compared with the age at death for the general population. Radiologists dying in the early 1930s were approximately 5 years younger than the average age at death of the general population. However, this difference in age at death had shrunk to zero by 1965.

A more recent study used two other physician groups as controls rather than the general population. Table

TABLE 37-2

Risk of Life Span Shortening as a Consequence of Occupation, Disease, or Various Other Conditions

Risky Condition	Expected Days of Life Lost
Being male rather than female	2800
Heart disease	2100
Being unmarried	2000
One pack of cigarettes a day	1600
Working as a coal miner	1100
Cancer	980
30 pounds overweight	900
Stroke	520
All accidents	435
Service in Vietnam	400
Motor vehicle accidents	200
Average occupational accidents	74
Speed limit increase from 55 to 65 mph	40
Radiation worker	12
Airplane crashes	1

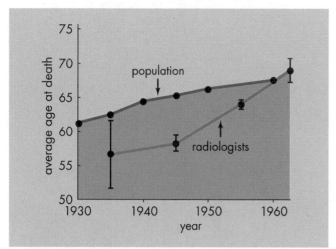

FIGURE 37-4 Radiation-induced life shortening is shown for American radiologists. The age at death in the radiologists has been less than that of the general population, but this difference has disappeared.

TABLE 37-3

Death Statistics for Three Groups of Physicians

Died During	Median Age at Death	Age-adjusted Deaths per 1000
1935 to 1944		
RSNA	71.4	18.4
ACP	73.4	15.4
AAOO	76.2	13.0
1945 to 1954		
RSNA	72.0	16.4
ACP	74.8	13.7
AAOO	76.0	11.9
1955 to 1958		
RSNA	73.5	13.6
ACP	76.0	11.4
AAOO	76.4	10.6

37-3 summarizes the results of this investigation. Two physician groups observed in this study were members of the Radiological Society of North America (RSNA) as the high-risk group and members of the American Academy of Ophthalmology and Otolaryngology (AAOO) as the low-risk group. Members of the American College of Physicians (ACP) represented an intermediate-risk group.

A comparison of the median age at death and age-adjusted death rates for these three physician specialties demonstrates a significant difference in age at death during the early years of radiology. This difference has disappeared in the contemporary practice of diagnostic imaging, presumably because of better attention to radiation protection through proper procedures and equipment design.

When these differences in mortality were first described, British investigators began looking for similar effects in British radiologists. None were found, which raises some questions about the validity and significance of the findings in American radiologists.

RISK ESTIMATES

The early effects of high-dose radiation exposure are usually easy to observe and measure. The late effects of low-dose radiation are also easy to observe, but it is nearly impossible to associate a particular late response with a previous radiation exposure. Consequently, precise dose-response relationships are often not possible. As a result, radiologists resort to **risk estimates.**

There are three types of risk estimates, and they each represent different statements of risk and have different dimensions.

Relative Risk

Relative risk involves estimating late radiation effects in large populations without having any precise knowledge of their radiation dose. The relative risk is computed by comparing the number of persons in the exposed population showing a given late effect with the number who developed the same late effect in an unexposed population.

$$\text{Relative Risk} = \frac{\text{Observed cases}}{\text{Expected cases}}$$

For instance, a relative risk of 1 would indicate no risk at all. A relative risk of 1.5 indicates that the frequency of the late response under observation is 50% higher in the irradiated population compared with the nonirradiated population.

Relative risk factors for radiation-induced late effects in humans range from 1 to 10. For the late effects of particular importance observed in human populations, most are reported in the range from 1 to 2.

Occasionally an investigation will result in a relative risk of less than 1. This would indicate that the exposed population receives some protective benefit, which is consistent with the hypothesis of radiation hormesis. However, the usual interpretation of such studies is that the results are not statistically significant either because of the small number of observations or because of inadequate identification of irradiated and control populations.

Question: In a study of radiation-induced leukemia after receiving diagnostic levels of radiation, 227 cases were observed in 100,000 persons so irradiated. The normal incidence of leukemia in the United States is 150 cases per 100,000. If this normal incidence was assumed to occur in a completely nonirradiated population, what would be the relative risk of radiation-induced leukemia?

Answer: Relative risk = $\dfrac{\text{Observed}}{\text{Expected}}$

$$= \dfrac{0.00227}{0.00150}$$

$$= 1.51$$

Excess Risk

Often when an investigation of human radiation response indicates the induction of some late effect, the magnitude of the effect will be reflected by the excess cases induced.

Excess risk = Observed cases − Expected cases

Leukemia, for instance, is known to occur spontaneously in nonirradiated populations. If the leukemia incidence in an irradiated population exceeds that which is expected, then the difference between the observed number of cases and the expected number would be excess risk.

The excess cases in this instance are assumed to be radiation induced. To determine the number of excess cases, one must be able to measure the observed number of cases in the irradiated population and compare them with the number that would have been expected on the basis of known population levels.

Question: Twenty-three cases of skin cancer were observed in a population of 1000 radiologists. The incidence in the general population is 0.5/100,000. How many excess skin cancers were produced in the population of radiologists?

Answer: Excess cases = Observed − Expected

$$= 23 - 0.005$$

$$\approx 23$$

Since none would be expected, all twenty-three cases represent risk.

Absolute Risk

If at least two different dose levels are known, then it may be possible to determine an absolute risk factor. Unlike the relative risk, which is a dimensionless ratio, the **absolute risk** has units of number of cases/10^6 persons/rad/year. Absolute-risk values range from approximately one to ten cases/10^6 persons/rad/year. Ten cases is the approximate absolute risk of death from all malignant disease.

To determine the absolute risk factor, one must assume a linear dose-response relationship. If the dose-response relationship is assumed nonthreshold, then only one dose level is required. The value of the absolute risk factor is equal to the slope of the dose-response relationship (Figure 37-5). The error bars on each data point indicate the fluctuation of the observation of response.

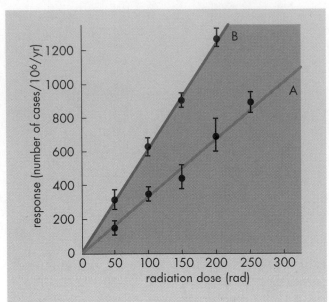

FIGURE 37-5 Slope of the linear, nonthreshold dose-response relationship is equal to the absolute risk. A and B show absolute risks of 3.4 and 6.2 cases/10^6 persons/rad/year, respectively.

Question: The absolute risk for radiation-induced breast cancer is considered to be six cases/10^6 persons/rad/yr for a 20-year at-risk period. If 100,000 women receive 100 mrad during mammography, what total number of cancers would be expected to be induced?

Answer: (Six cases/10^6 persons/rad/year)(10^5 persons) (0.1 rad)(20 year) = 1.2 cases

Question: There are approximately 300,000 American radiographers, and they receive an annual effective dose of less than 10 mrem. What is the expected number of annual deaths because of this occupational exposure?

Answer: (10 cases/10^6 persons/rad/year)(0.3×10^6) (0.01 rad) = (10 cases)(0.003)

$$= 0.03 \text{ cases/year}$$

Realize that death from malignant disease occurs in approximately 20% of the population.

RADIATION-INDUCED MALIGNANCY

All the late effects, including radiation induced malignancy, have been observed in experimental animals, and from these animal experiments dose-response relationships have been developed. At the human level these late effects have been observed, but often there are insufficient data to precisely identify the dose-response relationship. Consequently, some of the conclusions drawn regarding human responses are based in part on animal data.

Leukemia

When one considers radiation-induced leukemia in laboratory animals, there is no question that this response is real and that the incidence increases with increasing radiation dose. The form of the dose-response relationship is apparently linear and nonthreshold. The following human population groups have exhibited an elevated incidence of leukemia after radiation exposure: atom bomb survivors, radiotherapy patients, American radiologists, and children irradiated in utero.

Atom bomb survivors. Probably the greatest wealth of information that we have on radiation-induced leukemia in humans results from observations of the survivors of the atomic bombings of Hiroshima and Nagasaki. At the time of the bomb (**ATB**), approximately 300,000 persons were living in those two cities. Nearly 100,000 were killed from the blast and early effects of radiation. Another 100,000 persons received significant doses of radiation and survived. The remainder were unaffected because their radiation exposure was less than 10 rad.

After World War II, scientists of the Atomic Bomb Casualty Commission (**ABCC**), now known as the *Radiation Effects Research Foundation* (**RERF**), attempted to determine the radiation dose received by each of the atom bomb survivors in both cities. They first established the position of each individual ATB and estimated the dose to that survivor by considering not only distance from the hypocenter (the point at ground level where the bomb exploded) but also terrain, type of bomb, type of construction if the survivor were inside, and other factors that might influence dose.

A summary of the data obtained by these investigations is given in Table 37-4 and the data analysis is shown graphically in Figure 37-6. The spontaneous incidence of leukemia in the Japanese ATB was approximately 25 cases/10^6 persons/year. After high doses, the leukemia incidence is as much as 100 times that in the nonirradiated population. Even though there are large error bars at each dose increment, it is clear that the response appears linear, nonthreshold.

If, however, one expands the data in the low-dose region (e.g., below 200 rad), one could conclude that a

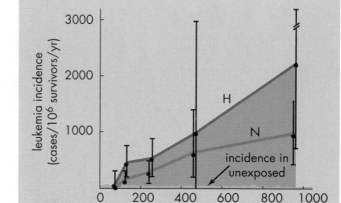

FIGURE 37-6 Data from the atomic bomb survivors of Hiroshima (H) and Nagasaki (N) suggest a linear, nonthreshold dose-response relationship.

threshold exists in the neighborhood of 50 rad. Nevertheless, neither this information nor other available information is interpreted to support a threshold response. Radiation-induced leukemia is considered linear, nonthreshold.

Figure 37-7 demonstrates the temporal distribution of the onset of leukemia in the atomic bomb survivors for the 40 years after the bombs. The data are presented as cases per 100,000 and include for comparison the leukemia rate in the population at large and in the nonexposed populations of the bombed cities. There was a rather rapid rise in leukemia incidence that reached a plateau after about 5 years. The incidence declined slowly for approximately 20 years when it reached the natural level experienced by the nonexposed.

Based on this analysis, radiation-induced leukemia is considered to have a latent period of 4 to 7 years and an at-risk period of approximately 20 years. The at-risk period is that time after irradiation during which one might expect the radiation effect to occur.

The data from the atomic bomb survivors show without a doubt that the radiation exposure to those survivors caused the later development of leukemia. It is interesting, however, to reflect on some additional aspects of these events. The first atomic bomb was dropped on Hiroshima; it was fueled with uranium, so the radiation dose was about equally distributed between gamma rays and neutrons. The Nagasaki bomb was a plutonium bomb. About 90% of its radiation was caused by gamma rays and only 10% by neutrons. Neutron radiation has a higher RBE than gamma rays, and this difference contributes to the difficulties in assessing the dose for each survivor.

TABLE 37-4

Summary of the Incidence of Leukemia in Atomic Bomb Survivors

	Hiroshima	Nagasaki	Total
Total number of survivors in study	74,356	25,037	99,393
Observed cases of leukemia	102	42	144
Expected cases of leukemia	39	13	52

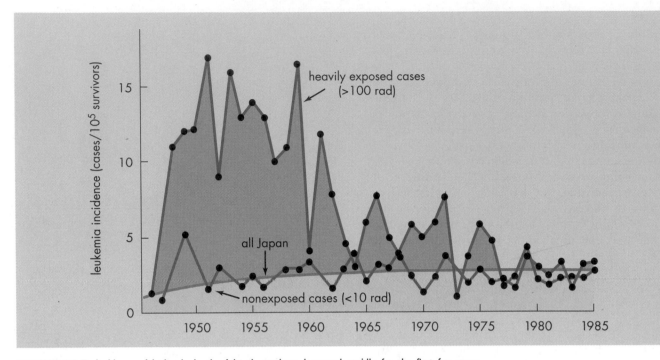

FIGURE 37-7 Incidence of leukemia in the A-bomb survivors increased rapidly for the first few years and has slowly declined since.

Of the 300,000 total resident population, 335 persons are estimated to have survived doses in excess of 600 rad. Through 1975 there had been only 144 cases of leukemia in the total exposed population. Acute leukemia and chronic **myelocytic leukemia** were observed most often in the atomic bomb survivors.

Taken to the final analysis, the data from the atomic bomb survivors pointed to an absolute risk of 1.5 cases/10^6 persons/rad/year. The overall relative risk based on the total number of observed leukemia deaths (144) versus the number of expected leukemia deaths (52) is approximately 2.8 : 1.

Radiologists. By the second decade of radiology, reports of pernicious anemia and leukemia in radiologists began to appear. In the early 1940s, several investigators had reviewed the incidence of leukemia in American radiologists and found it alarmingly high. These early radiologists functioned without the benefit of modern radiation protection devices and procedures, and many served as both radiation oncologists and diagnostic radiologists. In radiotherapy activities, they received substantial radiation exposures from radium applications. It has been estimated that some of these early radiologists received doses exceeding 100 rad/year (1 Gy/year).

One report of the death records of medical specialists dying between 1929 and 1943 showed that 8 out of 175 deaths in radiologists were caused by leukemia. In nonradiologist physicians there were 221 leukemia deaths in a total of 55,160 total deaths. These data indicate a relative risk of 10.3 : 1. In a more recent study covering the years 1948 to 1963 and based on a total of 12 leukemia cases in 425 radiology-related deaths, a relative risk of 4 : 1 was obtained. Currently, American radiologists do not exhibit an elevated incidence of leukemia when compared with other physician specialists.

It must be pointed out that a rather exhaustive study of mortality in radiologists in Great Britain covering the period from the turn of the century to 1960 did not show such an elevated risk of leukemia. The reasons for such a different experience between American and British radiologists is unknown. Some suggest that it is because the radiation therapy activities in Great Britain have always been attended by medical physicists, who presumably were more radiation safety conscious.

Ankylosing spondylitis patients. In the 1940s and 1950s, in Great Britain particularly, it was common practice to treat ankylosing spondylitis patients with radiation. Ankylosing spondylitis is an arthritic-like condition of the vertebral column. Such patients cannot walk upright or move except with great difficulty. For relief they would be given rather high doses of radiation to the spinal column, and the treatment was quite successful.

Patients who previously had to walk hunched over were able to stand erect. It was a permanent cure and remained the treatment of choice for approximately 20 years, until it was discovered that some who had been cured by radiation were dying from leukemia. The graphic results on the observations of these patients are shown in Figure 37-8. During the period from 1935 to

1955, 14,554 male patients were treated at 81 different radiation therapy centers in Great Britain. A review of the treatment records showed the dose to the bone marrow of the spinal column to range from 100 to 4000 rad (1 to 40 Gy). In this population, 52 cases of leukemia occurred.

The rate of leukemia in patients receiving more than 2000 rad was 17 cases/10,000 persons; in Great Britain the normal incidence of leukemia was 0.5 cases/10,000. The relative risk, therefore, is approximately 34:1. When one considers all 52 cases and compares the incidence of leukemia with that of the general population, the relative risk is 9.5:1.

The absolute risk can be obtained from these data by determining the slope of the best fit line through the data points (Figure 37-8). Such an analysis results in approximately 0.8 cases/10^6 persons/rad/year. If 95% confidence limits are placed on the data, one could not rule out the possibility of a threshold dose at approximately 300 rad.

Leukemia in other populations. There have been a number of studies designed to link leukemia incidence with environmental radiation. Natural background radiation levels increase in general with altitude and with latitude, but the range of levels observed is not sufficient to demonstrate a relationship with leukemia.

Other population groups that have provided evidence, both positive and negative, regarding the leukemia-inducing action of radiation are radium watch-dial painters, children receiving superficial x-ray

treatment, and some additional adult radiotherapy groups.

Cancer

What has been discussed regarding radiation-induced leukemia can be reported also for radiation-induced cancer. There is not quite as much human data concerning cancer as for leukemia; nevertheless, it can be said without question that radiation can cause cancer. Nearly all types of human cancer have been implicated as capable of being radiation induced. The relative risk factors and absolute risks are shown to be similar to those reported for leukemia. Many types of cancer have been implicated as radiation induced, and a discussion of the more important ones is in order.

It is difficult to ascribe any case of cancer to a previous radiation exposure, regardless of its magnitude, because cancer is so common. Approximately 20% of all deaths are caused by cancer; therefore any radiation-induced cancers are obscured. Leukemia, on the other hand, is a rare disease. That makes analysis of radiation-induced leukemia easier.

Thyroid cancer. Thyroid cancer has developed in three groups of patients whose thyroid glands were irradiated in childhood. The first two groups, called the *Ann Arbor series* and the *Rochester series,* consist of individuals who, in the 1940s and early 1950s, were treated shortly after birth for thymic enlargement. The thymus is a gland just below the thyroid gland that can enlarge shortly after birth in response to infection. At these facilities, radiation was often the treatment of choice. After a dose of up to 500 rad (5 Gy), the thymus gland would shrink so that all enlargement disappeared. No further problems were evident until up to 20 years later, when some of these patients began to develop thyroid nodules and some cases of thyroid cancer.

In the Ann Arbor series, several thousand children were involved. The dose to the thyroid gland was estimated to be 20 to 30 rad (200 to 300 mGy) and received mainly from scatter radiation from the adjacent useful beam to the thymus gland. Reasonable beam collimation was practiced.

In the Rochester series, there was a smaller number of cases, but the practice was to irradiate a rather large area so that the thymus gland and thyroid gland were equally irradiated. The estimated thyroid dose was approximately 300 rad (3 Gy).

The final group included 21 children who were natives of the Rongelap Atoll. In 1954, they were subjected to high levels of fallout during an atomic bomb test. The winds shifted during the test, carrying the fallout over an adjacent inhabited island rather than one that had been evacuated. These children received radiation doses to the thyroid gland from both external exposure and internal ingestion of about 1200 rad (12 Gy).

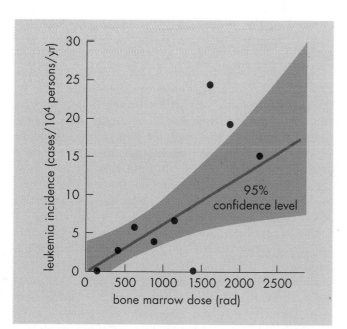

FIGURE 37-8 Results of observations of leukemia in ankylosing spondylitis patients treated with x-ray therapy suggest a linear, nonthreshold dose-response relationship.

If one computes the incidence of thyroid nodularity, considered **preneoplastic,** in these three groups and plots this incidence as a function of estimated dose, the result is that shown in Figure 37-9. Admittedly, the error bars on both the dose data and the incidence levels are large. Still, the implication of a linear, nonthreshold dose-response relationship is clear.

In a similar population of children irradiated for thymic enlargement, 24 thyroid carcinomas were reported in nearly 3000 irradiated patients. None was reported in 5000 nonirradiated siblings. The absolute risk factor was reported as 2.5 cases/10^6 persons/rad/year.

Bone cancer. Two population groups have contributed an enormous amount of data showing that radiation causes bone cancer. The first group consists of the radium watch-dial painters.

In the 1920s and 1930s, there were various small laboratories whose employees, mostly female, worked at benches painting watch dials with paint laden with radium sulfate. To prepare a fine point on the paintbrushes, the employees would touch the tip of the brush to the tongue. In this manner substantial quantities of radium were ingested.

Radium salts were used because the emitted radiation, principally alpha and beta particles, would continuously excite the luminous compounds so they would glow in the dark. Current technology uses harmlessly low levels of tritium (^{3}H) and promethium (^{147}Pm) for this purpose.

When ingested, radium behaves metabolically like calcium and deposits in bone structures. Because of radium's long half-life (1620 years) and alpha emission, these employees received radiation doses up to 50,000 rad (500 Gy) to bone. Seventy-two bone cancers in about 800 persons have been observed during a follow-up period in excess of 50 years. Analysis of these data has resulted in an overall relative risk of 122:1. The absolute risk is equal to 0.11 cases/10^6 persons/rad/year.

Another population to develop excess bone cancer is patients treated with radium salts for a variety of diseases from arthritis to tuberculosis. Such treatments were common practice in many parts of the world until about 1950.

Skin cancer. Skin cancer usually begins with the development of a radiodermatitis. Significant data have been developed from several reports of skin cancer induced in radiotherapy patients treated with orthovoltage (200 to 300 kVp) or superficial x-rays (50 to 150 kVp).

From these data we conclude that the latent period is approximately 5 to 10 years. Radiation-induced skin cancer follows a threshold dose-response relationship, but there is not enough data with which to develop absolute-risk values. When the dose delivered to the skin was in the range of 500 to 2000 rad (5 to 20 Gy), the relative risk of developing skin cancer was 4:1. If the dose were 4000 to 6000 rad (40 to 60 Gy) or 6000 to 10,000 rad (60 to 100 Gy), the relative risks were 14:1 and 27:1, respectively.

Breast cancer. In Chapter 23, some of the radiographic techniques used in mammography were discussed. The radiation dose to mammography patients is considered in a later chapter. At this time a discussion of the risk of radiation-induced breast cancer is considered.

A continuing controversy exists regarding the risk of radiation-induced breast cancer, and the implications of this controversy carry to breast cancer detection by x-ray mammography. The concern of such risk first surfaced in the middle 1960s after the published reports of breast cancer developing in tuberculosis patients.

Tuberculosis was for many years treated by isolation in a sanitarium. During the patient's stay, one mode of therapy was to induce an artificial pneumothorax in the affected lung, and this was done under fluoroscopy. Many patients received multiple treatments and up to several hundred fluoroscopic examinations. Precise dose determinations are not possible, but levels of several hundred rad would have been common. In some of these patient populations the relative risk for radiation-induced breast cancer were shown to be as high as 10:1.

One such population exhibited no excess risk. This finding, however, was explained as a consequence of the fluoroscopic technique. In the positive studies previously mentioned the patient faced away from the radiologist, toward the fluoroscopic x-ray tube, during exposure. In the study that reported negative findings, the patients were fluoroscoped facing the radiologist so that the radiation beam entered posteriorly. The breast tissue was exposed only to the low-intensity beam exiting the patient.

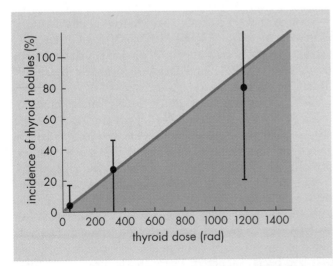

FIGURE 37-9 Radiation-induced preneoplastic thyroid nodularity in three groups of persons whose thyroid glands were irradiated in childhood.

Additional studies have produced results suggesting radiation-induced breast cancer developed in patients treated with x-rays for acute postpartum mastitis. The dose to these patients ranged from 75 to 1000 rad (0.75 to 10 Gy). The relative risk factor in this population was approximately 2.5:1.

Radiation-induced breast cancer has also been observed in the atomic bomb survivors. Through 1980, observations on nearly 12,000 women who received radiation doses to the breasts of 10 rad or more exhibited a relative risk of 4:1.

In some of these studies, only one breast was irradiated. In nearly every such case, breast cancer developed only in the irradiated breast. These patients have now been followed for up to 25 years. On the basis of all available data regarding radiation-induced breast cancer, the best estimate for absolute risk is six cases/10^6 persons/rad/year.

Lung cancer. Early in this century, it was observed that approximately 50% of the workers in the Bohemian pitchblende mines of Germany died of lung cancer. Lung cancer incidence in the general population was negligible by comparison. The dusty mine environment was considered to be the cause of this lung cancer. Now it is known that radiation exposure from radon in the mines contributed to the incidence of lung cancer in these miners.

Recently, observations of the American uranium miners active in the Colorado plateau in the 1950s and 1960s have also shown elevated levels of lung cancer. The peak of this activity occurred in the early 1960s when there were approximately 5000 miners active in nearly 500 underground mines and 150 open pit mines. Most of the mines were worked by less than ten men; therefore, for such a small operation, one could expect a lack of proper ventilation.

The radiation exposure in these mines occurred because of the high concentration of uranium ore. Uranium, which is radioactive with a very long half-life of 10^9 years, decays through a series of radioactive nuclides by successive alpha and beta emissions, each accompanied by gamma radiation.

One of the decay products of uranium is **radon** (^{222}**Rn**). This radionuclide is a gas that emanates through the rock to produce a high concentration in the air. When breathed, the radon can be deposited in the lung where it undergoes additional successive series of decay to a stable isotope of lead. During these subsequent decay actions, several alpha particles are released, and these result in a rather high local dose. Also, alpha particles are high-LET radiation and therefore have a high RBE.

To date more than 4000 uranium miners have been observed, and they have received estimated doses to lung tissue as high as 3000 rad, and on this basis the relative risk was approximately 8:1. Interestingly, ura-

nium miners who smoke have a relative risk of approximately 20:1.

The available data indicate a dose-response relationship that is linear, nonthreshold with an absolute risk of 1.3 cases/10^6 persons/rad/year.

Liver cancer. Thorium dioxide (ThO^2) in a colloidal suspension known as *Thorotrast* was widely used in diagnostic radiology between 1925 and 1945 as a contrast agent for angiography. Thorotrast was about 25% by weight ThO^2, and it contained several radioactive isotopes of thorium and its decay products. Radiation that was emitted produced a dose in the ratio of about 100:10:1 of alpha, beta, and gamma radiation, respectively.

The use of Thorotrast has been shown to be responsible for several types of carcinoma after a latent period of about 15 to 20 years. After extravascular injection, it is carcinogenic at the site of the injection. After intravascular injection, thorium dioxide particles are deposited in **phagocytic cells** of the **reticuloendothelial system** and are concentrated in the liver and spleen. Thorotrast long half-life and high alpha radiation dose has resulted in many cases of cancer in these organs.

TOTAL RISK OF MALIGNANCY
Three-Mile Island

From the basis of many of these observations on human population groups after exposure to low-level radiation, and considering all the risk estimates taken collectively for leukemia and cancer, a number of simplified conclusions can be made. The overall absolute risk for induction of malignancy is approximately 10 cases/10^6 persons/rad/year with the at-risk period extending for 20 to 25 years after exposure. This is approximately 200 deaths from radiation-induced malignancy after an exposure of 1 rad to 1,000,000 persons when all such cases occurring within 25 years of exposure are counted.

To make these values somewhat more meaningful, the celebrated Three-Mile Island incident can be considered. There are approximately 2,000,000 people residing within a 80-kilometer (50-mile) radius of Three-Mile Island. On the basis of our total population statistics, one would expect to observe approximately 330,000 cancer deaths in these persons. During the total period of the radiation incident, the average dose to persons living within a 160-kilometer (100-mile) radius was 1.5 mrad; to those within the 80-kilometer (50-mile) radius it was 8 mrad. Applying the upper limit estimate just cited, one can predict that the Three-Mile Island incident will result in no more than one additional malignant death as a result of this population radiation exposure.

BEIR Committee

The Committee on the Biologic Effects of Ionizing Radiation (BEIR), an arm of the National Academy of Sciences, has reviewed the data on late effects of low-dose, low-LET radiation. Their results are shown in Table 37-5.

The BEIR committee examined three situations. First, they estimated the excess mortality from malignant disease after a one-time accidental exposure to 10 rad that is highly unlikely in diagnostic imaging. Second, they considered the response to a dose of 1 rad/year for life. This situation is possible in diagnostic imaging but is certainly rare. Finally, they considered excess radiation-induced cancer mortality after a continuous dose of 100 mrad/year. This is considerably higher than that found for radiographers.

The dose-response relationship assumed to be true is the linear, nonthreshold model. These analyses showed an additional 800 cases of malignant-disease death in a population of 100,000 after 10 rad and an additional 550 after 100 mrad/year. These cases are in addition to the normal incidence of cancer death, which is approximately 19,000 per 100,000 persons. The BEIR Committee has further stated that because of the uncertainty in their analysis less than 1 rad/yr may not be harmful.

The BEIR Committee has also analyzed the available human data with regard to the age at exposure with a limited time of expression and whether the response was **absolute** or **relative**. If one is irradiated at an early age and the response is limited in time, the radiation-induced excess appears as a bulge on the age-response relationship (Figure 37-10). Childhood leukemia is a good example.

An **absolute age-response relationship** is shown in Figure 37-11. Here the increased incidence of cancer is a constant number of cases after a minimal latent period. Most subscribe to a **relative age-response relationship** in which the increased incidence of cancer is proportional to the natural incidence (Figure 37-12).

Perhaps the best way to present these radiation risk data is to compare them with other known causes of death. As one might imagine, there are volumes of tables that analyze risk. This information is presented in simplified form in Table 37-6. Note that in these common situations, risk from radiation exposure is near the bottom of the list. Actual occupational risk is even less,

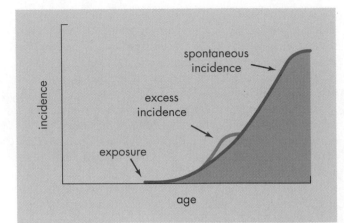

FIGURE 37-10 Exposure at an early age can result in an excess bulge of cancer after a latent period.

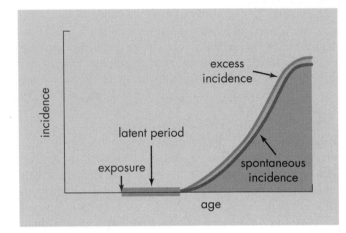

FIGURE 37-11 The absolute risk model predicts that excess radiation-induced cancer is constant for life.

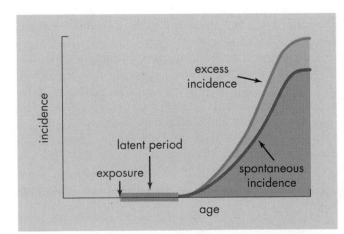

FIGURE 37-12 The relative risk model predicts that the excess radiation-induced cancer is proportional to the natural incidence.

TABLE 37-5		
BEIR Committee Estimated Excess Mortality from Malignant Disease in 100,000 Persons		
	Male	Female
Normal expectation	20,560	16,680
Excess cases		
Single exposure to 10 rad	770	810
Continuous exposure to 1 rad/year	2880	3070
Continuous exposure to 100 mrad/year	520	600

TABLE 37-6

Average Annual Risk of Death from Various Causes

Cause	Your Chance of Dying This Year
All causes (all ages)	1 in 100
20 cigarettes per day	1 in 280
Heart disease	1 in 300
Cancer	1 in 520
All causes (25 year old)	1 in 700
Stroke	1 in 1200
Motor vehicle accident	1 in 4000
Drowning	1 in 30,000
Alcohol (light drinker)	1 in 50,000
Air travel	1 in 100,000
Radiation, 100 mrad	**1 in 100,000**
Texas Gulf Coast hurricane	1 in 4,500,000
Being a rodeo cowboy	1 in 6,200,000

since radiographers use protective apparel during fluoroscopy and the radiation-risk estimate assumes whole-body exposure.

RADIATION AND PREGNANCY

Since the first medical applications of radiation, there has been concern and apprehension regarding the effects of radiation before, during, and after pregnancy. Before pregnancy, the concern is interrupted fertility. During pregnancy, concern is directed to the possible congenital effects in newborns. The postpregnancy concerns are related to the suspected genetic effects. All these effects have been demonstrated in animals, and some have been observed in humans.

Effects on Fertility

The early effect of high-level radiation on the interruption of fertility in both males and females has been discussed. There is ample evidence to show that such an effect does exist and is dose related. The effects of low-dose, long-term irradiation on fertility, however, are less well defined.

Animal data in this area are lacking. Those that are available indicate that, even when radiation is delivered at the rate of 100 rad per year, there is no noticeable depression in fertility.

There have been two national surveys of American radiologists, one reported in 1927 and the other in 1955. In each case a finding of depressed fertility and increased congenital abnormalities in the offspring of radiologists was reported. Both studies have been questioned because of their experimental methods. The conclusions reported are not generally accepted.

The health effects analysis of American radiographers mentioned earlier has indicated no effect on fertility. The number of births during a 12-year sampling period equaled the number expected.

Irradiation in Utero

Irradiation in utero concerns the following two types of exposures: (1) exposure of the radiation worker and (2) exposure of the patient. The recommended techniques and radiation control procedures associated with these exposed persons are considered fully in Chapter 40. At this time the biologic effects of such irradiation are considered.

Substantial animal data is available to describe rather completely the effects of relatively high doses of radiation delivered during various periods of gestation. Because the embryo is a rapidly developing cell system, it is particularly sensitive to radiation. With age the embryo (and then the fetus) becomes less sensitive to the effects of radiation, and this pattern continues into adulthood. After maturity, however, radiosensitivity increases with age. Figure 37-13 is a summary of the observed $LD_{50/30}$ in mice exposed at various times, which shows this aggregated radiosensitivity.

All observations point to the first trimester of pregnancy as the most sensitive period. Such findings are of particular concern because an x-ray exposure often occurs when pregnancy is unknown.

The effects of radiation in utero are time related and dose related. They include prenatal death, neonatal death, congenital abnormalities, malignancy induction, general impairment of growth, genetic effects, and mental retardation. Figure 37-14 is redrawn from studies designed to observe the effects of a 200 rad (2 Gy) dose delivered at various stages in utero in mice. The scale along the x-axis indicates the approximate comparable time in humans.

Within 2 weeks of fertilization, the most pronounced effect of a high radiation dose is prenatal death, which

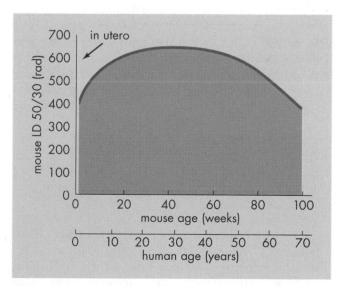

FIGURE 37-13 $LD_{50/30}$ of mice in relation to age at time of irradiation.

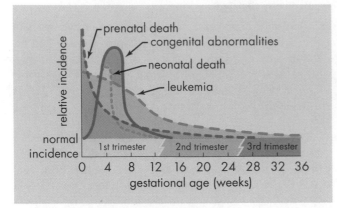

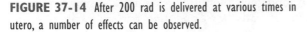

FIGURE 37-14 After 200 rad is delivered at various times in utero, a number of effects can be observed.

TABLE 37-7

Relative Risk of Childhood Leukemia after Irradiation in Utero by Trimester

Time of X-ray Examination	Relative Risk
First trimester	8.3
Second trimester	1.5
Third trimester	1.4
TOTAL	1.5

is manifested as a spontaneous abortion. Observations in radiotherapy patients have confirmed this effect but only after rather high doses.

On the basis of animal experimentation, it would appear that this response is very rare. Our best estimate is that a 10 rad (0.1 Gy) dose during the first 2 weeks will induce perhaps 0.1% spontaneous abortions. This is in addition to the 25% to 50% normal incidence of spontaneous abortions.

Fortunately, this response is of the all-or-none variety. Either there is a radiation-induced abortion or the pregnancy will carry to term with no ill effect. Indeed the first 2 weeks of pregnancy may be the safest.

During the period of **major organogenesis,** from the second through the tenth week, two effects are likely to occur. Early in this period, skeletal and organ abnormalities can be induced. As major organogenesis continues, congenital abnormalities of the central nervous system can be observed if the pregnancy is carried to term.

If the radiation-induced congenital abnormalities are severe enough, the result will be neonatal death. After a dose of 200 rad (2 Gy) to the mouse, nearly 100% of the fetuses suffered significant abnormalities. In 80%, it was sufficient to cause neonatal death. Such effects are rare after diagnostic levels of exposure and are essentially undetectable after radiation doses less than 10 rad (0.1 Gy). A dose of 10 rad (0.1 Gy) during this time is expected to increase the incidence of congenital abnormalities by 1% above the natural incidence. To complicate matters, there is approximately a 5% incidence of naturally occurring congenital abnormalities in the unexposed population.

Irradiation in utero at the human level has been associated with childhood malignancy by a number of investigators. Perhaps the most complete study of this effect was conducted by Alice Stewart and her co-workers in a project known as the *Oxford Survey,* a study of childhood malignancies, in England, Scotland, and Wales.

Nearly every case of such childhood malignancy in these countries since 1946 has been investigated. Each case was first identified and then investigated by way of interview with the mother, review of the hospital charts, and review of the physician records. Each case of childhood malignancy was matched with a control for age, gender, place of birth, socioeconomic status, and other demographic factors. The control was a child who matched with the case in all respects except the control did not have cancer or leukemia. The Oxford Survey is being continued at this time and has now considered more than 9000 cases and a like number of matched controls.

Although the Oxford Survey has reviewed all malignancies, it is the findings of radiation-induced leukemia that have been of particular importance. Table 37-7 shows the results of this survey in terms of relative risk. A relative risk of the development of childhood leukemia after irradiation in utero of 1.5 is significant. This indicates an increase of 50% over the presumed nonirradiated rate. The number of cases involved, however, is small.

The incidence of childhood leukemia in the population at large is approximately nine cases per 100,000 live births. According to the Oxford Survey, if all 100,000 had been irradiated in utero, perhaps 14 cases of leukemia would have resulted. Although these findings have been substantiated in several American populations, there is no consensus among radiation scientists that this effect after receiving such low doses is indeed real.

There are other effects after irradiation in utero that have been studied rather fully in animals and have been observed in some human populations. An unexpected finding in offspring of the atomic bomb survivors is mental retardation. Children of exposed mothers have performed poorly in IQ tests and have demonstrated poor scholastic performance in comparison with unexposed Japanese children. These differences are marginal yet significant. When assessed by test scores, measurable mental retardation is apparent in approximately 6% of all children. A 10-rad dose in utero is expected to increase this incidence by an additional 0.5%.

Radiation exposure in utero does retard the growth and development of the newborn. Irradiation in utero, principally during the period of major organogenesis, has been associated with microcephaly (small head) and, as just discussed, mental retardation. The human data bearing on these effects are obtained from patients irradiated medically, the atomic bomb survivors, and the residents of the Marshall Islands who were exposed to radioactive fallout in 1954 during weapons testing. For instance, the heavily irradiated children at Hiroshima are, on the average, 2.25 centimeters (0.9 inches) shorter, 3 kilograms (6.6 pounds) lighter, and 1.1 centimeters (0.4 inches) smaller in head circumference than members of the nonirradiated control groups.

These effects, as well as mental retardation, have been observed principally in those receiving doses in excess of 100 rad (1 Gy) in utero. The lack of appropriate and sensitive tests of mental function make it impossible to draw similar conclusions at doses below 100 rad (1 Gy).

A summary of the effects of irradiation in utero is shown in Table 37-8. There are the following four responses of concern to diagnostic imaging: (1) spontaneous abortion, (2) congenital abnormalities, (3) mental retardation, and (4) childhood malignancy. Spontaneous abortion is a concern because it is an all-or-none effect. Congenital abnormalities, mental retardation, and childhood malignancy are also a real concern, but it should be recognized that the probability of such a response after a fetal dose of 10 rad (0.1 Gy) is nil. Furthermore, 10 rad to the fetus is very rarely experienced in diagnostic imaging.

The form of the dose-response relationship for each of these effects is unknown. They do, however, appear to be linear and nonthreshold when based on doses greater than 100 rad (1 Gy). When large experimental animal populations were acutely exposed, the minimum reported dose for observing such effects as statistically significant was approximately 10 rad (0.1 Gy). There is no evidence at either the human or the animal level to indicate that the levels of radiation exposure currently experienced occupationally and medically are responsible for any such effects on growth and development.

Although efforts for protecting the unborn from the harmful effects of radiation are principally directed at diagnostic x-ray exposures, there must be an awareness of similar hazards from radioisotope examinations. For example, radioiodine is known to concentrate principally in the thyroid gland. After an administration of radioactive iodine, the dose to thyroid tissue is several orders of magnitude higher than the whole-body dose because of this organ concentration effect.

The thyroid gland begins to function at approximately 10 weeks of gestation, and, since radioiodine readily crosses the placental barrier from the mother's blood to the fetal circulation, radioiodine should be administered during pregnancy only in trace doses and before the 10-week gestation period. At any time thereafter the hazard of such an administration increases.

Genetic Effects

Unfortunately, the weakest area of knowledge in radiation biology is the area of radiation genetics. Essentially all the data indicating that radiation causes genetic effects have come from rather large-scale experiments with either flies or mice. There is no substantive data on humans.

Observations of the atomic bomb survivors have shown no radiation-induced genetic effects, and survivors are now into the third generation. Other human populations have likewise provided only negative observations. Consequently, in the absence of accurate human data, there is no choice but to rely on information from experimental laboratory studies.

In 1927 the Nobel prize-winning geneticist H.J. Muller from the University of Texas reported the results of his irradiation of *Drosophila*, the fruit fly. He irradiated mature flies before procreation and then measured the frequency of lethal mutations in the offspring. The radiation doses used were thousands of rad, but, as the data of Figure 37-15 show, the dose-response relationship for radiation-induced genetic damage is unmistakably linear, nonthreshold.

From Muller's studies, other conclusions were drawn. Radiation does not alter the quality of mutations but rather increases the frequency of those mutations that are observed spontaneously. Muller's data showed no dose rate or dose fractionation effects. Hence, he concluded that such mutations were single-hit phenomena.

It was principally on the basis of Muller's work that the National Council on Radiation Protection in 1932

TABLE 37-8

Summary of Effects After 10 Rad in Utero

Time of Exposure	Type of Response	Natural Occurrence	Radiation Response
0-2 weeks	Spontaneous abortion	25%	0.1%
2-10 weeks	Congenital abnormalities	5%	1%
2-15 weeks	Mental retardation	6%	0.5%
0-9 months	Malignant disease	8/10,000	12/10,000
0-9 months	Impaired growth and development	1%	nil
0-9 months	Genetic mutations	10%	nil

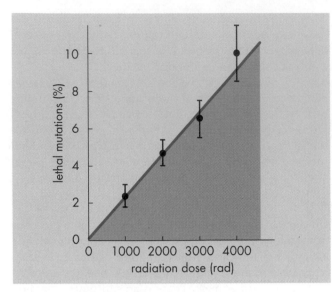

FIGURE 37-15 Irradiation of flies by H.J. Muller shows the genetic effects to be linear, nonthreshold. Note that the doses were exceedingly high.

lowered the maximum permissible dose and acknowledged officially for the first time the existence of nonthreshold radiation effects. Since that time, all radiation protection guides have assumed a linear, nonthreshold dose-response relationship.

The only other experimental work of any significance is that of Russell. Beginning in 1946, he commenced to irradiate a rather large mouse colony with radiation dose rates that varied from 0.001 to 90 rad per minute and total doses up to 1000 rad (10 Gy). These studies are continuing, and observations have now been made on over 8 million mice. The experiment requires the observation of seven specific genes that control readily recognizable characteristics such as ear shape, coat color, and eye color.

Russell's data show that a dose rate effect does exist, which would indicate that the mouse has some capacity to repair genetic damage. Significant differences between irradiation of males and of females were observed. He has confirmed the linear, nonthreshold form of the dose-response relationship and has not detected any types of mutations that did not occur naturally.

The average mutation rate per unit dose in the mouse is approximately fifteen times that observed in the fruit fly. Whether an increased sensitivity exists in humans relative to the mouse is unknown.

The concept of doubling dose has developed from these experimental studies. The doubling dose is that dose of radiation that will produce twice the frequency of genetic mutations as would have been observed without the radiation. The doubling dose in humans is estimated to lie in the range between 50 and 250 rad (0.5 and 2.5 Gy).

Some additional conclusions drawn from these experimental studies follow:

1. Radiation-induced mutations are usually harmful.
2. Any dose of radiation, however small, to a germ cell results in some genetic risk.
3. The frequency of radiation-induced mutations is directly proportional to dose so that a linear extrapolation of data obtained at high doses provides a valid estimate for low-dose effects.
4. The effect is dependent on the rate at which the radiation is delivered (protraction) and on the time between exposures (fractionation).
5. For most prereproductive life the female is less sensitive to the genetic effects of radiation than the male.
6. Most radiation-induced mutations are **recessive**. These require that the mutant genes be present in both the male and the female to produce the trait. Consequently, such mutations may not be expressed for many generations.
7. The frequency of radiation-induced genetic mutations is extremely low. It is approximately 10^{-7} mutation/rad/gene.

The significance of all this in daily practice for patients and radiation employees is considered next. First, it can be said with certainty that radiation-induced genetic mutations after the levels of exposure experienced in diagnostic imaging are essentially zero. The probability of such an effect is extremely low.

Under nearly all such exposures no action is required. However, should a high radiation dose be experienced (e.g., an excess of 10 rad), some protective action may be required. The prefertilized egg, in its various stages, exhibits a constant sensitivity to radiation. However, it also demonstrates some capacity for repair of genetic damage. If repair occurs, it is rapid in the female and delayed up to 60 days for the germ cell in the male.

SUMMARY

The late effect of radiation exposure is biologic damage that occurs over a long period of time after an exposure incident. Late effects can develop from high-dose, short-term exposure but the concern in diagnostic imaging is low-dose, intermittent exposures over a long period of time. Epidemiologic studies have been done concerning radiation exposure to large populations; however, there are problems: (1) the exact dose is usually not known and (2) the frequency of observable response is low.

Local tissues are affected by low-dose radiation. The late effects appear as nonmalignant changes in the skin. The skin develops a weathered, calloused, and discolored appearance. Chromosome damage in circulating lymphocytes and cataracts in the cornea of the eye have been observed as late effects of radiation exposure.

Humans can expect a reduced life span of 10 days for every rad of radiation exposure. However, with radiation protection practiced in diagnostic imaging departments, radiography is considered a safe occupation. Radiologists' risk factors have been studied extensively. Early in the century, radiologists were at risk because of exposure to unshielded equipment and lack of leaded barriers. However, in modern times, radiologists have no more risk of premature death than doctors in other medical specialities.

Because dose-response relationships are imprecise when observing late effects of radiation exposure, risk estimates are used to estimate radiation damage to populations. Relative risk is calculated when the population's exposure incident cannot be determined. Relative risk is computed by comparing the number of persons in the exposed population with late effects to the number in a unexposed population who developed the same condition. Excess risk determines the magnitude of the late effect because of the number of excess cases reported. Absolute risk is the calculation of the risk of death from radiation-induced malignant disease. The unit of absolute risk is the number of cases/10^6 persons/rad/year.

From the basis of many of the observations of radiation-induced malignancy in population groups after exposure to low-level radiation, a number of conclusions can be made. The overall absolute risk of developing malignant disease is 10 cases/1,000,000 persons/rad/year. The at-risk period extends from 20 to 25 years after exposure. This is approximately 200 deaths after exposure of 1 rad over 25 years of the population of 1,000,000.

The effects of low-dose, long-term irradiation in utero can include the following effects: prenatal death, neonatal death, congenital abnormalities, malignancy, impairment of growth, genetic effects, and mental retardation. However, these abnormalities are based on doses greater than 100 rad, with the minimum reported doses in animal experiments at 10 rad. There is no evidence at either the human or animal level to indicate the levels of radiation exposure currently experienced occupationally or medically are responsible for any such effects on fetal growth or development. It also can be said with certainty that radiation-induced genetic mutations at the levels of exposure used in diagnostic imaging are essentially zero.

REVIEW QUESTIONS

1. The late effects of radiation exposure can be produced by _____ doses delivered over long periods of time.

2. Describe the nonmalignant changes that occurred in the skin of early radiologists who performed fluoroscopy without lead protection.

3. Discuss the cases of radiation-induced cataracts reported in 1960. What was the population group?

4. What is the risk of life-span shortening for radiation workers? What is the risk of life-span shortening with heart disease?

5. What is the significance of the change in death statistics of American radiologists from the 1935-to-1944 time period to the 1955-to-1958 time period?

6. Write the formula for relative risk.

7. What is the absolute risk of three cases of leukemia developing per year in 100,000 persons after an average dose of 2 rad?

8. Write the formula for excess risk.

9. What is the unit of absolute risk?

10. Twenty million people in Scandinavia were exposed to an average 0.7 mrad as a result of Chernobyl. Assuming an absolute risk of 10 cases/10^6/rad/year over a 30-year period, how many malignancies will be induced?

11. Radiation-induced leukemia is considered to have a latent period of _____ years and an at-risk period of approximately _____ years.

12. What is the suspected reason that British radiologists did not have an elevated risk of leukemia compared with American radiologists?

13. Discuss the experience of radiation-induced leukemia in ankylosing spondylitis patients.

14. Why was the thymus gland irradiated in the Ann Arbor and Rochester series? What were the late effects of the thymus irradiation?

15. Discuss the way bone cancer developed in watch-dial painters in the 1920s and 1930s.

16. Explain the risk of radon gas to uranium miners.

17. During the period of the Three-Mile Island incident, what was the average dose to persons living within a 100-mile radius of the nuclear plant?

18. What are the effects on fertility from low-dose, long-term irradiation?

19. Refer to Table 37-7. What does the total relative risk of 1.5 mean?

20. Explain this statement: Most radiation-induced mutations are recessive.

Additional Readings

Dowd SB: The practice of radiobiology in the radiologic sciences, *Radiol Technol* 66(1):25 September-October, 1994.

Katz R: Dose, *J Radiat Res* 137(3):410 March, 1994.

Kumagai E, Tanaka R, Kumagai T, Onomichi M, Sawada S: Effects of long-term radiation exposure on chromosomal aberration in radiological technologists, *J Radiat Res* 31(3):270 September, 1990.

CHAPTER 38

Health Physics

OBJECTIVES

At the completion of this chapter the student will be able to:

1. Define health physics
2. List the cardinal principles of radiation protection and discuss the ALARA concept
3. Explain the meaning of NCRP and the concept of dose limits
4. Name the dose limits for occupational and nonoccupational workers for whole-body, skin, and extremities
5. Discuss the radiosensitivity of the stages of pregnancy
6. Describe the recommended management procedures for the pregnant radiographer and for the pregnant patient

OUTLINE

Definition of Health Physics
Cardinal Principles of Radiation Protection
    Minimize time
    Maximize distance
    Maximize shielding
Dose Limits
    Whole-body effective dose limits
    Equivalent dose limits for tissues and organs
Radiation Exposure to the Public
Educational Considerations
X-rays and Pregnancy
    Radiobiology of pregnancy
    The pregnant radiographer
    Management principles
    The pregnant patient
    What if?

Immediately after their discovery, x-rays were applied to the healing arts. It was recognized within months, however, that radiation could cause harmful effects. The first American fatality from radiation exposure was Thomas Edison's assistant, Clarence Dally. Since that time, a great deal of effort has been devoted to developing equipment, techniques, and procedures to control radiation levels and reduce unnecessary radiation exposure to radiation workers and to the public.

The cardinal principles for radiation protection are simplified rules to provide safety in radiation areas for occupational workers. In 1931 the first dose-limiting recommendations were made. Today the National Council on Radiation Protection and Measurement (NCRP) continuously reviews the recommended maximum permissible dose.

DEFINITION OF HEALTH PHYSICS

Health physics is concerned with providing radiation protection for the public and for persons working in radiation industries. The term *health physicist* was coined during the early days of the Manhattan Project (the secret wartime effort to develop the atomic bomb) to describe the group of physicists and physicians responsible for the radiation safety of persons involved in the production of atomic bombs. The health physicist thus can be a radiation scientist, an engineer, or a physician concerned with the research, teaching, or operational aspects of radiation safety in diagnostic imaging departments, in the nuclear industry, or in the public arena.

CARDINAL PRINCIPLES OF RADIATION PROTECTION

All health physics activity in diagnostic imaging is designed to minimize radiation exposure of patients and personnel. Three cardinal principles of radiation protection developed for nuclear activities find equally useful application in diagnostic radiology: time, distance, and shielding. By observing the following principles, radiation exposure can be minimized:

1. Keep the time of exposure to radiation as short as possible.
2. Maintain as large a distance as possible between the source of radiation and the exposed person.
3. Insert shielding material between the radiation source and the exposed person.

Minimize Time

The dose to an individual is directly related to the duration of exposure. If the time of exposure to radiation is doubled, the exposure will be doubled. The equation for this relationship is as follows:

$$\text{Exposure} = \text{Exposure rate} \times \text{Time}$$

Question: A radiation source has an exposure rate of 225 mR per hour (0.58 μC per kg-hr) at a position occupied by a radiation worker. If the worker remains at that position for 36 minutes, what will the total occupational exposure be?

Answer:

$$\text{Occupational exposure} = (225 \text{ mR/hr})\left(\frac{36 \text{ min}}{60 \text{ min/hr}}\right)$$
$$= 135 \text{ mR}$$

Question: A nuclear power plant worker is assigned a task in an area where the radiation exposure level is 600 mR per hour. If the allowable daily exposure is 50 mR, how long may the worker remain?

Answer:

$$\text{Time} = \text{Exposure} \div \text{Exposure rate}$$
$$= 50 \text{ mR} \div 600 \text{ mR/hr}$$
$$= \frac{1}{12} \text{ hour}$$
$$= 5 \text{ minutes}$$

During radiography the time of exposure is kept to a minimum to reduce motion blur. During fluoroscopy the time of exposure should also be kept to a minimum to reduce patient and personnel exposure.

Radiologists are trained to depress the fluoroscopic foot switch in an alternating fashion, sequencing **on-off** rather than continuous **on** during the course of the examination. A repeated up-and-down motion on the fluoroscopic foot switch permits a high-quality examination to be made with a considerably reduced exposure to the patient. The use of pulsed progressive fluoroscopy can reduce patient dose considerably.

The **5-minute reset timer** on all fluoroscopes reminds the radiologist that a considerable fluoroscopic time has elapsed. The timer records the amount of x-ray beam on-time. Most fluoroscopic examinations take less than 5 minutes. Only during difficult angiointerventional procedures should it be necessary to exceed 5 minutes of exposure time.

Question: A fluoroscope emits 4.2 R per minute (31 mC/kilogram-minute) at the tabletop for every milliampere of operation (4.2 R/mA-minute). What is the patient exposure in a barium enema examination that is conducted at 1.8 mA and requires 2.5 minutes of fluoroscopic time?

Answer:

$$\text{Patient exposure} = \left(\frac{4.2 \text{ R}}{\text{mA-minute}}\right)(1.8 \text{ mA})(2.5 \text{ minutes})$$
$$= 18.9 \text{ R}$$

Maximize Distance

As the distance between the source of radiation and a person increases, the radiation exposure decreases rapidly. The decrease in exposure is calculated using the inverse square law (see equation below) if the source of radiation can be considered a point source.

Most radiation sources are point sources. The x-ray tube target, for example, is a point source of radiation. The scattered radiation generated within a patient appears not to come from a point source but rather from an extended area. As a rule of thumb, even an extended source can be considered a point source if the distance from the source exceeds five times the source diameter.

Question: An x-ray tube has an output intensity of 2.6 mR/mAs (0.7 µC/kilogram-mAs) when operated at 70 kVp at 100-cm SID. What would be the radiation exposure 350 centimeters from the target?

Answer:

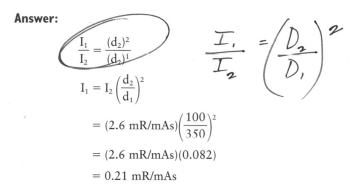

$$\frac{I_1}{I_2} = \frac{(d_2)^2}{(d_2)^1}$$

$$\frac{I_1}{I_2} = \left(\frac{D_2}{D_1}\right)^2$$

$$I_1 = I_2\left(\frac{d_2}{d_1}\right)^2$$

$$= (2.6 \text{ mR/mAs})\left(\frac{100}{350}\right)^2$$

$$= (2.6 \text{ mR/mAs})(0.082)$$

$$= 0.21 \text{ mR/mAs}$$

In radiography the distance from radiation source to patient is generally fixed by the type of examination. The radiographer is positioned behind a protective barrier in the control booth.

Even during fluoroscopy the radiographer can exercise good radiation protection procedures. Figure 38-1 shows the approximate radiation exposure levels at waist height during a fluoroscopic examination. The lines on the plot plan are called *isoexposure lines* and represent positions of equal exposure in the examining room. Point A indicates the normal position for a radiologist or a radiographer during a fluoroscopic examination. The exposure rate at this position is approximately 300 mR per hour (77 µC per kilogram-hr).

During portions of the examination, it might not be necessary for the radiographer to remain in that position. Two steps back, at position AN, the exposure rate is only 20 mR per hour (5 µC/kilogram-hour). This reduction in exposure does not follow the inverse square law, since the patient is an extended source of radiation during fluoroscopy because of scattered x-rays generated within the body. Therefore, during fluoroscopy, the radiographer should remain as far from the patient as practical.

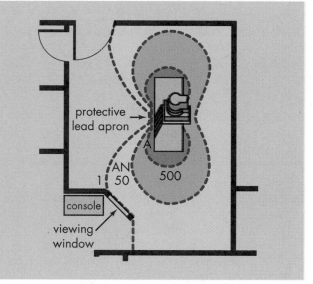

FIGURE 38-1 Typical isoexposure contours during fluoroscopic examination (mR/hour).

Question: Using the exposure levels shown in Figure 38-1, determine the approximate occupational exposure of a radiographer at position A and at a position AN, two steps farther back, during a fluoroscopic examination requiring 4 minutes, 15 seconds.

Answer: Occupational exposure equals

Position A: (300 mR per hour)(4.25 minutes)
(1 hour per 60 minutes) = 21.25 mR

Position AN: (20 mR per hour)(4.25 minutes)
(1 hour per 60 minutes) = 1.4 mR

Maximize Shielding

Positioning shielding between the radiation source and persons exposed greatly reduces the level of exposure. Shielding used in diagnostic imaging usually consists of lead, although often conventional building materials are used. The amount a protective barrier reduces radiation intensity can be estimated if the half-value layer (HVL) or the tenth-value layer (TVL) of the barrier material is known. The HVL is defined and discussed in Chapter 12.

The TVL is similarly defined. One TVL is the thickness of material that will reduce the radiation intensity to one tenth of its original value. Table 38-1 shows approximate HVL and TVL for lead and concrete for diagnostic x-ray facilities operated between 40 and 150 kVp. The following equation is the relationship between HVL and TVL.

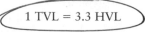

1 TVL = 3.3 HVL

TABLE 38-1

Approximate HVL and TVL of Lead and Concrete at Various Tube Potentials

	HVL		TVL	
Tube Potential	Lead (Millimeters)	Concrete (Inches)	Lead (Millimeters)	Concrete (Inches)
40 kVp	0.03	0.13	0.06	0.40
60 kVp	0.11	0.25	0.34	0.87
80 kVp	0.19	0.42	0.64	1.4
100 kVp	0.24	0.60	0.80	2.0
125 kVp	0.27	0.76	0.90	2.5
150 kVp	0.28	0.86	0.95	2.8

Question: When operated at 70 kVp, an x-ray machine has a radiation intensity of 3.6 mR/mAs (9 μC/kilogram-mAs) at a distance of 100 centimeters. How much shielding material (concrete and lead) would be required to reduce the intensity to less than 0.25 mR/mAs?

Answer: The amount of shielding material in the first or second column of the data below will reduce the beam intensity to the value in the third column.

Lead (millimeters)	Concrete (inches)	Beam intensity (mR/mAs)
0	0	3.60
0.15	0.33	1.80
0.30	0.67	0.60
0.45	1.00	0.45
0.60	1.33	0.23

Question: An x-ray machine is used strictly for chest radiography at 125 kVp. The useful beam is always pointed to a wall containing 0.8 millimeters of lead shielding. How much additional shielding will be required if the workload doubles?

Answer: When the workload doubles, so will the exposure on the other side of the wall. Therefore one HVL, or 0.27 millimeters of lead, will be necessary to reduce that exposure to its original level.

Usually, applications of the cardinal principles of radiation protection involve a consideration of all three. The typical problem involves a known radiation level at a given distance from the source. One can calculate the level of exposure at any other distance, behind any shielding, for any length of time. The order in which these calculations are made makes no difference.

Question: The operating kVp of a radiographic installation rarely exceeds 100 kVp. The output intensity is 4.6 mR/mAs (1.2 μC/kilogram-mAs) at 100 centimeters SID. The distance to a secretary's desk on the other side of the wall to which the x-ray beam is directed is 200 centimeters. The wall contains 0.96 millimeters of lead, and 300 mAs is antici-

pated daily. If the secretary is to be restricted to 2 mR exposure per week, how long each day may he or she remain at the desk?

Answer: Daily x-ray output at 100 cm =
(4.6 mR/mAs)(300 mAs) = 1380 mR

Daily output at 200 centimeters =
$(1380) (100/200)^2 = 345$ mR

Daily output behind 0.96 millimeters of lead, or 4 HVLs = 22 mR

= 110 mR per week

$$\text{Time allowed} = \frac{2 \text{ mR}}{110 \text{ mR/week}} =$$

0.018 week = 43 minutes

This analysis does not take into account the x-ray beam attenuation by the patient that is approximately 2 TVLs or 0.01 Therefore, the following is true:

Daily output behind 0.96 millimeters of lead and the patient = (110 mR)(0.01) = 1.1 mR

$$\text{Time allowed} = \frac{2 \text{mR}}{1.1 \text{ mR per week}} = 1.8 \text{ week (unlimited)}$$

Question: Suppose an analysis shows that if a secretary remains at his or her desk for more than 24 minutes each week, his or her dose limit will be exceeded. How much additional protective lead would be required?

Answer: Full occupancy is 40 hour ×
60 minutes/hour = 2400 minutes

$$\frac{2400 \text{ minutes}}{24 \text{ minutes}} = 100$$

The additional protection should reduce exposure to $\frac{1}{100}$ the present level. That is 2 TVLs or an additional 1.6 millimeters of lead.

DOSE LIMITS

A continuing effort of health physicists has been the description and identification of occupational dose limits. For many years a **maximum permissible dose (MPD)** was specified. The MPD was the maximum dose of radiation that, in light of current knowledge, would be expected to produce no significant radiation effects. At radiation doses below the MPD, no responses should occur. At the level of the MPD, the risk is not zero, but it is small—lower than the risks associated with other occupations and reasonable in light of the benefits derived.

Whole-Body Effective Dose Limits

The NCRP has assessed risk based on data from the BEIR Committee reports and reports of the National Safety Council (Table 38-2). The NCRP has also abandoned the terminology Maximum Permissible Dose for **Dose Limit (DL).** Current DLs are prescribed for various organs, as well as the whole body, and for various working conditions so that the lifetime risk from each years occupational radiation exposure does not exceed 10^{-4} year^{-1}.

The value 10^{-4} year^{-1} is the approximate risk of death to those working in safe industries. The NCRP Dose Limits are set to ensure that radiation workers have the same risk as those in safe industries.

Question: Suppose all 300,000 American radiographers receive the dose limit (5000 mrem) this year. How many would be expected to die prematurely?

Answer: $(300,000)(10^{-4}) = 30$

Of course radiographers actually receive much less exposure and therefore the expected mortality is closer to zero.

Particular care is taken to make certain that no **radiation worker** receives a radiation dose in excess of the DL. The DL is specified only for occupational exposure. It should not be confused with medical x-ray exposure received as a patient. Although patient dose should be kept low, there is no patient dose limit.

In 1902 the first dose limit, 50,000 mrem per week (500 mSv per week), was recommended. The current DL is 100 mrem per week (1 mSv per week). Through the years there has been a downward revision of the DL. The history of these continuing recommendations is given in Table 38-3 and is shown graphically in Figure 38-2.

In the early years of radiology the DL consisted of a single value considered the safe working level for whole-body exposure. It was based primarily on the known acute response to radiation exposure and presumed that a **threshold dose** existed. Today the DL is specified not only for whole-body exposure but also for partial-body exposure, organ exposure, and exposure of the general population, again excluding medical exposure as a patient and exposure from natural sources (Table 38-4).

These dose limits were first published by the NCRP in 1987 and further refined in 1993. They replace the previous MPDs, which had been in effect since 1959. These dose limits have been adapted by state and federal regulatory agencies and are now the law of the United States. Notice that SI units are preferred.

The basic annual DL remains the same—50 mSv per year (5000 mrem per year). Substantial changes were made in other specified DL values. The DL for the lens of the eye was raised to 150 mSv per year (15,000 mrem per year) and that for other organs to 500 mSv per year (50,000 mrem per year). The cumulative whole-body DL is now 10 mSv (1000 mrem) times one's age in years. The DL during pregnancy remains fixed at 5 mSv (500 mrem), but once pregnancy is declared the monthly exposure should not exceed 0.5 mSv (50 mrem).

TABLE 38-2	
Fatal Accident Rates in Various Industries	
Industry	Rate ($\times 10^{-4}$ year^{-1})
Trade	0.4
Manufacture	0.4
Service	0.4
Government	0.9
All Groups	0.9
Transport	2.2
Public utilities	2.2
Construction	3.1
Mining	4.3
Agriculture	4.4

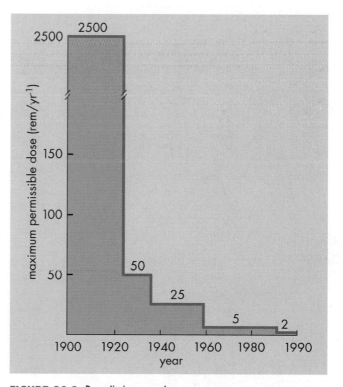

FIGURE 38-2 Dose limits over the past century.

TABLE 38-3

Historical Review of Dose Limits (DL) for Occupational Exposure

Year	Recommendation	Approximate Daily Dose Limit (Mrem)	Source
1902	Dose limited by fogging of a photographic plate after 7-minute contact exposure	10,000	Rollins
1915	Lead shielding of tube needed (no numerical exposure levels given)		British Roentgen Society
1921	General methods to reduce exposure		British X-Ray and Radium Protection Committee
1925	"It is entirely safe if an operator does not receive every 30 days a dose exceeding $1/100$ of an erythema dose."	200	Mutscheller
1925	10% of an SED* per year	200	Sievert
1926	One SED per 90,000 working hours	40	Dutch Board of Health
1928	0.000028 of an SED per day	175	Barclay and Cox
1928	0.001 of an SED per month 5 R per day permissible for the hands	150	Kaye
1931	Limit exposure to 0.2 R per day	200	Advisory Committee on X-ray and Radium Protection of the U.S.
1932	0.001 of an SED per month	30	Failla
1934	5 R per day permissible for the hands		Advisory Committee on X-ray and Radium Protection of the U.S.
1936	0.1 R per day	100	Advisory Committee on X-ray and Radium Protection of the U.S.
1941	0.02 R per day	20	Taylor
1943	200 mR per day is acceptable	200	Patterson
1959	5 rem per year, 5 (N − 18) rem accumulated	20	National Council on Radiation Protection and Measurements
1987	50 mSv per year, 10 × N mSv cumulative	20	National Council on Radiation Protection and Measurements
1991	20 mSv per year	8	International Commission on Radiation Protection

*SED, Skin erythema dose.

TABLE 38-4

1993 Dose Limits Rrecommended by the NCRP

A. Occupational Exposures	
1. Effective dose limit	
a. Annual	50 mSv (5000 mrem)
b. Cumulative	10 mSv × age (1000 mrem × age)
2. Equivalent annual dose limits for tissues and organs	
a. Lens of eye	150 mSv (15,000 mrem)
b. Skin, hands, and feet	500 mSv (50,000 mrem)
B. Public Exposures (Annual)	
1. Effective dose limit, continuous or frequent exposure	1 mSv (100 mrem)
2. Effective dose limit, infrequent exposure	5 mSv (500 mrem)
3. Equivalent dose limits for tissues and organs	
a. Lens of eye	15 mSv (1500 mrem)
b. Skin, hands, and feet	50 mSv (5000 mrem)
C. Education and Training Exposures (Annual)	
1. Effective dose limit	1 mSv (100 mrem)
2. Equivalent dose limit for tissues and organs	
a. Lens of eye	15 mSv (1500 mrem)
b. Skin, hands, and feet	50 mSv (5000 mrem)
D. Embryo-Fetus Exposures	
1. Total equivalent dose limit	5 mSv (500 mrem)
2. Equivalent dose limit in a month	0.5 mSv (50 mrem)
E. Negligible Individual Dose (Annual)	0.01 mSv (10 mrem)

Based on a linear, nonthreshold dose-response relationship, the current DLs are considered the level of exposure acceptable as an occupational hazard.

In practice, at least in diagnostic imaging, it is seldom necessary to exceed even one tenth the appropriate DL. Since the basis for the DL assumes a linear, nonthreshold dose-response relationship, all unnecessary radiation exposure should be avoided.

Occupational exposure is described as dose equivalent in units of millisieverts (mrem). Dose limits are specified as effective dose equivalent (H_E) or more recently as effective dose (E). This scheme has been adapted to be more precise in radiation protection. The following relationships describe this scheme:

Effective dose equivalent (H_E) =
   Weighting factor × Quality factor × Absorbed dose

Effective dose (E) = Radiation weighting factor (W_R) ×
      Tissue weighting factor (W_t) × Absorbed dose

Adoption of this scheme is progressing. For our purposes, effective dose (E) is the quantity of importance. It is expressed in mSv (mrem) and is the basis for our dose limits. As seen in Table 38-5, the radiation weighting factor (W_R) is LET dependent but is equal to one for types of radiation we use in medicine.

The tissue weighting factor (W_t) accounts for the relative radiosensitivity of various tissues and organs. These are shown in Table 38-6.

Practical implementation of these new dose limits and weighting factors does not change the previous approach. The dose limit is sufficiently high that rarely, if ever, will it be exceeded in diagnostic imaging.

With a collar-positioned monitor, a change in procedure is necessary to estimate effective dose (E). Since essentially all exposure to occupational workers occurs during fluoroscopy and the trunk is shielded by a lead apron, the response of the monitor on the collar overestimates the effective dose (E).

TABLE 38-5

Radiation Weighting Factor for Various Types of Radiation

Type and Energy Range	Radiation Weighting Factor (W_R)
X and γ rays, electrons	1
Neutrons, energy <10 keV	5
10 keV to 100 keV	10
>100 keV to 2 MeV	20
>2 MeV to 20 MeV	10
>20 MeV	5
Protons	2
Alpha particles	20

TABLE 38-6

Weighting Factors for the Various Tissues

Tissue	Tissue Weighting Factor (W_T)
Gonads	0.20
Active bone marrow	0.12
Colon	0.12
Lungs	0.12
Stomach	0.12
Bladder	0.05
Breasts	0.05
Esophagus	0.05
Liver	0.05
Thyroid	0.05
Bone surfaces	0.01
Skin	0.01

A conversion factor of 0.3 is applied to the monitor reported value to estimate (E). For a radiographer who does no fluoroscopy, the monitor response may be considered the effective dose.

Equivalent Dose Limits for Tissues and Organs

The whole-body DL of 50 mSv per year (5000 mrem per year) is an effective dose that takes into account the weighted average to various tissues and organs. In addition the NCRP identifies several specific tissues and organs with a specific dose limit.

Skin. Some organs of the body have a higher DL than the whole-body DL. The DL for the skin is 500 mSv per year (50,000 mrem per year). This is an increase from the earlier recommendation of 150 mSv per year (15,000 mrem per year).

This limit is not normally of concern in diagnostic imaging, since it applies to nonpenetrating radiation such as alpha and beta radiation and very soft x-rays. Radiographers exclusively engaged in soft tissue radiography or nuclear medicine are highly unlikely to sustain radiation exposures to the skin in excess of 10 mSv per year (1000 mrem per year).

Extremities. Radiologists often have their hands near the primary radiation beam, and therefore extremity exposure may be of concern. The DL for the extremities is the same as that for the skin, 500 mSv per year (50,000 mrem per year).

These radiation levels are quite high and under normal circumstances should not even be approached. For certain occupational groups, such as angiointerventional radiologists and nuclear medicine technologists, extremity personnel monitors may be provided. Such devices are worn on the wrist or the finger.

RADIATION EXPOSURE TO THE PUBLIC

The effective DL established for nonoccupationally exposed persons is one tenth of that for the radiation worker. Individuals in the general population are limited to 5 mSv per year (500 mrem per year) if the exposure is infrequent. If the exposure is frequent, such as hospital workers who may regularly pass by x-ray rooms, the DL is 1 mSv per year (100 mrem per year).

This is the DL that medical physicists use when computing the thickness of protective barriers. If a barrier separates an x-ray examining room from an area occupied by the general public, then the shielding is designed so that the annual exposure in the adjacent area cannot exceed 1 mSv per year (100 mrem per year). If the adjacent area is occupied by radiation workers, then the shielding must be sufficient to maintain an annual exposure level less than 10 mSv per year (1000 mrem per year). This approach to shielding derives from the 10 mSv × N cumulative dose limit.

Radiation exposure of the general population or individuals in the population is rarely measured because it is not necessary. Most diagnostic imaging personnel do not even receive this level of exposure.

EDUCATIONAL CONSIDERATIONS

There are several special situations associated with the whole-body occupational DL. Student radiographers under the age of 18 may not receive more than 1 mSv per year (100 mrem per year) during the course of their educational activities. This is included in and not in addition to the 1 mSv (100 mrem) permitted each year as a nonoccupational exposure. Consequently, student radiographers under the age of 18 may be engaged in departments of radiology, but their personnel exposure must be monitored and should remain below 1 mSv per year (100 mrem per year). Because of this, it is general practice not to accept underaged persons into schools of radiography unless their eighteenth birthday is only a few months away.

Even more changes in the recommended DL are on the way. Whatever changes are made are in keeping with **ALARA**. ALARA is an acromyn indicating a concept to maintain radiation exposures as low as reasonably achievable. The changes also acknowledge that radiographers can function efficiently even with these more restrictive dose-limiting recommendations. In 1991 the International Commission on Radiological Protection (ICRP) issued a number of recommendations, which includes an annual whole-body effective DL of 20 mSv (2000 mrem). Such a reduction is currently under consideration in the United States.

X-RAYS AND PREGNANCY

Two situations in diagnostic imaging require particular attention. Both are associated with pregnancy. There is heightened concern is for the pregnant radiographer and for the pregnant patient.

Radiobiology of Pregnancy

The severity of the potential response to radiation exposure in utero is both time related and dose related. This was discussed in Chapter 37. Unquestionably the most sensitive period to radiation exposure occurs before birth. Furthermore the fetus is more sensitive early in pregnancy. As a general rule, the higher the radiation dose, the more severe the radiation response will be.

Time dependence. The most critical time for irradiation is during the first 2 weeks when it is unlikely the expectant mother knows of her condition. In fact, this is the time during pregnancy when such irradiation results in only two responses.

The biologic response to irradiation during the first 2 weeks of pregnancy is resorption of the embryo or spontaneous abortion. No other type of response has ever been demonstrated in experimental animals after a radiation dose.

The time from approximately the second week to the eighth week of pregnancy is called *the period of major organogenesis*. During this time the major organ systems of the body are developing. If the radiation dose is sufficient, congenital abnormalities may result. Early in this interval, the most likely congenital abnormalities are associated with skeletal deformities. Later in this period, neurologic deficiencies are more likely to occur.

During the second and third trimesters of pregnancy, the responses previously noted are unlikely. Results of numerous investigations strongly suggest that if a response occurs after irradiation during the latter two trimesters, the only one possible would be the appearance during childhood of malignant disease such as leukemia or cancer. Malignant disease induction in childhood is also a possible response to irradiation during the first trimester.

These responses to irradiation during pregnancy require a very high radiation dose before there is significant risk of occurrence. No such responses would occur at less than 25 rad (250 mGy). Such dose levels are remote yet possible with patients who receive multiple x-ray examinations of the abdomen or pelvis. The dose of 25 rad or more is essentially impossible with radiographers. There are no other significant responses after irradiation in utero.

Dose dependence. As one might imagine, virtually no information is available at the human level to construct dose-response relationships for irradiation in utero. There is, however, a large body of data from animal irradiation, particularly rats and mice, from which relationships can be estimated. The statements that follow, although attributed to human exposure, represent estimates based on extrapolation from animal studies.

After an in utero radiation dose of 200 rad (2 Gy), it is nearly certain that each of the effects noted previously will occur. The likelihood, however, that an exposure of this magnitude would be experienced in diagnostic imaging is nil.

Spontaneous abortion after irradiation during the first 2 weeks of pregnancy is not likely to occur at radiation doses less than 25 rad (250 mGy). The precise nature of the dose-response relationship is unknown, but a reasonable estimate of risk suggests that 0.1% of all conceptions would be resorbed after a dose of 10 rad (100 mGy). The response at lower doses would be proportionately lower. Keep in mind, however, that the incidence of spontaneous abortion in the absence of radiation exposure is estimated to be in the 25% to 50% range.

When assessing the risk of inducing congenital abnormalities, one should be aware that in the absence of radiation exposure, approximately 5% of all live births exhibit a manifest congenital abnormality. A 1% increase in congenital abnormalities is estimated to follow a 10 rad (100 mGy) fetal dose and a proportionately lower increase at lower doses.

The induction of a childhood malignancy after irradiation in utero is difficult to assess. Risk estimates are even lower than those reported for spontaneous abortion and congenital abnormalities. The best approach to assessing risk of childhood malignancy is to use a relative risk estimate.

During the first trimester, the relative risk of childhood malignancy is in the range of 5 to 10; it drops to about 1.4 during the third trimester. The overall relative risk is accepted to be 1.5, a 50% increase over the naturally occurring incidence.

The Pregnant Radiographer

When a radiographer becomes pregnant, she should notify her supervisor. The pregnancy then becomes declared, and the DL becomes 0.5 mSv per month (50 mrem per month). The supervisor should then review the pregnant radiographer's previous radiation exposure history, since this will aid in deciding what protective actions are necessary.

The equivalent dose limit for the fetus is 5 mSv (500 mrem) for the period of pregnancy, a dose level that most radiographers will not reach. Although some may receive doses that exceed 5 mSv per year (500 mrem per year), most receive less than 1mSv per year (100 mrem per year). This is indicated with the personnel monitoring device that is positioned at the collar above the protective apron. The exposure at the waist under the protective apron will not normally exceed 10% of these values, and therefore, under normal conditions, specific protective action is not necessary.

Most lead aprons are 0.5-millimeter lead equivalent. These provide approximately 90% attenuation at 75 kVp, which is sufficient. One-millimeter lead equivalent protective aprons are available, but such thickness is not necessary, particularly in view of the additional weight of the apron. Back problems during pregnancy constitute a greater hazard than radiation exposure. The length of the apron need not extend below the knees, but wraparound aprons are preferred during pregnancy. A special effort should be made to provide an apron of proper size because of the weight.

It is reasonable to provide the pregnant radiographer with a second personnel monitoring device, which is positioned under the protective apron at waist level. The exposure reported on the second monitor should be maintained on a separate record and identified as exposure to the fetus. Do not allow the badges to be switched and the record confused. Additional or thicker lead aprons are not necessary.

The use of such an additional monitor shows consistently that exposures to the fetus are insignificant. Suppose, for instance, that a pregnant radiographer wearing a single radiation monitor at collar level receives 10 mSv (1000 mrem) during the 9-month period. The dose at waist level under a protective apron would be less than 10% of the collar dose, or 1 mSv (100 mrem). Because of attenuation by the maternal tissues overlying the fetus, the dose to the fetus would be approximately 30% of the abdominal skin dose, or 300 Sv (30 mrem). Consequently, when normal protective measures are taken, it is nearly impossible for a radiographer to approach the fetal DL.

When pregnancy is reported, regardless of the nature of the x-ray facilities or the radiographer's work experience, the supervisor should review acceptable practices of radiation protection. This review should emphasize the cardinal principles of radiation protection: minimize time, maximize distance, and use available shielding.

Management Principles

It should be clear that the probability of a damaging effect after any radiation exposure received in medicine is nil. A biologic response is very rarely expected and has not been observed in diagnostic imaging personnel for the past 50 years or so. It is essential for the director of diagnostic imaging to incorporate the following three steps into the radiation protection program: (1) new employee training, (2) periodic in-service training, and (3) counseling during pregnancy.

New employee training. The initial step for any administrative protocol dealing with pregnant employees involves orientation and training. During these orientation discussions, all female employees should be instructed as to their responsibility regarding pregnancy and radiation. Each radiographer should be provided with a copy of the facility radiation protection manual and other appropriate materials. This material might include a one-page summary of doses, responses, and proper radiation control working habits (see the box below).

The new employee should then be required to read and sign a form (see the box below), indicating that she has been instructed in this area of radiation protection. An important point to be made by signing this document is that the employee must notify her supervisor when she is pregnant or suspects she is pregnant.

In-service training. Every well-run diagnostic imaging service maintains a regular schedule of in-service training. Usually this training is conducted at monthly intervals but sometimes more often. At least twice each year such training should be devoted to radiation protection, and a portion of these sessions should be directed at the potentially pregnant employee.

The material to be covered in such sessions is outlined in the box to the left. Although it is good to review doses and responses, it is probably more appropriate to emphasize radiation control procedures. These, of course, affect the radiation safety of all radiographers, not just the pregnant radiographer.

A review of personnel monitoring records is particularly important. All too often radiographers are unaware of their radiation exposure because of their inability to interpret the radiation monitoring report. A helpful procedure is to post the most recent radiation monitoring report for all to see. The year-end report should be initialed by each radiographer, and the director of radiology should be sure that all radiographers understand the nature and magnitude of their annual exposure.

Through such training, imaging personnel will realize that their occupational exposure is minimal, usually much less than 10% of the DL. The following should be emphasized:

1. The effective DL is 50 mSv per year (5000 mrem per year)
2. Environmental background radiation is approximately 1 mSv per year (100 mrem per year)
3. Occupational exposures are closer to the latter than the former

---

Summary of Responses, Effects of Irradiation in Utero, and Protective Measures for the Pregnant Radiographer

Human responses to low-level x-ray exposure

Life-span shortening	10 days/rad
Cataracts	None below 200 rad
Leukemia	10 cases/10^6/rad
Cancer	100 cases/10^6/rad
Genetic effects	Doubling dose = 50 rad
Death from all causes	1:10,000/rad

Effects of irradiation in utero

0 to 14 days	Spontaneous abortion: 25% natural incidence; 0.1% increase/10 rad
2 to 8 weeks	Congenital abnormalities: 5% natural incidence; 1% increase/10 rad
Second to third trimester	Cell depletion: no effect at less than 50 rad; Latent malignancy: 4:10,000 natural incidence; 6:10,000/rad
0 to 9 months	Genetic effects: 10% natural incidence; 5×10^{-7} mutations/rad

Protective measures for the radiographer

Two personal radiation monitors
Dose limit: 500 mrem every 9 months, 50 mrem every month

New Employee Training Form

This is to certify that _____, a new employee of this diagnostic imaging facility, has received instructions regarding mutual responsibilities should she become pregnant during this employment.

In addition to personal counseling by _____, she has been given several documents dealing with pregnancy in diagnostic imaging to read. Furthermore, the additional reading material that follows is available in the departmental office:

1. *Review of NCRP radiation dose limit for embryo and fetus in occupationally-exposed women*, NCRP Report No. 53, Washington, DC: National Council on Radiation Protection and Measures, 1977.
2. *Medical radiation exposure of pregnant and potentially pregnant women*, NCRP Report No. 54, Washington, DC: National Council on Radiation Protection and Measures, 1977.
3. Wagner, LK et al, *Exposure of the pregnant patient to diagnostic radiation*, Philadelphia, 1985, JB Lippincott.
4. *The effects on populations of exposure to low levels of ionizing radiation*, Washington, DC: National Academy of Sciences, 1990.

I understand that should I become pregnant, it is my responsibility to inform my supervisor of my condition immediately so that additional protective measures can be taken.

_____
Employee

_____
Supervisor

_____
Date

Counseling during pregnancy. The next point for action on the part of the director of diagnostic imaging occurs when the radiographer declares her pregnancy. First the director should counsel the employee, including a review of her radiation exposure history.

In all likelihood a review of the employee's previous radiation exposure history will show a low-exposure profile. Those who wear the radiation monitor positioned at the collar, as recommended, and who are heavily involved in fluoroscopy, may receive an exposure greater than 5 mSv per year (500 mrem per year). Such employees, however, are protected by lead aprons so that exposure to the trunk of the body would not normally exceed 500 μSv (50 mrem per year).

This review of personnel radiation exposure is the appropriate time to emphasize that the DL during pregnancy is 5 mSv (500 mrem) and 0.5 mSv per month (50 mrem per month). Furthermore, it should be shown that this DL refers to the fetus and not to the radiographer. This level of 5 mSv (500 mrem) to the fetus during gestation is considered an absolutely safe radiation exposure level. In view of this discussion the director of diagnostic imaging should point out to the radiographer that an alteration in her work schedule is not essential.

For radiographers involved in radiation oncology, nuclear medicine, or ultrasound, a similar consultation and level of restriction as previously discussed is appropriate. In radiation oncology the pregnant radiographer may continue her normal work load but should not participate in brachytherapy applications.

In nuclear medicine the pregnant staff member should handle only small quantities of radioactive material. She should not elute radioisotope generators or inject millicurie quantities of radioactive material.

Ultrasonographers are not normally classified as radiation workers. A sizable portion of ultrasound patients, however, have previously been nuclear medicine patients and therefore become a potential source of exposure to the ultrasonographer. This possibility is remote, since the quantity of radioactivity is low. It may be advisable during the pregnancy to provide the ultrasonographer with a radiation monitor.

Finally the pregnant radiographer should be required to read and sign a form (see the box below), attesting to the fact that she has been given proper attention and that she understands that the level of risk associated with her employment is much less than that experienced by nearly all occupational groups.

The Pregnant Patient

Safeguards against accidental irradiation early in pregnancy are complex administrative problems. This situation is particularly critical during the first 2 months of pregnancy, when such a condition may not be suspected and when the fetus is particularly sensitive to radiation exposure. After a couple of months the risk of irradiating an unknown pregnancy becomes small because the patient is generally aware of her condition.

If pregnancy is known, then under some circumstances the radiographic examination should not be conducted. One should never knowingly examine a pregnant patient with x-rays unless a documented decision to do so has been made. When such an examination does proceed, it should be conducted with all of the previously discussed techniques for minimizing patient dose.

For many years, radiologists subscribed to the **10-day rule.** This rule was first stated in 1970 by the ICRP. It recommended that all x-ray examinations of the abdomen or pelvis of fertile women be performed only during the 10 days after the onset of menstruation. Be-

---

Acknowledgment of Radiation Risk During Pregnancy

I _____, do acknowledge that I have received counseling from _____, regarding my employment responsibilities during my pregnancy.

The reading material listed below has been made available to me to demonstrate that the additional risk during my pregnancy is much less than that for most occupational groups. I further understand that, although I may be assigned to low-exposure duties and provided with a second radiation monitor, these are simply added precautions and do not in any way convey that any assignment in this department is especially hazardous during pregnancy.

1. *Review of NCRP radiation dose limit for embryo and fetus in occupationally-exposed women,* NCRP Report No. 53, Washington, DC: National Council on Radiation Protection and Measures, 1977.
2. *Medical radiation exposure of pregnant and potentially pregnant women,* NCRP Report No. 54, Washington, DC: National Council on Radiation Protection and Measures, 1977.
3. Wagner LK et al, *Exposure of the pregnant patient to diagnostic radiation,* Philadelphia, 1985, J.B. Lippincott.
4. *The effects of populations of exposure to low levels of ionizing radiation,* Washington, DC: National Academy of Sciences, 1980.

Employee _____   Supervisor _____

Date _____

cause of our better understanding of the radiobiology of radiation and pregnancy, the 10-day rule is obsolete today. The risk of injury after irradiation in utero is small and the usual benefit so great that if the examination is clinically indicated, it should be performed.

When a pregnant patient must be examined, the examination should be done with precisely collimated beams and carefully positioned protective shields. Use of high-kVp technique is most appropriate in such situations. The administrative protocols that can be used to ensure that pregnant patients are not irradiated vary from simple to complex.

Elective booking. The most direct way to ensure against the irradiation of an unsuspected pregnancy is to institute **elective booking.** This requires that the clinician or radiologist determine the time of the patient's previous menstrual cycle. X-ray examinations in which the fetus is not in or near the primary beam may be allowed, but they should be accompanied by pelvic shielding.

Ideally the referring physician should be responsible for determining the menstrual cycle and for withholding the examination request if there is any question about the necessity of the examination. This may require a radiologist-sponsored educational program that can be easily conducted at regularly scheduled medical staff meetings.

Patient questionnaire. An alternative procedure is to have the patient herself indicate her menstrual cycle. In many diagnostic imaging departments the patient must complete an information form before examination. These forms often include questions such as "Are you or could you be pregnant?" and "What was the date of your last menstrual period?" The box below shows an example of such a simple yet effective patient questionnaire for protecting against irradiation of a pregnant patient.

Posting. If neither elective booking nor the request form seems appropriate to a diagnostic imaging service, an equally successful method is to post signs of caution in the waiting room. Such signs could read "Are you pregnant or could you be? If so, inform the radiographer," or "Warning—special precautions are necessary if you are pregnant," or "Caution—if there is any possibility that you are pregnant, it is very important that you inform the radiographer before you have an x-ray examination." Figure 38-3 is a helpful poster available from the Food and Drug Administration (FDA).

What If?

It has been estimated that fewer than 1% of all females referred for x-ray examination are potentially pregnant. If a pregnant patient escapes detection and is irradiated, however, what is the subsequent responsibility of the diagnostic imaging service? What follow-up should be in place?

The first step is to estimate the fetal dose. The medical physicist should be consulted immediately and requested to estimate the fetal dose. If a preliminary review of the examination techniques used (e.g., type of examination, kVp, and mAs) determines that the dose may have exceeded 1 rad (10 mGy), a more complete dosimetric evaluation should be conducted.

Table 38-7 presents representative radiation levels for many examinations. With a knowledge of the types of examinations performed and the techniques and apparatus used, the physicist can accurately determine the fetal dose. There are phantoms and dosimetry materials available to ensure that this determination can be made with confidence.

Once the fetal dose is known, the referring physician and radiologist should determine the stage of gestation at which the x-ray exposure occurred. With this infor-

---

X-ray Consent for Women of Child-bearing Age

X-ray examinations of abdomen and pelvis exposing the uterus to radiation are:

Abdomen (KUB)	Colon (barium enema)	Pyelograms (IVP and retrograde)
Stomach (UGI)	Gallbladder	Cystograms
Small intestine (SI)	Hips, sacrum, coccyx	Lumbar spine and pelvis

All nuclear medicine studies

The 10 days after onset of menstrual period are generally considered safe for x-ray examinations.

Onset of last menstrual period.   Date: _____   Date today: _____

I am pregnant	Yes _____	No _____	Don't know _____
I have had a hysterectomy	Yes _____	No _____	Don't know _____
I use an IUD	Yes _____	No _____	Don't know _____

I recognize that if I am pregnant and have radiation to the abdomen, there is a possibility of injury to the fetus. However, I understand that the likelihood of such injury is slight and that my physician feels that the information to be gained from this examination is important to my health. I therefore wish to have this x-ray examination performed now.

_____
Name of examination

_____
Witness   Signature of patient

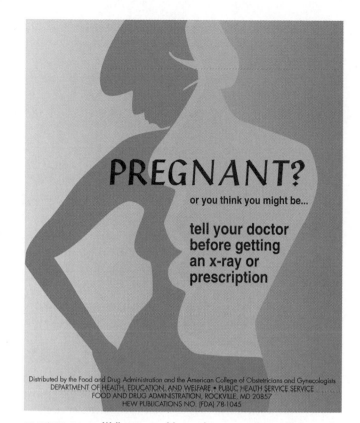

FIGURE 38-3 Wall posters with warnings concerning radiation and pregnancy are available from the National Center for Devices and Radiological Health. *(Courtesy FDA.)*

TABLE 38-7

Representative Entrance Exposures and Fetal Doses for Frequently Performed Radiographic Examinations with a 200-speed Image Receptor

Examination	Entrance Skin Exposure (mR)	Fetal Dose (mrad)
Skull (lateral)	70	0
Cervical spine (AP)	110	0
Shoulder	90	0
Chest (PA)	10	0
Thoracic spine (AP)	180	1
Cholecystogram (PA)	150	1
Lumbosacral spine (AP)*	250	80
Abdomen or KUB (AP)*	220	70
Intravenous pyelogram (IVP)*	210	60
Hip*	220	50
Wrist or foot	5	0

*Gonadal shields should be used if possible.

mation there are only two alternatives: suggest the patient to continue to term or suggest she terminate the pregnancy.

Few authoritative recommendations exist regarding when abortion is indicated. Since the natural incidence of congenital anomalies is approximately 5%, no such effects can reasonably be considered a consequence of diagnostic x-ray doses. Manifest damage to the newborn is unlikely at fetal doses below 25 rad (250 mGy), although some suggest that lower doses may cause mental developmental abnormalities.

In view of the available evidence a reasonable approach is to apply a 10- to 25-rad rule. Below 10 rad (100 mGy) a therapeutic abortion is not indicated unless there are additional risk factors involved. Above 25 rad (250 mGy) the risk of latent injury may justify a therapeutic abortion. Between 10 and 25 rad, one must carefully consider all the factors.

Fortunately, experience with such situations has shown that fetal doses have been consistently low. The fetal dose is usually in the 1 to 5 rad (10 to 50 mGy) range after a series of conventional x-ray examinations.

SUMMARY

Health physics is defined as radiation safety programs designed by radiation scientists, engineers, and physicians concerned with research, teaching, and operation aspects of radiation exposure. The three cardinal principles developed for nuclear and radiation workers are as follows: minimize time near the radiation source, maximize the distance from the radiation source, and include shielding to reduce radiation exposure.

The terminology *maximum permissible dose* has been replaced by the NCRP with *dose limit (DL)*. Dose limits are prescribed for various organs, the whole body, and various working conditions so that the lifetime risk of each year's occupational exposure does not exceed 10^{-4} per year^{-1}. The International Commission on Radiation Protection in 1991 determined a recommedation for the dose limit of radiation exposure to be 20 mSv per year. In 1993, recomendations were revised so the cumulative whole-body DL is now 10 mSv times one's age in years and the annual DL is 50 mSv. The DL during pregnancy remains at 5 mSv. In diagnostic imaging, however, it is seldom necessary to exceed one tenth the appropriate DL. Table 38-4 lists the recent dose-limit recommendations from the NCRP for occupational, public, educational, and embryo-fetus exposures. ALARA (as low as reasonably achievable) is the acronym that defines for occupational workers the principal concept of radiation protection.

The radiobiology of pregnancy requires particular attention for the pregnant radiographer and the pregnant patient. Irradiation during the first 2 weeks of pregnancy is the most critical. The response of spontaneous abortion occurs at doses of 10 to 25 rad or more. From the second to the eight week is the period of major organogenesis, and with irradiation of 200 rad it is nearly certain congenital abnormalities will occur. Severe irradiation during the last two trimesters of pregnancy may cause childhood malignant disease of leukemia or cancer. The pregnant radiographer should be provided with a second radiation monitoring device to be worn under the protective apron at waist level. The pregnant patient should not have a radiographic examination of the abdomen or pelvis unless a documented decision is made. The 10-day rule previously used stated radiographic examinations of women of child-bearing age should be performed only during the 10 days after the onset of menstruation. This rule is now obsolete. Elective booking, patient consent forms, and posting of education signs are now the established protocol for radiography of the pregnant patient.

If a patient is pregnant without knowledge of the imaging staff and has a radiographic examination performed, the following procedure is followed:

1. The medical physicist estimates fetal dose
2. The referring physicain and the radiologist determine the stage of gestation
3. Below 10 rad there is no evidence of risk; above 25 rad the risk of latent injury may suggest a therapeutic abortion; and between 10 and 25 rad requires careful consideration

REVIEW QUESTIONS

1. What wartime effort coined the term *health physicist?*
2. Write the exposure equation for the radiation dose and duration of exposure.
3. What is the function of the 5-minute reset timer on all fluoroscopy units?
4. What is the exposure rate at point A on the iso-exposure lines for the fluoroscopy room in Figure 38-2?
5. Define TVL.
6. A fluoroscope emits 3.5 R/mA minute at the table top for every mA of operation. What is the approximate patient exposure following a 3.2-minute fluoroscopic examination of 1.5 mA?
7. What are the three cardinal principles of radiation protection? How are they applied to diagnostic imaging?

8. Discuss the use of the term *maximum permissible dose.* What is the modern terminology for occupation exposure?
9. What does the value 10^{-4} yr^{-1} mean in regards to the NCRP Dose Limits?
10. Using Table 38-2, identify the industry with the most fatal accidents.
11. Review Table 38-3. According to 1959 dose recommendations, a 28-year-old radiographer would be allowed what accumulated dose? Using Table 38-4, what is the most recent annual dose-limit recommendation for that 28-year-old radiographer?
12. Define tissue weighting factor (W_t).
13. How do some radiation occupational groups such as nuclear medicine technologists monitor their extremity doses?
14. The effective DL established for nonoccupationally exposed persons is _____ that of the radiation worker.
15. What is the whole-body occupational DL for radiography students under 18 years old?
16. What is the embryo's response to irradiation above 25 rad during the first 2 weeks after conception?
17. During the period of major organogenesis of the fetus, what are the two responses to severe irradiation?
18. List the management protocol for the pregnant radiographer.
19. What information regarding radiation protection should be covered in regularly scheduled in-service training classes?
20. What is the procedure if a pregnant patient is irradiated accidentally?

Additional Reading

Dowd SB, Wilson B: Informed patient consent: a historical perspective, *Radiol Technol* 67(2):119 November-December, 1995.

Fung K: Lowering patient dose on single-phase x-ray units, *Radiol Technol* 66(3):159 January-February, 1995.

Israel MS: Electromagnetic radiation—parameters for risk assessment, *Rev Environ Health* 10(2):85 April-June, 1994.

Kline KB, Cope WB: ALARA overview system at Crystal River Unit 3 nuclear station, *Health Phys* 69(2):281 August, 1995.

Maharaj HP: Stray radiation from baggage x-ray equipment: results and implications, *Health Phys* 57(1):141 July, 1989.

39

Designing for Radiation Protection

OBJECTIVES

At the completion of this chapter the student will be able to:

1. Name the leakage radiation limit for x-ray tubes
2. List the beam-on indicators on the control panel
3. Indicate the nine radiation-protection aspects of radiographic equipment
4. List the nine radiation protection features of fluoroscopic equipment
5. Discuss the design of primary and secondary radiation barriers
6. Describe the design of the three types of radiation-detection dosimeters used in diagnostic imaging

OUTLINE

Design of X-ray Apparatus
 Diagnostic type of protective tube housing
 Control panel
Radiation-Protection Designs for X-ray Equipment
 Source-to-image receptor distance indicator
 Collimation
 Positive-beam limitation
 Beam alignment
 Filtration
 Reproducibility
 Linearity
 Exposure switch
 Mobile radiography exposure switch
 Fluoroscopic equipment

Design of Protective Barriers
 Primary barriers
 Secondary barriers
 Factors affecting barrier thickness
Radiation Detection and Measurement
 Gas-filled detectors
 Scintillation detectors
 Thermoluminescence dosimetry

A number of features of modern x-ray equipment designed to improve radiographic quality were discussed in previous chapters. Many of these features are also designed to reduce patient dose during x-ray examinations. For instance, proper beam collimation contributes to improved image contrast and is also effective in reducing patient dose. Filtration, on the other hand, is added to the x-ray beam only to reduce the patient dose.

More than 100 individual radiation-protection devices and accessories are associated with modern x-ray equipment. Some are characteristic of either radiographic or fluoroscopic assemblies, and some are determined by federal regulation for all diagnostic x-ray equipment. The list of devices required for all diagnostic x-ray equipment follow.

DESIGN OF X-RAY APPARATUS
Diagnostic-Type of Protective Tube Housing

Every x-ray tube must be contained within a protective housing that reduces the leakage radiation to less than 100 mR per hour (26 µC/kilogram-hour) at a distance of 1 meter from the housing.

Control Panel

The control panel must indicate the conditions of exposure and positively indicate when the x-ray tube is energized. These requirements are usually satisfied with kVp and mA meters. Also there are visible or audible signals indicating when the x-ray beam is on.

RADIATION-PROTECTION DESIGNS FOR X-RAY EQUIPMENT

Many aspects of radiation-protection designs of radiographic equipment are mandated by federal regulation. The designs that follow are required of all radiographic equipment.

Source-to-Image Receptor Distance Indicator

A source-to-image receptor distance (SID) indicator must be provided. It can be as simple as a tape measure attached to the tube housing or as advanced as laser lights, but it must be accurate to within 2% of the indicated SID.

Collimation

Light-localized variable-aperture rectangular collimators should be provided. The x-ray beam and light beam must coincide to within 2% of the SID. Cones and diaphragms may replace the collimator for special examinations. The attenuation of the useful beam by the collimator shutters must be equivalent to that attenuated by the protective housing.

Question: Most radiographs are taken at an SID of 100 centimeters. How much difference is allowed between the projection of the light field and the x-ray beam at the image receptor?

Answer: 2% of 100 centimeters = 2 centimeters

Positive-Beam Limitation

Automatic light-localized variable-aperture collimators were required on all but special equipment manufactured in the United States between 1974 and 1994. These positive-beam limitation (PBL) devices are no longer required but continue to be a part of most new radiographic equipment. They must be adjusted so that with any film size in use and at all standard SIDs the collimator shutters automatically provide an x-ray beam equal to the image receptor. The PBL must be accurate to 2% of the SID.

Beam Alignment

In addition to proper collimation, each radiographic tube head should be provided with a mechanism to ensure proper alignment of the x-ray beam and the film. It does no good to align the light field and the x-ray beam if the film is improperly aligned. An indicator light allows for tube/film alignment.

Filtration

All general-purpose diagnostic x-ray beams must have a total filtration (inherent plus added) of at least 2.5 millimeters aluminum when operated above 70 kVp. Radiographic tubes operated between 50 and 70 kVp must have at least 1.5 millimeters aluminum. Below 50 kVp, a minimum of 0.5 millimeters aluminum total filtration is required. X-ray tubes designed for mammography usually have 30 µm Mo or 60 µm Rh filtration, which is adequate below 50 kVp.

As discussed in Chapter 31, it is not normally possible to physically examine and measure the thickness of each component of total filtration. The measurement of half-value layer (HVL) and the relationship to total filtration is given in Table 31-3.

Question: The following data is obtained on a three-phase radiographic unit operating at 90 kVp, 100 mA, 100 ms. Is that sufficient filtration?

Added filtration (mm Al)	0	0.5	1.0	1.5	2.0	3.0	4.0	5.0
Exposure (mR)	87	74	65	56	49	39	31	25

Answer: When a plot is done of the given data it indicates an HVL of 3.4 millimeter aluminum. The minimum HVL that would indicate at least 2.5 millimeter aluminum total filtration is 3.1 millimeter aluminum. Therefore the filtration is adequate.

Reproducibility

For any given radiographic technique the output radiation intensity should be constant from one exposure to another. This is checked by making repeated exposures at the same technique and observing that the average variation in radiation intensity does not exceed 5%.

Linearity

When adjacent mA stations are used, for example, 100 and 200 mA, and exposure time is adjusted for constant mAs, the output radiation intensity must remain constant. Alternately, and perhaps better, the exposure time should remain constant, causing the mAs to increase in proportion to the increase in mA. This takes any inaccuracy in the exposure timer out of the analysis. The radiation intensity is expressed in units of mR/mAs, and the maximum acceptable variation is 10%.

Exposure Switch

It must not be possible to expose a radiograph while the radiographer stands inside the examination room. The radiographer must stand within a fixed protective barrier, usually the console booth. The exposure control should be fixed to the operating console and not to a long cord. The radiographer may be in the examination room during exposure but only if protective apparel is worn. However, some state laws prevent radiography personnel from standing with patients during exposure.

Mobile Radiography Exposure Switch

A protective lead apron should be assigned to each portable x-ray unit. The exposure switch of such a unit must allow the operator to remain at least 180 centimeters from the x-ray tube during exposure. Of course, while positioned at this minimum distance, the useful beam must be directed away from the radiographer and other medical personnel.

Fluoroscopic Equipment

The radiation protection features of fluoroscopic equipment are designed primarily to reduce patient and personnel exposure.

Source-to-skin distance. The source-to-skin distance must be not less than 38 centimeters on stationary fluoroscopes and not less than 30 centimeters on mobile fluoroscopes. Increasing the distance between the fluoroscopic tube and the patient results in reduced patient dose. The dose is reduced because of the corresponding decrease in the difference between the entrance and exit dose to the patient. Patient dose is higher when the fluoroscopic tube is close to the table top (Figure 39-1).

Primary protective barrier. The image-intensifier assembly serves as a primary protective barrier and must be 2-millimeters lead equivalent. It must be coupled with the x-ray tube and interlocked so that the fluoroscopic x-ray tube cannot be energized when in the parked position.

Filtration. The total filtration of the fluoroscope must be at least 2.5-millimeters aluminum equivalent. The table top, patient cradle, or other material positioned between the x-ray tube and the table top are included as part of the total filtration. When the filtration is unknown, the HVL should be measured. The minimum HVL reported in Table 31-2 must be met in order that adequate filtration may be assumed.

Collimation. The fluoroscopic x-ray beam collimators must be adjusted so that an unexposed border is visible on the television monitor when the input phosphor of the image intensifier is positioned 35 centimeters above the table top and the collimators are fully open. For automatic collimating devices, such an unexposed border should be visible at all heights above the table top, which the collimator shutters track automatically.

Exposure switch. The fluoroscopic exposure switch should be the dead-man type; that is, if the operator should drop dead, the exposure would be terminated—

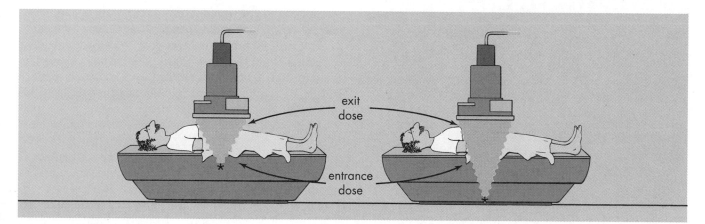

FIGURE 39-1 Patient entrance skin exposure is higher when the fluoroscopic x-ray tube is close to the table top.

unless, of course, he or she falls on the switch. The conventional foot pedal satisfies this condition.

Bucky slot cover. During fluoroscopy, the Bucky tray is moved to the end of the examining table, leaving an opening in the side of the table approximately 5-centimeters wide at gonadal level. This opening should be automatically covered by the Bucky slot cover, which has at least 0.25-millimeter lead equivalent.

Protective curtain. A protective curtain or panel of at least 0.25-millimeter lead equivalent should be positioned between the fluoroscopist and the patient. Figure 39-2 shows the typical isoexposure distribution for a fluoroscope. Without the curtain and Bucky slot cover, the exposure of radiology personnel is many times higher than the 100 mR per hour at 2 feet.

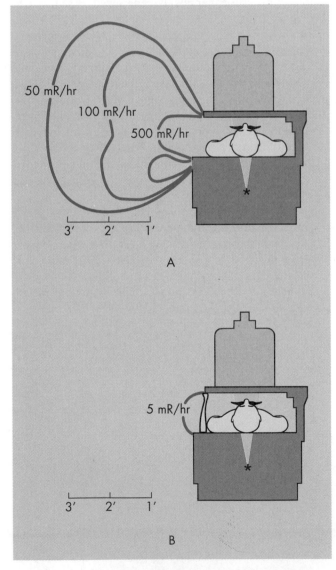

FIGURE 39-2 A, Isoexposure profile for an unshielded fluoroscope demonstrates the need for protective curtains and a Bucky slot cover. **B,** Exposure profile with these protective devices.

Cumulative timer. A cumulative timer that produces an audible signal or temporarily interrupts the x-ray beam when the fluoroscopic time has exceeded 5 minutes must be provided. This device is designed to make sure the radiologist is aware of the relative beam-on time during each procedure.

X-ray intensity. The intensity of the x-ray beam at the tabletop of a fluoroscope should not exceed 2.1 R per minute (0.54 mC/kilogram-minute) for each mA of operation at 80 kVp. If there is no optional high level control, the intensity must not exceed 10 R per minute (2.6 mC/kilogram-minute) during fluoroscopy. If an optional high level control is provided, the maximum table top intensity allowed is 20 R per minute (1.0 mC/kilogram-minute).

DESIGN OF PROTECTIVE BARRIERS

When designing diagnostic imaging departments or individual x-ray examination rooms, it is not sufficient to consider only general architectural characteristics described. Great attention must be given to the location of x-ray machines within the examination room and to the use of adjoining rooms. It is often necessary to insert protective barriers, usually sheets of lead, in the walls of x-ray examining rooms. If the diagnostic imaging facility is located on an upper floor, then it may be necessary to shield the floor as well.

A great number of factors are considered when designing a protective barrier. This discussion touches on only the fundamentals and some basic definitions. Any time new x-ray facilities are being designed or old ones renovated, a medical physicist must be consulted for assistance in designing proper radiation shielding.

Primary Barriers

For the purpose of designing protective barriers, three types of radiation are considered (Figure 39-3). Primary radiation is the most intense and therefore the most hazardous and the most difficult to protect against. Primary radiation is the useful beam. When a chest board is positioned on a given wall, it can be assumed that it will intercept the useful beam frequently. Therefore it is sometimes necessary to provide shielding directly behind the chest board in addition to that specified for the rest of the wall. Any wall to which the useful beam can be directed is designated a **primary protective barrier.**

Lead bonded to sheet rock or wood paneling is most often used as a primary protective barrier. Such lead shielding is available in various thicknesses, and it is specified for architects and contractors in units of pounds per square foot (lb/ft²). Rarely is it necessary to use in excess of 4 lb/ft² in a diagnostic room. Concrete, concrete block, or brick may be used instead of lead. As a rule of thumb, 4 inches of masonry is equivalent to $\frac{1}{16}$ inch of lead. Table 39-1 shows available lead thick-

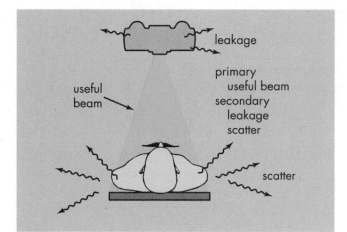

FIGURE 39-3 Three types of radiation: the useful beam, leakage radiation, and scatter radiation. All must be considered when designing the protective barriers for an x-ray room.

TABLE 39-1
Lead and Concrete Equivalents for Primary Protective Barriers

Lead			Concrete	
(Milli-meters)	(Inches)	(lb/ft²)	(Centi-meters)	(Inches)
0.4	1/64	1	2.4	1 3/8
0.8	1/32	2	4.8	1 7/8
1.2	3/64	3	7.2	2 7/8
1.6	1/16	4	9.6	3 3/4

nesses and equivalent thicknesses of concrete. The thinnest available shielding is 1 lb/ft², but because of some difficulties in fabrication, 2 lb/ft² lead is often no more costly.

Secondary Barriers

There are two types of **secondary radiation: scatter radiation** and **leakage radiation.** Scatter radiation results when the useful beam intercepts any object so that some x-rays are scattered. For the purpose of protective shielding calculations, the scattering object can be considered as a new source of radiation. During both radiography and fluoroscopy, the patient is the single most important scattering object. As a general rule of thumb, the intensity of scatter radiation 1 meter from the patient is 0.1% of the intensity of the useful beam at the patient.

Question: The output intensity of a radiographic unit at patient position is 410 mR (0.1 mC/kilogram) for a kidney, ureter, and bladder (KUB) examination. What will be the approximate radiation exposure 1 meter from the patient? 3 meters from the patient?

Answer: At 1 meter: 410 mR × 0.1% = 410 mR × 0.001

$$= 0.41 \text{ mR}$$

At 3 meters:

$$= 0.41 \text{ mR } (\tfrac{1}{3})^2$$

$$= 0.41 \text{ mR } (\tfrac{1}{9})$$

$$= 0.036 \text{ mR}$$

$$= 36 \text{ } \mu\text{R}$$

Leakage radiation is that radiation emitted from the x-ray tube housing in all directions other than that of the useful beam. If the tube housing is properly designed, the leakage radiation will never exceed the regulatory limit of 100 mR/hour (26 μC/kilogram-hour) at 1 meter. Although in practice, leakage radiation levels are much less than this limit, 100 mR per hour at 1 meter is used for barrier calculations.

Barriers designed to shield areas from secondary radiation are called **secondary protective barriers.** Secondary protective barriers are always less thick than primary protective barriers.

Lead is rarely required for secondary protective barriers because the computation usually results in less than 0.4 millimeter lead. In such cases, conventional gypsum board, glass, or lead acrylic is adequate. Many walls that are secondary protective barriers can be adequately protected with four thicknesses of 5/8-inch gypsum board. Control booth barriers are secondary protective barriers.

Remember: never direct the useful beam toward the control booth because it is a secondary barrier.

Four thicknesses of gypsum board and 1/2-inch plate glass may be all that is necessary. Sometimes glass walls 1/2- to 1-inch thick can be used for control booth barriers. Table 39-2 contains equivalent thicknesses for secondary protective barrier material.

Question: What percentage of the dose limit (100 mR per week) will be incident on a control booth barrier located 3 meters from the x-ray tube and patient? Assume the x-ray output is 3 mR/mAs and that the weekly beam-on time is 5 minutes at an average 100 mA, which is a generous assumption.

Answer: From scatter radiation the barrier will receive the following:

Total primary beam = 3 mR mAs × 100 mA × 5 m × 60 seconds per meter

$$= 90,000 \text{ mR}$$

Scatter radiation = 90,000 mR × 1/1000 × $(\tfrac{1}{3})^2$

$$= 10 \text{ mR}$$

TABLE 39-2

Equivalent Material Thicknesses for Secondary Barriers

Computed Lead Required (Millimeters)	Steel (Millimeters)	Glass (Millimeters)	Substitutes Gypsum (Millimeters)	Wood (Millimeters)
0.1	0.5	1.2	2.8	19
0.2	1.2	2.5	5.9	33
0.3	1.8	3.7	8.8	44
0.4	2.5	4.8	12	53

From leakage radiation, the barrier will receive the following:

$$\text{Leakage radiation at 1 meter} = 100 \text{ mR/hr} \times \frac{5}{60}\text{ hr}$$

$$= 8.3 \text{ mR}$$

$$\text{Leakage radiation} = 8.3 \text{ mR } (^1/_3)^2$$

$$= 0.9 \text{ mR}$$

$$\text{Total secondary radiation} = 10 \text{ mR} + 0.9 \text{ mR}$$

$$= 10.9 \text{ mR or } 11\%$$
$$\text{of the dose limit}$$

This analysis is representative of the clinical environment. The estimated exposure is to the control booth barrier, not to the radiographer. The composition of the barrier and the additional distance reduces radiographer exposure even more. This is the reason that personnel radiation exposure during radiography is very low. Radiographers get most of their exposure during fluoroscopy.

Factors Affecting Barrier Thickness

Many factors must be taken into consideration when calculating the required protective barrier thickness. A thorough discussion of these factors is beyond the scope of this book; however, a definition of each is useful for understanding the problems involved.

The thickness of a barrier naturally depends on the distance between the source of radiation and the barrier. The distance is that to the adjacent occupied area, not to the inside of the wall of the x-ray room. A wall along which an x-ray machine is positioned will probably require more shielding than the other walls of the room. In such a case the leakage radiation may be more hazardous than the scatter radiation or even the useful beam. It is usually desirable to position the x-ray machine in the middle of the room because then no single wall is subjected to especially intense radiation exposure.

The use of the area being protected is of principal importance. If the area were a rarely occupied closet or storeroom, the required shielding would be less than if it were an office or laboratory occupied 40 hours per week. This reflects the time of occupancy factor (T).

Table 39-3 reports the occupancy levels of various areas as suggested by the National Council on Radiation Protection and Measurements (NCRP).

An area occupied primarily by diagnostic imaging personnel and patients is called a *controlled area.* The design limits for a controlled area require that the barrier reduce the exposure rate in the area to less than 100 mR per week (26 μC/kilogram-week). An **uncontrolled area** can be occupied by anyone, and therefore the maximum exposure rate allowed in such an area is 2 mR per week (0.5 μC/kilogram-week). Consequently a wall protecting an uncontrolled area must have nearly two tenth-value layers (TVL) more lead than one protecting a controlled area.

Question: A wall protecting a controlled area contains 0.8 millimeters lead. If the area is converted to an uncontrolled area, approximately how much additional lead will be required?

Answer: The controlled dose limit of 10 mR per week is achieved with 0.8 millimeters lead. The HVL, assuming 100 kVp, single phase, is approximately 0.25 lead. Therefore an additional 0.25 lead will achieve 5 mR per week. An additional 0.5 lead will achieve 2.5 mR per week. Perhaps an additional 0.6 millimeters lead should be added to the existing 0.8 millimeters lead for a total of 1.4 millimeters lead.

The shielding required for an x-ray examining room depends on the level of radiation activity in that room.

TABLE 39-3

Levels of Occupancy of Areas that may be Adjacent to X-ray Rooms, as Suggested by the NCRP

Occupancy	Area
Full	Work areas (e.g., offices, laboratories, shops, wards, nurses' stations), living quarters, children's play areas, occupied space in nearby buildings
Frequent	Corridors, restrooms, elevators, with operators, unattended parking lots
Occasional	Waiting rooms, stairways, unattended elevators, janitors' closets, outside areas

The greater the number of examinations performed each week, the thicker the shielding required. This characteristic is called *workload (W)* and has a unit of milliampere-minutes per week (mA-min/wk). A busy, general purpose x-ray room may have a workload as high as 500 mA-minutes per week. Rooms in private offices have workloads of less than 100 mA-minutes per week.

For combination radiographic/fluoroscopic (R/F) rooms, usually only the radiographic workload need be considered for barrier calculations. When the fluoroscopic x-ray tube is energized, a primary barrier in the form of the fluoroscopic screen always intercepts the useful beam. Consequently the primary barrier requirements are always much less for fluoroscopic beams than for radiographic beams.

The percentage of time during which the x-ray beam is on and directed toward a particular wall is called the *use factor (U)* for that wall. The NCRP recommends that walls be assigned a use factor of $\frac{1}{4}$ and the floor a use factor of 1. Many studies have shown these recommendations to be high. Many medical physicists suggest that primary barriers are a misnomer because the useful beam is always intercepted by the patient, the image receptor, and the radiographic equipment. Walls, in a certain way, are always secondary barriers.

If an x-ray room has a special design, other use factors may be assigned. A room designed strictly for chest radiography has one wall with a use factor of 1. All others have a use factor of 0 for primary radiation and thus would be considered secondary radiation barriers. The ceiling is nearly always considered a secondary protective barrier. The use factor for secondary barriers is always 1, since leakage and scatter radiation are present 100% of the time that the tube is energized.

The final consideration in the design of an x-ray protective barrier is the penetrability of the x-ray beam. For protection calculations, kVp is used as the measure of penetrability. Most modern x-ray machines are designed to operate at up to 150 kVp. Most examinations, however, are conducted at an average of 75 kVp. An operating potential of 100 kVp is usually assumed. It is more likely for the protective barrier to be too thick than too thin.

Measurements of radiation exposure outside the x-ray room always result in weekly levels far less than that anticipated by calculation. The total on-beam time is always less than assumed. The average kVp is usually closer to 75 kVp than to 100 kVp. The calculations do not account for the fact that the patient and image receptor always intercept the useful beam. Although calculations are intended to result in a dose limit of 100 mR per week or 2 mR per week outside the x-ray room, rarely will the actual exposure exceed one tenth of that dose limit.

RADIATION DETECTION AND MEASUREMENT

Instruments are designed either to detect radiation or to measure radiation or both. Those designed for detection generally operate in the **pulse** or **rate** modes used to indicate the presence of radiation. In the pulse mode, radiation is indicated by a ticking, chirping, or beeping sound. In the rate mode the instrument response is measured in mR per hour or R per hour. Those designed to measure the intensity of radiation usually operate in the **integrate** mode. They accumulate the signal and respond with a total exposure of mR or R. Such application is called *dosimetry,* and the measuring devices are called *dosimeters.*

The earliest radiation detection device was the photographic emulsion, and it is still the primary means of radiation detection and measurement. Film has two principal applications in diagnostic imaging. Film is used in making the radiograph, and film is used as a personnel radiation monitor called a *film badge.*

Table 39-4 lists currently available radiation detection and measurement devices along with some of their principle characteristics and uses.

The following three types of radiation detection devices other than film badges are important to diagnostic imaging: (1) gas-filled radiation detectors, of which there are three types—ionization chambers, proportional counters, and Geiger-Muller detectors used to measure radiation intensity and detect radioactive contamination; (2) thermoluminescence dosimeters (TLD) used for patient and personnel monitoring; and (3) scintillation detectors, the imaging device used in the gamma

TABLE 39-4

Radiation Detection and Measuring Device Characteristics and Uses

Device	Characteristics and Uses
Photographic emulsion	Limited range, sensitive to radiation Personnel monitoring, imaging film.
Ionization chamber	Wide range, accurate, portable. Survey for fields greater than 1 mR per hour.
Proportional counter	Laboratory instruments, accurate, sensitive to radiation. Assay of radionuclides.
Geiger-Muller counter	Limited to less than 100 mR per hour, portable. Personnel monitoring, stationary monitoring.
Thermoluminescence dosimetry	Wide range, accurate, sensitive. Personnel monitoring, stationary area monitoring.
Scintillation detection	Limited range, very sensitive, stationary or portable instruments. Photon spectroscopy, imaging.

camera in nuclear medicine and in some computed tomography (CT) scanners.

Gas-Filled Detectors

The following three types of gas-filled detectors are used: ionization chambers, proportional counters, and Geiger-Muller (G-M) detectors. Although they are different in response characteristics, each is based on the same principle of operation.

As radiation passes through gas, it ionizes atoms of gas in its path. The electrons released in ionization are detected as a signal proportional to radiation intensity. This ionization of gas is the basis of these gas-filled radiation detectors. Consider the gas-filled detector shown in Figure 39-4. It consists of a cylinder filled with air or other gas.

Along the central axis of the cylinder is positioned a rigid wire called the *central electrode*. If a voltage difference occurs between the central electrode and the wall, electrons will be liberated in the chamber. These electrons form an electric signal either as a pulse of electrons or as a continuous current. This electric signal is then amplified and measured. Its intensity is proportional to the radiation intensity that caused it.

In general the larger the chamber, the more gas molecules there are available for ionization and, therefore, the more sensitive the instrument. A high sensitivity means that an instrument can detect very low radiation intensities.

The **region of recombination** is the stage (R) in Figure 39-5 in which the electrons released in ionization recombine. As the voltage is increased, a level will be reached, usually between 100 to 300 volts, in which every electron released in ionization will be attracted to the central electrode and collected. This performance curve is known as the *ionization region* and is indicated by I in Figure 39-5. The **proportional region** (P) results from an increase in primary ionization that causes secondary ionization and a rather large electron pulse for each ionization. Proportional counters are sensitive instruments that are used primarily as stationary laboratory instruments for the assay of small quantities of radioactivity. Proportional counters are useful in their ability to detect the difference between alpha and beta radiation.

The fourth region of the voltage response curve for the gas-filled chamber is the **Geiger-Muller (G-M) region.** This is the region in which Geiger counters operate. In the GM region the voltage across the ionization chamber is sufficiently high that, when a single ionizing event occurs, a cascade of secondary electrons causes a brief, yet violent, chain reaction. This results in a large electron pulse.

A **quenching agent** is added to the filling gas of the Geiger counter to return the counter after the first ionizing event to its original condition. The minimum time between ionizations that can be detected is known as the *revolving time.*

Geiger counters are extensively used for contamination control in nuclear medicine laboratories. They are used to detect the presence of radioactive contamination on work surfaces and laboratory apparatus. If equipped with an audio amplifier and speaker, the crackle of individual ionizations can be heard. The Geiger counter does not have a very wide range. Most instruments are limited to less than 110 mR per hour.

If the voltage across the gas-filled chamber is further increased, electrons produced from ionization will produce a continuous current or signal from the chamber. In this condition the instrument is useless for the detection of radiation. This region is known as the *region of continuous discharge (CD)* in Figure 39-5.

Of the number of different types of ion chambers, the most familiar is the portable instrument in Figure 39-6. This is used mainly for area surveys measuring a wide range of radiation intensities from 1 mR per hour to

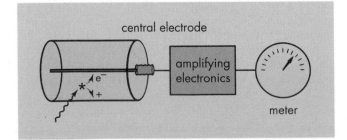

FIGURE 39-4 The gas-filled detector consists of a cylinder of gas and a central collecting electrode. By maintaining a voltage between the central electrode and the wall of the chamber, electrons produced in the ionization can be collected and measured.

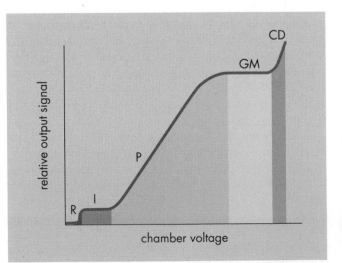

FIGURE 39-5 The intensity of the signal from a gas-filled detector increases in stages as the voltage across the chamber increases.

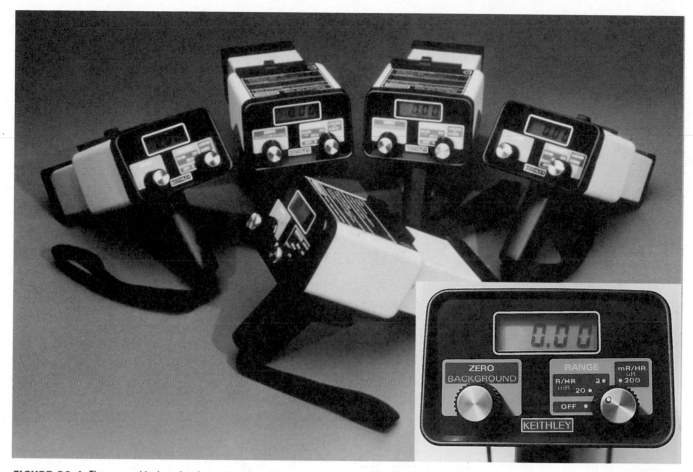

FIGURE 39-6 These portable ion chamber survey instruments are useful for radiation surveys when exposure levels are in excess of 1 mR per hour. *(Courtesy of Keithly Instruments, Inc.)*

several thousand R per hour. It is the instrument of choice for measuring radiation intensity around a fluoroscope, areas with radionuclide use, the vicinity around patients with therapeutic quantities of radioactive materials, and areas outside of protective barriers.

A more accurate ion chamber is shown in Figure 39-7. This is used for precise calibration of the output intensity of diagnostic x-ray units. Figure 39-8 is another version of a precision ion chamber that is used daily in nuclear medicine laboratories to assay quantities of radioactive material.

Scintillation Detectors

Scintillation process. Scintillation detectors are used in diagnostic imaging in the gamma camera in nuclear medicine and in some detector arrays in CT scanners.

The scintillation process occurs when a flash of light is emitted from the absorption of ionizing radiation. The amount of light emitted is proportional to the amount of energy absorbed by the material. Only those materials with a particular crystalline structure will

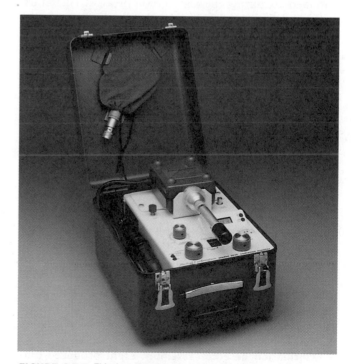

FIGURE 39-7 This ion chamber dosimeter is used for accurate measurement of diagnostic x-ray beams. *(Courtesy Radcal Corp.)*

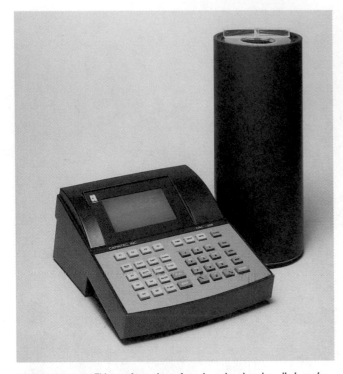

FIGURE 39-8 This configuration of an ion chamber is called a *dose colibrator.* It is used in nuclear medicine to accurately measure quantities of radioactive material used. *(Courtesy Capintec, Inc.)*

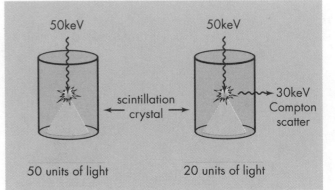

FIGURE 39-9 During scintillation, the quantity of light emitted is proportional to the amount of energy absorbed in the crystal.

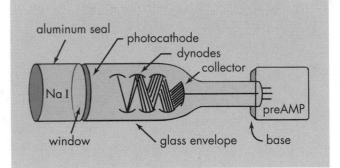

FIGURE 39-10 Scintillation detector assembly characteristic of the type used in a portable survey instrument.

scintillate. At the atomic level, the process involves the rearrangement of valence electrons into traps. The return of the electron from the trap to its normal position is immediate during the scintillation process. The return of the valence electron causes a flash of energy to be emitted.

Consider the two photon interactions diagrammed in Figure 39-9. If a 50-keV photon underwent photoelectric absorption in the crystal, all the energy would reappear as light. If the photon underwent Compton scattering and 30 keV of the energy was absorbed, then a proportionally lower quantity of light would be emitted in the scintillation event.

Many types of liquids, gases, and solids can respond to ionizing radiation with scintillation. By far the most widely used scintillation phosphors are the inorganic crystals: thallium-activated sodium iodide (NaI:Tl) or thallium-activated cesium iodide (CsI:Tl). The **activator atoms** of thallium are impurities grown into the crystal to control the spectrum of the light emitted and to enhance its intensity. The NaI:Tl crystals are incorporated into gamma cameras. CsI:Tl is the phosphor incorporated into the fluoroscopy image-intensifier tubes as the input phosphor. Both of these types of phosphors are used in CT scanner detector arrays.

Scintillation detector assembly. Light produced during scintillation is emitted isotropically, with equal intensity in all directions. When used as a radiation detector,

scintillation crystals are enclosed in aluminum that has a polished inner surface in contact with the crystal. This allows the light flash to be reflected internally to the face of a crystal called a ***window***. The crystal needs to be sealed because scintillation crystals are **hydroscopic,** which means they absorb moisture. Swollen and cracked crystals produce an interface that absorbs the scintillation.

Figure 39-10 shows the basic components of a scintillation detector assembly that is representative of the type used as a portable survey instrument. The detector portion of the assembly is the NaI:Tl crystal contained in an aluminum hermetic seal. The photomultiplier (PM) converts the light flashes from the scintillator into electric pulses.

The PM tube is an electron vacuum tube that contains the following elements: the **glass envelope,** the **window of the tube,** the **optical coupling,** and the **photocathode.** The glass envelope provides structural support for the internal elements and maintains the vacuum inside the tube. The window of the tube is the portion of the glass envelope that is coupled to the scintillation crystal. An optical coupling allows light emitted from the scintillator to be transmitted to the interior of the tube with minimum loss. As light passes from the crystal into the tube, it hits a metal coating called the *photocathode,* which consists of a cesium, antimony, and bismuth compound. The photocathode emits electrons when illuminated, a process called *photoemission.* The number of electrons emitted from the photocathode is directly proportional to the intensity of the incident light.

The photoelectrons are then accelerated through a series of platelike elements called *dyodes.* The electron pulse is amplified by secondary electron emission. The last element is a collecting electrode called a *collector,* which absorbs the electron pulse and conducts it to a **preamplifier.** The preamplifier provides an initial stage of pulse amplification.

The overall result of scintillation detection is that a single photon interaction produces a burst of light, which produces a photoelectron emission, which is amplified to produce a large electron pulse. The size of the electron pulse is proportional to the energy absorbed by the crystal from the incident photon.

Scintillation detectors are sensitive devices for detecting x-rays and gamma rays. The detector is sensitive to radiation intensities as low as single photon interactions. As a result, scintillation detectors are useful as portable radiation detectors to monitor the presence of contamination and low levels of radiation.

Thermoluminescence Dosimetry

Thermoluminescence occurs when materials are heated and emit visible light. In the early 1960s, Cameron and his co-workers at the University of Wisconsin experimented with some thermoluminescent materials. They discovered materials that glowed even more brightly after heating when they were exposed to ionizing radiation. This radiation-induced thermoluminescence has been developed into a sensitive and accurate method of radiation dosimetry for personnel monitoring. It is also used for recording patient dose during radiation therapy procedures.

The basic principles of thermoluminescence dosimetry (TLD) (Figure 39-11) are discussed in the following paragraphs.

After irradiation, the TLD phosphor is placed on a special dish called a *planchet* to be analyzed in a TLD analyzer. The temperature of the planchet is carefully controlled. Directly viewing the planchet is a PM tube. The output signal from the PM tube is amplified and displayed on a meter or a chart recorder. Figure 39-12 is a cutaway illustration of a commercially available TLD analyzer.

Glow curve. As the temperature of the planchet is increased, the amount of light emitted by the TLD increases in an irregular manner. Figure 39-13 shows the light output from lithium fluoride (LiF) as the temperature increases. There are several prominent peaks in the graph that result from electron transitions in the

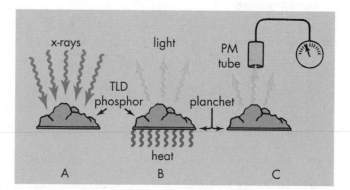

FIGURE 39-11 TLD is a multistep process. **A,** Exposure to ionizing radiation, **B,** Subsequent heating, **C,** Measurement of the intensity of the emitted light.

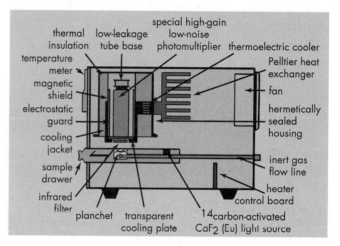

FIGURE 39-12 Cutaway illustration of a representative TLD analyzer. *(Courtesy of Harshaw Chemical Company.)*

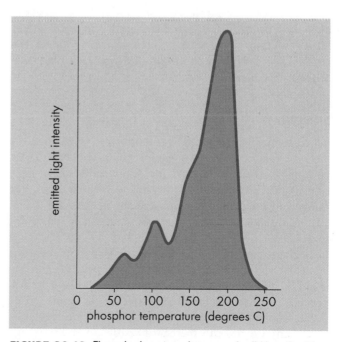

FIGURE 39-13 Thermoluminescence glow curve for lithium fluoride.

TABLE 39-5

Thermoluminescent Phosphors and Their Characteristics and Applications

	Lithium Fluoride	Lithium Borate	Calcium Fluoride	Calcium Sulfate
Composition	LiF	$Li_2B_4O_7$:Mn	CaF_2:Mn	$CaSO_4$:Dy
Density $\times$ 103 (kg/m³)	2.64	2.5	3.18	2.61
Atomic number	8.2	7.4	16.3	15.3
Temperature of main peak (degrees centigrade)	195	200	260	220
Principal use	Patient and personnel dosimetry	Research	Environmental monitoring	Environmental monitoring

TL crystals. This graph is known as a *glow curve*. Each TL material has a specific glow curve. Both the height of the highest temperature peak and the total area under the curve are directly proportional to the energy deposited in the TLD by ionizing radiation. The TLD analyzers are electronic instruments designed to measure the height of the glow curve or the area under the curve.

Types of TLD material. Many materials, including some body tissues, exhibit the property of radiation-induced thermoluminescence. Materials that are used for TLD are generally inorganic crystals. Lithium fluoride is the most widely used TLD material. With an atomic number of 8.2, it has x-ray absorption properties similar to soft tissue; thus LiF is considered a **tissue equivalent dosimeter.** LiF can measure as low as 10 mrad (0.1 mGy) and as high as 10 rad (100mGy), with accuracy better than 5%. Table 39-5 lists some thermoluminescent phosphors, their characteristics, and their applications.

The TLD is reusable. When irradiated, the energy absorbed by the TLD remains stored until released as visible light by heat analysis. The heating restores the crystal to its original condition and makes it ready for another exposure.

SUMMARY

More than 100 individual radiation protection devices and accessories are associated with modern x-ray equipment. This chapter discusses the radiation protection devices that are common for all radiographic and fluoroscopic equipment. Many of the devices are federally mandated to be provided by equipment manufacturers.

Leakage radiation emitted by the x-ray tube during exposure must be contained by a protective tube housing. The limit of leakage must be no more than 100 mR per hour (26 µC per hour) at a distance of 1 meter from the housing. The control panel must indicate exposure by either kVp and mA meters or visible and audible signals.

The following are radiation protection requirements for radiographic equipment:

1. **SID.** An SID indicator must be provided, which must be accurate within 2% of the indicated SID.
2. **Collimation.** A light-localized variable-aperture rectangular collimator should be provided. The light field and the x-ray beam must coincide to within 2% at the standard SID.
3. **PBL.** Positive-beam limitation or automatic collimators were required to be installed in x-ray equipment up until 1994. They are no longer required; however, they are still often used. The PBL must be accurate, with no more than 2% variation at the standard SID.
4. **Beam alignment.** Proper alignment must be ensured between the x-ray tube and the radiographic film. Diligence in aligning the tube and x-ray film helps reduce repeated radiographs.
5. **Filtration.** Total filtration must be 2.5-millimeter aluminum equivalent when operated above 70 kVp. A tube operated between 50 and 70 kVp must have at least 1.5-millimeter aluminum equivalent. Below 50 kVp, for example, in mammography tubes, 0.5-millimeter aluminum equivalent is required.
6. **Reproducibility.** Output intensity must not exceed a 5% variation from one exposure to another.
7. **Linearity.** A 10% variation in output radiation intensity is allowed between mA stations when testing for linearity.
8. **Exposure switch.** The exposure switch on the operating console must be fixed and not have a long cord. The fixed switch prevents the radiographer from being exposed to radiation in the examination room.
9. **Mobile unit exposure switch.** The exposure switch on the mobile x-ray unit must extend at least 180 centimeters from the x-ray tube during exposure so personnel can stand a maximum distance from the tube and beam.

The following are radiation protection devices designed for fluoroscopic equipment:

1. **Source-to-skin distance.** The source-to-skin distance on stationary fluoroscopes must be not less than 38 centimeters and on mobile fluoroscopic units, not less than 30 centimeters.
2. **Primary protective barrier.** The image-intensifier assembly serves as a primary protective barrier and must be 2-millimeter lead equivalent.
3. **Filtration.** The total filtration of the fluoroscope must be at least 2.5-millimeter aluminum equivalent.
4. **Collimation.** Fluoroscopic beam collimators must be adjusted so that an unexposed border is visible on the television monitor when the image intensifier is positioned 35 centimeters above the table top.
5. **Exposure switch.** The fluoroscopic exposure switch must be a dead-man type, which means if the fluoroscopy operator were incapacitated and removed his or her foot from the switch, the fluoroscopy beam would terminate.
6. **Bucky slot cover.** The slot where the Bucky tray moves is covered automatically by 0.25-millimeter lead equivalent.
7. **Protective curtain.** A protective curtain between the fluoroscopy operator and the patient must be 0.25-millimeter lead equivalent.
8. **Cumulative timer.** Audible signal must sound indicating 5 minutes of fluoroscopic beam-on time.
9. **X-ray intensity.** The intensity of the beam at the table top should not exceed 2.1 R per minute (0.54 mC/kilogram per minute) for each mA of operation at 80 kVp.

Great attention is given to the design of radiographic rooms, to the placement of x-ray machines, and to the use of adjoining rooms. There are two types of protective barriers: primary barriers and secondary barriers. Primary barriers intercept the primary beam and must be lead bonded to Sheetrock, usually 4 lbs/ft². This amount of leaded Sheetrock is equivalent to 1.6 millimeters or $\frac{1}{16}$-th inch of lead. Concrete of $3\frac{3}{4}$ inches would allow equivalent protection. Secondary barriers protect personnel from scatter and leakage radiation. Secondary protective barriers usually use materials other than lead because the lead equivalent is 0.4 millimeters. Barrier thickness depends on a number of factors: the distance between the source of radiation and the barrier; the occupancy factor; the workload; and the penetrability of the x-ray beam (100 kVp is usually assumed).

Dosimeters are instruments designed to detect and measure radiation. Other than photographic emulsion, there are three types of highly accurate devices for measuring radiation. The gas-filled detectors are the ionization chamber, the proportional counter, and the Geiger-Muller counter. Two other devices used to detect and measure radiation are the thermoluminescence dosimeter and scintillation detector.

REVIEW QUESTIONS

1. What is the regulatory limit of leakage radiation from the x-ray tube during an exposure?
2. What do audible and visible signals indicate on the radiographic control console?
3. List and describe the nine devices used for radiation protection on radiographic equipment.
4. What is the result if the x-ray beam and the film are not properly aligned?
5. What filtration is used for mammography equipment operated below 50 kVp?
6. How are reproducibility and linearity different when measuring the intensity of the x-ray beam?
7. What characteristics of fluoroscopic equipment are designed for radiation protection?
8. How can filtration be measured if the amount of inherent and added filtration is unknown?
9. Name the three types of radiation exposure that are of concern when designing protective barriers.
10. During both radiography and fluoroscopy, the _____ is the single most important scattering object.
11. Using Table 39-2, identify the millimeters of glass required for a secondary barrier if the required lead equivalent is 0.4 millimeters.
12. List the four factors that are taken into consideration when designing a barrier for a radiographic room.
13. Define controlled area and uncontrolled area.
14. What are the units of workload in an x-ray examination room?
15. Explain the use factor (U) as it relates to a wall in a radiographic room.
16. Why is the use factor for secondary barriers always 1?
17. Name the three gas-filled dosimeters.
18. Discuss the properties of TLD that make it suitable for personnel monitoring.
19. Which modality of diagnostic imaging uses scintillation detection as a radiation detection process?
20. What are the two most widely used scintillation phosphors?

Additional Reading

Dowd SB: The basics of radiation protection for hospital workers, *Hosp Top*, 69:31 1991.

Greenspan BS, O'Mara RE: Low-level radioactive waste, *Appl Radiol* 22(9):8 September, 1993.

Proposed recommended practices: reducing radiological exposure in the practice setting, *AORN J*, 58(3):599 September, 1993.

40

Radiation Protection Procedures

OBJECTIVES

At the completion of this chapter the student will be able to:

1. Discuss the units and concepts of occupational exposure
2. Indicate the three ways that patient dose is reported
3. Describe the radiation doses in mammography and CT
4. Discuss the ways to reduce occupational exposure, especially during fluoroscopy and mobile radiography
5. Explain the three personnel monitors and where they are placed on the body
6. Discuss the reports coming from personnel monitoring programs
7. List the thicknesses of protective apparel
8. Discuss the procedure for holding patients during an x-ray examination
9. Describe the four cases of screening x-rays that are no longer performed unless indicated
10. Discuss how repeat examinations, radiographic technique, and the image receptor affect patient exposure dose
11. Explain when to shield a patient

OUTLINE

Occupational Exposure
Patient Dose
  Estimation of patient dose
  Patient dose in special examinations
Reduction of Occupational Exposure
  Personnel monitoring
  Personnel monitoring report
  Protective apparel
  Position
  Patient holding

Reduction of Unnecessary Patient Dose
  Unnecessary examinations
  Repeat examinations
  Radiographic technique
  Image receptor
  Patient positioning
  Specific area shielding

edical physicists work hard to minimize occupational exposure to diagnostic imaging personnel. Additionally, physicists try to reduce the radiation dose to patients during x-ray examinations. Radiation exposure of radiologists and radiographers is measured with personnel monitoring devices. Patient dose is usually estimated by conducting simulated x-ray examinations with human phantoms.

If radiation control procedures are adopted, occupational exposure and patient dose can be kept acceptably low. Health physicists subscribe to ALARA, which is an acronym that means maintain all radiation exposure as low as reasonably achievable.

■ ■ ■ ■ ■ ■ ■ ■ ■ ■ ■ ■ ■ ■ ■ ■ ■ ■

OCCUPATIONAL EXPOSURE

Radiation dose is measured in units of rad (gray) or millirad. Radiation exposure is measured in roentgens (coulomb per kilogram) or milliroentgens. When the exposure concerns radiographers and radiologists (occupational workers), the proper unit is the rem (sievert) or millirem. The rem is the unit of effective dose and is used for radiation protection purposes. Although **exposure, dose,** and **effective dose** have precise and different meanings, they are often used interchangeably in diagnostic imaging because they have approximately the same numerical value.

When properly used, exposure (R) refers to radiation intensity in air. Dose (rad) measures the radiation energy absorbed as a result of a radiation exposure during patient examinations. Effective dose (rem) identifies the biologic effectiveness of the radiation energy absorbed. The rem unit is usually applied to occupationally exposed persons.

Although the dose limit for imaging personnel is 50 mSv per year (5000 mrem per year), experience has shown that considerably lower exposures than this should be routine. The occupational exposure of imaging personnel engaged in general x-ray activity should not normally exceed about 5 mSv per year (500 mrem per year).

Radiologists generally receive slightly higher exposures than radiographers. This is because the radiologist receives most of his or her exposure during fluoroscopy, and the radiologist is usually closer to the radiation source and the patient during such procedures. Table 40-1 reports the results of an analysis of the annual occupational radiation exposure of 584,000 medical radiation workers. Clearly the radiation exposures are low.

Unquestionably the highest occupational exposure of diagnostic x-ray personnel occurs during fluoroscopy and portable radiography. During radiographic exposures, the radiologist is rarely present, and the radiographer should be positioned behind a protective barrier.

TABLE 40-1

Occupational Radiation Exposure to 584,000 Medical Radiation Workers

Exposure Category	Value
Average whole-body dose	70 mrem
Those receiving less than minimum detectable dose	53%
Those receiving less than 100 mrem per year	88%
Those receiving greater than 5000 mrem per year	0.05%

When protective barriers are not available, such as during portable examinations, the portable x-ray machine should be equipped with an exposure cord long enough to allow the radiographer to leave the immediate examination area. The radiographer should wear a protective apron for each portable examination.

During fluoroscopy, both radiologist and radiographer are exposed to relatively high levels of radiation. Personnel exposure, however, is directly related to the x-ray beam-on time. With care, personnel exposures are acceptably low.

Question: A barium enema examination requires $2\frac{1}{2}$ minutes of fluoroscopic x-ray beam time. If the radiographer is exposed to 250 mR per hour what will be his or her occupational exposure?

Answer:
$$\text{Exposure} = \text{Exposure rate} \times \text{Time}$$
$$= 250 \text{ mR per hour} \times 2.5 \text{ minutes}$$
$$= 250 \text{ mR per hour} \times 0.0417 \text{ hour}$$
$$= 10.4 \text{ mR}$$

Remote fluoroscopy results in low personnel exposures because personnel are usually not in the examination room adjacent to the patient. Some fluoroscopes have the x-ray tube over the table and the image receptor under the table. This geometry offers some advantage to image quality, but personnel exposures are higher because the secondary radiation levels are higher. This condition should be kept in mind during portable fluoroscopy. It is best to position the x-ray tube under the patient during portable fluoroscopy (Figure 40-1).

Personnel engaged in angiointerventional procedures often receive higher exposures than do those in general imaging practice because of longer fluoroscopic exposure times. The frequent absence of an intensifier-tower protective curtain and the extensive use of cineradiography also contribute to higher personnel exposure.

Extremity exposure during fluoroscopy may be significant. Even with protective gloves, exposure of the

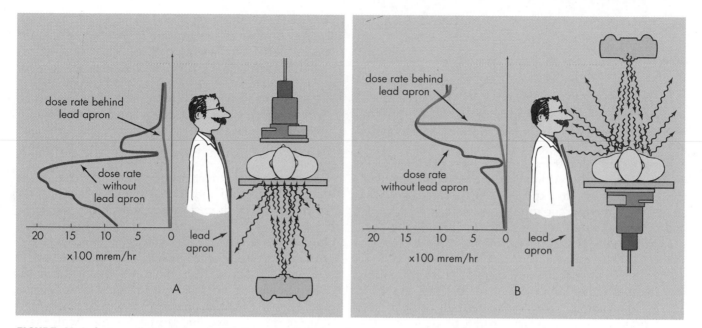

FIGURE 40-1 Scatter radiation during portable fluoroscopy is **A,** low when the x-ray tube is under the table and **B,** more intense with the x-ray tube over the patient. *(Courtesy Stephen Balter.)*

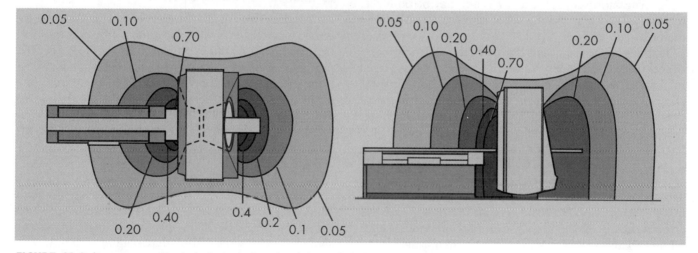

FIGURE 40-2 Isoexposure profiles in both the horizontal and the vertical planes for a typical CT operation. *(Courtesy General Electric Medical Systems.)*

forearm can approach the applicable dose limit of 500 mSv per year (50 rem per year) if care is not taken. Without protective gloves, excessive hand exposures are possible, and extremity monitoring must be provided.

Personnel exposures associated with mammography are low because the low kVp of operation results in reduced scatter radiation. Usually a long exposure cord and a conventional wall or window wall are sufficient to provide adequate protection. Rarely does a room used strictly for mammography require protective lead shielding. Dedicated mammography x-ray units have personnel protective barriers made of lead glass, lead acrylic, and even plate glass as an integral component. Such barriers are totally adequate.

Personnel exposures in computed tomography (CT) facilities are low. Since the CT x-ray beam is finely collimated and only secondary radiation is present in the scan room, the radiation levels are low compared with those experienced in fluoroscopy. Figure 40-2 shows the isoexposure profiles for both the horizontal and vertical planes of a typical CT scanner. These data are usually reported as milliroentgen per scan to show that personnel can be permitted to remain in the room during scanning. Protective apparel should always be worn in such situations.

Question: It is necessary for a radiographer to remain in the CT room at midtable position during a 20-scan examination. What would be the occupational exposure if no protective apron were worn?

Answer: From Figure 40-2, assume an exposure of 0.1 mR per scan.

Occupational exposure =
0.1 mR per scan × 20 scans = 2 mR

Nursing personnel and others working in the operating room and in intensive care units are sometimes exposed to radiation from portable x-ray machines and C-arm fluoroscopes. Although these persons are often anxious about such exposures, many studies have shown that their occupational exposure is near zero and certainly is nothing for concern. It is usually not necessary to provide radiation monitors for such personnel.

Personnel radiation monitors are not necessary during portable radiography except for the radiographer and anyone routinely required to restrain or hold patients. Personnel who regularly operate or are in the immediate vicinity of a C-arm fluoroscope should wear radiation monitors in addition to protective apparel. During C-arm fluoroscopy, the x-ray beam may be on for a relatively long time and the beam can be pointed in virtually any direction.

It should never be necessary for diagnostic x-ray personnel to exceed 50 mSv per year (5000 mrem per year). In smaller hospitals, emergency centers, and private clinics, occupational exposures rarely exceed 5 mSv per year (500 mrem per year). Average exposures in most facilities are less than 1 mSv per year (100 mrem per year).

PATIENT DOSE

The exposure of patients to medical x-rays is commanding increased attention for two reasons.

First the frequency of x-ray examination is increasing among all age groups at a rate of between 6% and 10% per year in the United States. This rate of increase is exceeded in many other countries. This indicates that physicians are relying more and more on x-ray diagnosis to assist them in patient care even when accounting for the newer imaging modalities. This is to be expected. X-ray diagnosis is considered much more accurate today than in the past. More rigorous training programs required of radiologists and radiographers and improvements in diagnostic x-ray equipment allow for more difficult, but more substantive, x-ray examinations. Efficacy and diagnostic accuracy are much improved.

Second, there is increasing concern among public health officials and radiation scientists regarding the risk associated with medical x-ray exposure. Acute effects on superficial tissues after angiointerventional procedures are reported with increasing frequency. The possible late effects of diagnostic x-ray exposure are of concern not because such exposures are high but because of unnecessary radiation exposure. If attention is given to good radiation control practices, the same level of diagnostic information can be obtained with lower radiation and therefore with reduced risk.

Estimation of Patient Dose

Patient dose from diagnostic x-rays is generally reported in one of three ways. The exposure to the entrance surface, or **entrance skin exposure (ESE)**, is most often reported because it is easy to measure. The **gonadal dose** is important because of the possible genetic responses to medical x-ray exposure. The dose to the gonads is not difficult to measure or estimate. The dose to the **bone marrow** is important because bone marrow is the target organ believed responsible for radiation-induced leukemia.

Table 40-2 presents some representative values of ESE and gonadal dose for various x-ray examinations. The mean marrow dose for each procedure is also presented. Note that these are only approximate values and should not be used to estimate patient dose at any facility. In any given x-ray facility, actual doses delivered may be considerably different. Efficiency of x-ray pro-

TABLE 40-2				
Representative Radiation Quantities from Various Diagnostic X-ray Procedures				
Examination	Technique (kVp/mAs)	Entrance Skin Exposure (mrad)	Mean Marrow Dose (mrad)	Gonad Dose (mrad)
Skull	76/50	200	10	<1
Chest	110/3	10	2	<1
Cervical spine	70/40	150	10	<1
Lumbar spine	72/60	300	60	225
Abdomen	74/60	400	30	125
Pelvis	70/50	150	20	150
Extremity	60/5	50	2	<1
CT (head)	125/300	3000	20	50
CT (pelvis)	124/400	4000	100	3000

duction and image receptor speed are the most important variables.

These values do provide for relative dose comparisons among various radiographic examinations. Doses during fluoroscopy are too dependent on technique, equipment, and beam-on time to be easily estimated. Usually such doses must be measured.

Entrance skin exposure. Exposure to the skin (ESE) is most often referred to as the *patient dose*. It is widely used because it is easy to measure and because reasonably accurate estimates can be made in the absence of measurements.

The measurement technique uses thermoluminescence dosimeters (TLDs). The size, sensitivity, and accuracy of TLDs make them very satisfactory patient radiation monitors. A small grouping or pack of three to ten TLDs can be easily taped to the patient's skin in the center of the x-ray field. Since the response of the TLD is proportional to exposure and dose, the TLD can be used to measure all radiation levels in diagnostic imaging. With proper laboratory technique, the results of such measurements will be accurate to within 5%.

Two rather straightforward methods for estimating ESE are available in the absence of patient measurements. The first requires the use of a nomogram such as that shown in Figure 40-3. This figure contains a family of curves from which one can estimate the output intensity of a radiographic unit if the technique is known or can be assumed. The output intensity of different x-ray machines varies widely, so the use of this nomogram method is only good to perhaps ±50%.

To use this nomogram, one must first know the total filtration in the x-ray beam. This is usually available from the medical physics report, but if not, 3 millimeters aluminum is a good estimate. Next, identify the kVp and mAs of the intended examination. Draw a vertical line rising from the value of total filtration until it intersects with the kVp of the examination. From this intersection, draw a horizontal line to the left until it intersects the mR/mAs axis. The resulting mR/mAs value is the approximate output intensity of the radiographic unit. Multiply this value times the examination mAs to obtain the approximate patient exposure.

Question: With reference to Figure 40-3, estimate the skin dose from a lateral skull film taken at 66 kVp, 150 mAs, with a radiographic unit having 2.5-millimeters aluminum total filtration.

Answer: Estimate the intersection between a vertical line rising from 2.5 millimeters aluminum and a horizontal line through 66 kVp. Extend the horizontal line to the y-axis and read 3.8 mR/mAs.

3.8 mR/mAs × 150 mAs = 570 mR

= 0.570 mrad

A better approach requires that a medical physicist construct a nomogram such as that shown in Figure 40-4 for each radiographic unit. A straight edge between any kVp and mAs will cross the ESE scale at the correct mR value.

Question: Using the nomogram of Figure 40-4, what is the ESE when this radiographic unit is used at 66 kVp, 150 mAs?

Answer: The line is drawn as shown and crosses the ESE scale at 1800 mR.

A third method for estimating ESE requires that one know the output intensity for at least one operating condition. During the annual or special radiation control survey and calibration of an x-ray facility, the medical physicist will measure this output intensity, usually in units of mR/mAs at 80 centimeters, the approximate source-to-skin distance (SSD), or at 100 centimeters, the SID. At 70 kVp, radiographic output intensity varies from about 2 to 10 mR/mAs at 80-centimeters SSD.

With this calibration value available, one would first make adjustment for a different SSD by using the inverse square law.

Question: The output intensity of a radiographic unit is reported as 3.7 mR/mAs (1 μC/kilogram-

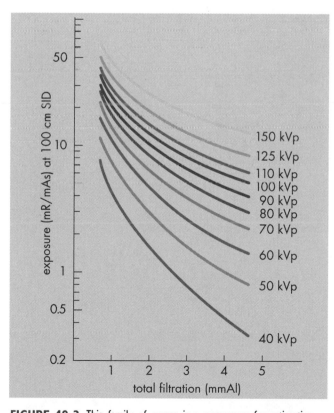

FIGURE 40-3 This family of curves is a nomogram for estimating output x-ray intensity from a single-phase radiographic unit. *(Courtesy John R. Cameron.)*

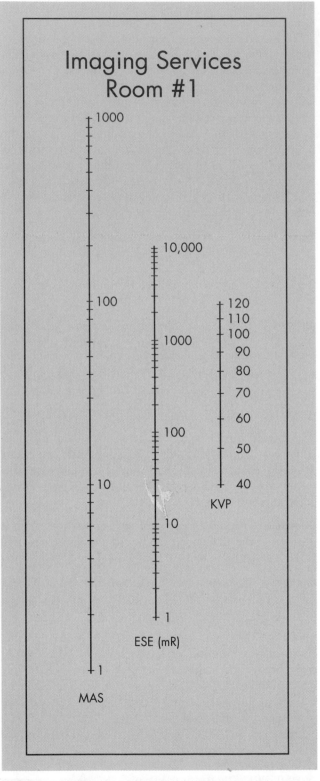

FIGURE 40-4 This type of nomogram is very accurate but must be fashioned individually for each radiographic unit. *(Courtesy Michael D. Harpen.)*

mAs) at 100-centimeters SID. What is the intensity at 75-centimeters SSD?

Answer: At 75-centimeters SSD the intensity will be greater by $(^{100}/_{75})^2 = (1.32)^2 = 1.78$

3.7 mR/mAs $\times$ 1.78 = 6.6 mR/mAs

Knowing the ESE, the kVp and mAs of the examination can be calculated. Output intensity varies according to the square of the kVp.

Question: The output intensity at 70 kVp and 75-cm SSD is 6.6 mR/mAs (1.8 μC/kilogram-mAs). What is the output intensity of 76 kVp?

Answer: At higher kVp the output intensity is greater by the square of the kVp or:

$(76/70)^2 = (1.08)^2 = 1.18$

6.6 mR/mAs $\times$ 1.18 = 7.8 mR/mAs

The final step in estimating ESE is to multiply the output intensity in mR/mAs by the examination mAs, since they are proportional.

Question: If the radiographic technique for an IVP calls for 80 mAs, what is the skin dose when the output intensity is 7.8 mR/mAs (2.1 μC/kilogram-mAs)?

Answer: 7.8 mR/mAs $\times$ 80 mAs = 624 mR

= 0.624 mR

Normally, one would combine each of these steps into a single calculation.

Question: The output intensity for a radiographic unit is 4.5 mR/mAs (1.2 μC/kilogram-mAs) at 70 kVp and 80 centimeters. If a lateral skull film is taken at 66 kVp, 150 mAs, what will the skin dose at an 80-centimeters SSD be? What would the skin dose at a 90-centimeters SSD be?

Answer: At 80-centimeters SSD:

$$\text{Dose} = (4.5 \text{ mR/mAs})\left(\frac{66 \text{ kVp}}{70 \text{ kVp}}\right)^2(150 \text{ mAs})$$

= 600 mR

$\approx$ 600 mrad

At 90-centimeters SSD:

$$\text{Dose} = (600 \text{ mrad})\left(\frac{80}{90}\right)^2$$

= 474 mrad

ESE in fluoroscopy is much more difficult to estimate because the radiation field moves and sometimes varies in size. If the field were of one size and stationary, ESE would be directly related to exposure time. It is usually satisfactory, in the absence of measurements, to estimate fluoroscopic ESE at 4 R/mAs. Stated differently, for the average fluoroscopic examination, one can assume an ESE of 4 R per minute.

Question: A fluoroscopic procedure requires 2.5 minutes at 90 kVp, 2 mA. What is the approximate ESE?

Answer: ESE = (4 R/minute)(2.5 minute)

$$= 10 \text{ R}$$

Mean marrow dose. The hematologic effects of radiation are rarely, if ever, experienced in diagnostic imaging. It is appropriate, however, that radiographers understand the mean marrow dose, which is one measure of patient dose during diagnostic procedures. The mean marrow dose is the average radiation dose to the entire active bone marrow. For instance, if during a particular examination, 50% of the active bone marrow were in the primary beam and received an average dose of 25 mrad (250 μGy), the mean marrow dose would be 12.5 mrad (125 μGy).

Table 40-2 includes the approximate mean marrow dose in adults for various types of diagnostic x-ray examinations. In children, these levels would generally be less because the active bone marrow is more uniformly distributed and because the radiographic techniques used are considerably less. Table 40-3 shows the distribution of active bone marrow in the adult, and this will give some clue as to which diagnostic x-ray procedures involve exposure to large amounts of bone marrow.

In the United States the mean marrow dose from diagnostic x-ray examinations averaged over the entire population is approximately 100 mrad per year (1 mGy per year). Such a dose never results in the hematologic responses described in Chapter 36.

Genetically significant dose. Measurements and estimates of gonad dose are important because of the suspected genetic effects of radiation. Although the gonad dose from diagnostic x-rays is low for each individual, it may have some significance in terms of population effects.

The population gonad dose of importance is the **genetically significant dose (GSD)**, the radiation dose to the population gene pool. The GSD is defined as the gonad dose which, if received by every member of the population, would be expected to produce the total genetic effect on the population as the sum of the individual doses actually received. Thus it is a weighted-average gonad dose. It takes into account those persons who are irradiated and those who are not and averages the results. The GSD can only be estimated through large-scale epidemiologic studies. It is estimated using the following expression:

$$\text{GSD} = \frac{\Sigma \times D \times N_X \times P}{\Sigma \times N_I \times P}$$

Σ is the mathematic symbol that means to add values, D is the average gonad dose per examination, N_X is the number of persons receiving x-ray examinations, N_T is the total number of persons in the population, and P is the expected future number of children per person.

For computational purposes, therefore, the GSD considers the age, gender, and expected number of children for each person so examined. It also acknowledges the various types of examinations and the gonadal dose per examination type.

Estimates for GSD have been conducted in many different countries (Table 40-4). The estimate reported by the U.S. Public Health Service is 20 mrad (200 μGy). Thus this is a genetic radiation burden over and above the existing average background radiation level of approximately 40 mrad (400 μGy).

Patient Dose in Special Examinations

Dose in mammography. Because of the considerable application of x-rays for examination of the female breast and the concern for the induction of breast cancer by radiation, it is imperative that radiographers have

---

TABLE 40-3

Distribution of Active Bone Marrow in Adults

Anatomic Site	Percent of Bone Marrow
Head	10
Shoulders and upper humeri	8
Sternum	3
Ribs	11
Cervical vertebrae	4
Thoracic vertebrae	13
Lumbar vertebrae	11
Sacrum	11
Pelvis and upper femora	29
TOTAL	100

TABLE 40-4

Estimated GSD Caused by Diagnostic X-ray Examination

Population	GSD (mrad)
Denmark	22
Great Britain	12
Japan	27
New Zealand	12
Sweden	72
United States	20

some understanding of the radiation doses involved in such examinations.

Screen-film mammography currently is the only acceptable technique. Direct-exposure film and xeromammography are things of the past. Entrance skin exposures of approximately 800 mR per view (8 mGy per view) are experienced with screen films. Increasing tube potential much beyond 30 kVp degrades the image unacceptably in screen-film mammography, and therefore further dose reductions by technique manipulation are unlikely. Faster films and screens, however, may make even lower-dose screen-film mammography possible.

Radiographic grids are now employed in most screen-film mammography examinations. Grid ratios of 3:1 and 4:1 are most popular. The contrast enhancement produced by using such grids is significant, but so is the increase in patient dose. Patient dose is increased by approximately two times with the use of such grids.

The values stated for patient dose in mammography can be misleading. Because of the low x-ray energies used in mammography, the dose falls off very rapidly as the beam penetrates the breast. If the ESE for a craniocaudad view is 800 mR (8 mGy), the dose to the midline of the breast may be only 100 mrad (1 mGy). The biologic effect of such an examination is presumed to be more closely associated with the total energy absorbed by glandular tissue.

It is known that the risk of an adverse biologic response from mammography is small. Certainly, it is nothing for a patient to be concerned about. Any possible response, however, is related to the average radiation dose to glandular tissue and not the skin dose. **Glandular dose** (D_g) varies in a complicated way with variations in x-ray beam quality and quantity. For screen-film mammography, D_g is approximately 15% of the entrance skin exposure.

Specification of an ESE can also be misleading when one considers a two-view examination such as that used for screening (Figure 40-5). Consider an examination consisting of craniocaudad and mediolateral oblique views. The craniocaudad and the mediolateral oblique views produce an ESE of 800 mR each. It would be incorrect to describe this total examination procedure as resulting in an ESE of 1.8 R. Skin exposures from different projections cannot be added. Radiographers must either specify the skin exposure for each view or attempt to estimate the total D_g.

To estimate the total D_g, radiographers can make the approximation that the contribution from each view will be 15% of the skin dose. Consequently the total glandular dose would be the sum of the contribution from each of the craniocaudad and mediolateral oblique views (0.15 × 800 = 120 mrad) (1.2 mGy). The total glandular dose would therefore be 240 mrad (2.4 mGy). Total glandular dose should not exceed 100 mrad per

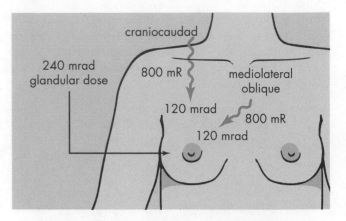

FIGURE 40-5 Two mammographic exposures result in a total glandular dose that is the sum of the individual glandular doses.

view with nongrid screen film mammography and 300 mrad per view with a grid.

From this discussion, it would seem that patient dose in mammography can be considerably reduced if the number of views is restricted. The axillary view should not be done routinely. For screening programs, no more than two views are advisable.

Dose in CT scanning. An important consideration in CT scanning, as with any x-ray procedure, is not only the skin dose but the distribution of dose during the scan.

On the basis of skin dose, CT is comparable with other diagnostic procedures. The skin dose delivered to a patient by a series of contiguous CT scans is somewhat higher than that delivered by a single skull or abdominal radiographic view. A typical radiographic head or body examination, however, often involves several views. Thus the dose from CT is roughly equivalent to the cumulative dose produced by a series of radiographic views. Furthermore, for most CT examinations, considerably less tissue volume is irradiated than in conventional radiography. The CT dose is significantly less than most fluoroscopic procedures.

As was pointed out in Chapters 29 and 30, CT differs in many important ways from other x-ray examinations. A regular x-ray film can be likened to a photograph taken with a flash: the patient is floodlighted with x-rays to directly expose the image receptor, whether it is film or an image intensifier. On the other hand, CT scans the patient with a fine-collimated beam of x-rays. This difference in delivery also means that the **dose distribution** from CT is different from radiographic procedures.

Part of the dose efficiency of CT is because of the precise collimation of the x-ray beam. Scatter radiation interferes with radiography and increases patient dose while reducing contrast resolution. Because CT uses narrow, well-collimated x-ray beams, scatter radiation is significantly reduced and contrast resolution significantly improved. Thus a larger percentage of the x-rays contribute usefully to the image.

The precise collimation used in CT means that only a well-defined volume of tissues is irradiated during each scan. The ideal x-ray beam for CT would have sharp boundaries. There would be no overlap between adjacent scans. Thus, aside from a minimum contribution caused by scatter, the dose delivered to a patient from a series of ideal adjacent CT scans would be the same as from a single scan.

Figure 40-6 illustrates how this ideal situation, however, cannot be attained in practice. The size of the focal spot of the x-ray tube blurs the sharp boundaries of the section. In addition, the beam is not precisely parallel, and some spreading occurs as the beam traverses the scan field.

If a series of adjacent scans is performed with an automatically indexed patient couch, the couch movement must be precise. If it moves too much between scans, some tissue will be missed. If it moves too little, some tissue in each scan will be overexposed.

Finally, and perhaps most important, if the prepatient collimators are too wide, tissues near the interface of each scan may receive twice the dose that they otherwise should. It is essential that CT collimators be periodically monitored for proper adjustment. Thus, in practice, a series of adjacent scans delivers a slightly higher dose than a single scan because of the overlapping dose profiles.

Dose is more uniformly distributed in CT than in radiography. Typical skin doses range from 1000 to 3000 mrad (10 to 30 mGy) during head scans and 2000 to 6000 mrad (20 to 60 mGy) during body scans. These values are only approximate and vary widely depending on the type of CT scanner and the examination technique. Because the CT beam is well collimated, the area of irradiation can be precisely controlled. Thus, radiosensitive organs such as the eyes can be selectively avoided.

Shields for protection from the primary x-ray beam in CT are of little use. Not only does the metal from these shields produce terrible artifacts in the image, but the rotational scheme of the x-ray source greatly reduces their effectiveness as well. The patient, however, can effectively be shielded from the low levels of scatter radiation as long as the direct x-ray beam does not intersect the shield.

Patient dose during spiral CT is somewhat more difficult to assesss than the dose during conventional CT. At a pitch of 1:1 the patient dose is about the same. At a higher pitch the dose is reduced compared with conventional CT and at a lower pitch it is increased.

As with any radiographic procedure, many factors influence patient dose. For CT the following generally holds true:

$$\text{Patient dose} = k \times \frac{IE}{\sigma^2 \times w^3 \times h}$$

In this equation, k is a conversion factor, I is beam intensity in mAs, E is average beam energy in keV (approximately 0.45 kVp), σ is system noise, w is pixel size, and h is slice thickness.

Note that, as with radiography, patient dose is proportional to the beam intensity. It is also directly proportional to the average beam energy. The other factors of the equation above are variables that are unique to CT scanning. Sigma (σ) is the noise. This is equivalent to quantum mottle in screen-film radiography and

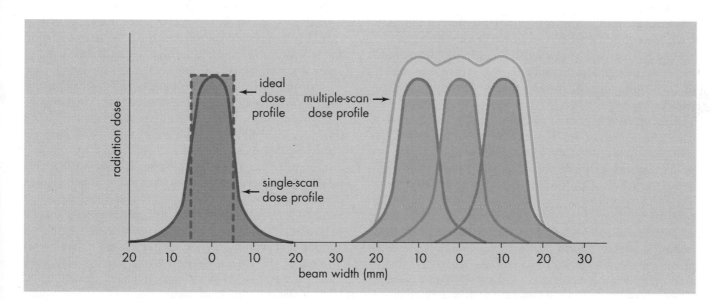

FIGURE 40-6 Patient dose distribution in CT is complicated because the profile of the x-ray beam cannot be made sharp.

represents random statistical variations in the CT numbers. The w stands for the pixel size, one of the determinants of spatial resolution. The last factor, h, is the slice thickness. A decrease in either the noise, pixel size, or slice thickness while the other factors remain constant results in increased patient dose.

All other factors being equal, a low-noise, high-resolution CT image results in higher patient dose. The challenge in CT, as indeed with all x-ray imaging, is not so much to deliver fantastically good resolution and low noise but to use the x-ray beam efficiently, producing the best possible image at a reasonable dose to the patient.

REDUCTION OF OCCUPATIONAL EXPOSURE

The radiographer can do much to minimize the occupational radiation exposure of other imaging personnel. Most equipment characteristics, technique changes, and administrative procedures designed to minimize patient dose will also reduce occupational exposure.

In diagnostic imaging, at least 95% of the radiographer's occupational radiation exposure comes from fluoroscopy and portable radiography. Attention to the cardinal principles of radiation protection (time, distance, and shielding) and ALARA (as low as reasonably achievable) is the most important aspect of occupational radiation control.

During fluoroscopy, the radiologist should minimize x-ray beam-on time. This can be done by careful technique, which includes intermittent activation of the fluoroscopic views rather than one long period of x-ray beam-on time. It is a common radiation protection practice to maintain a log of fluoroscopy time by recording the x-ray beam-on time using the 5-minute reset timer.

During fluoroscopy, the radiographer should step back from the table when his or her immediate presence and assistance is not required. The radiographer should also take maximum advantage of all protective shielding, including apron, curtain, Bucky slot cover, and the radiologist.

Each portable x-ray unit should have a protective apron assigned to it. The radiographer should wear such an apron during all portable examinations and maintain maximum distance from the source. The exposure cord on a portable x-ray unit must be at least 1.8 meters long. The primary beam should never be pointed at the radiographer or other nearby personnel.

During radiography, the radiographer is positioned behind a control-booth barrier. These barriers are usually considered secondary barriers because they only intercept leakage and scatter radiation. Consequently, leaded glass and leaded gypsum board are all that are needed for such barriers. The useful beam should never be directed toward the control booth barrier.

Other work assignments in diagnostic imaging, such as scheduling, darkroom duties, and filing, result in essentially no occupational radiation exposure.

Personnel Monitoring

Radiologists and radiographers are routinely exposed to ionizing radiation. The level of exposure depends on the type of activity in which they are engaged. Determining the quantity of radiation they receive requires a program of personnel monitoring. *Personnel monitoring* refers to procedures instituted to estimate the amount of radiation received by individuals who work in a radiation environment.

Personnel monitoring is required when there is any likelihood that an individual will receive more than one tenth of the dose limit. Most clinical diagnostic imaging personnel, therefore, must be monitored; however, it is usually not necessary to monitor diagnostic imaging secretaries and file clerks. Furthermore, it is usually not necessary to monitor operating room personnel, except perhaps those routinely involved in cystoscopy and C-arm fluoroscopy.

The personnel monitor offers no protection against radiation exposure. It simply measures the quantity of radiation to which the monitor was exposed and therefore is used as an indicator of the exposure of the wearer. There are basically three types of personnel monitors in use in diagnostic imaging: film badges, thermoluminescence dosimeters, and pocket ionization chambers.

Regardless of the type of monitor, it is essential that it be obtained from a certified laboratory. In-house processing of radiation monitors should not be attempted.

Film badges. Film badges came into general use during the mid-1940s and have been widely used in diagnostic imaging ever since. Film badges are specially designed devices in which a small piece of film similar to dental radiographic film is sandwiched between metal filters inside a plastic holder. Figure 40-7 is a view of several typical radiation monitors.

The film incorporated into a film badge is special radiation dosimetry film that is particularly sensitive to ionizing radiation. The optical density on the exposed and processed film is proportional to the exposure received by the film badge.

Carefully controlled calibration, processing, and analyzing conditions are necessary for the film badge to accurately measure occupational exposure. Usually, exposures less than 10 mR (2.6 μC per kilogram) are not measured by film badge monitors, and the film badge vendor will report only that a minimum exposure (M) was received. When higher exposures are received, they can be accurately reported.

The metal filters, along with the window in the plastic film holder, allow estimation of the x-ray energy. Usually the filters are made of aluminum and copper. If

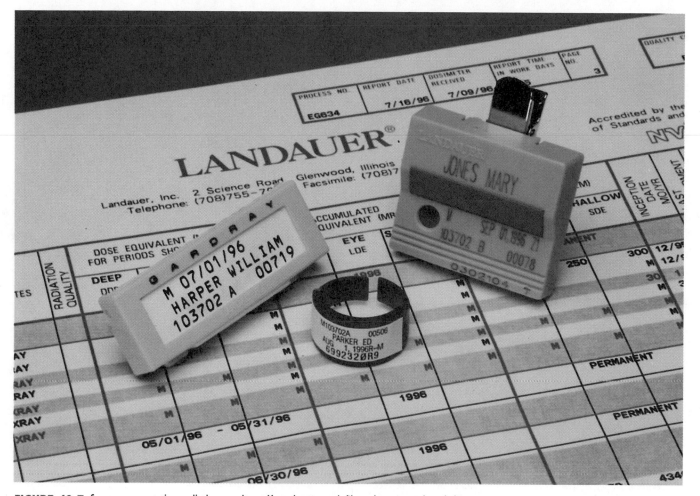

FIGURE 40-7 Some representative radiation monitors. Many have metal filters incorporated to help identify the type of radiation and its energy. *(Courtesy R.S. Landauer Jr. & Co.)*

the radiation exposure is a result of penetrating x-rays, the image of the filters on the processed film will be faint and there may be no image at all of the window in the plastic holder. If the badge is exposed to soft x-rays, the filters will be well imaged and the optical densities under the filters will allow estimation of the x-ray energy.

Often the filters to the front of the badge differ in shape from the filters to the back of the badge. Radiation that had entered through the back of the badge would normally indicate that the person wearing the badge was exposed to considerably higher levels of x-radiation than indicated, since the x-rays would have penetrated through the body before interacting with the film badge. For this reason, film badges must be worn with their proper side to the front.

Several advantages of film badge personnel monitors continue to make them popular. They are inexpensive, easy to handle, not difficult to process, reasonably accurate, and have been in use for several decades.

Film badge monitors also have disadvantages. Since they incorporate film as the sensing device, they cannot

be worn for long periods because of fogging caused by temperature and humidity.

Film badge monitors should never be left in an enclosed car or other area where excessive temperatures may occur. The fogging produced by elevated temperature and humidity will result in a falsely high evaluation of exposure. Consequently, film badge monitors should not be worn for longer than 1 month.

Thermoluminescence dosimeters. The sensitive material of the TLD monitor (Figure 40-8) is lithium fluoride (LiF) in crystalline form, either as a powder or more often as a small chip approximately 3 millimeters square and 1 millimeter thick. When exposed to x-rays, the TLD absorbs energy and stores it in the form of excited electrons in the crystalline lattice. When heated, these excited electrons fall back to their normal orbital state with the emission of visible light. The intensity of visible light is measured with a photomultiplier tube and is proportional to the radiation dose received by the crystal. This sequence was described in detail in Chapter 39.

The TLD monitoring device has several advantages over film. It is more sensitive and more accurate than a

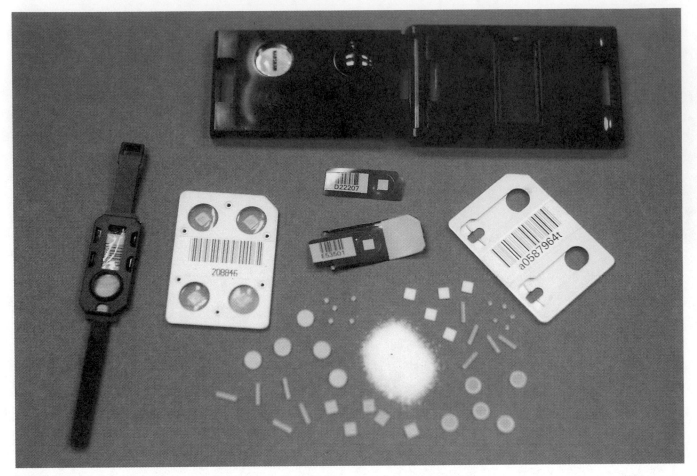

FIGURE 40-8 TLDs are available as chips, disks, rods, and powder. They are used for area and environmental radiation monitoring and especially for occupational radiation monitoring. *(Courtesy · Bicron NE.)*

film badge monitor. Properly calibrated TLD monitors can measure exposure as low as 5 mR (1.3 μC per kilogram). The TLD monitor does not suffer from loss of information after exposure to excessive heat or humidity. Consequently, they can be worn for intervals up to 3 months at a time.

The primary disadvantage of TLD personnel monitoring is cost. The price of a typical TLD monitoring service is perhaps twice that of film badge monitoring. If the frequency of monitoring is quarterly, however, the cost is about the same.

Pocket ionization chambers. Pocket ionization chambers are small devices measuring approximately 2 centimeters in diameter by 10 centimeters long and are designed to be clipped onto wearing apparel like a writing pen. Pocket ionization chambers are available in several different ranges, but the one usually used in diagnostic imaging has a range of 0 to 200 mR (0 to 50 μC per kilogram).

The use of a pocket ionization chamber can be somewhat time consuming. Before it is used, the chamber must be charged to a predetermined voltage so that

the scale reading indicates 0. As the chamber is exposed to radiation during the day, the charge is neutralized. An additional analysis of the chamber voltage at the end of the day indicates the radiation exposure to the chamber.

Pocket ionization chambers are not used frequently in diagnostic imaging. Their use requires daily identification of personnel exposures. A manipulation of the charging and reading mechanism is required daily. They are often used for a day or so to monitor nonimaging personnel such as nurses.

Pocket ionization chambers are reasonably accurate and sensitive, but they do have a limited range. Should exposure to an individual exceed the range of the dosimeter, the precise level of exposure would never be known. Pocket ionization chambers are fairly expensive and can be easily damaged.

Where to wear a personnel monitor. Much discussion and research in health physics have gone into providing precise recommendations about where a radiographer should wear the film badge. The official publications of the National Council on Radiation Protection and Measurements (NCRP) offer little assistance in this regard. They suggest that the radiographer consult a qualified expert. Qualified experts are medical physicists who are diplomats of either the American Board of Medical Physics (ABMP), the American Board of Diagnostic imaging (ABR), or the American Board of Health Physics (ABHP).

Many radiographers wear their personnel monitors in front at the waist or chest level because it is convenient to clip the badge over a belt or a shirt pocket. If the radiographer is not involved in fluoroscopic procedures, these locations are acceptable.

If the radiographer participates in fluoroscopy, then the personnel monitor should be positioned on the collar above the protective apron. The dose limit of 5000 mrem per year (50 mSv per year) refers to the effective dose (E). It has been shown that during fluoroscopy, when a protective apron is worn, exposure to the collar region is approximately 20 times greater than that to the trunk of the body beneath the protective lead apron. So, if the personnel monitor is worn beneath the protective apron, it will record a falsely low exposure and will not indicate what could be a hazardous exposure to unprotected body parts.

Nearly all state radiation control programs recommend or require that the personnel radiation monitor be worn at collar level. This is the official recommendation of the Council of Radiation Control Program Directors (CRCPD).

In some clinical situations, it may be advisable to wear more than one personnel monitor. This is not normally necessary for diagnostic radiographers. Two exceptions exist. The abdomen should be monitored during pregnancy. The extremities should be monitored during angiointerventional procedures during which the radiologist's hands are in close proximity to the useful beam. Nuclear medicine radiographers should wear extremity monitors when handling radioactive material.

Personnel Monitoring Report

State and federal regulations require that the results of the personnel monitoring program be recorded in a precise fashion and maintained for review. Monitoring periods and the associated exposure records must not exceed a calendar quarter. Quarterly, monthly, or weekly reports are acceptable, but records reflecting longer periods of time are not.

The personnel radiation monitoring report must contain a number of specific items of information (Figure 40-9). The first column lists the employee name. The second column is an identification number assigned to the radiation worker and monitor. The third column identifies the type of monitor. Additional personal data required include birthdate, social security number, and gender.

The exposure data that must be included on the form are the current exposure, the cumulative quarterly exposure, and the cumulative annual exposure. Separate radiation monitors, for example, extremity monitors, would be identified separately from the whole-body monitor.

Occasionally, if a personnel exposure involves low-energy radiation, a dose to the skin might occur that is greater than the dose of penetrating radiation. In such a case the skin dose is separately identified. There are areas of the report for neutron radiation exposure to accommodate nuclear reactor and particle accelerator workers.

When one changes employment, the total radiation exposure history must be transferred to the records of the new employer. Consequently, when one leaves employment, one should automatically receive a report of the previous total radiation exposure history at that facility. Such a report should be given automatically; if it is not, it should be requested.

When establishing a personnel radiation monitoring program, the supplier of the monitor should be informed of the type of radiation facility involved. That information will influence the method of calibration of the monitors and the control monitors.

The **control monitor** is used to measure the background exposure during transportation, handling, and storage. It should never be stored in or adjacent to a radiation area. It should be kept in a distant room or office.

All monitors should be returned to the supplier together and in a timely fashion so they can be processed together. Lost or inadvertently exposed monitors must be evaluated and an estimate of the true exposure recorded. Unless there are unusual circumstances, the estimate can be made by averaging the previous 6-month exposures.

Protective Apparel

The control console is usually positioned behind fixed protective barriers during diagnostic radiographic procedures. It is not normally so positioned during fluoroscopy or portable radiography. In these instances, protective apparel must be worn.

Protective gloves and aprons are available in many sizes and shapes. They are usually constructed of lead-impregnated vinyl. Some protective garments are impregnated with tin rather than lead because tin has some advantages over lead as a shielding material in the diagnostic range of x-ray energies.

The normal thicknesses for protective apparel are 0.3, 0.5, and 1 millimeter of lead equivalent. The garments themselves are much thicker than these dimensions, but they provide shielding equivalent to that thickness of pure lead (Table 40-5).

Of course, maximum exposure reduction is obtained with the 1-millimeter lead equivalent garment, but an

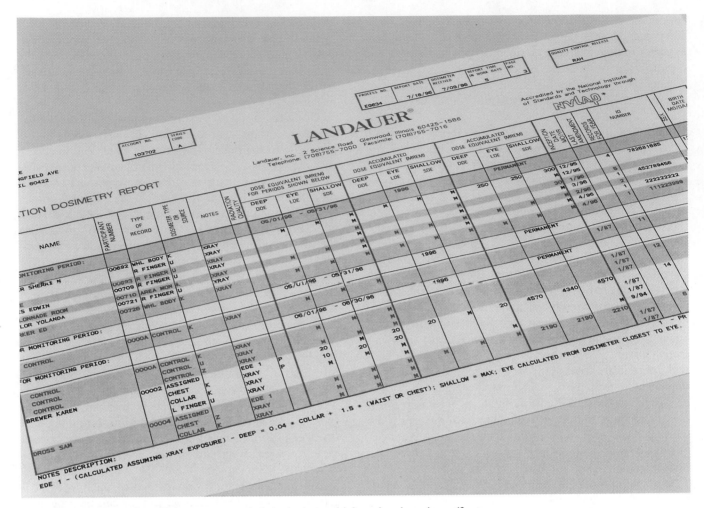

FIGURE 40-9 Personnel monitoring report must include the items of information shown here. *(Courtesy R.S. Landauer Jr. & Co.)*

TABLE 40-5

Some Physical Characteristics of Protective Lead Aprons

Equivalent Thickness (mm Pb)	Weight (lb)	Percent Attenuation				
		60 kVp	80 kVp	100 kVp	120 kVp	140 keV
0.3	3-10	99	97	94	92	58
0.5	6-15	99	99	96	95	70
1.0	12-25	99	99	98	97	79

apron of this material can weigh as much as 11 kilograms (25 pounds). The wearer could be exhausted by end of the fluoroscopic schedule just from having to carry the protective apron. The x-ray attenuation at 80 kVp for 0.3-millimeter lead equivalent and 1-millimeter lead equivalent is 97% and 99%, respectively. Most diagnostic imaging departments find 0.5-millimeter lead equivalent protective garments a workable compromise between unnecessary weight and desired protection.

Protective aprons for angiointerventional suites should be of the wrap-around type. During these procedures, there can be a lot of personnel movement and some, such as an anesthesiologist, may even have their back to the source.

When not in use protective apparel must be stored on properly designed racks. If they are continuously folded or heaped in the corner, cracks can develop. At least once a year aprons and gloves should be fluoroscoped to be sure that no such cracks appear. If fluoroscopy is not available, high kVp radiography (e.g., 120 kVp/10 mAs) may be used.

Position

During fluoroscopy, all personnel should remain as far from the patient as possible. After loading spot films, the radiographer should take a step or two back from the table when his or her presence is not required. The radiologist should be trained to use the deadman's foot switch sparingly. Naturally, when x-ray beam-on time is high, the radiation exposure to patient and personnel will be proportionately high.

Patient Holding

Many patients referred for x-ray examination are not physically able to support themselves. Examples are infants, the elderly, and the incapacitated. Diagnostic imaging personnel should never be used to hold these patients. Mechanical restraining devices should be available. Otherwise, a relative or friend accompanying the patient should be asked to help. As a last resort, other hospital employees such as nurses and orderlies may be used occasionally to hold patients but never diagnostic imaging employees.

When it is necessary to have another person hold the patient, protective apparel must be provided to that person. An apron and gloves are necessary, and the holder should be carefully positioned and instructed so that he or she is not exposed to the useful beam.

REDUCTION OF UNNECESSARY PATIENT DOSE

Many sources of unnecessary patient dose exist over which the radiographer has considerable control. Unnecessary patient dose is defined as any radiation dose that is not required for the patient's well-being or proper management and care.

Unnecessary Examinations

The radiographer has practically no control, however, over what some consider the largest source of unnecessary patient dose, that is, the unnecessary x-ray examination. This is almost exclusively the radiologist's responsibility.

Unfortunately, this source of unnecessary patient dose presents a serious dilemma for the radiologist and the clinician. Many x-ray examinations are knowingly requested when the yield of helpful information may be extremely low or nonexistent. When such an examination is performed, the benefit to the patient in no way compensates for the radiation dose.

If the examination is not performed, the clinician and radiologist may be severely criticized and then sued if the patient's ultimate management results in failure, even though the examination in question would have contributed little, if anything, to effective patient management. In such situations the radiologist is caught in the middle.

Routine x-ray examinations should not be performed when there is no precise medical indication. Substantial evidence shows that such examinations are of little benefit because they are not cost-effective and the disease detection rate is very low. Examples of such cases follow:

1. **Mass screening for tuberculosis.** General screening has not been found effective, and better methods of tuberculosis testing are now available. Some x-ray screening in high-risk groups (e.g., medical and paramedical personnel), in service personnel posing a potential community hazard (e.g., food handlers or teachers), and in special occupational groups (e.g., miners and workers having contact with beryllium, asbestos, glass, or silica) may be appropriate. Screening in these groups is for diseases other than tuberculosis.
2. **Hospital admissions.** Chest x-ray examinations for routine hospital admission when there is no clinical indication of chest disease should not be performed. Among patients who would be candidates for such examinations are those admitted to the pulmonary or surgical service or elderly patients.
3. **Preemployment physicals.** Chest and lower back x-ray examinations are not justified because knowledge gained about previous injury or disease is nil.
4. **Periodic health examinations.** Many physicians and health care organizations promote annual or biannual physical examinations. Certainly, when such an examination is conducted on an asymptomatic patient, it should not include x-ray examination, especially a fluoroscopic examination.

Repeat Examinations

One area of unnecessary examination that the radiographer can influence considerably is that of repeat examinations. The frequency of repeat examinations has been variously estimated to range as high as 10% of all examinations. In the typical busy hospital facility, repeat examinations will not normally exceed 4%. Examinations with the highest retake rates are lumbar spine, thoracic spine, KUB, and abdomen.

Some repeat examinations are caused by equipment malfunctions. Most are caused by radiographer error. Studies of causes of repeat examinations have shown that improper positioning and poor radiographic technique resulting in a film too light or too dark are primarily responsible for retakes. Motion and improper collimation are responsible for some retakes. Infrequent errors that contribute to repeat examinations are dirty screens, use of improperly loaded cassettes, light leaks, chemical fog, artifacts caused by a dirty processor, wrong projection, grid errors, and multiple exposure (Figure 40-10).

Radiographic Technique

In general the use of high-kVp technique will result in reduced patient dose. Increasing the kVp is always as-

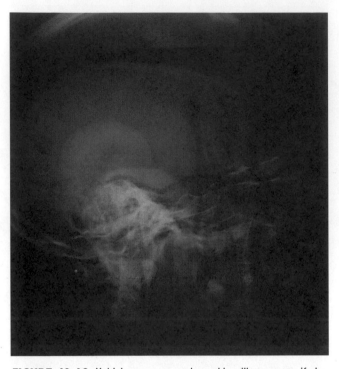

FIGURE 40-10 Multiple exposures such as this will not occur if the radiographer is careful. *(Courtesy Dianne DeVos.)*

sociated with a reduction in mAs to obtain an acceptable radiographic optical density, and this in turn results in a reduced exposure. This occurs because the patient dose is linearly related to the mAs, but it is related to the kVp by approximately the square.

Question: A lateral skull radiograph is obtained at 64 kVp, 80 mAs and results in an ESE of 400 mR (4 mGy). If the tube potential is increased to 74 kVp (15% increase) and the mAs reduced by half to 40 mAs, the optical density will remain the same. What will the new skin dose be?

Answer: Dose $= (400 \text{ mR})\left(\dfrac{40 \text{ mAs}}{80 \text{ mAs}}\right)\left(\dfrac{74 \text{ kVp}}{64 \text{ kVp}}\right)^2$

$= (400 \text{ mR})(0.5)(1.34)$

$= 267 \text{ mR}$

Of course the radiologist must be the final judge of radiographic quality. Increasing kVp even slightly may result in images that are too flat for proper interpretation by the radiologist. An area of radiography where high-kVp technique is becoming widely accepted is examination of the chest.

Proper collimation is essential to good radiographic technique. Positive-beam limitation (PBL) does not prevent the radiographer from reducing the field size still further by collimation. By using collimation, not only does one reduce the patient dose, but the image quality will be improved as well because scatter radiation will also be reduced.

Image Receptor

The image receptor should be selected first for the type of examination and second for the radiation dose necessary to provide a quality image. The fastest-speed screen-film combination consistent with the nature of the examination should be used. It should be kept in mind that the screen speed, in general, controls the patient dose.

Rare-earth and other fast screens should be used when possible. Routine application of such screens in orthopedic, chest, and magnification radiography is appropriate. In general, 200- to 400-speed systems are now used.

Patient Positioning

When examining the upper extremities or breast, especially with the patient in a seated position, care should be taken so that the useful beam does not intercept the gonads. The patient should be positioned lateral to the useful beam, and a protective apron should be provided as a shield.

Specific Area Shielding

X-ray examinations result in a partial-body exposure, although most radiation protection guides and radiation response information are based on whole-body exposure. The partial-body nature of the x-ray examination is controlled by proper beam collimation and the use of specific area shielding.

Use of specific area shielding is indicated when a particularly sensitive tissue or organ is in or near the useful beam. The lens of the eye, breasts, and the gonads are frequently shielded from the primary radiation beam. There are two kinds of specific area shielding devices: the **contact shield** and the **shadow shield.**

Lens shields are always of the contact type. The contact shielding device is positioned directly on the patient. Gonad shields, on the other hand, can be of either the contact or the shadow type.

Breast shields are recommended for use during scoliosis examinations. Such examinations often use an AP projection, which subjects the juvenile breasts to primary beam irradiation. The PA projection, however, is equally satisfactory, since magnification is of little importance. The PA projection results in a breast dose of only about 1% of the AP projection.

Figure 40-11 shows some examples of contact gonad shields. When such contact shields are not purchased commercially, a properly cut piece of protective material is perfectly adequate. Shapes such as hearts, diamonds, triangles, and squares have been used effectively, especially for children.

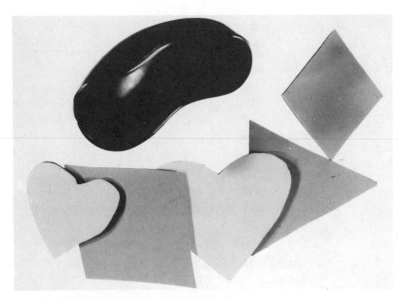

FIGURE 40-11 Examples of useful gonad shields.

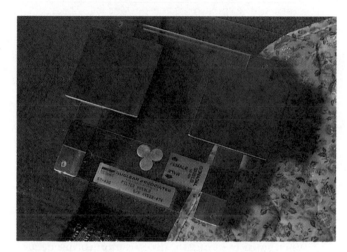

FIGURE 40-12 Shadow shield. *(Courtesy Nuclear Associates, Inc.)*

An example of the shadow shield is shown in Figure 40-12. This type of shield is equally as effective as the contact shield and is more acceptable for use with adult patients. Use of such devices, however, requires careful attention on the part of the radiographer. The shield must shadow the gonads without interfering with adjacent tissue. Improper positioning of the shadow shield can result in a repeat examination and increased patient dose.

The subject of gonad shielding is sufficiently important to require emphasis. Its use should be governed by the following concepts:

1. Gonad shielding should be considered for all patients, especially children and those who are potentially reproductive.
2. Gonad shielding should be used when the gonads lie in or near the useful beam.
3. Proper patient positioning and beam collimation should not be relaxed when gonad shields are in use.

4. Gonad shielding should only be used when it does not interfere with obtaining the required diagnostic information.

SUMMARY

Although the dose limit for occupational workers is 50 mSv per year, most radiographic personnel should not receive more than 5 mSv per year. Radiologists generally receive a higher dose because of their exposure during fluoroscopy, which brings them closer to the radiation source.

Patient dose from diagnostic x-rays is generally recorded in one of the following three ways: (1) ESE, (2) mean marrow dose, or (3) gonadal dose. Thermoluminescence dosimeters are the monitor of choice for patient radiation dose. Knowing the output intensity of at least one x-ray and the SSD, the medical physicist can estimate the ESE for patient examinations. For fluoroscopic examinations, the ESE can be estimated at 4 R per minute. Patient dose to the bone marrow can be calculated by determining what percent of the active bone marrow is in the primary beam and using this percent to calculate the average dose. The gonadal dose is measured in terms of population effects. The genetically significant dose is a gonadal dose if received by every member of the population would be expected to produce a total genetic effect. This total genetic effect is the sum of the individual doses actually received.

For mammography, patient dose should not exceed 100 mrad per view with nongrid screen film and 300 mrad per view with a grid. The patient dose in CT is approximately equivalent to the cumulative dose produced by a series of radiographic views. Part of the usefulness of CT is that a larger percentage of the beam contributes to the image because of the precise collimation compared with radiography.

Because 95% of occupational exposure comes from fluoroscopy and mobile radiography, the radiographer should follow these guidelines for reducing occupational exposure:

1. During mobile radiography, wear an apron, maintain maximum distance from the source, and never direct the primary beam toward radiography or other personnel.
2. During fluoroscopy, step back from the table if not needed and use shielding, including an apron, thyroid shield, curtain, Bucky slot cover, and the radiologist.
3. During radiography, stand behind the control booth and never direct the primary beam toward the control-booth barrier.

Personnel monitoring is required when there is any likelihood that an individual will receive more than one fourth the dose limit. The various personnel radiation monitors are: (1) film badges, (2) thermoluminescence dosimeters, and (3) pocket ionization chambers. Film badges are widely used because they are inexpensive, accurate, and have been used for many years. The TLDs can be worn for up to 3 months at a time, but the film badges must be changed every month. The pocket ionization chamber requires daily identification of exposure. For general use the radiographer should wear the personnel monitor at waist or chest level; however, during fluoroscopy, the monitor is worn on the collar outside the protective apron. Occupational exposure data is printed on an exposure report on a regular basis, usually monthly. The data that must be included on the report is current exposure, cumulative quarterly exposure, and cumulative annual exposure.

Protective apparel must always be worn when the radiographer cannot stand behind a protective barrier during an exposure. Radiographers and occupational workers should never be used to hold patients during an exposure.

The radiographer has no control over what is considered to be the largest source of unnecessary patient exposure: unnecessary x-ray examinations. Screening x-rays such as chest x-rays for TB screening, routine chest x-rays for hospital admissions, pre-employment x-ray examinations, and x-rays for asymptomatic patients during annual physicals are no longer performed.

Use of specific area shielding is indicated when sensitive tissue or a sensitive organ is in or near the primary beam. Gonadal shielding should be considered for all patients of reproductive age and when the gonads are in line with or near the primary beam. Even though shields may be used, proper patient positioning and collimation should be used. Finally, gonadal shielding should only be used when it does not interfere with the required diagnostic information.

REVIEW QUESTIONS

1. Name the units of radiation dose, radiation exposure, and effective dose.
2. What is the dose limit for diagnostic imaging personnel? Why do radiologists receive slightly higher exposure than radiographers?
3. During what two examination procedures does the highest radiation dose occur for diagnostic imaging personnel?
4. What are the two reasons that medical radiation exposure to patients is commanding increased attention?
5. List the three ways patient dose is reported.
6. Using Table 40-2, identify the mean marrow dose for a CT of the head and for a skull x-ray.
7. For an average fluoroscoping examination, the entrance skin exposure of the patient is _____.
8. Using Table 40-3, radiographic examination of which anatomic site would result in the greatest bone marrow dose?
9. Define GSD. What is the estimated GSD caused by diagnostic x-ray examination?
10. Why are measurements of gonadal dose important?
11. Why is ESE not used in values stated for patient dose in mammography?
12. What is the difference between skin dose in CT versus skin dose in routine radiography?
13. What is the required length of the exposure cord on the mobile radiographic unit?
14. When must personnel radiation monitoring occur?
15. When did film badges come into use? Describe the design of film badges. How are they to be worn, and where are they placed on the body?
16. List the exposure data that must be included in the personnel monitoring report.
17. Name the thicknesses of protective apparel. What thickness is required to attenuate 94% of the x-ray beam at 100 kVp?
18. What is the procedure for holding patients during an x-ray examination?
19. What are the four types of screening x-rays that are no longer performed?
20. List the four concepts of patient shielding during x-ray examinations.

Additional Reading

Dowd SB: The basics of radiation protection for hospital workers, *Hosp Top* 69:31 1991.

Dowd SB, Wilson B: Informed patient consent: a historical perspective, *Radiol Technol* 67(2):119 November-December, 1995.

Fung K: Lowering patient dose on single-phase x-ray units, *Radiol Technol* 66(3):159 January-February, 1995.

Kramer GH, Meyerhof DP: The Canadian national calibration reference centre for invivo monitoring: thyroid monitoring. Sources of errors in thyroid monitoring of occupationally exposed personnel, part 2, *Can J Med Radiat Technol* 25(1):21 March, 1994.

Larson BJ et al: Radiation exposure during fluoroarthroscopically assisted anterior cruciate reconstruction, *Am J Sports Med* 23(4):462 July-August, 1995.

Appendix A

Sources for Supplementary Teaching Materials

Advanced Health Education Center
102 Portland
Houston, Texas 77006

American Association of Physicists in Medicine
335 East 45th Street
New York, New York 10017

American College of Medical Physics
1891 Preston White Drive
Reston, Virginia 22091

American College of Radiology
1891 Preston White Drive
Reston, Virginia 22091

American Society of Radiologic Technologists
1500 Central Avenue S.E.
Albuquerque, New Mexico 87123

Center for Devices and Radiological Health
5600 Fishers Lane
Rockville, Maryland 20857

Eastman Kodak Company
Radiography Markets Division
343 State Street
Rochester, New York 14650

E.I. du Pont de Nemours & Co., Inc.
Photo Products Department
Wilmington, Delaware 19898

General Electrical Medical Systems
P.O. Box 414
Milwaukee, Wisconsin 53201

Liebel-Flarsheim Company
2111 East Galbraith Road
Cincinnati, Ohio 45215

Mallinckrodt Inc.
P.O. Box 5840
St. Louis, Missouri 63134

Medical Technology Management Institute
P.O. Box 26337
Milwaukee, Wisconsin 53226-0337

National Council on Radiation Protection and
  Measurements
7910 Woodmont Avenue, Suite 1016
Bethesda, Maryland 20814

Philips Medical Systems, Inc.
710 Bridgeport Avenue
Shelton, Connecticut 06484

Picker International
595 Miner Road
Highland Heights, Ohio 44143

Radiological Society of North America, Inc.
1415 West 22nd Street, Tower B
Oak Brook, Illinois 60521

Siemens Medical Systems, Inc.
186 Woods Avenue South
Iselin, New Jersey 08830

U.S. Nuclear Regulatory Commission
Office of Information
Washington, D.C. 20555

Victoreen, Inc.
6000 Cochran Road
Cleveland, Ohio 44139-3395

Important Dates in the Development of Modern Radiology

Date	Event
1895	Roentgen discovers x-rays.
1896	First medical applications of x-rays in diagnosis and therapy are made.
1900	The American Roentgen Society, the first American radiology organization, is founded.
1901	Roentgen receives the first Nobel Prize in physics.
1905	Einstein introduces his theory of relativity and the famous equation $E = mc^2$.
1907	The Snook interrupterless transformer is introduced.
1913	Bohr theorizes his model of the atom, featuring a nucleus and planetary electrons.
1913	The Coolidge hot-filament x-ray tube is developed.
1917	Cellulose nitrate film base is widely adopted.
1920	Several investigators demonstrate the use of soluble iodine compounds as contrast media.
1920	The American Society of Radiologic Technology is founded.
1921	The Potter-Bucky grid is introduced.
1922	Comptom describes the scattering of x-rays.
1925	The First International Congress of Radiology is convened in London.
1928	The roentgen is defined as the unit of x-ray intensity.
1929	Forssmann demonstrates cardiac catheterization . . . on himself.
1929	The rotating anode tube is introduced.
1930	Tomographic devices are shown by several independent investigators.
1937	The International Committee on X-ray and Radium Protection officially defines the roentgen.
1942	Morgan exhibits an electronic phototiming device.
1942	First automatic film processor (Pako) is introduced.
1948	Coltman develops the first fluoroscopic image intensifier.
1951	Multidirectional tomography (polytomography) is introduced.
1953	The rad is officially adopted as the unit of absorbed dose.
1956	Xeroradiography is demonstrated.
1956	First automatic roller transport film processing (Eastman Kodak) is introduced.
1963	Kuhl and Edwards demonstrate single-photon emission computed tomography (SPECT) imaging.
1965	Ninety-second rapid processor introduced (Eastman Kodak).
1966	Diagnostic ultrasound enters routine use.
1972	Rare-earth radiographic intensifying screens are introduced.
1973	Hounsfield completes development of first computed tomographic (CT) scanner (EMI, Ltd).
1973	Damadian and Lauterbur produce first magnetic resonance images (MRI).
1979	Mistretta demonstrates digital fluoroscopy.
1980	First commercial superconducting MR imager is introduced.
1981	The International System of Units (SI) is adopted by ICRU.
1982	Picture archiving and communications systems (PACS) become available.
1983	First tabular grain film emulsion (Eastman Kodak) is developed.
1984	Laser-stimulable phosphors for direct digital radiographs appear.
1988	Clinical application of a superconducting quantum interference device (SQUID) is demonstrated.
1990	Last xeromammography system is produced.

Appendix C

Answers to Review Questions

CHAPTER 1

1. Anything that occupies space.
2. The ability to do work.
3. True.
4. Weight is the mass of an object in a gravitational field.
5. Potential energy is the capacity to do work because of the position of an object. Kinetic energy is the energy of motion. Chemical energy is the energy released in a chemical reaction. Electrical energy is the work done when an electron moves through a wire. Thermal energy is the kinetic energy of molecules. Nuclear energy is the energy contained in the nucleus of an atom. Electromagnetic energy is the energy of the electromagnetic spectrum including x-rays, microwaves, light, and radio waves.
6. Sunlight and sound.
7. X-rays can ionize matter.
8. Ionization occurs when radiation passes close enough to an orbital electron, causing it to escape from its orbit. The escaping electron is a negative ion, and the atom remaining is a positive ion.
9. Radon.
10. The rad is the measurement of ionizing dose to humans and is called the gray (Gy) in international units.
11. 11%.
12. The Crookes tube.
13. X-rays were discovered by accident. Roentgen's contemporaries had observed x-rays but had not recognized their significance. Roentgen studied his discovery with such enthusiasm that within a month he had described all the properties that are recognized today.
14,. The risk of radiation exposure in modern diagnostic imaging departments is minimal.
15. Skin damage, hair loss, and low red-cell count.
16. As low as reasonably achievable.
17. Exposure must have specific benefit. All exposure should follow ALARA. Doses should not exceed limits for appropriate circumstances.
18. Filtration, collimation, intensifying screens, protective barriers, protective apparel, and gonadal shielding.
19. Glass plates were used as x-ray image receptors until WWI, when cellulose nitrate flexible film began to be used. This quickly became a better product than the original glass plate.
20. The Coolidge tube was a vacuum tube that allowed the x-ray intensity and energy to be accurately selected. The Snook transformer provided a high-voltage power supply to power the Coolidge tube.

CHAPTER 2

1. 10^5.
2. Roentgen (c/kg), rad (gray), rem (seivert), curie (becquerel).
3. .1 R $\times$ 2.58 $\times$ 10^{-4} (conversion factor) = 2.58 $\times$ 10^{-5} C/kg.
4. 4.05 $\times$ 10^3.
5. 2^3.
6. 24.93 $\times$ 10^{-12}.
7. $1\frac{7}{15}$.
8. $1\frac{3}{7}$.
9. .003.
10. .42.
11. 6.586.
12. x = 1.875.
13. $x = \dfrac{d - c}{ab}$.
14. 15.6 m/gallon.
15. 288 mR.

CHAPTER 3

1. 1.1 m^3.
2. 250 in^3.
3. 12.5 m/s.
4. 7 m/s.
5. 44.
6. 0.1 ft/sec.
7. 4.5 m/s^2.
8. 770 N.
9. 24,540 N.
10. 735 N (on Earth), 122 N (on moon).
11. 135 J.
12. 3.0 kgm^2/s^3.
13. 32 watts.
14. 88.2 ft-lbs (J).
15. −426.6° F.
16. 25° C.
17. 26.6° C.

CHAPTER 4

1. c) atom.
2. The atom is the smallest part of an element that has all the properties of that element.
3. The periodic table.
4. Neils Bohr.
5. Atoms of various elements combine to form molecules.

6. A chemical compound is a measurable quantity of one type of molecule. NaCl.
7. Electron, proton, and neutron are the fundamental particles.
8. The atomic number is the number of protons in the nucleus, which in a neutral atom is equal to the number of electrons in the shells. Atomic mass number is the number used to express the mass of an atom. The mass number of an electron is 0, and the mass number of protons and neutrons is 1.
9. Hydrogen ($^1_1$H) has 1 proton and 1 electron. Helium ($^4_2$He) has 4 protons and neutrons and 2 electrons. Lithium ($^7_3$Li) has 7 protons and neutrons and 3 electrons. Uranium ($^{238}_{92}$U) has 238 protons and neutrons and 92 electrons.
10. Electrons exist only in certain shells or energy levels that are associated with binding energies.
11. Atoms cannot be ionized by changing the number of protons in the nucleus because that changes the atom into another element.
12. An electron is removed from its shell surrounding the nucleus. The electron becomes the negative ion, and the remaining atom becomes the positive ion.
13. The valence of an element.
14. See any of 29 transitional elements in the Periodic Table in Figure 4-4.
15. Electrons are negatively charged, and protons in the nucleus are positively charged. The basic law of electricity states that opposite charges are attracted to each other.
16. An alpha particle consists of two protons and two neutrons bound together and emitted from the nucleus. A beta particle is electron-like and ejected from the nucleus of the atom.
17. The half-life of a radioisotope is the period of time required for a quantity of radioactivity to be reduced to one-half its original value.
18. ^{14}C is fixed in petrified trees and decays in time. The dating of the tree can be determined by the remaining radioactivity of the carbon.
19. Particulate and electromagnetic radiation.
20. Photons have no mass and no charge.

CHAPTER 5
1. Bundles of energy, the speed of light.
2. 186,400 miles per second.
3. Velocity = frequency × wavelength.
4. Wavelength and frequency are inversely proportional at a given velocity.
5. $\frac{I_1}{I_2} = \left(\frac{d_2}{d_1}\right)^2$. The intensity of electromagnetic radiation is inversely proportional to the square of the distance of the object from the source.
6. 11 mlm.
7. Reduced by one-fourth, increased by a factor of four.
8. The unit of frequency.
9. Visible light; x-radiation; and radiofrequency.
10. 1 keV to 50 MeV.
11. The only difference is their origin. X-rays form from the electron cloud, and gamma rays come from the nucleus.
12. Wave-particle duality.
13. The partial absorption of energy.
14. 30 to 150 kVp.

15. 1.69×10^{19} Hertz.
16. Matter can be neither created or destroyed.
17. Energy can be neither created or destroyed.
18. 6.24×10^{18} eV.
19. $E = mc^2$.

CHAPTER 6
1. To convert electric energy into electromagnetic energy of the x-ray beam.
2. Positive (proton) and negative (electron).
3. An object is electrified when it has too few or too many electrons.
4. Contact, friction, and induction.
5. The Earth.
6. The coulomb (C). 1 C = 6.3×10^{18} electron charges.
7. Unlike charges attract, like charges repel. Electrostatic force is directly proportional to the product of the charges and inversely proportional to the square of the distance between them. When an object becomes electrified, the electric charges are distributed throughout the object. Electric charges are concentrated along the sharpest curvature of the surface.
8. The unit of electric potential is the volt.
9. Electric conductors are matter through which electrons flow easily. Electric insulators are matter that inhibits the flow of electrons.
10. A semiconductor is a material that under some conditions behaves as an insulator and in other conditions it behaves as a conductor. Semiconductors led to the development of microchips, which is the basis for the present explosion in computer technology.
11. An electric circuit is a closed path of controlled electron flow.
12. The voltage across the total circuit or any portion of that circuit is equal to the current times the resistance.
13. 44 Ohms.
14. For the formulas for series circuits see Figure 6-14. For the formulas for parallel circuits see Figure 6-15.
15. Direct current is the flow of electrons in one direction along the conductor. Alternating current is the oscillation of electrons back and forth along a circuit.
16. 17.6 kW.
17. 1 A of current flowing through an electric potential of 1 V.
18. The study of electricity is important to understanding the x-ray tube circuit.

CHAPTER 7
1. Magnetism is of increasing importance in radiography because of the increasing use of magnetic resonance imaging as part of routine diagnostic medical procedures.
2. Lodestone was discovered in Magnesia, Western Turkey, and was used to point the way to water.
3. Any charged particle in motion will create a magnetic field.
4. An accumulation of many atomic magnets with their dipoles aligned creates a magnetic domain.
5. Magnets are classified according to the origin of the magnetic property.
6. Naturally occurring magnets, artificially induced permanent magnets, and electromagnets.
7. An electromagnet consists of a wire wrapped around an iron core.
8. Dimagnetic.
9. Ferromagnetic.

10. Gadolinium.
11. Magnetic susceptibility is the degree to which materials can be magnetized.
12. Magnetism, electrostatics, gravity, strong nuclear force, and weak nuclear interaction.
13. North pole and south pole.
14. The force created by a magnetic field is proportional to the product of the magnetic pole strengths divided by the square of the distance between them.
15. Gauss and Tesla. One Tesla (T) = 10,000 gauss (G).
16. Like magnetic poles repel, and unlike magnetic poles attract.
17. The law of magnetic induction, which states a ferromagnetic material can be made magnetic by placing it in the magnetic field lines of a magnet.
18. When rubbed on a sweater a comb attracts lightweight objects such as paper.
19. If the magnetic domains of an object are all aligned in the same direction, the object will act as a magnet.
20. A hydrogen ion is a strong magnetic dipole because of the unpaired electron, but in a hydrogen molecule the magnetic domains cancel each other out so there is no magnetic dipole.

CHAPTER 8

1. c.
2. Orested fashioned a long straight wire supported near a freely rotating compass. Without current flowing through the wire, the compass pointed North as one might expect. When current passed through the wire, however, the compass needle pointed towards the wire. Thus, electrons flowing through a wire produce a magnetic field around that wire.
3. A coil of wire.
4. The direction of the magnetic field lines surrounding a wire can be determined by using the right-hand rule. When gripping the wire with the right hand, the thumb points in the direction of the current flow. The fingers will curl in the direction of the magnetic field lines.
5. An electromagnet is a ferromagnetic material wrapped in a coil of wire.
6. Faraday's law says an electric current will be induced to flow in a circuit if some part of that circuit is in a changing magnetic field. Lenz' law says the induced current will flow in a direction such that it opposes the action that induces it.
7. The magnitude of induced currents depends on the strength of the magnetic field, the velocity of the magnetic field as it moves past the conductor, the angle of the conductor in relation to the magnetic field, and the number of turns in the conductor.
8. Mutual induction is the process of inducing a current flow through a secondary coil by passing a varying current through a primary coil.
9. See Figure 8-15.
10. In an electric generator a coil of wire is placed in a strong magnetic field between two poles of a magnet.
11. See Figure 8-14.
12. The induction motor contains a rotor and stators. The external electromagnets (stators) are energized in sequence, producing a changing magnetic field. The rotor begins to rotate, trying to bring its magnetic field into alignment. Thus, the rotor rotates continuously.

13. Transformer law for voltage: $\dfrac{V_s}{V_p} = \dfrac{N_s}{N_p}$

   Transformer law for current: $\dfrac{I_s}{I_p} = \dfrac{N_p}{N_s}$

14. 2.4 A.
15. 1,200 V.
16. Hysteresis.
17. Autotransformer.
18. Rectification.
19. *Therm* refers to heat. *Ion* refers to a charged particle. *Emission* means to give off.
20. Semiconductors sometimes behave as conductors and sometimes behave as insulators in their ability to conduct electricity.

CHAPTER 9

1. Radiographic unit, fluoroscopic unit, image intensifier.
2. X-rays can pass through.
3. Cassette, grid.
4. Extremity x-rays.
5. Table tilt of 80 degrees to the foot and 20 degrees to the head.
6. Line compensation control, mA, time, kVp, and photo-timing controls.
7. 20 V.
8. Supplies precise voltage to the filament circuit and to the high-voltage circuit. It is much safer to vary low voltage and increase it to the kilovolt level than to increase low voltage and then vary its magnitude.
9. Single winding has primary and secondary connections along its length.
10. The voltage to be monitored before an exposure.
11. .33 mAs.
12. 18 mAs.
13. Precision resistors.
14. Primary side.
15. Synchronous timers.
16. A device that measures the amount of radiation reaching the image receptor.
17. A high-voltage generator converts low supply voltage to kilovoltage of the proper waveform. A high-voltage transformer steps up the voltage in relation to the coil windings.
18. To produce direct current.
19. Single-phase is 100%; three-phase, twelve pulse is 4%; three-phase, six pulse is 13%; and high frequency is less than 3%.

CHAPTER 10

1. Ceiling support consists of rails mounted over the radiographic table; floor-to-ceiling support has a single column with rollers; floor mount system has the x-ray tube mounted on a column supported on the floor; fluoroscopy tube is mounted underneath the x-ray table; C-arm is a mobile fluoroscopy unit; and mobile radiography unit.
2. Source-to-image receptor distance.
3. Leakage radiation.
4. 30 to 50 cm long and 20 cm in diameter.
5. Because of the use of metal envelope tubes.
6. Formation of an electron cloud around the filament in preparation for acceleration toward the target.
7. Vaporization of the tungsten filament. 1% to 2% thorium added to the filament prolongs tube life.

8. It condenses the electron beam to a small area.
9. Space charge.
10. Small focal spots are used for increased spatial resolution. Large focal spots are used when techniques produce high heat.
11. Anode is positive; cathode is negative.
12. Stationary anodes serve low tube current and low power uses. Rotating anodes are needed in most cases when high-intensity beams are required.
13. Electrical conductor; mechanical support; and thermal conductor. Copper, molybdenum, and graphite.
14. High atomic number results in high-efficiency x-ray production; tungsten efficiently dissipates heat; and tungsten has a high melting point that withstands high tube current.
15. See Figure 10-13.
16. 3400 rpm.
17. The anode is driven by an induction motor.
18. See Figure 10-16.
19. Radiation intensity on the cathode side of the x-ray beam is higher than that on the anode side. In general, radiographers position the cathode side of the x-ray tube over the thicker part of the anatomy.
20. Three exposures, three seconds apart, 200 mA, 1 second, 80 kVp. Tube failure is caused by single excessive exposure, causing pitting of the anode, bearing failure from heat overload, and vaporization of the filament.

Answers to Tube Rating Chart Questions
1. 840 Hu
2. 23,693 HU
3. Approximately 80 kVp

CHAPTER 11

1. By increasing the kVp.
2. 1.28×10^{-14} J.
3. 0.56.
4. 1 to 3 cm. Half the velocity of light.
5. 99% of the kinetic energy of projectile electrons is converted to heat.
6. See Figure 11.3. Characteristic radiation is formed from the removal of an inner-shell electron.
7. 66.71 keV.
8. K-shell characteristic x-rays are energetic and penetrating.
9. See Figure 11-5. Braking of projectile electrons by the nucleus.
10. 0 to 70 keV.
11. Bremsstrahlung.
12. The spectrum describes the output of the x-ray tube.
13. Minimum.
14. 0.0124 nm.
15. Integration is the addition of the number of x-rays from each energy level over the entire spectrum.
16. A change in mA is directly proportional to change in the amplitude of x-ray emission at all energies; a change in kVp affects both the amplitude and position of the x-ray emission spectrum; added filtration increases quality of the beam; as the atomic number of the target material increases, high-energy x-rays increase; three-phase vs. single-phase power is equivalent to doubling the mAs.
17. A 15% increase in the kVp factor is equivalent to doubling the mAs factor.
18. 50 to 150 kVp.
19. 23 to 32 kVp. Low-energy characteristic x-rays.
20. To harden the x-ray beam, that is, to remove the low-energy x-rays from the beam.

CHAPTER 12

1. Tube output = x-ray quantity; penetrability = quality of the beam.
2. Roentgens (R), radiation exposure.
3. 50 mAs = 50 mC; 1 C = 6.25×10^{18}; 3.13×10^{17} electrons will interact with the target.
4. 2×10^{15} electrons.
5. 23.5 mR.
6. a) 48 mR, b) 39 mR.
7. 15%; reduction.
8. Radiation intensity from an x-ray tube varies inversely with the square of the distance from the target.
9. To reduce the number of low-energy x-rays that reach the patient.
10.

Increasing	Effect on Quantity of the X-ray Beam	Effect on Optical Density
mAs	Increases	Increases
kVp	Increase is proportional to square of ratio of kVp	Increases
Distance	Reduces by the square of the ratio of distance	Reduces
Filtration	Reduces	Reduces

11. X-ray quantity is directly proportional to mAs.
12. Hard x-rays have high penetrability; soft x-rays have low penetrability.
13. The HVL of the x-ray beams refers to the thickness of absorbing material necessary to reduce the x-ray intensity to half of its original value.
14. Increasing kVp and increasing filtration.
15. Aluminum is used because it is efficient at removing low-energy x-rays and because it is available, inexpensive, and easily shaped into filters.
16. A light field is used with leaded leaves that can change and limit the light and radiation field.
17. Thick portion shadowing the toes and the thin portion over the heel.
18. Yes.
19.

Increasing	Effect on X-ray Quality	Effect on Optical Density
mAs	None	Increases
kVp	Increases	Increases
Distance	None	Reduces
Filtration	Increases	Reduces

CHAPTER 13

1. The wavelength of the radiation.
2. Classical scattering.
3. The energy of the incident x-ray and the energy of the ejected electron.
4. Compton interaction.

5. False. The atomic number of matter has no effect on Compton scattering. It is most likely to occur with outer shell electrons and loosely bound electrons.
6. In general, Compton scattering decreases as x-ray energy increases; however, there is an increase in Compton scattering in relation to photoelectric effect as energy increases.
7. The photoelectric effect is an x-ray absorption interaction in which the x-rays are not scattered but are totally absorbed. An electron or photoelectron is then removed from the atom.
8. Pair production.
9. As x-ray energy increases, there is an increase of Compton scattering in relation to the photoelectric effect.
10. 10 MeV.
11. Differential absorption is the characteristic of producing a radiographic image; it results from the difference between x-rays absorbed photoelectrically and those not absorbed at all.
12. An x-ray is 6.5 times more likely to interact with bone than muscle.
13. See Table 13-6.
14. See Table 13-6.
15. The quantity of matter per unit volume.
16. The total reduction in the number of x-rays remaining in an x-ray beam following penetration through a given thickness of tissue.
17. Absorption plus scattering.
18. Remnant radiation.
19. 1890 times more probable.
20. Above 90 kVp.

CHAPTER 14
1. Duplitized.
2. See Figure 14-1.
3. The base maintains its size and shape during use and processing so the image is not distorted. This property is called dimensional stability.
4. Original film was glass. During WWI glass became unavailable, and cellulose nitrate was substituted. Later because of the inflammability of cellulose nitrate, cellulose triacetate was used. In the 1960s polyester base was introduced and has become the base of choice.
5. Silver bromide (Z = 35) and silver iodide (Z = 47).
6. See the formula on p. 167. The arrow pointing down indicates that silver bromide is precipitated out of solution.
7. The concentration of silver halide crystals determines film speed.
8. Proprietary secret.
9. Silver (positive ions), bromide (negative ions), and iodine (negative ions) are in a crystal lattice, with the greatest amount of positive ions in the center of the crystal and the negative ions along the edges. Free electrons from stimulation by x-rays or light migrate and form metallic silver at the crystal's sensitivity speck. The metallic silver will be developed into black grains; unradiated crystals are inactive. The information contained in the light-activated and nonactivated crystals is the latent image.
10. Light photons from the intensifying screen cause photo-electric and Compton interactions to occur with the silver halide crystals in the film emulsion.
11. 20 × 35 cm.
12. Direct-exposure film.
13. Early 1970s.

14. Panchromatic film is sensitive to the whole light spectrum. Orthochromatic film is green and blue-sensitive.
15. Lanthanum oxybromide and barium strontium sulfate.
16. If there is improper matching, the image-receptor speed will decrease and patient dose will increase.
17. The image receptor may not operate optimally at very long or very short exposure times.
18. For use with blue-sensitive film. For use with green-sensitive film.
19. Mammography screen film has an emulsion on one side only.
20. a) Temperature is less than 68° F, b) humidity is between 40% to 60%, c) shelf-life is indicated as an expiration date on the box of film.

CHAPTER 15
1. 1956.
2. Eastman Kodak Company.
3. Answers will vary.
4. See Table 15-1.
5. Water.
6. The latent image is converted into the manifest image.
7. Silver ions reduced to metallic silver.
8. Synergism.
9. Hydroquinone.
10. Alkali compounds of sodium carbonate and sodium hydroxide are caustic to your skin.
11. To prevent oxidation of the developer by the air. When the developing agent has been oxidized, it turns a brownish color.
12. Depletion of the hardener (glutaraldehyde) in the developer solution.
13. Refers to the permanence of the radiograph.
14. To stop development of the emulsion.
15. Hypo retention in the film emulsion.
16. Reduced time was compensated for by increasing developer temperature and increasing the concentration of developer chemicals.
17. The feed tray receives the film, entrance rollers grip the film and begin its trip through the processor, the rollers and racks transport the film through the wet chemistry tanks and through the drying chamber, and finally the film is dropped into the receiving bin.
18. The longer dimension should be fed first with the shorter dimension along the side rail of the feed tray.
19. 95° F.
20. Mammography film has extended processing time to 3 minutes to increase image contrast and to lower patient dose.

CHAPTER 16
1. Less than 1%.
2. Intensifying screens convert the energy of the x-ray beam into visible light.
3. Because double-emission film is placed between the two intensifying screens.
4. The phosphor layer emits light during stimulation by x-rays.
5. Afterglow would continue to expose the emulsion of the film after x-ray interaction, causing fog.
6. Before 1972, phosphors were calcium tungstate, zinc sulfide, and barium lead sulfate. After 1972, phosphors in rare earth screens were gadolinium, lanthanum, and yttrium.

7. Protective coating, phosphor layer, reflective layer, and base.
8. Reflective layer.
9. Sturdy, flexible base; does not discolor with age; chemically inert; and no impurities.
10. Visible light that is emitted in response to outside stimulation is called luminescence.
11. If visible light is emitted only during stimulation, the process is fluorescence. If visible light continues to be emitted after stimulation, the process is called phosphorescence.
12. X-ray absorption, screen conversion efficiency, image noise, and spatial resolution.
13. The intensification factor compares nonscreen exposures with screen-film exposures in relation to patient dose reduction. See the formula on p. 193.
14. Phosphor composition, phosphor thickness, reflective layer, dye, crystal size, and concentration of phosphor crystals.
15. See Figure 16-4.
16. Conversion efficiency.
17. Quantum mottle is the term used to describe the mottled or noisy appearance of an image that has been exposed by a limited number of x-ray photons.
18. Better.
19. Screens and film are selected for compatability. The film emulsion sensitivity has to match the intensifying screen spectral output. For phosphors and emission color, see Table 16-2.
20. Handle film and screens carefully, clean screens only with products recommended by the screen manufacturer, and test film-screen contact to examine for areas of blurring.

CHAPTER 17

1. Remnant radiation that passes through the patient without interacting and remnant radiation that is scattered in the patient by Compton interaction.
2. 52%.
3. Kilovoltage.
4. a) 53%, b) increased contrast at 70 kVp, c) increased Compton interaction, which is scattered in the patient increasing patient dose.
5. Collimators and grids.
6. Scatter radiation.
7. Increased.
8. Mammography.
9. Restricting the x-ray beam reduces patient dose and improves image contrast.
10. It is a lead-lined metal plate attached to the x-ray tube head.
11. To reduce patient dose and improve image quality.
12. X-ray tube, extension cone, and image-receptor alignment.
13. Scatter of the useful beam in the cone tip.
14. Off-focus radiation.
15. On the clear plastic exit surface of the collimator.
16. Positive beam-limiting devices.
17. Usually adjustment of the mirror or lamp is required.
18. Never.

CHAPTER 18

1. More than half.
2. Increased absorption of low-energy x-rays.
3. a) Number of shades of gray and the difference between light and dark areas on the image. b) Increased scatter decreases contrast.
4. The grid to reduce scatter radiation.
5. μ
6. 12.5:1.
7. a) See the formula on p. 217 b) 45 lines/cm.
8. 2:1 or 4:1.
9. Easy to shape and relatively inexpensive.
10. The ratio of the contrast of a radiograph made with the grid to the contrast of a radiograph made without a grid.
11. 2.24.
12. 2.
13. The ratio of transmitted primary radiation to transmitted scatter radiation.
14. Contrast improves with reduction of scatter radiation, and high ratio grids remove more scatter.
15. See Figures 18-7 and 18-11.
16. 6.5 cm around the edges of the radiograph.
17. Crossed.
18. See Figures 18-14 to 18-17.
19. Moving grids remove grid lines.
20. 8:1, 90 kVp, 8:1, 90 kVp.

CHAPTER 19

1. Radiographic quality.
2. Resolution.
3. Objects of similar subject contrast.
4. Fluctuation, optical density.
5. Randomness of x-ray interaction with the intensifying screen phosphors.
6. Low noise, high resolution-slow image receptors/high noise, low resolution-fast image receptors.
7. a) Processing quality control and b) equipment quality control.
8. Sensitometry—step wedge or step-wedge image; densitometry—device for reading OD of step-wedge increments.
9. To ensure that each x-ray is developed with the same processing parameters.
10. Answers will vary.
11. OD = 2; gray.
12. High, lower.
13. 2.5.
14. Factors affecting the degree of development are the composition of the chemical solutions, the degree of agitation of solutions, the development time, and the development temperature.
15. A = 66 R^{-1}; B = 22 R^{-1}.
16. Magnification, distortion, and focal spot blur.
17. Approximately 72 inches; approximately 40 inches.
18. Large SID and small OID.
19. Thickness of the object and the position of the object.
20. Patient thickness, tissue mass density, tissue atomic number, object shape, and kilovoltage.
21. See Table 19-3.

CHAPTER 20

1. Beam quality, penetrability.
2. Quantity.
3. One coulomb.
4. 100%, double.
5. Changes in mA change only the number of electrons flowing across the tube.

6. To minimize patient exposure and to minimize motion blur.

7. 100 mA at 1 second-long exposure time for breathing technique or use of small focal spot; 200 mA at ½ second-short exposure time or small focal spot; 400 mA at ¼ second. Short exposure time minimizes motion blur.

8. 200 mA.

9. Single-phase—$\frac{1}{120}$ second; three-phase and high frequency equipment—1 ms.

10. 486 mAs.

11. Glen Files in 1945.

12. Large focal spots for routine use; small focal spots for fine-detail radiography (extremities) or magnification radiography.

13. 2.5 mm Al.

14. Single-phase, three-phase, and high frequency.

15. Half-wave and full-wave—100% ripple; three-phase, 6 pulse—14% ripple; three-phase, 12 pulse—4% ripple; high-frequency—less than 1%.

16. An increase in kVp increases x-ray beam quantity and quality.

17. An increase in mAs increases x-ray beam quantity and causes no change in x-ray beam quality.

18. High-voltage generation increases x-ray beam quality and quantity.

19. Added filtration decreases x-ray beam quantity and increases x-ray beam quality.

20. Answers will vary.

CHAPTER 21

1. Patient factors, image quality factors, and exposure technique factors.

2. A sthenic patient is average, and technique charts are based on this patient. A hyposthenic patient requires less technique. A hypersthenic patient requires more technique. An asthenic patient requires much less technique.

3. Radiolucent pathology requires less technique. Radiopaque pathology requires more technique.

4. Calipers.

5. See pathology in Table 21-3 under "radiopaque", white.

6. Patient request form or ask patient or referring physician.

7. Optical density, contrast, image detail, and distortion.

8. $OD = \log_{10} \times \dfrac{I_o}{I_t}$

9. Black to clear OD range is from 3 to 0.2

10. Optical density increases directly with mAs.

11. 30%.

12. Decreases.

13. The difference in optical density between adjacent anatomic structures. High contrast—bone and soft tissue; low contrast—kidney and muscle.

14. Penetrability.

15. Long, low; short, high.

16. Use the smallest appropriate focal spot and the longest standard SID, and place the anatomic part as close to the image receptor as possible.

17. Elongation means the part imaged is larger than normal. Foreshortening means the part imaged appears smaller than normal.

18. MAs, kVp, focal-spot size, patient positioning.

19. Variable kVp chart—kVp varies with patient thickness. Fixed-kVp chart—optimum kVp is selected and mAs varies

with part thickness. High kVp chart—for fluoroscopy and chest radiography using fixed high kVp and variation of mAs with patient thickness. Automatic exposure chart—a post-patient phototimer determines the exposure.

20. Fluoroscopy and chest radiography. 80 kVp for Bucky/grid radiography and 60 kVp for screen-film table top radiography.

CHAPTER 22

1. Anatomical structures may be superimposed on conventional radiographs. Tomography "separates" anatomic planes.

2. Tomography blurs anatomic structures lying outside the object plane by using the moving x-ray tube. Only the object lying within the fulcrum plane is properly imaged.

3. CT and MRI.

4. 1 cm. Kidneys, ureters, and bladder.

5. Linear, circular, elliptical, hypocycloidal, and trispiral.

6. Tube and Bucky need to be attached and moved synchronously.

7. Fulcrum—imaginary pivot point around which the tube and image receptor move. Object plane—anatomy in the fulcum that will be clearly imaged. Tomographic angle—angle of movement of the tube and image receptor.

8. The tomographic angle determines the section thickness. The larger the tomographic angle, the thinner the tomographic section.

9. By blurring the anatomy above and below the area of interest and removing the superimposed anatomy.

10. More.

11. Reduced patient dose.

12. Mandible and teeth.

13. Grid lines must be oriented in the same direction as the tube movement.

14. Making two radiographs of the same object and viewing them stereoscopically. Identifying foreign bodies and identifying calcified lesions in thick body sections.

15. Calculation is equal to the interpupillary distance of the viewer.

16. SID × 0.1 = tube shift. Radiographs should be exposed with the central ray shifted to either side of the midline equal to the tube shift calculation.

17. Stereoscopes using lenses are needed to view the two radiographs.

18. For vascular and neuroradiology studies.

19. 24 mm.

20. Increased patient dose.

CHAPTER 23

1. Mammography is designed to enhance the differential absorption of very similar tissues.

2. He developed a successful technique using low kVp, high mAs, and direct exposure film.

3. ACR—American College of Radiology. MQSA—Mammography Quality Standards Act.

4. Diagnostic mammography is performed on patients with symptoms or elevated risk factors. Screening mammography is performed on asymptomatic women.

5. Annually.

6. Fibrous, glandular, and fat.

7. Calcific deposits in ductal and connective tissue.

8. At low x-ray energy (24 to 28 kVp) photoelectric absorption becomes increasingly more frequent than Compton scattering.

9. Reduces motion blur, separates overlying tissue, creates uniform thickness, improves contrast resolution, improves spatial resolution, and reduces radiation dose.
10. Tungsten, molydenum, or rhodium.
11. .6 to .1 mm focal spots are needed to image microcalcifications.
12. Tungsten target with a rhodium filter.
13. 4:1 to 5:1 grid ratio with 30 lines per cm grid frequency.
14. 1½.
15. Blurring from poor film-screen contact.
16. Screen.
17. Closest.
18. Spatial resolution will be better.
19. 60, 70.
20. Three.

CHAPTER 24

1. A series of monitoring and evaluation tests used by personnel to evaluate and maintain high quality standards in mammography.
2. Quality assurance and continuous quality improvement.
3. See Table 24-1.
4. Processor quality control.
5. Radiologist.
6. Radiographer.
7. Base plus fog is the OD recorded from the unexposed area of the sensitometry strip.
8. Contrast.
9. Image receptor speed.
10. Using materials and method suggested by the screen manufacturer. Weekly.
11. Higher luminance levels than conventional viewboxes.
12. Covering of the illumination so no extraneous light from the viewbox enters the radiologist's eyes.
13. Fiber, speck, and mass.
14. Fiber—1.0 with entire length visible; speck group—1.0 with four or more specks visible; mass—1.0 if a density difference is seen with a generally circular border.
15. See Figure 24-12.
16. Fixer.
17. Phantom film is half covered and left on the darkroom counter top for two minutes with the safelights turned on. The fog differences on the phantom film are then recorded.
18. Not exceeding 0.05.
19. Wire mesh device.
20. 25 to 40 pounds of compression.

CHAPTER 25

1. Thomas Edison. Zinc cadmium sulfide.
2. See Figure 25-2.
3. Rods are sensitive to dim light; cones are sensitive to bright light. Visual acuity is greater in bright light. Photopic vision is daylight vision. Scotopic vision is night vision.
4. See Table 21-1.
5. See Figure 25-4.
6. Photoemission is emission of electrons after stimulation by light. Thermionic emission is emission of electrons following heat stimulation.
7. See Figure 25-6.
8. 6345 is the brightness gain.
9. Reduction of brightness at the periphery.
10. Thermionic emission.

11. The 525-line system of the television monitor can only resolve 2 line pairs per mm.
12. Patient, image intensifier.
13. Patient dose.
14. To aid the radiologist in viewing dynamic images of anatomy.
15. Spot film.

CHAPTER 26

1. Arteriography is the imaging of contrast-filled vessels. Cardiac catherization is the inserting of catheters into the coronary arteries for imaging.
2. Using a stylet, guidewire, and catheter, arterial access is made without surgery of the vessel.
3. Femoral.
4. Guidewires allow the safe introduction of the catheter into the vessel.
5. J-tip catheter for obstructed vessel, headhunter (H1) catheter for femoral approach to the brachiocephalic vessels, Simmons catheter for the curved approach to the celiac axis, and the Cobra (C2) for the renal and mesenteric arteries.
6. To establish rapport and to obtain informed consent.
7. Bleeding at the puncture site.
8. Thrombolysis—declotting a vessel; embolization—vascular occlusion to stop bleeding.
9. 1 MHU.
10. Radiographer R.T.(R) (CV)—sets up runs; interventional radiologist—performs the procedure; radiology nurse—monitors patient; and anesthesiologist—administers medication and monitors patient.
11. 1.0 mm to 0.3 mm. Neuroangiography.
12. Table movement is computer-controlled when imaging from the abdomen to the feet with a contrast injection.
13. Cardiac catheterization, angiography.
14. 7.5 to 60 frames per second. 4 images per second.
15. One exposure is obtained before the injection of contrast.

CHAPTER 27

1. Computers have the extensive ability to make decisions.
2. Patient scheduling and tracking; x-ray console, and any imaging modality.
3. Abacus.
4. ASCC—automatic sequence controlled calculator; ENIAC—electronic numerical integrator and calculator, UNIVAC—universal automatic computer.
5. Calculators handle arithmetic functions, computers handle arithmetic and logic functions.
6. Transistors made possible the "stored program" computer.
7. Microcomputer—smallest computer (PC); minicomputer—larger and more flexible for many applications; mainframe computer—for very large applications and uses multiple microprocessors.
8. Hardware—CPU and the input and output devices; software—computer programs that tell the hardware what to do.
9. CPU—supervises all the components of the computer system; control unit—identifies route of entry and directs data to arithmetic or memory unit; arithmetic unit—holds numbers that are involved in numeric and logic calculations; memory unit—obtains and stores programs and data and transfers data between input and output devices; input/ouput devices—allow user to communicate with the

computer; video display terminal—keyboard and CRT; secondary memory storage—floppy disk or CD-ROM; printers—output can be transferred to printed form; and modem—allows data transmission between computers.

10. Bit—single binary digit; byte—bits grouped in bunches of eight; and word—two bytes.
11. System software—operating system; applications program—programs to perform a specific task.
12. See Table 27-4 and pp. 351-353.
13. 307.
14. 40,096,000 bits.
15. Operating system.
16. Allows programmers to write instructions in a form approaching human language rather than the ones and zeros of machine language.
17. "C."
18. System programs.
19. Batch—processing from mainframe computers; on-line systems—transactions are processed immediately (example, ATM); time-sharing systems—using passwords to share a computer network; and real-time systems—special purpose operating systems that provide rapid management of system hardware (example, processing data for imaging modalities).
20. Mainframe computer.

CHAPTER 28
1. CT, MRI, and computed tomography.
2. The computer technology needed to handle large quantities of data generated.
3. The layout of cells in rows and columns. The range of values over which a system can respond is the dynamic range.
4. For digital fluoroscopy, image subtraction techniques; for digital radiography, enhanced radiographic contrast due to reduced scatter from the fan-beam collimation.
5. Atomic number and mass density.
6. Larger.
7. 65,536.
8. 2^5 or 32 shades of gray.
9. Windowing is postprocessing of the image by the operator using the computer. Window level identifies the type of tissue being imaged. Window width determines the gray scale rendition of that tissue.
10. Though DF operates at current measured in hundreds of mA, the tube is not constantly energized. It operates like a rapid film changer, obtaining images at intervals.
11. 1024 gray scales.
12. See Figure 28-14.
13. Interlace mode—two fields of 262½ lines read in 1/60 second; progressive mode—camera tube sweeps the target continuously from top to bottom in 33 milliseconds.
14. Because of the current always flowing in any electric circuit, there is always a background electronic noise.
15. Temporal subtraction refers to a number of computer-assisted techniques whereby an image obtained at one time is subtracted from an image obtained later. Energy subtraction uses two different beam energy levels to provide a subtraction image. With energy subtraction, complex equipment is needed; however, motion artifacts are reduced compared to temporal subtraction.
16. Fan-beam collimation.
17. See Figure 28-24.

18. Subtraction, edge enhancement, windowing, highlighting, panning, scrolling, and zoom.
19. The network is the manner in which computers can be connected to interact with each other. CT imager, radiologists' offices, and archiving workstation.
20. Teleradiology.

CHAPTER 29
1. Godfrey Hounsfield.
2. Axial—perpendicular to the long axis of the body; translation—the sweep of the source-detector assembly across the body; reconstruction—computer processing of a large number of projections.
3. See Table 29-3.
4. X-ray tube, detector array, high-voltage generator, patient couch, and mechanical supports for each component.
5. Instantaneous power capacity must be high. X-ray tube failure.
6. 1 to 8 detectors per centimeter or 1 to 5 detectors per degree.
7. To restrict the volume of tissue irradiated.
8. Prepatient and postpatient collimators. One collimator is placed over the patient, and one is placed under the patient. Improper adjustment results in unnecessary radiation dose.
9. Low-Z material such as carbon fiber. Automatic indexing changes the patient position automatically without the operator entering the examination room.
10. 30,000 equations must be solved simultaneously, so an ultra-high-speed, large-capacity computer is required. Humidity less than 30% relative humidity, temperatures below 20° C.
11. 0.2 mm³.
12. Collimation.
13. In excess of 100 kVp. 1 to 5 seconds.
14. CT number or Hounsfield unit.
15. Blood.
26. See Figure 29-20.
17. Spatial resolution of the system.
18. Higher.
19. 7.7 lp/cm.
20. Contrast resolution—distinguish material of one composition from another without regard to size or shape; system noise—percent of standard deviation of a large number of pixels obtained from a water bath scan; linearity—a test plotting the CT number versus linear attenuation coefficient, which indicates malalignment or malfunction of the CT scanner; spatial uniformity—when the water bath is scanned, the pixel values should be constant in all regions of the reconstructed image.

CHAPTER 30
1. Less expensive.
2. Estimate of a value between two known values. Interpolation algorithm is estimated image data interpolated from other data within the same plane.
3. Reduction of artifacts compared to interpolation at 360 degrees; 180-degree interpolation results in improved z-axis resolution and greatly reformatted saggital and coronal views.
4. $$\frac{\text{Couch movement (in mm/sec) each 360-degree rotation}}{\text{collimation}}.$$
5. 48 cm.

6. $\dfrac{\text{Collimation} \times \text{pitch} \times \text{scan time}}{\text{Gantry rotation time}}$.

7. 3.0:1.

8. In a slip ring gantry system, power and electrical signals are transmitted through stationary rings within the gantry, eliminating the need for electrical cables that make continuous rotation impossible.

9. High heat capacity and high cooling rates.

10. Efficiency is improved.

11. Examination time, couch travel, pitch, and collimation.

12. Lung calcifications and CT angiography.

13. Transverse images are stacked to form a 3-D data set.

14. MIP is the simplest form of 3-D imaging; it provides excellent differentiation of vasculature from surrounding tissue.

15. See Table 30-4.

CHAPTER 31

1. Quality assurance—organization wide program to continually monitor and evaluate the quality of patient care (e.g., outcome analysis of radiologist's diagnosis). Quality control—a program that monitors and evaluates instrumentation and equipment (e.g., processor QC).

2. The Ten Step Monitoring Process is implemented to make sure a health care organization has a commitment to provide high-quality services and care to patients.

3. Acceptance testing, routine performance evaluation, and error correction.

4. Medical physicist, radiologist, and QC radiographer.

5. See Table 31-1.

6. By millimeters of aluminum.

7. With misalignment, anatomy will be missed and unintended anatomy will be irradiated. Plus or minus 2%.

8. Measuring of the light intensity of viewboxes.

9. Plus or minus 4%.

10. The pinhole camera, the star pattern, and the slit camera.

11. Exposure timer accuracy.

12. 6,600.

13. Linearity—ability of a radiographic unit to produce a constant radiation output for multiple combinations of mA and exposure time. Reproducibility—expectation that the radiographic factors chosen by the radiographer will have the same output from exposure to exposure. Variation of linearity is plus or minus 10%; variation of reproducibility is plus or minus 5% radiation output.

14. Wire mesh test.

15. Determined by the manufacturer.

16. Annually.

17. 3 to 5 rad/minute (30 to 50 mGy/minute).

18. Spatial resolution is assessed by imaging an edge to get an edge-response function. Medical physicists often use an image bar pattern or a hole pattern.

19. See Table 31-8.

20. To ensure processed films are of consistently high quality.

CHAPTER 32

1. Artifacts can interfere with radiologists' diagnoses.

2. To indicate trends in poor film quality.

3. See Figures.

4. Foreign optical density on a radiograph that is not caused by superimposition of anatomy by the primary beam.

5. During radiographic exposure, during processing, and when handling film before and after processing.

6. Patient motion blurring, position errors, incorrect radiographic technique.

7. Encourage patient cooperation.

8. Radiographers mix up exposed and unexposed cassettes.

9. Roller marks, chemical fog, and pi lines.

10. A term used to mean all types of chemical stain.

11. When the turn-around assembly of the processor is sprung or improperly positioned.

12. Revolution of one roller.

13. Produced in the developer tank from irregular or dirty rollers.

14. Light leaks in the darkroom, light leaks from warped cassettes, and radiation fog from film being left in the exam room.

15. Kink marks.

16. Buildup of electrons.

17. Crown, tree, and smudge.

18. A yellowish stain.

CHAPTER 33

1. Radiation hormesis.

2. Atomic.

3. Its chemical-binding properties change. Ionization results in breakage of the molecule or relocation of the atom within the molecule.

4. Early effect—radiation response that occurs within minutes or days after radiation exposure. Late effect—radiation response that is not observable for months or years after radiation exposure.

5. See Table 33-2.

6. Robert Hooke.

7. Watson and Crick.

8. Eighty percent of the human body is composed of water.

9. The concept of the relative constancy of the internal environment of the human body.

10. Provide support and structure to the human body.

11. Provide fuel for human cell metabolism.

12. Deoxyribonucleic acid, ribonucleic acid.

13. Nucleus, cytoplasm.

14. DNA.

15. Channel or series of channels that allow the nucleus to communicate with the cytoplasm.

16. 1 Mrad (10 kGy).

17. Prophase, metaphase, anaphase, and telephase or M, G_1, S, G_2.

18. See Figure 33-13.

19. Lymphoid tissue, bone marrow, and gonads.

20. Muscle and nerve cells.

CHAPTER 34

1. Bergonie and Tribondeau. 1) Stem cells are radiosensitive; 2) younger tissue is more radiosensitive; 3) when there is high metabolic activity, radiosensitivity is also high; and 4) as proliferation rate and growth rate for cells and tissue increase, radiosensitivity increases also.

2. The amount of energy deposited per unit mass.

3. The rate at which energy is transferred from ionizing radiation to soft tissue.

4. 3.0 keV/μm.

5. Relative biologic effectiveness—as LET increases, the ability to produce biologic damage from radiation increases also.

6. Protracted doses are delivered continuously over a long time. Fractionated doses are many equal doses given by regular time intervals.

7. To increase the radiosensitivity of tumors that have a poor blood supply.

8. $OER = \dfrac{\text{Dose necessary under anoxic conditions to produce a given effect}}{\text{Dose necessary under aerobic conditions to produce the same effect}}$

   Biologic tissue is more sensitive when irradiated in an oxygenated state.

9. See Figure 34-3.
10. Existing in an artificial environment outside the host organism.
11. Atrophy.
12. Sensitizing agents.
13. Halogenated pyrimidines, methotrexate, actinomycin D.
14. Sulfhydryl group.
15. No. They are toxic to humans.
16. Mathematical relationship between radiation dose and the magnitude of the observed response.
17. The response is directly proportional to the dose.
18. A large response will result from a very small radiation dose.
19. Threshold—below the threshold dose, no response is expected. Nonthreshold—any dose regardless of its size is expected to produce a response.
20. Because diagnostic imaging is exclusively concerned with the late effects of radiation exposure.

CHAPTER 35
1. In vivo—in the living cell, in vitro—outside the living cell.
2. Main-chain scission, cross-linking, and point lesions. See Figure 35-1.
3. Main-chain scission reduces the viscosity of solution.
4. Point lesions.
5. Catabolism—molecular nutrients are broken down into smaller molecular units and energy is released. Anabolism—systesis or construction of macromolecules from smaller molecules.
6. S phase.
7. Terminal deletion, dicentric formation, and ring formation.
8. See Figure 35-2.
9. See Figure 35-7.
10. 80%.
11. $H_2O + \Uparrow \rightarrow HOH^+ + e^-$
12. An uncharged molecule containing a single unpaired electron in the outermost shell. Highly reactive.
13. Direct.
14. Indirect effect.
15. For a cell to die following irradiation, its target molecule must have been inactivated.
16. See Figure 35-10.
17. Colony.
18. See Figure 35-12. Radiation interacts randomly with matter.
19. $S = N/N_o = e^{-D/D_{37}}$
20. $S = N/N_o = 1 - (1 - e^{-D/D_0})^n$

CHAPTER 36
1. The sequence of events following high-level radiation exposure leading to death within days or weeks. Lethality.
2. 300 rad.
3. Greater than 5000 rad.

4. Manifest illness stage, gastrointestinal syndrome.
5. Latent period.
6. Acute clinical symptoms that occur within hours of the exposure and continue for a few days.
7. Hematologic, gastrointestinal, and neuromuscular.
8. Latent period.
9. Generalized infection, electrolyte imbalance, and dehydration.
10. 1000-5000 rad. Three to five days.
11. Electrolyte imbalance and infection.
12. Elevated fluid level in the brain results in increased intracranial pressure, vasculitis of the brain, and meningitis.
13. Dose of radiation to the whole body that will result in death within 30 days to 50% of the subjects irradiated.
14. Non-linear, threshold dose.
15. 300 rad, 600 rad.
16. The newt.
17. See Figure 36-4. Female—oocyte in the mature follicle. Male—spermatogonial stem cells.
18. Hemopoietic cells.
19. The basal cell, the stem cell, is the lowest layer of cells in the epidermis. As they mature, they migrate to the surface of the skin where they are slowly lost and replaced by new cells.
20. Lymphocytes and spermatogonia.

CHAPTER 37
1. Low.
2. Callused, discolored, and weathered appearance of the hands.
3. Several hundred cases of radiation-induced cataracts have been reported. Cyclotron physicists.
4. 12 days. 2,100 days.
5. Median age of death was increased, and deaths per thousand were decreased because there was better attention to radiation protection through proper procedures and equipment design.
6. $\text{Relative risk} = \dfrac{\text{Observed cases}}{\text{Expected cases}}$
7. 15 cases/10^6 persons/rad/year.
8. Excess risk = Observed cases − Expected cases
9. Number of cases/10^6 persons/rad/year.
10. 4.2.
11. 4 to 7 years, 20 years.
12. Radiation therapy in Great Britain is attended by medical physicists, who are, in general, more radiation safety conscious.
13. Patients were given high doses of radiation to the spinal cord, which was found to increase the relative risk of leukemia for this group.
14. For thymus gland enlargement. Thyroid cancer.
15. Luminous compounds that contained radium sulfate were used to paint watch dials. To prepare a fine tip on paint brushes, the employees would touch the tip of the brush with their tongue and ingest radium. Once ingested, radium behaved like calcium and was deposited in bone but emitted alpha particles, whereupon the employees developed bone cancer.
16. Radon is a decay product of uranium, and uranium miners with improper ventilation risk lung cancer.
17. 1.5 mrad.
18. There is no noticeable depression in fertility.

19. An increase of 50% over the nonirradiated rate.
20. To produce the trait, the mutant genes must be present in both male and female. Consequently, such mutations may not be evident for many generations.

CHAPTER 38

1. The Manhattan Project.
2. Exposure = Exposure rate × Time.
3. Reminds the radiologist that a considerable fluoroscopic time has elapsed.
4. 300 mR/hr.
5. Tenth value layer.
6. 4.32 R.
7. Time, distance, and shielding. Minimize time during exposure, maximize distance from the source, and place a shield or barrier between the source and the operator.
8. MPD was the maximum dose expected to produce no significant radiation effects. Dose limit is the modern term.
9. The value is the approximate risk of death.
10. Agriculture.
11. 50 rem. 50 mSv (5 rem).
12. Accounts for the relative radiosensitivity of various tissues and organs.
13. Use of extremity personnel monitors.
14. One tenth.
15. 1 mSv/year.
16. Resorption of the embryo.
17. Skeletal deformities and neurologic deficiencies.
18. Notify supervisor, use wrap around lead apron, provide second monitoring device positioned under the apron at waist level, and review safe radiation practices.
19. See box on p. 504.
20. Estimate fetal dose and determine stage of gestation then consider the 10 to 25 rad rule.

CHAPTER 39

1. 100 mR/hr.
2. The beam is on.
3. SID with 2% error; collimation within 2% error of the indicated SID; PBL accurate to 2% of the SID; beam alignment; filtration of 2.5 mm AL when operated above 70 kVp; reproducibility of output intensity; linearity of output intensity; exposure switch permanently fixed in back of a secondary shield; mobile unit with a 180 cm exposure switch cord; and mobile unit with an apron assigned to it.
4. Unnecessary exposure.
5. 30 μm MO or 60 μm Rh.
6. Reproducibility—for any given radiographic technique, the output intensity should be constant from one exposure to another. Linearity—output of mAs increases in proportion to the increase in mA.
7. Source to skin distance must be not less than 38 cm on stationary fluoroscopes and not less than 30 cm on mobile fluoroscopy units; image-intensifier is a primary protective barrier and must be 2 mm Pb equivalent, total filtration must be 2.5 mm Al; collimation must be sufficient so that an unexposed border is visible on the monitor; unit should have dead-man exposure switch; Bucky slot cover should automatically cover the area with 25 mm Pb equivalent; a protective curtain should be positioned between the source and the operator; after 5 minutes of fluoroscopy time an audible signal temporarily interrupts the beam on; and the x-ray intensity at tabletop level should not exceed 2.1 R/min for each mA of operation at 80 kVp.
8. Half-value layer must be determined.
9. Primary radiation, scatter radiation, and leakage radiation.
10. Patient.
11. 4.8 mm.
12. Barrier thickness, occupancy factor, use factor, and beam penetrability.
13. A controlled area is occupied by diagnostic imaging personnel and patients. An uncontrolled area is occupied by anyone.
14. Milliampere-minutes per week.
15. The percentage of time the x-ray beam is on and directed toward a particular wall.
16. Leakage and scatter radiation are present 100% of the time the tube is energized.
17. Ionization chambers, proportional counters, and Geiger-Muller counters.
18. Small size and reuseable.
19. Nuclear medicine.
20. Thallium-activated sodium iodide and thallium-activated cesium iodide.

CHAPTER 40

1. Radiation dose—rad (gray); radiation exposure in air—roentgen (coulomb per kilogram); and effective dose—rem (sievert).
2. 500 mrem/year (5 mSv/yr). The radiologist is nearer the source of exposure during most fluoroscopic procedures.
3. Fluoroscopy and mobile radiography.
4. Frequency of x-ray examination is increasing and increasing concern among public health officials and radiation scientists regarding the risk associated with medical x-ray exposure.
5. ESE, gonadal dose, and bone marrow dose.
6. 20 mrad. 10 mrad.
7. 4 R/minute.
8. Lower limb girdle (pelvis).
9. Genetically significant dose, the radiation dose to the population gene pool. See Table 40-4.
10. Because of the suspected genetic effects of radiation exposure.
11. Any possible biologic response in mammography is related to the average radiation dose to the glandular tissue, not the skin dose.
12. The dose from CT is roughly equivalent to the cumulative dose produced by a series of radiographic views.
13. 1.8 m long.
14. When it is likely an individual will receive one-quarter of the dose limit.
15. Mid-1940s. See Figure 40-7. Film badges are worn with their proper sides to the front and are worn at waist or chest level.
16. Current exposure, cumulative quarterly exposure, and cumulative annual exposure.

17. 0.25, 0.5, and 1 mm of lead equivalent. 1 mm (see Table 40-5).
18. Radiology personnel should never be used to hold patients during an x-ray examination.
19. TB screening chest x-rays, hospital admission chest x-rays, preemployment physical x-rays, and x-rays during annual physicals on healthy individuals.
20. Gonadal shielding is required on children and reproductive-age patients, gonadal shielding is required when gonads lie in or near the useful beam, proper patient positioning and collimation is never relaxed, and gonadal shielding is only used when it does not interfere with obtaining the proper diagnostic information.

Glossary

Units are shown in parenthesis, e.g., (Joules), (mHz), (m/s).

Absorbed dose Quantity of radiation in rad or gray (Gy).

Absorption Removal of x-rays from a beam.

Activator Chemical, usually acetic acid in the fixer and sodium carbonate in the developer, to neutralize the developer and to swell the gelatin.

Afterglow Phosphorescence.

Algorithm Computer-compatible equation.

Alpha particle Ionizing radiation having two protons and two neutrons emitted from nucleus of a radioisotope.

Alternating current Oscillation of electricity in both directions of a conductor.

American Association of Physicists in Medicine (AAPM) Scientific society of medical physicists.

American College of Medical Physicists (ACMP) Professional society of medical physicists.

American College of Radiology (ACR) Professional society of radiologists and medical physicists.

American Society of Radiologic Technologists (ASRT) Scientific and professional society of radiographers.

Anode Positive side of the x-ray tube, contains the target.

Anthropomorphic Human characteristics.

Area beam X-ray beam pattern usually shaped as a square or rectangle used in conventional radiography and fluoroscopy.

Artifact Unintended optical density on a radiograph or other film-type image receptor.

Atomic mass number (A) Number of protons and the number of neutrons in the nucleus.

Atomic number (Z) Number of protons in the nucleus.

Attenuation Reduction in radiation intensity as a result of absorption and scattering.

Autotransformer Transformer located in the operating console that controls kVp.

Average gradient Measure of radiographic contrast.

Axial Perpendicular to the long axis of the body.

Beta particle Ionizing radiation with characteristics of an electron; emitted from nucleus of a radioisotope.

Bremsstrahlung x-rays X-rays resulting from interaction of the projectile electron with a target nucleus; braking radiation.

Bucky factor Ratio of incident to transmitted radiation through a grid; ratio of patient dose with and without a grid.

Cathode Negative side of the x-ray tube; contains the filament and focusing cup.

Characteristic curve Graph of optical density versus log relative response; H & D curve.

Characteristic x-rays X-rays produced following ionization of inner-shell electrons; characteristic of the target element.

Classical scattering Scattering of x-rays with no loss of energy.

Clearing agent Chemical, usually ammonium thiosulfate, added to the fixer to remove undeveloped silver bromine from the emulsion.

Collimation Restriction of the useful x-ray beam to reduce patient dose and improve image contrast.

Collimotor Device to restrict x-ray beam size.

Commutator Device that converts an AC generator to a DC generator.

Compensating filter X-ray beam filter designed to make the remnant beam more uniform in intensity.

Compton effect Scattering of x-rays resulting in ionization and loss of energy.

Conduction Transfer of heat by molecular agitation.

Conductor Material that allows heat or electric current to flow.

Contrast Range of shades of gray on an image.

Contrast improvement factor Ratio of radiographic contrast with a grid to that without a grid.

Convection Transfer of heat by the movement of hot matter to a colder place.

Conversion efficiency Rate at which x-ray energy is transformed into light in an intensifying screen.

Coolidge tube This type of vacuum tube in use today allows x-ray intensity and energy to be separately and accurately selected.

Crookes tube Forerunner of modern fluorescent, neon, and x-ray tubes.

Crossover rack Device in an automatic processor that transports film from one tank to the next.

CRT Cathode ray tube; a television picture tube.

Densitometer Device that measures optical density.

Developing agent Chemical, usually phenidone, hydroquinone, or Metol, that reduces exposed silver ions to atomic silver.

Diaphragm Device to restrict x-ray beam size.

Differential absorption Different degrees of absorption in different tissues that results in image contrast and formation of the x-ray image.

Diode Vacuum tube with two electrodes.

Direct current Flow of electricity in only one direction in a conductor.

Distortion Unequal magnification.

Dose equivalent Quantity of radiation absorbed by radiographers (rem or Sv).

Dynamic range Range of values that can be displayed by an imaging system; shades of gray.

Effective atomic number Weighted average atomic number of tissue.

Electrification Process of adding or removing electrons from a substance.

Electrode Electrical terminal or connector.

Electromagnet Solenoid with an iron core resulting in an intensified magnetic field.

Electromagnetic radiation X-rays, gamma rays, and some nonionizing radiation.

Electromagnetic spectrum Continuum of electromagnetic energy.

Electromotive force Electric potential; measured in volts (V).

Electrostatics Study of fixed or stationary electric charge.

Element Consists of atoms having the same structure and reacting the same chemically.

Energy Ability to do work; measured in joules (J).

Exponent Superscript or power to which ten is raised in scientific notation.

Exposure Quantity of radiation intensity; (R or C/kg).

Extinction time Time required to turn off the x-ray tube.

Fan beam X-ray beam pattern used in CT and DR; projected as a slit.

Filament That part of the cathode that emits electrons resulting in a tube current.

Film graininess Distribution of silver halide grains in an emulsion.

Filtration Removal of low-energy x-rays from the useful beam with aluminum or other metal.

Fluorescence Emissions of visible light only during stimulation.

Fluoroscope Device used to image moving anatomic structures with x-rays.

Focal spot Region of anode target where electrons interact to produce x-rays.

Focused grid Radiographic grid constructed so that the grid strips converge on an imaginary line.

Focusing cup Metal shroud surrounding the filament.

Fog Unintended optical density on a radiograph that reduces contrast because of light or chemical contamination.

Force That which changes the motion of an object; a push or a pull.

Grid Device to reduce the intensity of scatter radiation in the remnant x-ray beam.

Grid cutoff Absence of optical density on a radiograph because of unintended x-ray absorption in a grid.

Grid frequency Number of grid lines per inch or cm.

Grid ratio Ratio of grid height to grid strip separation.

Guide shoe Device in an automatic processor for steering film around bends.

Half-value layer (HVL) Thickness of absorber necessary to reduce an x-ray beam to half its original intensity.

Hardener Chemical, usually potassium glutaraldehyde alum in the fixer, to stiffen and shrink the emulsion.

Heel effect Absorption of x-rays in the heel of the target, resulting in reduced x-ray intensity to the anode side of the central axis.

Hertz Unit of frequency; cycles or oscillations each second of a simple oscillating motion.

High-contrast resolution Ability to image small objects having high subject contrast; spatial resolution.

Houndsfield unit (HU) Scale of CT numbers used to judge the nature of tissue.

Image intensifier Electronic device that amplifies a fluoroscopic image to reduce patient dose.

Inertia Property of matter that resists its change in motion.

Insulator Material that inhibits the flow of electricity.

Intensification factor Ratio of exposure without screens to that with screens to produce the same optical density.

Intensifying screen Sensitive phosphor that converts x-rays to light to shorten exposure time and reduce patient dose.

Interrogation time Time during which the signal from an image detector is sampled.

Ion Electrically charged particle.

Ionization Removal of an electron from an atom.

Ionizing radiation Radiation capable of ionization.

Isobar Atoms having the same number of nucleons but different numbers of protons and neutrons.

Isomer Atoms having the same number of protons and neutrons but a different nuclear energy state.

Isotone Atoms having the same number of neutrons.

Isotope Atoms having the same number of protons.

Isotropic Equal intensity in all directions.

Kinetic energy Energy of motion.

Lag Phosphorescence.

Latent image An unobservable image stored in the silver halide emulsion; made manifest by processing.

Lateral decentering Improper positioning of grid resulting in cutoff.

Latitude Range of x-ray exposure over which a radiograph is acceptable.

Leakage radiation Secondary radiation emitted through the tube housing.

Line focus Projection of an inclined line into a surface resulting in a smaller size.

Low-contrast resolution Ability to image objects with similar subject contrast.

Luminescence Emission of visible light.

Mammography Radiographic examination of the breast using low kVp.

Mass Quantity of matter (kg).

Matrix Array of numbers in rows and columns.

Matter Anything that occupies space and has form or shape.

Misregistration Misalignment of two or more images because of patient motion between image acquisition.

Modulation transfer function (MTF) Mathematical procedure for measuring resolution.

Molecule Structure formed of atoms of various elements.

Molybdenum X-ray tube target material for use in mammography.

Monoenergetic One energy; single energy photon.

Mutual induction Producing electricity in a secondary coil or wire by passing an AC current through a nearby primary coil.

Node One of many stations or terminals of a computer network.

Nucleon Proton or neutron.

Off-focus radiation X-rays produced in the anode but not at the focal spot.

OID Object-to-image receptor distance.

Optical density Degree of blackening of a radiograph.

Orthochromatic Blue- or green-sensitive film; usually exposed with rare earth screen.

Penetrability Ability of an x-ray to penetrate tissue; range in tissue; x-ray quality.

Penetrometer Aluminum step wedge.

Penumbra Image blur as a result of the size of the focal spot; geometric unsharpness.

Phosphorescence Emission of visible light during and after stimulation.

Photoconductor Material that conducts electrons when illuminated.

Photodiode Solid-state device that converts light into an electric current.

Photoelectric effect Absorption of an x-ray by ionization.

Photomultiplier tube Electron tube that converts visible light into an electrical signal.

Photon Smallest quantity of electromagnetic radiation; an x-ray, gamma ray, or light.

Photostimulation Emission of visible light following excitation by laser light.

Phototimer Automatic exposure control device.

Pixel Picture element; cell of a digital image matrix.

Polyenergetic Many energies; a spectrum of energies.

Power Time rate at which work is done (W).

Preservative Chemical additive, usually sodium sulfide, that maintains chemical balance of the developer and the fixer.

Processing Chemical treatment of the emulsion of a radiographic film to change latent image to manifest image.

Protective housing Lead-lined metal container into which the x-ray tube is fitted.

Quantum detection efficiency (QDE) Rate at which x-rays interact with a phosphor.

Quantum mottle Radiographic noise produced by the random interaction of x-rays with an intensifying screen.

Quantum theory Physics of matter smaller than an atom and of electromagnetic radiation.

Radiation Energy emitted and transferred through matter.

Radiation quality Relative penetrability of an x-ray beam determined by its average energy; usually measured by HVL or kVp.

Radiation quantity Intensity of radiation; usually measured in mR.

Radiation (thermal) Transfer of heat by emission of infrared electromagnetic radiation.

Radioactive half-life Time for a radioisotope to decay to one half its activity.

Radioactivity Quantity of radioactive material; curies (Ci) or becquerel (Bq).

Radiofrequency (RF) Electromagnetic radiation having frequencies from 0.3 kHz to 300 GHz; MRI employs RF in the range of approximately 1 to 100 mHz.

Radiological Society of North America (RSNA) Scientific society of radiologists and medical physicists.

Radiolucent Tissue or material that transmits x-rays and appears dark on a radiograph.

Radiopaque Tissue or material that absorbs x-rays and appears bright on a radiograph.

Radon Colorless, odorless naturally occurring radioactive gas.

Reconstruction time Time after completion of examination for the computer to present a digital image.

Rectification Conversion of AC to DC.

Relay Electrical devices based on electromagnetic induction that serves as a switch.

Replenishment Replacement of developer and of fixer in the automatic processing of film.

Resolution Ability to image objects with fidelity.

Rotor Rotating part of electromagnetic induction motor located inside the glass envelope.

Scalar Quantity or measurement that has only magnitude.

Scanned projection radiography Generalized method of making a DR; used in CT for precision localization.

Screen lag Phosphorescence.

Selectivity Ratio of primary radiation to scattered radiation transmitted through grid.

Self-induction Magnetic field produced in a coil of wire that opposes the AC current being conducted.

Semiconductor Material that can serve both as a conductor and as an insulator of electricity.

Sensitivity Ability of an image receptor to respond to x-rays.

Sensitometry Study of the response of an image receptor to x-rays.

SID X-ray source-to-object.

Sinusoidal Simple motion; a sine wave.

SOD Source-to-object distance.

Solenoid Helical winding of current-carrying wire that produces a magnetic field along the axis of the helix.

Space charge Electron cloud near the filament.

Spatial frequency Measure of resolution (lp/mm or lp/cm).

Spatial resolution High-contrast resolution.

Spectrum Graphic representation of the range over which a quantity extends.

Speed Term used to loosely describe the sensitivity of film to x-rays.

Spinning top Device to check exposure timers.

Spot film Static image in small-format image receptor taken during fluorscopy.

SSD Source-to-skin distance.

Stator Stationary coil windings located in the protective housing but outside the x-ray tube glass envelope; part of the electromagnetic induction motor.

Structure mottle Distribution of phosphor crystals in an intensifying screen.

Subtraction A method of removing overlying anatomy to better view small anatomy such as vessels in angiography.

Target Region of the anode struck by electrons emitted by the filament.

Tenth value layer (TVL) Thickness of absorber necessary to reduce an x-ray beam to one tenth its original intensity; 3.3 HVLs.

Tesla (T) SI unit of magnetic field strength; a frequently used unit is gauss (G), 1 T = 10,000 G.

Thermal energy Energy of molecular motion; heat; infrared radiation.

Thermionic emission Emission of electrons from a heated surface.

Transaxial Across the body; transverse.

Transcription The process of constructing mRNA.

Transfer An addition of an amino acid during translation.

Transformer Electrical device operating on the principle of mutual induction to change the magnitude of current and voltage.

Transformer Electrical device to alter the magnitude of kVP or mA.

Translation The process of forming a protein molecule from mRNA.

Transverse Across the body; axial.

Tungsten Metal element that is the principal component of the cathode and the anode.

Turnaround assembly Device in an automatic processor for reversing the direction of film.

Turns ratio Quotient of the number of turns in the secondary coil to the number of turns in the primary coil.

Useful beam Primary radiation used to form the image.

Valence electrons Electrons in the outermost shell.

VDT Video display terminal.

Vector Quantity or measurement that has magnitude, unit, and direction.

Voxel Three-dimensional pixel.

Wavelength Distance between similar points on a sine wave; length of one cycle.

Weight Force caused by the acceleration of gravity on a mass.

Window Thin section of glass envelope through which the useful beam emerges.

Work Product of the force on an object and the distance over which the force acts (J).

Index

A

Abacus, 342
Abdomen
   computed tomography of, 378
   fixed kilovoltage technique chart for, 273
Absolute age-response relationship, 488
Absolute risk, 482, 488
Absorbed dose, 6
Absorption, 159-160
   differential, 155-159
   grid interspace material and, 217
   intensifying screen and, 193, 194
   rare-earth screen and, 198-199
   wave model of electromagnetic radiation, 51
Absorption blur, 246
Acceleration, 21-22
Acceleration of gravity, 23
Acceptance testing, 408
Accident rates, 499
Acetic acid, 182
Action/reaction, 22, 23
Activator atom, 518
Activator in fixing agent, 182
Active trace, 329
Acute radiation lethality, 464-467
Acute radiation syndrome, 464
Added filtration, 135, 145
Addition of fractions, 15
Adenine, 433
Adhesive layer of x-ray film, 166
Adipose tissue in breast, 295
Aerial oxidation, 181
Aerobic, term, 443
Afterglow, 190, 192
Age, radiosensitivity and, 443-444
Age-response function, 458
Air
   computed tomography numbers, 387
   as contrast medium, 160-161
   effective atomic number, 154
   mass density, 158
Air filtration, 227
Air-gap technique, 226-227
ALARA acronym, 8, 502
Algebra, 16-17
Alignment
   of camera lens in fluoroscopy, 328
   of image receptor, 269-270
Alignment coil, 327
Alkali compound, 181

Alkali metals, 30
Alnico, 71
Alopecia, 6
Alpha emission, 37-39
Alpha particle, 38, 40-41
Alternating current, 65-66
   generator, 81
   rectification, 84
   transformer and, 83
Aluminum
   atomic number and K-shell electron binding energy, 153
   characteristics of, 33
   as conductor, 61
   filtration and, 255
   as grid interspace material, 217
Aluminum chloride, 182
Amber filter, 171
Ambient, 445
American Registry of Radiologic Technologists, 11
Amino acids, 432
Ammeter, 64, 78
Ampere, 63
Amplifier tube, 11
Amplitude, 44-45, 100
Anabolism, 432, 450
Analog computer, 343, 344
Analog-to-digital converter, 365-366
Anaphase, 436-437
Anatomically programmed radiography, 275
Anemia, 6
Angiography, 227, 333
Angiointerventional radiology, 333-340
   angiointerventional suite, 335-339
   basic principles, 334-335
   occupational exposure, 524-525
   types of procedures, 334
Angiointerventional suite, 335-339
Angioplasty, 334
Ankylosing spondylitis, 484-485
Ann Arbor series, 485
Annulus, 381
Anode, 84, 113-118
   cooling chart, 122-123
   electron-target interaction, 127-131
   glass envelope, 108
Anorexia, radiation sickness and, 465
Antibody, 432
Antigen, 432
Antihalation coating, 172
AOT film changer, 338, 339

Aperture diaphragm, 209-210
Aplastic anemia, 7
Application programs, 349-350
APR; *see* Anatomically programmed radiography
Apron, 535-536
Archival quality, 182, 314, 316
Archiving in digital imaging, 372-374
Area x-ray beam, 358, 371
Arithmetic unit of computer, 345
Array processor, 354, 385
ARRT; *see* American Registry of Radiologic Technologists
Arterial access, 334
Arteriography, 334, 335
Artifact, 419-424
    exposure, 420, 421
    generation of, 390
    handling and storage, 422-423
    improper handling and, 174
    misregistration, 368
    processing, 420-422
    ring, 381
Artificial intelligence, 342
Assembler computer program, 349
Asthenic patient, 259
Asymmetric screen, 200, 201
Ataxia, radiation sickness and, 466
Atherosclerosis, 334
Atom, 4, 28-42
    activator, 518
    in body composition, 431
    coherent scattering, 150
    combination of atoms, 31-32
    Compton effect, 150-151
    effective atomic number, 154
    fundamental particles, 32, 33
    historical background, 29-31
    nomenclature, 32-34
    radioactivity, 37-39
    structure, 34-37
    types of ionizing radiation, 39-42
Atom bomb survivors, 483-484
Atom smasher, 32
Atomic clock, 21
Atomic mass, 29-30
Atomic mass number, 32, 33
Atomic mass unit, 32
Atomic number, 30, 33
    differential absorption and, 159
    effect on x-ray emission spectrum, 135
    K-shell electron binding energy and, 153
    of phosphor layer of intensifying screen, 190, 199
    subject contrast and, 246
Atrophy, 444, 467
Attenuation, 51-52, 159-160
Attraction and repulsion, 72
Authentic logic unit, 345
Automatic exposure
    chart, 270
    controls, 98, 300
    systems, 413
    techniques, 272-275
Automatic processing, 178, 179, 183-186
Automatic sequence controlled calculator, 343
Autosome, 473
Autotransformer, 83-84, 94
Average gradient, 235
Average velocity, 21

Axial tomography, 378
Axis, 16-17, 77
    aperture diaphragm and, 210

B

Background electronic noise, 365
Backscatter radiation, 151, 152, 196
Backup timer, 411
Bandpass, 330
Bandwidth, 330
Bar magnet, 78
Barium
    atomic number and K-shell electron binding energy, 153
    characteristics of, 33
    as contrast medium, 160
    effective atomic number, 154
    in fluoroscopic contrast studies, 37
    high-kilovoltage technique chart for, 272
    mass density, 158
    in phosphor layer of intensifying screen, 190
Barium platinocyanide, 6, 9, 190
Basal cell, 467
Base
    of intensifying screen, 191
    of x-ray film, 166
Base density, 233
Base plus fog, 231, 307-310
Base quantities, 20
Baseline mammographic examination, 293
BASIC, 349, 351-352
Batch processing, 342, 353
Battery, 64, 76
Baud, 349
Beam alignment, 510, 520
Beam penetrability, 252
Beam-restricting devices, 208-213
    aperture diaphragm, 209-210
    collimator filtration, 213
    scatter radiation and, 215-216
    variable-aperture collimator, 211-213
Beam-splitting mirror, 328
Becquerel, 13, 14
BEIR Committee, 487-489
Berenstein catheter, 335
Beryllium
    characteristics of, 33
    in mammography x-ray tube, 298
Beta emission, 37-39
Beta particle, 41
Binary number system, 350-351
Binding energy, 129
    atomic number and, 153
    intensifying screen phosphors and, 199
Biologic effectiveness factor, 14
Biology, human; *see* Human biology
Biopsy, 334
Biplane imaging, 338
Bipolar, term, 69
Bit, 345, 349
Bladder weighting factor, 501
Blanked electron beam, 329
Bleeding, 335
Blood
    computed tomography numbers, 387
    radiation effects, 470-471
Blue-dot CRT phosphor, 172
Blue-sensitive film, 169, 171

Body composition, 259, 260, 430-439
   cell, 434-437
   cell theory, 430-431
   molecular, 432-434
   tissues and organs, 437-439
Body habitus, 259
Bohr atom, 30, 31
Bone
   computed tomography numbers, 387
   differential absorption, 157
   effective atomic number, 154
   mass density, 158
   radiation-induced cancer, 486
   scatter radiation and, 207
   weighting factor, 501
Bone marrow
   mean lethal dose, 458
   radiation effects, 470-471
   weighting factor, 501
Bone marrow dose, 526
Bootstrap, 350
Borosilicate in mammography x-ray tube, 298
Bow-tie filter, 145
Brachiocephalic vessels, 334, 335
Breakup, 398
Breast
   cancer, 293-294
     radiation-induced, 486-487
   self-examination, 293
   shield, 538
   weighting factor, 501
Bremsstrahlung radiation, 130, 297-298
Bremsstrahlung x-ray spectrum, 132, 133
Brightness gain, 325
British system of measurement, 21
British thermal unit, 122
BTU; *see* British thermal unit
Bubblejet printer, 348
Bucky diaphragm, 222
Bucky factor, 218, 219
Bucky grid, 216, 222
Bucky slot cover, 92, 512, 521
Bucky tray, 92
Buffering agent
   in developer, 180, 181
   in fixing agent, 182
Bus, 344
Byte, 349

C

Calcium
   atomic number and K-shell electron binding energy, 153
   characteristics of, 33
   mass density, 158
Calcium tungstate, 9
   in phosphor layer of intensifying screen, 190
   screen-film combinations and, 196-198
Calculator, 343
Calibrated, term, 98
Caliper, 259
Calorie, 24-25
Camera
   in angiointerventional radiology, 337-338
   in fluoroscopy, 327-328
   laser, 348
   photo-spot, 331
Cancer, radiation-induced, 485-487

Candela, 325
Capacitor, 64, 98
Capacitor discharge generator, 103-104
Carbohydrates, 433
Carbon
   atomic number and K-shell electron binding energy, 153
   characteristics of, 33
   ionization of, 37
Carbon fiber in cassette, 196
C++, 349, 352-353
C-arm unit, 108, 109
C2 catheter, 334, 335
Cardiac catheterization, 172-173, 334
Cassette, 166, 196
   exposure artifact and, 420
   intensifying screen in, 190
   tomography, 283
Cassette-loaded spot film, 330-331, 412
Catabolism, 432, 450
Cataract, radiation exposure-induced, 478-480
Catheter in angiointerventional radiology, 334-335
Cathode, 84, 110-113
   electron-target interaction, 127-131
   glass envelope, 108
Cathode ray, 6-7, 30
Cathode ray tube, 172, 329, 346
CD-ROM, 348
Ceiling support, 108, 109
Celiac axis, 334, 335
Cell, 434-437
   mean lethal dose, 458
   recovery from radiation damage, 444
   target theory, 453-454
Cell cycle, 458, 459
   radiation effects, 473-474
Cell cycle time, 458
Cell division, 436
Cell of battery, 76
Cell proliferation, 436
Cell survival kinetics, 454-460
Cellular radiobiology, 449-462
   cell survival kinetics, 454-460
   direct and indirect effect, 453
   irradiation of macromolecules, 450-452
   radiolysis of water, 452-453
   target theory, 453-454
Cellulose nitrite, 166
Cellulose triacetate, 166
Celsius scale, 24-25
Central axis
   linear grid cutoff and, 220
   off-level error, 223-224
Central electrode, 516
Central nervous system syndrome, 466
Central processing unit, 344-345
Central ray, 117-118, 120, 212
Centrifugal force, 36
Centripetal force, 36
Cerebral angiography, 227
Cerebrospinal fluid, 387
Cesium
   as input phosphor, 324
   measurement of time, 21
CGS system of measurement, 21
Character generator, 347
Characteristic curve, 231-232
   contrast and, 234-237

Characteristic curve, cont'd
  speed and, 237-238
Characteristic radiation, 128-130
  photoelectric effect and, 153
Characteristic x-ray emission spectrum, 132
Charge-coupled device
  in digital fluoroscopy, 365-369
  in mammography, 301
Chelates, 181
Chemical agents enhancing radiosensitivity, 444
Chemical compound, 31
Chemical element, 34
Chemical energy, 4
Chemical fog, 182, 420, 422
Chemical symbol, 32-34
Childhood malignancy, 503
Chip, 344
Choke coil, 80
Chromatid, 437
Chromatid deletion, 473
Chromium alum, 182
Chromosome
  damage from radiation, 451-452, 471-475, 478
  mitosis and, 436-437
Cine camera, 337-338
Cine film, 172-173, 174
Cinefluorography, 172-173
Circuit
  filament, 97
  inverter, 103
  x-ray, 105
Circular tomographic movement, 285
Circulation system in automatic processing, 185
Classical scattering, 150
Cleanup properties of grid, 216
Clinical tolerance, 468
Cloning, 455
Closed-circulation system in automatic processing, 185
Closed-core transformer, 83
Coast time, 115
COBOL, 352
Cobra catheter, 334, 335
Code of ethics, 8
Codon, 435
Coefficient of correlation, 414-415
Coherent scattering, 150
Collector, 519
Collimation, 9
  automatic-exposure techniques, 274
  in computed tomography, 384, 385, 531
  fan beam, 369
  quality control, 409-410
  radiation protection designs, 510, 511, 520, 521
  reduced patient dose and, 538
  scale of contrast and, 268
Collimator, 145
  filtration, 213
  positive beam-limiting, 410
  scatter radiation and, 205, 206
Colon weighting factor, 501
Colony, 455
Committee on Biologic Effects of Ionizing Radiation, 487-489
Common denominator, 15
Communication system in digital imaging, 372-374
Commutator ring, 81
Compact disk with read only memory, 348
Compensating filter, 145, 146

Compiler computer program, 349
Compression check, 317, 318
Compression device
  in cassette, 196
  to improve spatial resolution, 208
Compression, mammographic, 208, 295, 296
Compton electron, 151, 168-169
Compton scattering, 150-151, 152
  image contrast and, 215
  remnant radiation and, 205
  soft tissue and, 295
Computed fluoroscopy, 358
Computed radiography, 358, 359, 371-372
Computed tomography, 11, 377-394
  collimation, 384, 385
  computer, 385-386
  filter, 145
  gantry, 383-384, 385
  high-voltage generator, 384-385
  historical perspective, 378
  image matrix, 386-387
  image quality, 388-392
  image reconstruction, 387-388
  laser film, 172
  occupational exposure, 525
  operational modes, 379-382
  patient dose, 530-532
  patient positioning and support couch, 385
  principles of operation, 378-379
  quality control, 413-417
  spiral, 395-406
    advantages and limitations, 404, 405
    image characteristics, 402-404
    patient dose, 531
    scan principles, 396-399
    scanner design, 399-401
    technique selection, 401-402
Computed tomography numbers, 387, 393
Computer, 341-355
  binary number system, 350-351
  in computed tomography, 385-386
  in digital fluoroscopy, 365-366
  hardware, 344-347
  hexadecimal number system, 351-353
  historical background, 342-344
  processing methods, 353-354
  secondary memory devices, 347-349
  software, 349-350
Computer languages, 350-351
Computer program, 349
Concrete
  effective atomic number, 154
  half-value layer and tenth-value layer, 498
  mass density, 158
  as primary protective barrier, 512-513
Condenser, 64
Conduction of heat, 25, 120
Conductor, 61-62
Cone cutting, 210
Cones, 210-211, 212, 323-324
Conic filter, 145
Connective tissue, 438
Conservation of energy, 24
Conservation of momentum, 23
Constant of proportionality, 54
Contact shield, 538
Contiguous slice, 386

Continuous ejection spectrum, 131
Continuous quality improvement, 306
Contrast, 167, 170
    characteristic curve and, 234-237
    densitometry and, 231
    high subject, 259
    radiographic technique and, 265-268
    scatter radiation and, 215-216
    in tomography, 286
Contrast agents, 71, 160-161
    in angiointerventional radiology, 335
    effective atomic number, 154
    mass density, 158
Contrast improvement factor, 218
Contrast index, 307
Contrast perception, 323
Contrast resolution, 230, 326, 360
    in computed tomography, 390-391
    quality control, 415
Control-booth barrier, 532
Control console in computed tomography, 385-386
Control film, 307
Control grid in fluoroscopy, 329
Control monitor, 535
Control panel, 510
Control unit of computer, 345
Controlled area, 514
Convection of heat, 25, 120
Conversion efficiency, 193, 198, 199-200
Conversion factor, 325
Coolidge tube, 7, 10, 110
Coordinates, 17
Copper
    anode, 113
    characteristics of, 33
    as conductor, 61
Cornea, 323
Coronal view, 397
Cosmic ray, 5
Couch in angiointerventional radiology, 337
Couch incrementation, 415
Coulomb/kilogram, 13-14
Coulomb's law, 60, 72
Covalent bonding, 32
CPU; see Central processing unit
CQI; see Continuous quality improvement
Cracks, 115, 116
Crookes' tube, 6-7
Cross-linking, 450
Crossed grid, 220-222
Crossing over, 437
Crossover, 170, 171, 300
Crossover rack, 185
CRT imaging, 172
Cryogen, 25
Cubic relationships, 154-155
Cubic-spline interpolation, 397
Cumulative timer, 512, 521
Curie, 14
Current
    filament, 111-112
    milliampere second and, 253-254
    transformer law for, 83
Curtain effect, 420, 422
Cut-film changer, 338
Cyclotron, 478-479
Cylinder in spiral computed tomography, 400

Cytogenetics, 451, 471-475
Cytoplasm, 433, 434
Cytosine, 433

D
Daily processor control chart, 309
Dalton atom, 29-30
Darkroom, 171, 307
Darkroom fog, 316
Daylight processing, 186-187
Death, acute radiation lethality, 464-467
Decimal, 16
Decimal system, 14-15
Deflection coil, 327
Denominator, 15
Densitometer, 231-232
Densitometry, 231-234
Density, 158-159, 260
Density difference, 307-310
Dental radiography
    aperture diaphragm in, 210
    panoramic tomography, 286, 287
Deoxyribonucleic acid, 433, 434, 435
    ionization of, 6
    radiation effects, 451-452
    synthesis of, 436-437, 450-451
Derived quantities, 20
Dermis, 467
Desktop publishing, 348
Desquamation, 468
Destructive pathology, 260
Detail, 230, 269
Detective quantum efficiency, 194
Detector assembly in computed tomography, 383-384, 385, 401
Developing agent, 180
Development of film, 180-182
Development fog, 181
Development temperature, 236-237
Development time, 236
Diagnoses, 230
Diagnostic mammography, 293
Diagnostic x-ray, 53
Diarrhea, radiation sickness and, 465
Dicentrics, 473
Dichroic stain, 420, 422
Differential absorption, 155-159
Diffraction x-ray, 53
Digital computer, 343, 344
Digital fluoroscopy, 361-369
    charge-coupled device, 365-369
    high voltage generator, 362-365
    video system, 365
Digital imaging, 357-376
    dynamic range, 360-361, 362, 363
    fluoroscopy, 361-369
    historical development, 358-359
    image matrix, 359-360
    picture archiving and communication system, 372-374
    radiography, 369-372
Digital radiography, 369-372
Digital subtraction angiography, 358
Digital vascular imaging, 358
Digital videoangiography, 358
Digitizer, 372
Dilation of iris, 323
Dimagnetic, term, 71
Dimensional stability, 166

Diode, 64, 108, 519
Dipolar, term, 69
Dipole, 71, 72
Direct current, 65-66
   generator, 81
Direct current motor, 82
Direct effect, 453, 454
Direct-exposure film, 168-169, 171-172, 294
   intensifying screen and, 196-198
Direct memory access, 345
Direct square law, 254
Directly proportional fraction, 16
Dirty roller, 420
Disaccharides, 433
Disk
   in angiointerventional radiology, 336
   for computed tomography image storage, 386
   in spiral computed tomography, 400
Display system in digital imaging, 372-373
Dissection, J-tip guidewire and, 334
Distance, 8, 254
   radiation protection and, 497
Distance maintenance law, 254
Distortion, 240-242, 243
   radiographic technique and, 269-270
Division of fractions, 15
DL; *see* Dose limit
DMA; *see* Direct memory access
DNA; *see* Deoxyribonucleic acid
Dose, 20, 524, 526-532
   cell survival kinetics, 454-460
   estimation of, 526-529
   grid and, 225-226
   image receptor and, 538
   pregnancy and, 502-503
   quality control, 416
   radiographic technique, 537-538
   repeat examinations, 537, 538
   in special examinations, 529-532
   specific area shielding, 538-539
   unnecessary examinations, 537
Dose calibrator, 518
Dose equivalent, 20
Dose limits, 498-501
Dose profile, 416
Dose-response relationships, 444-446
Dosimeter, 515
Dosimetry, 515
Dot matrix printer, 348
Double-capacity processor, 416
Double-contrast examination, 161
Double-emulsion film, 166, 190
Double-helix configuration, 433, 435
Drive subsystem in automatic processing, 185
Dry cell, 76
Dryer system in automatic processing, 186
Drying in film processing, 182-183
Dual-focus tube, 112
Duplicating film, 172
Duplitized x-ray film, 166
Dynamic RAM, 346
Dynamic range, 360-361, 362, 363, 365
Dyskinetic motion, 368

E

EBCT; *see* Electron beam computed tomography
Eddy current, 83

Edge enhancement in digital imaging, 373
Edge response function, 388, 415
Effective dose, 524
Effective dose limit, 500
Effective focal spot, 116-117, 243
Effectiveness ratio, 444
Elective booking, 506
Electric charge, 57-58
Electric-charge concentration, 61
Electric-charge distribution, 61
Electric circuit, 62-65
Electric current, 61
   Faraday's law, 78
   generator, 80-81
   Lenz' law, 79
   motor, 81-82
   thermionic emission, 84
   transformer law, 83
Electric field, 60
Electric force, 72
Electric generator, 80-81
Electric ground, 58
Electric motor, 81-82
Electric potential, 61
Electric power, 66-67
Electrical conductor, 113
Electrical energy, 4-5
Electrical system in automatic processing, 186
Electricity, 56-67
   electrodynamics, 61-67
   electrostatics, 57-61
   magnetism and, 76-78
Electrification, 58-60
Electrified, term, 58
Electrodynamics, 61-67
Electrolytic paste, 76
Electromagnet, 71, 77
Electromagnetic energy, 5
Electromagnetic force, 76
Electromagnetic induction laws, 78-80
Electromagnetic radiation, 5, 39, 40, 41, 43-55
   electromagnetic spectrum, 48-50
   matter and energy, 54-55
   photons, 44-48
   wave-particle duality, 50-54
Electromagnetic spectrum, 48-50
Electromagnetism, 75-87
   electricity and magnetism, 76-78
   electromagnetic force, 76
   electromechanical and electronic devices, 80-86
   laws of electromagnetic induction, 78-80
Electromechanical devices, 80-86
Electromotive force, 61, 76
Electron, 32, 33
   arrangement, 35-37
   Compton, 151
   electric charge, 57-58
   electron-target interaction, 127-131
   energy equivalence, 54
Electron beam computed tomography, 382
Electron binding energy, 35, 36-37
Electron gun in fluoroscopy, 327
Electron optics, 324
Electron spin, 69
Electron volt, 48
Electronic devices, 80-86
Electronic numerical integrator and calculator, 343

Electronic timer, 98
Electrostatic focusing lens, 324-325
Electrostatic force, 60
Electrostatic grid in fluoroscopy, 327
Electrostatics, 57-61
Elemental mass, 30
Elements, 29
Elliptical tomographic movement, 285
Elongation of image, 269-270
Embolization, 334
Embryo exposure, 489-491, 500
Emulsion of x-ray film, 156, 167
Emulsion pickoff, 420
Endocrine glands, 432
Endoplasmic reticulum, 434
Energy, 4-5, 24
    attenuation, 51-52
    Compton effect and, 151
    conservation of, 24, 54
Energy equivalence of electron, 54
Energy levels, 31, 35
Energy subtraction, 366, 368-369
ENIAC, 343
Entrance skin dose, 412, 413
Entrance skin exposure, 252, 526, 527-529
Enzymes, 432
Epidemiologic studies of radiation exposure, 478
Epidermis, 467
Epilation, 468
Epithelium, 438
EPROM; *see* Erasable-programmable read-only memory
Equivalent dose limits, 501
Erasable-programmable read-only memory, 346
Error correction, 408
Erythema, 6, 468
Erythrocyte, 470
ESE; *see* Entrance skin exposure
Esophagus weighting factor, 501
Essences, 29
Examination table, 94
EXCEL, 353
Exponent, 13, 14-15
Exponential attenuation, 160
Exposed crystal, 180, 181
Exposure, 20, 251-257, 524
    characteristic curve and, 231
    dose limits, 500
    grid ratio and, 217
    programmed, 274-275
    of radiographic film, 170-171
    radiographic rating chart, 121-122
Exposure artifact, 420, 421
Exposure factors, 252-254
Exposure linearity, 411
Exposure rate, 412
Exposure reproducibility, 411-412
Exposure switch, 511-512, 520, 521
Exposure-technique factors, 270-275
Exposure time, 92, 252-253
    long, 120-121
    quality control, 411
    radiation protection and, 497
    single excessive, 120
Exposure timer, 97-99
Extended processing, 186
Extension cones and cylinders, 210-211, 212
External filtration, 132

Extinction time, 103, 365
Extrafocal radiation, 118, 119
Extrapolation, 396-398
    cell survival kinetics, 457
    of dose-response relationships, 446
Extremities
    equivalent dose limits, 501
    radiographic technique and, 259
Eye, 323-324
    dose limits, 500
    radiation-induced cataracts, 478-480

F
Face plate of fluoroscopic camera, 327
Fahrenheit, 25f
Falling-load generator, 254
Falling-load milliampere, 97
Fan beam collimation, 369
Fan x-ray beam, 358, 371, 380
Faraday's Law, 78-79
Fast-access system, 416
Fat
    computed tomography numbers, 387
    effective atomic number, 154
    mass density, 158
    soft tissue radiography, 293
Fatty acid, 433
Feed tray in automatic processing, 183
Femoral artery, 334
Ferromagnetic material, 69-70, 73
Fertility after radiation exposure, 469, 489
Fetus exposure, 489-491
    dose limits, 500, 503, 507
    response to ionizing radiation, 430
Fiber optics in fluoroscopy, 328
Field of view
    in computed tomography, 387
    in digital imaging, 360
15% peak kilovoltage rule, 134-135, 261
Fifth-generation CT scanner, 382, 393
Filament, 84, 110-111
    circuit, 97
    current, 111-112
    vaporization, 121
Film, 165-176
    in angiointerventional radiology, 339
    artifacts, 419-424
        exposure, 420
        handling and storage, 422-423
        processing, 420-422
    characteristics of, 169-171
    factors in image quality, 230-238
        contrast and characteristic curve, 234-237
        latitude, 238
        quality control, 230-231
        sensitometry and densitometry, 231-234
        speed and characteristic curve, 237-238
    film construction, 166-167
    formation of latent image, 167-169
    handling and storage, 174-175
    processing of, 177-188
        alternative methods, 186-187
        automatic, 178, 179
        components of automatic processor, 183-186
        development, 180-182
        drying, 182-183
        fixing, 182

Film, cont'd
  processing of, cont'd
    hand, 178
    sequence of steps, 178-179
    washing, 182
    wetting, 179
  remnant radiation and, 166
  sensitometry and densitometry, 231-234
  storage, 174-175
  types of, 171-174, 176
Film badge, 515, 532-533
Film bin, 174
Film changer, 338
Film contrast, 234
Film emulsion, 156
Film fog, 156
Film graininess, 230
Film illuminator, 412
Film-screen combination changes, 238
Film-screen contact, 196, 412
Film speed, 237 238
Filtered back projection, 387
Filtered ion chamber, 410
Filtered photo diode, 410
Filtration, 8-9, 255
  air, 227
  collimator, 213
  effect on x-ray emission spectrum, 135
  external, 132
  in mammography, 298-300
  quality control, 409
  radiation protection designs, 510, 511, 520, 521
  x-ray quality and, 144-147
  x-ray quantity and, 142
Fingernail artifact, 42
First-generation CT scanner, 379, 380, 393
525-line system, 330
5-minute reset timer, 496
Five-percent rule, 268
Five-pin test, 391, 392
Fixed kilovoltage technique chart, 270, 272
Fixer solution, 178
Fixing, 182
Flip-flop semiconductor storage, 345
Floor-mount system, 108, 109
Floor-to-ceiling support system, 108, 109
Floppy disk, 347
Fluorescence, 6, 192
Fluorescent screen, 330
Fluoroscope, 9
Fluoroscopic table, 94
Fluoroscopic unit, 92
Fluoroscopy, 11, 322-332
  before angiointerventional radiology, 339
  digital, 361-369
    charge-coupled device, 365-369
    high voltage generator, 362-365
    video system, 365
  filter in, 145
  historical background, 322
  image intensification, 324-326
  image monitoring, 326-330
  occupational exposure during, 524-525
  personnel positioning during, 536-537
  quality control, 412-413
  radiation protection designs for equipment, 511-512
  radiation protection during, 497

Fluoroscopy, cont'd
  spot filming, 330-331
  visual physiology in, 322-324
  x-ray tube, 108
Flux gain, 325
Fly wheel, 369
Focal spot, 116
  in angiointerventional radiology, 336
  in magnification radiography, 290
  in mammography, 298
  sharpness of image and, 269
Focal-spot blur, 242-244
Focal-spot size, 254-255, 410
Focused grid, 222, 225
Focusing coil, 327
Focusing cup, 111, 112
Fog density, 233
Force, 22, 23
  centripetal and centrifugal, 36
  electromagnetic, 76
  electromotive, 61, 76
  electrostatic, 60
  fundamental, 72
  magnetic, 73-74
Foreign body stereoradiography, 286
Foreshortened image, 242, 270
FORTRAN, 351
Fourth-generation CT scanner, 381-382, 393
Fovea centralis, 323
Fraction, 15-16
Fractionation, 443
Free radicals, 453
Frequency
  grid, 217
  photon, 45
Friction, 22
Fringe lines, 73
Fruit fly studies, 491-492
Fulcrum, 282
Full-wave rectification, 101-102, 256
Full-wave rectified x-ray generator, 223
Full width at half maximum, 399
Fundamental particles, 32, 33

G
Gadolinium, 71
  in phosphor layer of intensifying screen, 190
  in rare-earth screen, 198
Gamma ray, 38
  electromagnetic radiation, 41
  production of, 50
Gantry
  in computed tomography, 383-384, 385
  in spiral computed tomography, 400
Gas detector, 384, 385
Gas-filled detectors, 516-517
Gastrointestinal syndrome, 465-466
Gauss, 73
Gauss' law, 72
Gear-reduction assembly, 185
Geiger-Muller counter, 515, 516
Geiger-Muller region, 516
Gelatin buildup, 420
Gelatin in x-ray film, 167
Gender, radiosensitivity and, 444
Generation time, 458
Generator, 99-102

Generator, cont'd
in angiointerventional radiology, 337
in computed tomography, 384-385
in digital fluoroscopy, 362-365
falling-load, 254
high-frequency, 103-104
in mammography, 302
in spiral computed tomography, 401
Genetic cell, 436
Genetic effects of radiation, 451-452, 491-492
Genetically significant dose, 529
Geometric factors in radiographic quality, 238-244
distortion, 240-242, 243
focal-spot blur, 242-244
heel effect, 244
magnification, 239-240, 241
object position, 242, 243
Geometric unsharpness, 244
Germ cell, 469-470
Glandular dose, 530
Glass envelope, 108-110, 518
in fluoroscopic television camera, 327
Glass, thickness for secondary protective barrier, 514
Gloves, 535-536
Glow curve, 519-520
Glutaraldehyde, 181
Glycerol, 433
Glycogen, 433
Gold, 33
Gonadal dose, 526
Gonads
local damage from radiation, 469-470
shielding, 9, 538, 539
weighting factor, 501
Gradient
densitometry and, 231
film contrast and, 235
Granulocyte, 470
Granulocytopenia, 471
Granulocytosis, 471
Graph, 16-17
Graphite, anode, 113
Gravitational field, 24
Gravitational force, 72
Gravitational potential energy, 24
Gravity, 22-23
Gray, 6, 13-14
Gray matter, 387
Greek atom, 29, 30
Green-dot CRT phosphor, 172
Green-sensitive film, 169, 171
Grenz ray, 53, 468
Grid, 92, 214-228
alternative to grid use, 226-227
cleanup of scatter radiation, 216
construction, 216-218
in fluoroscopy, 327
image contrast and, 215-216
mammographic, 300
patient dose and, 225-226
performance, 218-219
problems, 223-225
scatter radiation and, 205, 206, 215-216
selection, 225
in tomography, 286
types, 219-223
Grid-controlled tube, 111

Grid cutoff, 219
Grid factor, 218, 219
Grid frequency, 217
Grid lines on radiograph, 222
Grid ratio, 216-217, 228
Group, 36
GSD; see Genetically significant dose
Guanine, 433
Guide shoe, 184
Guide-shoe marks, 420, 422
Guidewire in angiointerventional radiology, 334
Gypsum, thickness for secondary protective barrier, 514

H
H and D curve, 231
H1 catheter, 334, 335
Hair loss, 468
Halation, 172
Half-life, 38-39
Half-life layer, 39
Half-value layer, 92, 142, 143-144, 497-498
Half-wave rectification, 101, 255-256
Half-wave rectified x-ray generator, 223
Halogens, 30
Ham operator, 49-50
Hand processing, 178
Handling and storage artifacts, 422-423
Handling and storage of film, 174-175
Hard disk, 347
Hard x-ray, 142, 145
Hardener
in developer, 180, 181
in fixing agent, 182
Hardening of x-ray beam, 135
Hardware, 344-345
Headhunter tip catheter, 334, 335
Health physics, 495-508
cardinal principles, 496-498
dose limits, 498-501
educational considerations, 502
radiation exposure to public, 501-502
x rays and pregnancy, 502-507
Heat, 24-25
electron-target interaction, 127-128
handling and storage of film, 174
Heat unit, 122-123
Heavy grid, 219
Heel effect, 117, 118, 244
in mammography, 298, 299
Hematologic syndrome, 465
Hemopoietic system, 470-471
Heparin in J-tip guidewire coating, 334
Hertz, 45, 48
Hexadecimal number system, 351-353
High-contrast radiograph, 234, 266
High-energy physics, 478
High-frequency generator, 103-104, 256
High-frequency grid, 219
High-frequency x-ray unit, 252-253
High kilovoltage chart, 270, 272
High-lighting in digital imaging, 373
High-ratio grid, 216-217, 219
High-speed rotor, 115
High subject contrast, 259
High-voltage generator, 92, 99-102, 255-256
in angiointerventional radiology, 337
in computed tomography, 384-385

High-voltage generator, cont'd
  in digital fluoroscopy, 362-365
  in spiral computed tomography, 401
High-voltage transformer, 100
Histogram, 386
Hit, single-hit chromosome aberration, 473
Hole, 85
Homeostasis, 432
Horizontal resolution in fluoroscopy, 330
Horizontal retrace, 329
Hormones, 432
Horsepower, 24
Hospital admission, 537
Hot-cathode x-ray tube, 10
Hot light, 234
Hounsfield unit
  in computed tomography, 386, 393
  in digital imaging, 359
Housing cooling chart, 123-124
HU; *see* Heat unit
Human biology, 429-440
  composition of body, 430-439
    cell, 434-437
    cell theory, 430-431
    molecular, 432-434
    tissues and organs, 437-439
  response to ionizing radiation, 430, 431
Humidity, handling and storage of film, 174
Hybrid subtraction, 366, 369
Hydrated, term, 433
Hydrogen, 153
Hydrogen peroxide, 453
Hydroperoxyl radical, 453
Hydrophilic polymers, 334
Hydroquinone, 180
Hydroscopic crystal, 518
Hyperbaric, term, 443
Hypersthenic patient, 259
Hypo retention, 182, 422
Hypocycloidal tomographic movement, 285
Hyposthenic patient, 259
Hypoxic, term, 443
Hysteresis, 83

I

I/O devices, 346
ICRP; *see* International Council of Radiation Protection
ICRU; *see* International Commission on Radiologic Units
Ideal gas-filled detector, 384
Illumination in fluoroscopy, 322-323
Image; *see* Radiographic image
Image acquisition time in digital fluoroscopy, 365
Image blur, 194, 195
Image detail, 269
Image integration, 367
Image intensification in fluoroscopy, 324-326
Image intensifier, 92
Image intensifier tower, 108
Image-intensifier tube, 324-325
Image matrix
  in computed tomography, 386-387
  in digital fluoroscopy, 365
  in digital x-ray procedures, 359-360
Image noise, 193-194
Image quality factors, 260-270
  in computed tomography, 388-392
  contrast, 265-268

Image quality factors, cont'd
  distortion, 269-270
  image detail, 269
  optical density, 260-265
  in spiral computed tomography, 402-404
Image receptor, 98, 166
  alignment, 269-270
  in angiointerventional radiology, 337
  mammographic, 300-301
  radiographic quality and, 247
  reduced patient dose and, 538
Image receptor speed, 192
Image reconstruction in computed tomography, 379, 387-388
Image storage
  in computed tomography, 386
  in digital imaging, 374, 375
Immersion time, 310
Improper fraction, 15
In-service training, 504
In vitro experiments, 444
In vivo experiment, 450
Incident radiation, 98
Indirect effect, 453, 454
Induction coil, 10
Induction, magnetic, 72-73
Induction motor, 82
Inertia, 22
Infrared emission, 25
Infrared light, 48
Inherent filtration, 145, 255
Initiation time, 103
Inkjet printer, 348
Inplane resolution, 402
Input device of computer, 345, 346
Input operation, 346
Input phosphor, 324
Insulator, 61-62
Integrated circuit, 344
Integration, 133
Intensification factor, 192, 193
Intensifying screen, 9, 189-203
  care of, 201-202
  characteristics of, 192-194
  construction of, 190-191
  luminescence, 191-192
  quality control, 412
  scale of contrast and, 268
  screen-film combinations, 194-201
    cassette, 196
    compatibility, 194-196
    direct-exposure film, calcium-tungstate screens, and rare-earth systems, 196-198
    rare earth, 198-200
    recent developments, 200, 201
  sharpness of image and, 269
Interlace, 330
Interlace *versus* progressive node, 365
Intermittent slice, 386
International Commission on Radiologic Units, 13
International Council of Radiation Protection, 8
International System of measurement, 21
Interphase, 436-437
Interphase death, 444
Interpolation algorithm, 396-398
Interpreter computer program, 349
Interpupillary distance, 287
Interrogation time, 365

Interspace material of grid, 216, 217
Inverse square law, 47-48, 60, 142, 254, 527-528
Inverse voltage, 101
Inversely proportional fraction, 16
Inverter circuit, 103
Iodine
    atomic number and K-shell electron binding energy, 153
    characteristics of, 33
    as contrast medium, 160
    effective atomic number, 154
    mass density, 158
Ion pair, 5, 35, 453
Ionic bonding, 32
Ionization, 5, 35
Ionization chamber, 98, 515, 516-517
    pocket, 534
Ionization potential, 37
Ionization region, 516
Ionizing radiation, 5-11
    electromagnetic spectrum, 50
    human response to, 430, 431
    linear energy transfer, 442, 443
    medical x-ray, 6-11
    natural sources, 5-6
    types of, 39-42
    units of, 13-14
Iris, 323
Iron, 33
Irradiation
    in utero, 489-491
    of macromolecules, 450-452
Isobar, 34
Isochromatid, 473
Isoexposure lines, 497
Isoexposure profile, 525
Isomer, 34
Isotone, 34
Isotope, 33
    krypton, 21

J

J-tip guidewire, 334
Joint Commission on Accreditation of Healthcare Organizations, 408
Joule, 23, 54
Joystick, 362

K

K absorption edge, 369
K-shell absorption edge, 199
K-shell electron, 128-129
    binding energy, 153
    rare-earth screen and, 198-199
Karyotype, 472-473
Kelvin, 25
Keyboard, 346-347
Kilobyte, 349
Kilogram, 21
Kilovolt, 13
Kilovoltage, 92, 132
    adjustment, 96
    calibration quality control, 410-411
    contrast and, 248
    effect on x-ray emission spectrum, 134-135
    in fluoroscopy, 326-327
    intensity of scatter and, 215
    in mammography, 295

Kilovoltage, cont'd
    penetrability and, 266
    radiographic technique and, 261, 265
    remnant radiation and, 205
    scale of contrast and, 268
    scatter radiation and, 205, 206
    subject contrast and, 246, 247
    x-ray quality and, 144, 252
    x-ray quantity and, 141
Kilowatt, 105
Kinetic energy, 4, 24, 127
    photoelectric effect and, 153
Kinetics
    cell survival, 454-460
    of chromosome aberration, 474-475
Kink mark, 422, 423
Knee, variable kilovoltage technique chart for, 270
Krypton isotope, 21
kVP; see Kilovoltage

L

L-shell electron, 129
Lanthanum, 190, 198
Large focal spot, 112-113
Large-scale integration, 344
Laser-beam modulation, 172
Laser camera, 348
Laser disk, 347-348
Laser film, 172, 173
Laser localizer, 415
Laser printer, 173, 348
Latent image
    formation of, 167-169
    processing of, 177-188
        alternative methods, 186-187
        automatic, 178, 179
        components of automatic processor, 183-186
        development, 180-182
        drying, 182-183
        fixing, 182
        hand, 178
        sequence of steps, 178-179
        washing, 182
        wetting, 179
Latent-image center, 169
Latent period in acute radiation lethality, 464-465
Lateral decentering, 224
Lateral dispersion, 329
Latitude, 170, 238
Law of Bergonie and Tribondeau, 442
Law of conservation of energy, 54
Law of conservation of matter, 54
Laws of Motion, 22
$LD_{50/30}$, 466-467
Lead
    atomic number and K-shell electron binding energy, 153
    characteristics of, 33
    effective atomic number, 154
    in grid, 217-218
    half-value layer and tenth-value layer, 498
    mass density, 158
    thickness for secondary protective barrier, 514
Lead shielding, 512-513
Leakage radiation, 108, 513-514
Length, 20, 21
Lens coupling, 328
Lens of eye, 323

Lens of eye, cont'd
    dose limits, 500
    shield for, 538
Lenz' Law, 79
Leukemia, 7, 483-485
    after irradiation in utero, 490
    minimum population sample, 478
Leukopenia, 464
Lexan, 392
Life-span shortening, 480-481
Light fog, 422
Light, handling and storage of film, 174
Light-localizing variable-aperture collimator, 145, 211, 212, 255
Light-stimulated phosphorescence, 371
Lightning, 58, 59
Limiting resolution, 389
Line compensation, 92, 94
Line-focus principle, 116-117
Line pair, 389
Line-pair test pattern, 194, 195
Line pairs per millimeter, 194
Linear
    nonthreshold dose-response relationship, 474, 501
    nonthreshold model, 446
    quadratic dose-response relationship, 445, 446
    threshold model, 445
Linear attenuation coefficients, 387
Linear dose-response relationships, 444-445
Linear energy transfer, 442, 443, 454, 459-460
Linear parallel grid, 219-223
Linear scale, 17
Linear tomography, 282-284, 285
Linearity
    in computed tomography, 391, 392
    quality control, 414-415
    radiation protection designs, 511, 520
Lipids, 432-433
Lithium fluoride, 520
Liver
    radiation-induced cancer, 487
    weighting factor, 501
Lodestone, 69
Log of relative exposure, 232
Logarithmic scale, 17
Logic functions, 343
LOGO, 353
Long-cone technique, 240
Long gray scale, 238
Long-scale contrast, 246, 266
Low contrast, 266
Low-osmolality contrast media, 335
Low-ratio grid, 226
Luminescence, 191-192
Lung
    computed tomography numbers, 387
    effective atomic number, 154
    mass density, 158, 159
    radiation-induced cancer, 487
    weighting factor, 501
Lye, 181
Lymph nodes, 470-471
Lymphocyte, 470
Lymphoid tissue, 470-471
Lymphopenia, 471
Lysosome, 434-435

M

mA; *see* Milliampere
Macromolecule, 432, 450-452
Macros, 353
Magnesium oxide, 191
Magnet
    bar, 78
    classification of, 70-71
    electromagnet, 77
Magnetic core of computer, 345
Magnetic dipole, 69
Magnetic disk for secondary memory, 347
Magnetic domain, 69
Magnetic field, 76-77
Magnetic force, 72, 73-74
Magnetic lines of induction, 72-73
Magnetic moment, 69
Magnetic resonance imaging, 11
    electromagnetic spectrum, 49
    of eye, 323
    laser film in, 172
    radiation used in, 39
Magnetic sink, 73
Magnetic susceptibility, 71
Magnetic tape
    for computed tomography image storage, 386
    for secondary memory, 348
Magnetism, 68-74
    classification of magnets, 70-71
    electricity and, 76-78
    magnetic laws, 71-73
Magnetite, 69
Magnification, 239-240, 241
Magnification factor, 239, 289
Magnification mammography, 301-302
Magnification radiography, 239, 289-291
Magnitude, systems of measurement, 21
Main-chain scission, 450
Main memory of computer, 345
Mainframe computer, 344
Major peak kilovoltage, 96
Malignancy
    radiation-induced, 482-487
    total risk of, 487-489
Mammography, 293-319
    breast cancer, 293-294
    charged couple device, 301
    compression during, 208, 295, 296
    film, 172
    filtration, 298-300
    focal spot, 298
    grids, 300
    history and development, 293
    image receptors, 300-301
    intensifying screen, 195
    low-ratio grid for, 226
    magnification, 301
    occupational exposure, 525
    patient dose in, 529-530
    photo timers, 300
    quality control, 306-321
        daily tasks, 307-310
        quality control team, 306-307
        quarterly tasks, 313-316
        semiannual tasks, 316-317

Mammography, cont'd
quality control, cont'd
weekly tasks, 310-313
source-to-image receptor distance, 240
target composition, 296-298
x-ray machine, 93
Mammography Quality Standards Act, 306
Manifest illness stage in acute radiation lethality, 464-465
Manifest image, 168
Mark 1, 343
Mask mode, 366-367
Masking, 310
Mass, 4-5, 20
in mammography, 311
standard of measurement, 21
Mass density, 158-159
radiographic technique and, 259
subject contrast and, 245-246
Mass equivalence of photon, 54
Mass screening for tuberculosis, 537
Mathematics, 14-16
Matrix of intensities, 359-360
Matter, 4-5
atom, 28-42
combination of atoms, 31-32
fundamental particles, 32, 33
historical background, 29-31
nomenclature, 32-34
radioactivity, 37-39
structure, 34-37
types of ionizing radiation, 39-42
electrostatics, 57-61, 62
law of conservation, 54
magnetism, 69-70
x-ray interaction with, 149-161
attenuation, 159-160
classical scattering, 150
Compton effect, 150-151, 152
differential absorption, 155-159
pair production, 155
photodisintegration, 155, 156
photoelectric effect, 151-155
radiologic contrast agents, 160-161
Maximum available power, 105
Maximum differential absorption, 156
Maximum intensity projection, 402-404
Maximum permissible dose, 498-499
Maxwell's field theory of electromagnetic radiation, 73
Mean deviation of computed tomography values, 386
Mean lethal dose, 457, 458
Mean marrow dose, 529
Mean solar day, 21
Mean survival time, 467
Measurement
standards of, 20-21
systems of, 21
units of, 20
Mechanical energy, 24
Mechanical timer, 97-98
Mechanics, 21-27
quantum, 31
Mediastinum, 145
Medical physicist, 306-307
Medical x-ray, 6-11
basic radiation protection, 7-9

Medical x-ray, cont'd
development of modern radiography, 9-11
discovery of, 6, 7
reports of radiation injury, 6-7
Megavoltage x-ray, 53
Meiosis, 436, 437
Memory module, 345
Memory unit of computer, 345-346
Meningitis, radiation sickness and, 466
Mental retardation, 591
Mesenteric artery, 334, 335
Messenger ribonucleic acid, 433, 436
Metabolism, 432
Metal envelope, 110
Metaphase, 436-437
Meter, 21, 48
Metol, 180
Microcalcifications in breast cancer, 295
Microcomputer, 344
Microfocus tube, 254-255
Microprocessor, 342
Microswitch, 183
Microwave radiation, 50
Mid-density, 307-310
Milliampere, 13, 92
quantity and, 252
Milliampere second, 253-254
affect on x-ray emission spectrum, 133-134
contrast and, 248-249
control, 96-97
grid ratio and, 228
optical density and, 261, 263-264
x-ray quality and quantity and, 140-141, 252
Milliamperes timer, 98
Minicomputer, 344
Minification gain, 325
Minimum line spacing, 194
Minimum wavelength, 133
Minor peak kilovoltage, 96
MIP; see Maximum intensity projection
Misregistration artifact, 368
Mitochondria, 434
Mitosis, 436-437
MKS system of measurement, 21
Mobile radiography exposure switch, 511
Modem, 348-349
Modulation of video signal, 329
Modulation transfer function, 388-389, 415
Molecular composition of body, 432-434
Molecular radiobiology, 449-462
cell survival kinetics, 454-460
direct and indirect effect, 453
irradiation of macromolecules, 450-452
radiolysis of water, 452-453
target theory, 453-454
Molecule, 4, 31, 32
Molybdenum
anode, 113
atomic number and K-shell electron binding energy, 153
characteristics of, 33
effective atomic number, 154
in mammographic x-ray tube, 296-298, 299-300
mass density, 158
Momentum, 23
Monitoring

Monitoring, cont'd
in angiointerventional radiology, 335
digital fluoroscopic system, 364
fluoroscopic image, 326-330
processor, 417
Monosaccharides, 433
Motion, 22
Motion blur, 283-284
Motion unsharpness, 246-247
Mouse, computer, 362
Moving grid, 222-223
MPD; *see* Maximum permissible dose
MPR; *see* Multiplanar reformation
Mrad, 6
Multidirectional tomography, 285, 286
Multifield image intensification, 326
Multiformat camera, 172, 173
Multihit chromosome aberrations, 473-474
Multiplanar reformation, 402
Multiplication of fractions, 15
Multitarget, single hit model, 455, 456-457
Muscle, 438
· computed tomography numbers, 387
effective atomic number, 154
mass density, 158
soft tissue radiography, 293
Mutation, genetic, 451-452
Mutual induction, 80
Myelocytic leukemia, 484

N

N-type semiconductor, 85
National Council on Radiation Protection and Measurements, 7-9, 499
Natural convection, 25
Natural magnet, 70
NCRP; *see* National Council on Radiation Protection and Measurements
Negative acceleration, 22
Negative charge, 57
Negative ion, 5
Nephrotomography, 378
Nervous tissue, 438
Network in digital imaging, 373, 374
Neuron, 438
Neutron, 32, 33
New employee training, 503-504
Newton, 22
Newton's law, 22-23, 72
Nitrogen, 153
Noble gases, 30
Node of network, 373
Noise, 193-194, 230
in computed tomography, 391
quality control, 414
Nomogram, 140, 527, 528
Non-ionizing radiation, 39
Nonhydroscopic, term, 217
Nonlinear
nonthreshold dose-response relationship, 474
nonthreshold model, 445
threshold model, 445
Nonlinear dose-response relationships, 445
Nonscheduled maintenance, 417
Nonscreen film, 169
Nonthreshold form, 472
North pole, 71

Nuclear energy, 5
Nuclear medicine, 14
Nucleic acids, 433
Nucleolus, 434
Nucleon, 32
Nucleotide, 433
Nucleus, 31, 433, 434
Nuclide, 37
Number systems, 14-17
Numerator, 15
Numeric prefixes, 13
Nutated, term, 382
Nylon, 392

O

Object-oriented programming, 353
Object plane, 282
Object position, 242, 243
Object thickness, 240-242
Object-to-image distance, 240
focal-spot blur and, 243-244
in magnification radiography, 289-290
Objective lens, 328
Occupational exposure, 501, 524-526
dose limits, 500
radiation-induced cataracts, 479-480
reduction of, 532-537
Off-center error, 224
Off-focus error, 224-225
Off-focus radiation, 118, 119, 211
Off-level error, 223-224
Ohm, 63
Ohm's law, 63
OID; *see* Object-to-image distance
On-line systems, 353
Oocyte, 469
Oogonia, 469
Oogonium, 436
OOP; *see* Object-oriented programming
Opaque, term, 52
Open circulation system in automatic processing, 185-186
Open filament, 121
Operating console, 92-99, 385-386
Operating system of computer program, 349
Optical coupling, 518
Optical density, 98, 158, 180, 232-234
characteristic curve, 231
grid cutoff and, 220
image quality and, 260-265
scatter radiation and, 215
Optical disk, 347-348
Optical scanner, 348
Ordered pair, 17
Organ system, 438
Organic molecules, 432
Organogenesis, 490, 502
Organs, 437-439
equivalent dose limits, 501
Origin of axes, 16-17
Orthochromatic film, 169
Orthovoltage x-ray, 53, 467-468
Oscillating grid, 222-223
Oscilloscope, 410
Outcome analysis, 408
Outer-shell electron, 191
Output intensity, 140, 527-528
Output operation, 346

Output phosphor, 325
Ovary, 469
Overexposure, 261, 262
Overlapping images, 402, 403
Ovum, 469
Oxygen
    atomic number and K-shell electron binding energy, 153
    characteristics of, 33
Oxygen effect, 443, 454
Oxygen enhancement ratio, 443, 459-460

P

P-n junction semiconductor, 85
P-type semiconductor, 85
Pair production, 155
Pan in digital imaging, 373
Panchromatic film, 169-170
Panoramic tomography, 286, 287
Parallel circuit, 64, 65
Paramagnetic material, 71
Parenchymal, term, 439
Particle accelerator, 32, 478-479
Particle model, 52-54
Particulate radiation, 39, 40-41
Pascal, 349, 352
Pathology, radiographic technique and, 259-260
Patient, 259-260
    care performed by radiographer, 10
    holding during x-ray, 537
    motion of, 247
    pregnant, 505-506
    preparation for angiointerventional radiology, 335
    quality assurance of care, 408
    repeat examinations, 537, 538
    unnecessary radiographic examinations, 537
Patient positioning
    automatic-exposure techniques, 273-274
    in computed tomography, 385
    distortion and, 270
    exposure artifact and, 420
    radiation protection and, 536-537
    radiographic quality and, 247
    reduced patient dose and, 538
Patient thickness
    radiographic quality and, 245
    radiographic technique and, 259
Penetrability, 142, 252
    kilovoltage and, 266
Penetrometer, 231-232
Pentium microprocessor, 344, 345
Penumbra, 244
Peptide bonds, 432
Percutaneous transluminal angioplasty, 334
Periapical exposure, 240, 241
Period, 36
Periodic health examination, 537
Periodic table of elements, 30, 31
Permanent magnet, 70-71
Personal computer, 343, 344
Personnel
    in angiointerventional suite, 335-336
    monitoring of, 532-535
Personnel monitoring report, 535, 536
pH, 181
Phagocytic cell, 487
Phantom, 98, 206
    for contrast resolution quality control, 415

Phantom,, cont'd
    five-pin, 391, 392
    in mammography quality control, 311-313
Phenidone, 180
Phosphor layer of intensifying screen, 190, 197
Phosphorescence, 192
Photo-fluoroscent image, 412-413
Photo-multiplier sensing device, 98
Photo-spot camera, 331
Photo timer, 98-99, 274
    mammographic, 300
    quality control, 411
Photo timing, 92, 274
Photocathode, 324, 518-519
Photoconductive layer, 328
Photodisintegration, 155, 156
Photoelectric effect, 151-155
Photoemission, 324, 519
Photographic effect, 168
Photographic emulsion, 515
Photometer, 412
Photometric analysis, 412
Photon, 41, 44-48
    interaction with silver-halide crystal, 168-169
    mass equivalence, 54
    x-ray interaction with matter, 149-161
        attenuation, 159-160
        classical scattering, 150
        Compton effect, 150-151, 152
        differential absorption, 155-159
        pair production, 155
        photodisintegration, 155, 156
        photoelectric effect, 151-155
        radiologic contrast agents, 160-161
Photostimulable phosphor, 371-372
Phototopic vision, 323
Physician's viewing console in computed tomography, 386
Physics of radiation, 1-87
    atom, 28-42
        combination of atoms, 31-32
        fundamental particles, 32, 33
        historical background, 29-31
        nomenclature, 32-34
        radioactivity, 37-39
        structure, 34-37
        types of ionizing radiation, 39-42
    definitions and mathematics review, 12-18
    electricity, 56-67
        electrodynamics, 61-67
        electrostatics, 57-61
    electromagnetic radiation, 43-55
        electromagnetic spectrum, 48-50
        matter and energy, 54-55
        photons, 44-48
        wave-particle duality, 50-54
    electromagnetism, 75-87
        electricity and magnetism, 76-78
        electromagnetic force, 76
        electromechanical and electronic devices, 80-86
        laws of electromagnetic induction, 78-80
    ionizing radiation, 5-11
        medical x-ray, 6-11
        natural sources, 5-6
    magnetism, 68-74
        classification of magnets, 70-71
        magnetic laws, 71-73
    matter and energy, 4-5

Physics of radiation, cont'd
  mechanics, 21-27
  standards of measurement, 20-21
  systems of measurement, 21
  units of measurement, 20
Pi lines, 420, 422
Pigtail catheter, 334, 335
Pinhole camera, 410
Pipeline processor, 354
Pitch, 398
Pits, 115, 116
Pixel
  binary number system, 351
  in computed tomography, 386
  in digital imaging, 359
Planar analysis, 386
Planchet, 519
Planck's constant, 53-54
Plaque, J-tip guidewire and, 334
Plastic fiber as grid interspace material, 217
Platelets, 470
Platinum-iridium bar, 20
Plexiglas, five-pin AAPM phantom, 392
Pluripotential stem cell, 470
Pneumoencephalography, 160
Pocket ionization chamber, 534
Point lesion, 450
Point mutation, 452
Point source, 497
Poisson distribution, 455
Polarity, 102
Polyester base
  of film, 166-167
  of intensifying screen, 191
Polyethylene, five-pin AAPM phantom, 392
Polysaccharides, 433
Polystyrene, five-pin AAPM phantom, 392
Portable fluoroscopy unit, 108
Portable x-ray machine, 93
Positioning
  exposure artifact and, 420
  grid problems, 223-225
Positive-beam limitation, 510, 520
Positive beam-limiting collimator, 212, 410
Positive charge, 57
Positive electrode in battery, 76
Positive ion, 5
Positron emission tomography, 11
Postpatient collimation, 380-381
Potassium alum, 182
Potassium bromide, 167, 181
Potassium iodide, 181
Potential energy, 4, 24, 61
Potter-Bucky diaphragm, 222
Potter-Bucky grid, 10-11
Power, 24
Power rating, 104-105
Pre-DNA synthesis phase, 436
Preamplifier, 519
Precursor cell, 438
Predetector collimation, 380-381
Preemployment physical, 537
Pregnancy, 502-507
  irradiation in utero, 489-491
  radiation effects on fertility, 489
Preneoplastic thyroid nodularity, 486
Prepatient collimation, 381

Prereading voltmeter, 96
Preservative
  in developer, 180, 181
  in fixing agent, 182
Preventive maintenance, 414, 417
Primary coil, 80
Primary connection, 94
Primary protective barrier, 511, 512-513, 521
Primary x-ray
  grid cutoff and, 219-220
  grid interspace material and, 216
Primordial follicle, 469
Principal quantum number, 36
Printer, 348
Probability of interaction formula, 157
Processing artifact, 420-422
Processing methods of computer, 353-354
Processing of radiograph, 169, 177-188
  alternative methods, 186-187
  automatic, 178, 179
  components of automatic processor, 183-186
  contrast and characteristic curve, 236-237
  development, 180-182
  drying, 182-183
  fixing, 182
  hand, 178
  sensitometry and densitometry, 231-234
  sequence of steps, 178-179
  washing, 182
  wetting, 179
Processor quality control, 307-310, 416-417
Prodromal syndrome in acute radiation lethality, 464-465
Programmed exposure, 274-275
Progressive *versus* interlace node, 365
Projectile electron, 128, 130
Projection in computed tomography, 378-379
Proper fraction, 15
Prophase, 436-437
Proportion, 16
Proportional counter, 515, 516
Proportional region, 516
Protective apparel, 9, 412, 535-536
Protective barriers, 9, 512-515
Protective coating of intensifying screen, 190
Protective curtain, 512, 521
Protective housing, 108, 110, 510
Proteins, 432
  nucleic acids and, 433, 434
  synthesis of, 435-436, 450-451
Proton, 32, 33, 57-58
Protraction, 443
Public exposure, 500, 501-502
Puck film changer, 338-339
Purines, 433
Pyrimidines, 433

Q

Quality, 92, 133, 142-147, 229-250
  definitions, 230
  factors affecting, 144-147
  film factors, 230-238
    contrast and characteristic curve, 234-237
    latitude, 238
    quality control, 230-231
    sensitometry and densitometry, 231-234
    speed and characteristic curve, 237-238
  geometric factors, 238-244

Quality, cont'd
 geometric factors, cont'd
  distortion, 240-242, 243
  focal-spot blur, 242-244
  heel effect, 244
  magnification, 239-240, 241
  object position, 242, 243
 half-value layer and, 143-144
 image factors, 260-270
  in computed tomography, 388-392
  contrast, 265-268
  distortion, 269-270
  image detail, 269
  optical density, 260-265
  in spiral computed tomography, 402-404
 image receptors and, 247
 patient positioning and, 247
 penetrability and, 142
 selection of technique factors, 248-249
 subject factors, 244-247
Quality assurance, 306, 408
Quality control, 407-418
 in computed tomography, 413-416
 definition, 408
 film artifacts and, 420
 film factors, 230-231
 in film processing, 174
 in fluoroscopy, 412-413
 in mammography, 306-321
  daily tasks, 307-310
  quality control team, 306-307
  quarterly tasks, 313-316
  semiannual tasks, 316-317
  weekly tasks, 310-313
 processor, 416-417
 radiation and light field testing, 212
 radiographic, 408-412
 three steps of, 408
 in tomography, 413
Quantity, 92, 133
 factors affecting, 140-142
 milliampere and, 252
 output intensity, 140
Quantum, 44
Quantum mechanics, 31
Quantum mottle, 193, 198, 230
Quantum theory, 52-54
Quenching agent, 516
QuickBASIC, 352
Quotient, 15

R

Rad, 6, 13-14
Radiation, 3-11
 backscatter, 151, 152
 bremsstrahlung, 130
 characteristic, 128-130
 detection and measurement, 515-520
 early effects, 430, 463-476
  acute radiation lethality, 464-467
  cytogenetic, 471-475
  hematologic, 470-471
  local tissue damage, 467-470
 electromagnetic, 5, 39, 40, 41, 43-55
  electromagnetic spectrum, 48-50
  matter and energy, 54-55
  photons, 44-48

Radiation, cont'd
 electromagnetic, cont'd
  wave-particle duality, 50-54
 extrafocal, 118, 119
 handling and storage of film, 174-175
 incident, 98
 ionizing, 5-11
  electromagnetic spectrum, 50
  human response to, 430, 431
  linear energy transfer, 442
  medical x-ray, 6-11
  natural sources, 5-6
  types of, 39-42
  units of, 13-14
 late effects, 430, 477-494
  epidemiologic studies, 478
  life-span shortening, 480-481
  local tissue effects, 478-480
  pregnancy and, 489-492
  radiation-induced malignancy, 482-487
  risk estimates, 481-482
  total risk of malignancy, 487-489
 leakage, 108
 matter and energy, 4-5
 non-ionizing, 39
 off-focus, 118, 119, 211
 particulate, 39, 40-41
 remnant, 160, 166, 205
  intensifying screen and, 190
 scatter, 204-213
  beam-restricting devices, 208-213
  factors affecting, 205-208
  grid and, 214-228; see also Grid
 terminology and definitions, 13-14
 thermal, 25
Radiation absorbed dose, 13-14
Radiation dose response relationships, 444-446
Radiation Effects Research Foundation, 483
Radiation equivalent man, 14
Radiation exposure, 6-7, 92, 133, 140
 basic radiation protection, 7-9
 characteristic curve and, 231
 early effects, 463-476
  acute radiation lethality, 464-467
  cytogenetic, 471-475
  hematologic, 470-471
  local tissue damage, 467-470
 factors affecting, 140-142
 measurements outside x-ray room, 515
 output intensity, 140
Radiation fog, 182, 422
Radiation protection, 495-508, 523-541
 basic concepts, 7-9
 cardinal principles, 496-498
 designing for, 509-521
  protective barriers, 512-515
  radiation detection and measurement, 515-520
  x-ray apparatus, 510
  x-ray equipment, 510-512
 dose limits, 498-501
 educational considerations, 502
 health physics, 495-508
 occupational exposure, 524-526
 patient dose, 526-532
  estimation of, 526-529
  image receptor and, 538
  radiographic technique, 537-538

Radiation protection, cont'd
  patient dose, cont'd
    repeat examinations, 537, 538
    in special examinations, 529-532
    specific area shielding, 538-539
    unnecessary examinations, 537
  patient holding, 537
  personnel monitoring, 532-535
  personnel monitoring report, 535, 536
  positioning, 536-537
  protective apparel, 535-536
  radiation exposure to public, 501-502
  x-rays and pregnancy, 502-507
Radiation weighting factor, 501
Radio frequency, 49-50
Radio reception, 78-79
Radioactive decay, 37
Radioactive decay law, 38
Radioactive disintegration, 37
Radioactive gas, 5
Radioactive half-life, 38-39
Radioactivity, 20, 37-39
Radiobiology, 441-448
  biologic factors affecting radiosensitivity, 443-444
  Law of Bergonie and Tribondeau, 442
  molecular and cellular, 449-462
    cell survival kinetics, 454-460
    direct and indirect effect, 453
    irradiation of macromolecules, 450-452
    radiolysis of water, 452-453
    target theory, 453-454
  physical factors affecting radiosensitivity, 442-443
  radiation dose-response relationships, 444-446
Radiographer
  clinical skills, 10
  dose limits, 499
  life-span shortening risks, 480
  occupational exposure, 524
  personnel monitoring, 532-535
  pregnant, 503-504
  quality assurance and, 306
  specialist in angiointerventional radiology, 336
Radiographic density, 260
Radiographic exposure, 251-257
  equipment characteristics, 254-256
  exposure factors, 252-254
Radiographic film, 165-176
  characteristics of, 169-171
  factors in image quality, 230-238
    contrast and characteristic curve, 234-237
    latitude, 238
    quality control, 230-231
    sensitometry and densitometry, 231-234
    speed and characteristic curve, 237-238
  film construction, 166-167
  formation of latent image, 167-169
  handling and storage, 174-175
  processing of, 177-188
    alternative methods, 186-187
    automatic, 178, 179
    components of automatic processor, 183-186
    development, 180-182
    drying, 182-183
    fixing, 182
    hand, 178
    sequence of steps, 178-179
    washing, 182

Radiographic film, cont'd
  processing of, cont'd
    wetting, 179
  remnant radiation and, 166
  sensitometry and densitometry, 231-234
  types of, 171-174, 176
Radiographic image, 162-276
  beam-restricting devices, 208-213
  digital, 357-376
    dynamic range, 360-361, 362, 363
    fluoroscopy, 361-369
    historical development, 358-359
    image matrix, 359-360
    picture archiving and communication system, 372-374
    radiography, 369-372
  equipment characteristics, 254-256
  exposure factors, 252-254
  grid, 214-228
    alternative to grid use, 226-227
    cleanup of scatter radiation, 216
    construction, 216-218
    patient dose and, 225-226
    performance, 218-219
    problems, 223-225
    scatter radiation and image contrast, 215-216
    selection, 225
    types, 219-223
  intensifying screen, 9, 189-203
    care of, 201-202
    characteristics of, 192-194
    construction of, 190-191
    luminescence, 191-192
    screen-film combinations, 194-201
  processing of latent image, 177-188
    alternative methods, 186-187
    automatic, 178, 179
    components of automatic processor, 183-186
    development, 180-182
    drying, 182-183
    fixing, 182
    hand, 178
    sequence of steps, 178-179
    washing, 182
    wetting, 179
  quality, 229-250
    contrast and characteristic curve, 234-237
    definitions, 230
    distortion, 240-242, 243
    focal-spot blur, 242-244
    heel effect, 244
    image receptors and, 247
    latitude, 238
    magnification, 239-240, 241
    object position, 242, 243
    patient positioning and, 247
    selection of technique factors, 248-249
    sensitometry and densitometry, 231-234
    speed and characteristic curve, 237-238
    subject factors, 244-247
  radiographic film, 165-176
    characteristics of, 169-171
    film construction, 166-167
    formation of latent image, 167-169
    handling and storage, 174-175
    remnant radiation and, 166
    types of, 171-174, 176
  scatter radiation, 204-208

Radiographic image, cont'd
  technique, 258-276
    contrast, 265-268
    distortion, 269-270
    exposure-technique factors, 270-275
    image detail, 269
    optical density, 260-265
    patient factors, 259-260
Radiographic noise, 193-194, 230
Radiographic quality, 229-250
  definitions, 230
  film factors, 230-238
    contrast and characteristic curve, 234-237
    latitude, 238
    quality control, 230-231
    sensitometry and densitometry, 231-234
    speed and characteristic curve, 237-238
  geometric factors, 238-244
    distortion, 240-242, 243
    focal-spot blur, 242-244
    heel effect, 244
    magnification, 239-240, 241
    object position, 242, 243
  image receptors and, 247
  patient positioning and, 247
  selection of technique factors, 248-249
  subject factors, 244-247
Radiographic quality control, 408-412
Radiographic rating chart, 121-122
Radiographic technique, 258-276
  exposure-technique factors, 270-275
  image quality factors, 260-270
    contrast, 265-268
    distortion, 269-270
    image detail, 269
    optical density, 260-265
    patient factors, 259-260
  reduction of unnecessary patient dose, 537-538
Radiographic technique chart, 104, 270
Radiographic unit, 92
Radioisotopes, 37-39
Radiologic physics, see Physics of radiation
Radiologist, 532-535
Radiolucency of tissue, 259, 260
Radiolucent, term, 52, 53, 156
Radiolysis of water, 452-453
Radionuclides, 5, 37
Radiopacity of tissue, 259, 260
Radiopaque, term, 52, 53, 156
Radiopaque grid material, 216
Radioprotectors, 444
Radiosensitive molecule, 432
Radiosensitivity
  biologic factors affecting, 443-444
  Law of Bergonie and Tribondeau, 442
  physical factors affecting, 442-443
Radiosensitizers, 444
Radon, 5, 487
RAM; see Random access memory
Random access memory, 345-346
Rapid film changer, 338
Rapid processing, 186
Rapid serial exposure, 98
Rare earth, 198
Rare-earth intensifying screen, 9, 196-198
Raster pattern, 329, 330
Ratio, 15-16

Ratio, cont'd
  grid, 216-217
  turns, 83, 100
Rayleigh scattering, 150
RBE; see Relative biologic effectiveness
Read-only memory, 345-346
Read-write memory, 346
Real-time systems, 354
Reciprocal roentgens, 237-238
Reciprocal translocation, 473-474
Reciprocating grid, 222-223
Reciprocity law, 170-171
Reconstruction of image
  in computed tomography, 379, 387-388
  in spiral computed tomography, 402
Reconstruction time, 385
Recording of macros, 353
Rectification, 84, 100-102
  full-wave, 101-102, 256
  half-wave, 101, 255-256
Rectifier, 84-85
Red blood cell, 470
Red filter, 171
Redox reaction, 180
Reducing agent, 180
Reduction division, 437
Reduction in film development, 180
Reflection, wave model of electromagnetic radiation, 51
Reflective layer of intensifying screen, 191
Refraction, 48
Region of continuous discharge, 516
Region of interest
  in computed tomography, 391
  in digital imaging, 361
Region of recombination, 516
Registers of memory unit of computer, 345
Reject analysis form, 315
Relative age-response relationship, 488
Relative biologic effectiveness, 442, 459-460
Relative risk, 481-482, 488
Relativity, 5, 54, 128
Rem, 14
Remasking, 367
Remnant radiation, 160, 166, 205
  intensifying screen and, 190
Remote terminal, 349
Renal artery, 334, 335
Repeat analysis, 313-315
Replenishment rate, 183-184
Replenishment system in automatic processing, 185
Repopulation of cells, 444
Reproducibility, radiation protection designs, 511, 520
Repulsion and attraction, 72
Reregistration, 368
Resistor, 64
Resolution, 230
  in digital x-ray procedures, 360
  of radiographic film, 167
Resorption of embryo, 502
Restrainer in developer, 180, 181
Reticuloendothelial system, 487
Retina, 323
Revolutions per minute, 115
Revolving time, 516
Rhenium
  atomic number and K-shell electron binding energy, 153
  mass density, 158

Rhenium, cont'd
   target, 114, 115
Rheostat, 64
Rhodium, 296-298, 299-300
Ribonucleic acid, 433-434, 450-451
Ribosome, 434
Right-hand rule, 77
Ring artifact, 381
Risk estimates, 481-482
RJE system, 353
RNA; *see* Ribonucleic acid
Rochester series, 485
Rods, 323-324
Roentgen, 13-14, 140
   reciprocal, 237-238
ROI; *see* Region of interest
Roll-film changer, 338
Roller marks, 420, 422
Roller subassembly in automatic processing, 184
ROM; *see* Read-only memory
Rotate-nutate scanner, 382
Rotating anode, 113, 114-115
Rotor, 115
Routine performance evaluation, 408
Ruthenium, 33

S

S-type dose-response relationship, 445
Saccharides, 433
Safelight, 171
Sagittal view, 397
Saturation current, 112
Scalar, 21
Scale of contrast, 266
Scan beam digital radiography, 358
Scan time, 385
Scanned projection radiography, 359, 369-370, 371
Scatter radiation, 204-213
   beam-restricting devices, 208-213
   factors affecting, 205-208
   grid and, 214-228
      alternative to grid use, 226-227
      cleanup of scatter radiation, 216
      construction, 216-218
      image contrast and, 215-216
      patient dose and, 225-226
      performance, 218-219
      problems, 223-225
      selection, 225
      types, 219-223
   secondary protective barriers and, 513-514
Scattered x-ray, 151
Scheduled maintenance, 417
Scientific notation, 14
Scintillation detection, 515, 517-519
Scintillation detector, 383-384
Scintillation detector assembly, 518
Scintillation process, 517-518
Scotopic vision, 323
Screen film, 169
Screen-film combinations, 194-201
   cassette, 196
   compatibility, 194-196
   direct-exposure film, calcium-tungstate screens, and rare-earth systems, 196-198
   mammographic, 300-301
   quality control, 412

Screen-film combinations, cont'd
   rare earth, 198-200
   recent developments, 200, 201
Screen-film contact, 201
   in mammography quality control, 316-317
Screen lag, 192
Screen speed, 192
Screening
   mammography, 293
   tuberculosis, 537
Scroll in digital imaging, 373
Second-generation CT scanner, 379-380, 393
Secondary coil, 80
Secondary electron, 151, 168-169
Secondary memory, 346
Secondary memory devices, 347-349
Secondary protective barrier, 513-514
Section sensitivity profile, 399
Section thickness, 282, 284
Seivert, 13, 14
Seldinger needle, 334
Selectivity of grid, 218-219
Self-induction, 80
Self-rectification, 101
Sella turcica, 211
Semiconductor, 61-62, 85
Semiconductor memory, 345
Semilogarithmic graph, 17, 231
Sensitivity, 230
   speed and, 237-238
Sensitivity profile, 381, 415
Sensitivity speck, 167
Sensitometry, 231-234
Sequestering agent
   in developer, 180, 181
   in fixing agent, 182
Serial changer, 338-339
Series circuit, 64, 65
Sex chromosome, 473
Shaded surface display, 404
Shadow shield, 538, 539
Shadowgraph, 238
Sharpness of image, 269
Shelf life of radiographic film, 175
Shell, 34, 35-36
Shell-type transformer, 84
Shielding, 8, 497-498, 538-539
Short gray scale, 238
Short-scale contrast, 246, 266
Shoulder of characteristic curve, 231
SI unit, 13, 73
SID; *see* Source-to-image receptor distance
Sigmoid-type dose-response relationship, 445
Signal plate of fluoroscopic camera, 327-328
Signal-to-noise ratio, 365
Significant figure, 16
Silver, 33
Silver bromide crystals, 167
Silver-halide crystals, 167, 168-169
Silver nitrate, 167
Simmons catheter, 335
Simple linear interpolation, 397
Simultaneous multifilm tomography, 282
Sine wave, 44, 45, 46
Single-hit chromosome aberration, 473
Single-phase power, 102, 136-137, 252-253
Single stroke grid, 222

Single-target, single-hit model, 455-456
Sinusoidal movement, 44
Skin
    dose limits, 500
    equivalent dose limits, 501
    local damage from radiation, 467-468, 478
    mean lethal dose, 458
    radiation-induced cancer, 486
    weighting factor, 501
Skin erythema dose, 468
Slice thickness, 381, 415
Slip-ring technology
    fifth-generation CT scanner and, 382
    in spiral computed tomography, 399-400
Slit camera, 410
Slope, 17
Sludge deposit, 420
Small focal spot, 112-113
Smudge static, 422, 423
Snook transformer, 7, 10
SNR; see Signal-to-noise ratio
Sodium carbonate, 181
Sodium hydroxide, 181
Sodium sulfite, 181, 182
Soft tissue
    Compton scattering and, 295
    differential absorption, 157
    mammography and, 293-295
    mass density, 159
    photoelectric effect and, 154
    scatter radiation and, 207-208
Soft x-ray, 142
Software, 349-350
Solenoid, 77, 78
Solid-state diode, 86
Solid-state microchip, 85
Solid-state rectifier, 85
Solid state timer, 99
Solvent
    in developer, 179, 180
    in fixing agent, 182
Somatic cell, 436
Source-to-image receptor distance, 108
    in aperture diaphragm, 210
    focal-spot blur and, 243
    linear grid cutoff and, 220
    magnification and, 239-240, 289-290
    optical density and, 261
    radiation protection requirements, 520
    in stereoradiography, 287-288
    x-ray quantity and, 142
Source-to-image receptor distance indicator, 510
Source-to-skin distance, 511, 521
South pole, 71
Space charge, 112
Space-charge effect, 112
Space-charge limited, term, 112
Spatial distortion, 242
Spatial frequency, 389
Spatial resolution, 194, 195, 230, 360
    in angiointerventional radiology, 337
    in computed tomography, 388-390
    in fluoroscopy, 330
    in mammography, 300-301
    quality control, 415
Spatial uniformity, 391-392
Special quantities, 20

Speciality film, 172
Speck group, 311
Spectral matching, 169-170, 175, 190
    screen-film combinations and, 196-198
Spectral response, 166, 169
Speed, 21, 230
    characteristic curve and, 237-238
    densitometry and, 231
    of radiographic film, 167, 170
    of screen, 192
Speed index, 307
Spermatocyte, 469
Spermatogonia, 469
Spermatogonium, 436
Spermatozoa, 469
Spindle, 437
Spindle fiber, 437
Spinning top, 99, 411
Spiral computed tomography, 395-406
    advantages and limitations, 404, 405
    image characteristics, 402-404
    patient dose, 531
    scan principles, 396-399
    scanner design, 399-401
    technique selection, 401-402
Spiral scan pitch ratio, 398-399
Spiral scanning, 386
Spleen, 470-471
Split-dose technique, 458
Spontaneous abortion, 502, 503
Spot film, 173-174
Spot-film exposure, 412-413
Spot filming, 330-331
SSD; see Shaded surface display
Standard deviation of computed tomography values, 386, 391
Standard scientific notation, 13
Standards, 20
Star pattern, 410
Starch, 433
Static artifact, 422, 423
Static electricity, 58
Static RAM, 346
Stationary anode, 113, 114
Stator, 82, 115
Steel, thickness for secondary protective barrier, 514
Stem cell, 438, 467
    cytogenetic damage to, 472
    pluripotential, 470
Step-down transformer, 83
Step-up transformer, 83
Step-wedge filter, 145-147
Stepping capability of patient couch, 337
Stereoradiography, 286-289
Stereoscope, 286
Sthenic patient, 259
Stomach weighting factor, 501
Stop bath, 178, 182
Storage
    of film, 174-175
    system in digital imaging, 374, 375
Storage artifact, 422-423
Stored electric energy, 76
Straight-line portion, 231
Stroboscopic effect, 223
Stromal, term, 439
Structure mottle, 230
Subatomic particle, 29

Subcutaneous layer of skin, 467
Subject contrast, 234, 244-245
Subject radiopacity, 145
Sublethal radiation damage, 444, 457-458
Subtraction film, 172
Subtraction image, 362
Subtraction in digital imaging, 373
Subtraction of fractions, 15
Sugar, 433
Supercoating, 166
Superconduction super collider, 32
Superconductivity, 62
Superficial x-ray, 53
Superimposition, 368
Supervoltage x-ray, 53
Support couch, 385
Supporting tissue, 438
Switch, 64
Synchronized cells, 459
Synchronous motor of cine camera, 338
Synchronous spinning top, 411
Synchronous timer, 98
Synergism, 180
Synthesis, 450
System noise in computed tomography, 391
System programs, 346
Systems Internationale des Units, 13
Systems software, 349

T

Tabular grain, 170
Target, 113, 115
    electron-target interaction, 127-131
    in fluoroscopy, 327, 328
    mammographic, 296-298
    material effect on x-ray emission spectrum, 135
Target number, 457
Target theory, 453-454
Technique guides, 270-272, 273
Teleradiology, 373
Television field, 329
Television frame, 330
Television monitoring system in fluoroscopy, 327-330
Television picture tube, 329
Telophase, 436-437
Temperature-control system in automatic processing, 185
Temperature for development, 236-237
Temporal subtraction, 366-368
Temporary magnet, 73
10 day rule, 505-506
Tenth-value layer, 497-498
Terminal software, 348-349
Terrestrial radiation, 5
Tesla, 73
Testis, 469-470
Theory of relativity, 5, 54, 128
Thermal conductor, 113
Thermal energy, 5
Thermal printer, 348
Thermal radiation, 25
Thermionic emission, 84, 110, 324
Thermistor, 185
Thermocouple, 185
Thermoluminescence dosimetry, 515, 519-520, 527, 533-534
Thermometer, 25
Thickness

Thickness, cont'd
    of patient, 259
    section, 282, 284
Third-generation CT scanner, 380-381, 393
Thomson atom, 30-31
Thoriated tungsten, 110-111
Thorotrast, 487
Three-Mile Island, 487
Three-phase power, 102-104, 136-137, 252-253, 256
Threshold dose, 457, 458, 499
Threshold phenomenon, 456
Thrombocyte, 470-471
Thrombocytopenia, 471
Thrombolysis, 334
Throughput, 408
Thymine, 433
Thymus, 470-471
Thyroid
    radiation-induced cancer, 485-486
    weighting factor, 501
Tilting patient examination table, 94
Time, 8, 20
    development, 236
    extinction, 103
    initiation, 103
    milliampere second and, 253-254
    radiation protection and, 496
    standard of measurement, 21
    x-rays and pregnancy, 502
Time interval difference mode, 367-368
Time-sharing systems, 353-354
Timer, 97-99
    5-minute reset, 496
    quality control, 411
Timing circuit, 97-98
Tin, 33
Tissue, 437-439
    biologic factors affecting radiosensitivity, 443-444
    cellular radiobiology, 449-462
        cell survival kinetics, 454-460
        direct and indirect effect, 453
        irradiation of macromolecules, 450-452
        radiolysis of water, 452-453
        target theory, 453-454
    computed tomography numbers, 387
    differential absorption, 157
    dose limits, 500
    equivalent dose limits, 501
    imaged with changing pitch, 398-399
    intensity of scatter and, 215
    Law of Bergonie and Tribondeau, 442
    local damage from radiation, 467-470, 478-480
    mass density, 159
    photoelectric effect and, 154
    physical factors affecting radiosensitivity, 442-443
    pixel values and, 359
    radiation dose-response relationships, 444-446
    scatter radiation and, 207-208
    subject contrast and, 245-246
    weighting factors, 501
Tissue equivalent dosimeter, 520
Titanium dioxide, 191
Toe gradient, 235
Toe of characteristic curve, 231
Tomographic angle, 282, 284
Tomographic layer, 284

Tomographic x-ray machine, 93
Tomography, 282-286
    linear, 282-284, 285
    motion unsharpness and, 246
    multidirectional, 285, 286
    panoramic, 286, 287
    quality control, 413
    zonography, 286
Trackball, 362
Transaxial image, 378, 379
Transfemoral selective coronary angiography, 334
Transfer ribonucleic acid, 433, 436
Transformer, 82-84
    high-voltage, 100
    self-induction and, 80
    symbol and function, 64
Transformer law for current, 83
Transformer law for voltage and current, 83
Transistor, 64, 343, 344
Transitional elements, 36
Translation
    in computed tomography, 378
    of genetic code, 450
    in scanned projection radiography, 370
Transmission, wave model of electromagnetic radiation, 51
Transparent, term, 52
Transport-rack subassembly, 184-185
Transport system in automatic processing, 183-185
Transverse image, 378, 379
Tree static, 422, 423
Trifield tube, 326
Trispiral tomographic movement, 285
Trough filter, 145, 146
Tuberculosis, 537
Tungsten
    for anode, 113
    atomic number and K-shell electron binding
        energy, 153
    characteristic x-rays of, 130, 132
    characteristics of, 33
    effective atomic number, 154
    in mammographic x-ray tube, 296-298, 299-300
    mass density, 158
    thoriated, 110-111
Turnaround assembly, 185
Turns ratio, 83, 100
TVL; see Tenth-value layer
Two-position exposure switch, 115

U

Ultrasound, 11, 39
Ultraviolet light, 48-49
Uncontrolled area, 514
Underexposure, 261, 262
Undifferentiated cell, 438
Uniformity, quality control, 414
Unit
    electric charge, 57-58
    systems of measurement, 21
UNIVAC, 343
Universal automatic computer, 343
Unsharpness, 283-284
Upside-down grid error, 225
Uranium, 33
Urologic x-ray machine, 93
Use factor, 515

V

Vacuum tube, 10
Vacuum-tube rectifier, 84-85
Valve tube, 100-102
Vaporization of filament, 121
Variable-aperture collimator, 211-213, 255
Variable kilovoltage technique chart, 270, 271-272
Variable resistance, 98
Vascular stent, 334
Vasculitis, radiation sickness and, 466
Vector, 17, 21
Velocity, 21
    kinetic energy and, 127
    photon, 44-45
Ventriculography, 160
Vertical resolution in fluoroscopy, 330
Vertical retrace, 329-330
Very large-scale integration, 344
Video display terminal, 172, 346-347
Video film, 172
Video system in digital fluoroscopy, 365
Vidicon television camera, 327-328
Vignetting, 326
Virtual reality, 289
Visibility of detail, 230, 269
Visible light, 48-49, 50-52, 53
Vision, 323-324
Visual acuity, 323
Visual Basic, 353
Visual C++, 353
Visual checklist, 313, 314
Visual imaging, electromagnetic spectrum, 49
Volt, 61, 63
Voltage, 61, 83
Voltage diode, 410
Voltage rectification, 100-102
Voltage ripple, 104, 137
Voltage waveform, 136-137
Voltaic pile, 76
Voltmeter, 64
Volumetric quantitative analysis, 386
Voxel, 386-387

W

Warm-up procedure, 120
Washing in film processing, 182
Water
    in body composition, 432
    in circulation system in automatic processing, 185
    computed tomography numbers, 387
    as conductor, 61
    in film processing, 179
    five-pin AAPM phantom, 392
    radiolysis of, 452-453
Watt, 24, 66-67
Wave equation, 46
Wave-particle duality, 50-54
Waveform
    alternating current, 66
    direct current, 65-66
    high frequency generator circuit voltage, 103
    influence on x-ray emission spectrum, 136-137
    unrectified voltage, 100
Waveguide in electron beam computed tomography, 382
Wavelength, 21
    minimum, 133

Wavelength, cont'd
  photon, 45-46
Wedge filter, 145, 146
Weight, 4, 22-23
Weighting factor, 501
Wet-pressure sensitization, 422
Wetting, 178, 179
White blood cell, 470
White light, 49
White matter, 387
Whole-body effective dose limits, 499-501
Whole number, 14
Window, 108, 518
Window level, 361, 362
Window of fluoroscopic camera, 327
Window tube, 518
Window width, 361
Windowing, 361, 373
Windows applications, 353
Wire-mesh device, 201-202
Wood, thickness for secondary protective barrier, 514
Work, 23
Workload, 515

X

X-axis, 16-17
X chromosome, 473
X-ray
  application of, 53
  electromagnetic radiation, 41
  electromagnetic spectrum, 49
  half-value layer and tenth-value layer, 498
  interaction with matter, 149-161
    attenuation, 159-160
    classical scattering, 150
    Compton effect, 150-151, 152
    differential absorption, 155-159
    pair production, 155
    photodisintegration, 155, 156
    photoelectric effect, 151-155
    radiologic contrast agents, 160-161
  production of, 50, 126-138
    added filtration and, 135
    affect of milliampere, 133-134
    effect of peak kilovoltage, 134-135
    effect of target material, 135
    electron-target interaction, 127-131
    emission spectrum, 131-133
    influence of voltage waveform, 136-137
X-ray beam field size, 205-207
X-ray cassette, 92, 108
X-ray circuit, 105
X-ray conversion efficiency, 190

X-ray detector, 401
X-ray emission, 139-148
  quality, 92, 133, 142-147
    factors affecting, 144-147
    half-value layer and, 143-144
    penetrability and, 142
  quantity, 92, 133
    factors affecting, 140-142
    output intensity, 140
X-ray emission spectrum, 131-133
X-ray head unit, 209-210
X-ray intensity, 512, 521
X-ray room, 8, 94
X-ray tube, 92, 107-125
  in angiointerventional radiology, 336-337
  anode, 113-118
  cathode, 110-113
  in computed tomography, 383
  electricity and, 56-67
    electrodynamics, 61-67
    electrostatics, 57-61
  external structure, 108-110
  failure of, 118-121
  focal-spot size, 254-255
  housing, 103, 108-110, 510
  mammographic, 296-297
  movement during multidirectional tomography, 286, 287
  protective design, 510
  rating chart, 121-124
  in spiral computed tomography, 396, 397, 400-401
X-ray tube-detector assembly, 370-371
X-ray unit, 91-106
  high-voltage generator, 99-102
  mammographic, 295-301
  operating console, 92-99
  output intensity, 140
  power rating, 104-105
  single-phase power, 102
  three-phase power, 102-104
Xeroradiography, 294

Y

Y-axis, 16-17
Y chromosome, 473
Yellow light, 47
Yttrium, 190, 198

Z

Z-axis resolution, 401-402
Zinc cadmium sulfide, 9
Zinc sulfide, 190
Zonography, 286
Zoom in digital imaging, 373

Conversion Tables

Length

Unit	Equivalent in Meters
1 centimeter (cm)	10^{-2}
1 micron (μm)	10^{-6}
1 nanometer (nm)	10^{-9}
1 angstrom (Å)	10^{-10}
1 mile (mi)	1609

Mass-energy*

Electron Volts	Joules	Kilograms	Atomic Mass Units
1.0	1.60×10^{-19}	1.78×10^{36}	1.07×10^{-9}
6.24×10^{18}	1.0	1.11×10^{17}	6.69×10^{9}
5.61×10^{32}	8.99×10^{13}	1.0	6.02×10^{23}
9.32×10^{8}	1.49×10^{-10}	1.66×10^{27}	1.0

*(1 J = 10^7 ergs; 4.19 J = 1 calorie; 1 BTU = 1.06×10^{10} ergs.)

Time

Years	Days	Hours	Minutes	Seconds
1	365	8.75×10^3	5.26×10^5	3.15×10^7
	1	24	1.44×10^3	8.64×10^4
		1	60	3.6×10^3
			1	60